ARTIFICIAL INTELLIGENCE IN MEDICINE

Studies in Health Technology and Informatics

Editors

Volume 10

Earlier published in this series

Vol. 1, CEC DG XIII/F AIM (Ed.), Data Protection and Confidentiality in Health Informatics
Vol. 2, J. Noothoven van Goor and J.P. Christensen (Eds.), Advances in Medical Informatics
Vol. 3, H. Bouma and J.A.M. Graafmans (Eds.), Gerontechnology
Vol. 4, M. Di Rienzo, G. Mancia, G. Parati, A. Pedotti and A. Zanchetti (Eds.), Blood Pressure and Heart Rate Variability
Vol. 5, A. Pedotti (Ed.), Electrophysiological Kinesiology
Vol. 6, G.J.E. De Moor, C. McDonald, J. Noothoven van Goor (Eds.), Progress in Standardization in Health Care Informatics
Vol. 7, J.E.W. Beneken and V. Thévenin (Eds.), Advances in Biomedical Engineering
Vol. 8, E. Fleck, H. Hansen, B. Mahr and H. Oswald (Eds.), Open Systems in Medicine
Vol. 9, E. Ballabio, I. Placencia-Porrero and R. Puig de la Bellacasa (Eds.), Rehabilitation Technology

ISSN: 0926-9630

Artificial Intelligence in Medicine

Proceedings of the 4th Conference on
Artificial Intelligence in Medicine Europe,
3–6 October 1993, Munich

Edited by

S. Andreassen, R. Engelbrecht and J. Wyatt

IOS Press
1993
Amsterdam • Oxford • Washington • Tokyo

ISBN 90 5199 141 X
ISSN 0926-9630
Library of Congress Catalog Card Number: 93-061133

Publisher:

IOS Press
Van Diemenstraat 94
1013 CN Amsterdam
Netherlands

Sole distributor in the UK and Ireland:

IOS Press/Lavis Marketing
73 Lime Walk
Headington
Oxford OX3 7AD
England

Distributor in the USA and Canada:

IOS Press, Inc.
P.O. Box 10558
Burke, VA 22009-0558
USA

Distributor in Japan:

Kaigai Publications, Ltd.
21 Kanda Tsukasa-Cho 2-Chome
Chiyoda-Ku
Tokyo 101
Japan

PRINTED IN THE NETHERLANDS

TABLE OF CONTENTS

Foreword

Keynote Addresses

Model Based Reasoning

Strategies for Medical Reasoning

Strategies for Medical Reasoning - Applications

Strategies for Medical Reasoning - ICU Applications

Strategies for Medical Reasoning - Patient Management

Knowlwdge Representation - Protocols

Knowledge Representation - Terminology

Knowledge Acquisition, Representation & Learning

Applications Based on Neural Nets

(* poster or demo presentations)

Foreword

This volume contains the proceedings of the 4th International Conference on Artificial Intelligence in Medicine, which will be held in Munich, Germany, 3 - 6 October 1993. The conference is organized by AIME, the European Society for Artificial Intelligence in Medicine Europe. Previous international conferences were held in Marseille (1987), London (1989), and Maastricht (1991).

AIME was established in 1986 to foster fundamental and applied research in artificial intelligence and in symbolic information processing techniques for medical care and medical research Artificial Intelligence in medicine is a special field of Medical Informatics and deals with the enhancement of medical information systems by knowledge based components and new paradigms.

AIME 93 is hosted by the German National Centre for Environmental and Health Research (GSF) and supported by both the working group on "Expert Systems" of the German Society for Medical Informatics, Biometry, and Epidemiology (GMDS) and the national research project on Medical Knowledge Bases MEDWIS. The GSF-MEDIS Institute and the GSF conference service have taken most of the organizational burden on their shoulders.

AIME 93 will show recent scientific results presented in oral contributions, posters and demonstrations. The informatical topics range from "A priori probabilities" to "Validation" and the clinical topics from "Abdomen" to "Ventilation". The tutorials, which are both methodological and user-oriented, will constitute and important element of the conference.

The present proceedings contain 60 contributions to AIME 93 and cover all presentations which are part of the scientific programme, among the 2 keynotes, 26 oral presentations with an average of 12 pages, 38 poster presentations and demonstrations with an average of 4 pages. The papers were each selected and reviewed by at least two members of the international programme committee. We are very thankful for the trouble they have taken. Their recommendations were sent to the authors and incorporated in the final texts. They also helped us shape the structure of the conference.

The papers are mainly grouped around the two subject areas of "Knowledge acquisition and representation" and "Strategies for medical reasoning" which form the backbone of most of the theoretical work in the field. It was encouraging to see that many papers also describe applications of AI systems in medicine and that many of these have reached a remarkable degree of maturity. AI technology is passing the threshold between research-oriented feasibility studies and recognized clinical applications. AIME 93 will show both the research of understanding the principles of medical knowledge and medical reasoning and the development of methodologies and tools for professional design, realization, and implementation of knowledge-based systems.

Many people - too many to name all of them here - have contributed to the solid preparation of this conference. We wish to thank them all as they have done this job in addition to their usual work, especially Volker Böhm, Lydia Janke, and Wolfgang Moser, whose considerable efforts have paved the way for AIME 93.

Steen Andreassen, Rolf Engelbrecht and Jeremy Wyatt (Editors)
October 1993

Proceedings editors

Steen Andreassen, Rolf Engelbrecht, Jeremy Wyatt

International Program Committee

Chair: Steen Andreassen, University of Aalborg

Pedro Barahona, Lisboa
Rolf Engelbrecht, Munich
Mario Fieschi, Marseille
Torgny Groth, Uppsala
Roman Hovorka, London
Peter Hucklenbroich, Munich
Johan van der Lei, Rotterdam
Peter McNair, Copenhagen
Vassilis Moustakis, Heraklion
Pirkko Nykänen, Tampere
Kristian Olesen, Aalborg
Rory O'Moore, Dublin
Francesco del Pozo, Madrid
Michael M. Richter, Kaiserslautern
Mario Stefanelli, Pavia
Jan Talmon, Maastricht
Thomas Wetter, Heidelberg
Ove Wigertz, Linköping
Jeremy Wyatt, London
Pieter Zanstra, Nijmegen

Local Organising Committee

Chair: Rolf Engelbrecht, GSF-Forschungszentrum für Umwelt und Gesundheit

Volker Böhm
Thomas Diedrich
Karl-Heinz Englmeier
Norbert Gerzer
Lothar Gierl
Claudia Hildebrand
Lydia Janke
Elke Kühnel
Wolfgang Moser
Manfred Schnabel
Thomas Waschulzik

Tutorials

Chair: Jeremy Wyatt, Imperial Cancer Research Fund

Editors

Steen Andreassen
Department of Medical Informatics and Image Analysis,
Institute of Electronic Systems,
Universitity of Aalborg,
Fredrik Bajersvej 7D, 9220 Aalborg, Denmark

Rolf Engelbrecht
GSF-Forschungszentrum für Umwelt und Gesundheit GmbH,
MEDIS-Institut für Medizinische Informatik und Systemforschung,
Neuherberg, Postfach 1129, 85758 Oberschleißheim, Germany

Jeremy Wyatt
Imperial Cancer Research Fund,
Biomedical Informatics Unit,
Lincoln´s Inn Fields,
PO Box 123, London WC2A 3PX, United Kingdom

Keynote Addresses

Artificial Intelligence in Medecine
S. Andreassen et al. , Eds.
IOS Press, 1993

In Pursuit of Time's Arrow: Temporal Reasoning in Medical Decision Support

Michael G. Kahn, M.D., Ph.D.

Division of Medical Informatics, Department of Medicine, Washington University School of Medicine, St. Louis, Missouri USA

1. TIME'S ARROW

Philosophers have long debated the structure and properties of time [1, 2]. Is time real? Is it infinite or bounded? Is time linear, branching, or circular? Is it constructed from discrete or dense points or intervals? Time's Arrow refers time as an endless unidirectional river of past, present, and future events. Clinicians frequently describe a patient's medical history in terms of past-present-future chronicles – sequences of key events spread out over a simple time line. Therapeutic choices or prognostic statements usually are described using similar terms – anticipated outcomes placed on a hypothetical future time line. Although we experience time in a sequential or "flow-like" manner, it is clear that humans reason about temporal concepts with more complexity than simple past-present-future linear chronologies. The purpose of this paper is to examine how three representative medical expert systems have encoded non-linear temporal structures and reasoning strategies.

2. REVISITING THE PAST

Most medical phenomena recur. Illnesses reappear, symptoms return, treatments start, stop, and resume. Frequently, events from one clinical episode provide key patient-specific insights about what might transpire during a later episode. Thus, the ability to reason about recurring events is an essential aspect of temporal problem-solving.

VM, a ventilator-management program developed by Fagan, is one of the first symbolic decision-support programs to represent temporal knowledge explicitly [3]. VM uses a state-based temporal model to encode changes in parameter values and expectations over time. Transitions between states are represented explicitly in a state-transition network (Figure 1). Note the two arrows marked with the asterisk. In the absence of these state-transitions, VM's temporal model allows only a linear sequence of unique states. The bidirectional arrow between *CMV Ventilation* and *Assist Ventilation* allows the system to cycle repeatedly between these two states – a two-state temporal cycle. The arrow between *T-Piece Ventilation* and *Volume Ventilation* permits more complex cycles among four ventilator states. Note that although VM allows temporal cycles as a valid topology, the program has no mechanism for recognizing that the subsequent episodes of a state have been preceded by previous episodes of the same state. Thus VM's *representation* of time is more complex than its *reasoning* about time.

3. RELIVING THE PAST

As time passes, new information may become available, causing us to reconsider previous conclusions. Russ uses the term *hindsight* to describe the ability of a system to revise its conclusions based on newly acquired data [5].

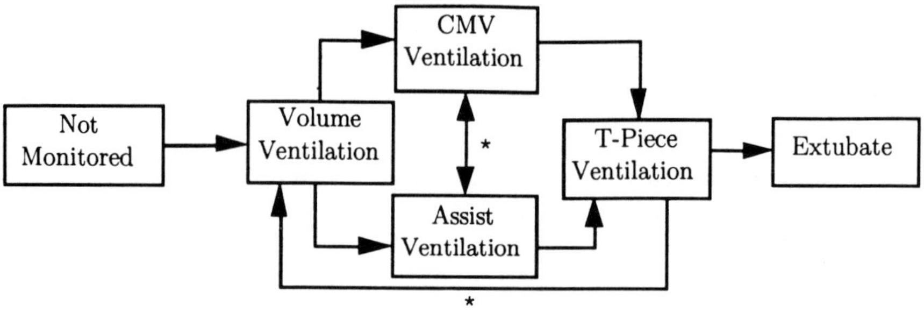

Figure 1: The state-transition graph from the VM system. Transitions marked with the asterisk permit VM to represent state cycles (Adapted from [4, pg. 79]).

The Temporal Control Structure (TCS) by Russ performs hindsight re-evaluation of past conclusions. TCS reasons by fragmenting time into homogeneous intervals [5]. A homogeneous interval is one during which no new events start or stop; events form the boundaries between successive homogeneous intervals. During a homogeneous interval, a reasoning system does not need to consider the effects of the sudden appearance of a new event or context. Reasoning within homogeneous intervals is performed by user-defined modules called process instances. To reason about changes between intervals, adjoining modules may exchange memory variables (Figure 2).

To support the re-evaluation of past conclusions, TCS contains a truth-maintenance system which maintains context dependencies between data and conclusions within each homogeneous interval. New input data may result in the retraction of conclusions within an interval. Memory variables permit these changes to modify previous intervals. These changes may propagate backward in time through the entire TCS process chain. Once completed, inferences about the past have been changed in response to the new contemporary information. Thus TCS "revisits" the past whenever information from the present causes previous conclusions to be revised.

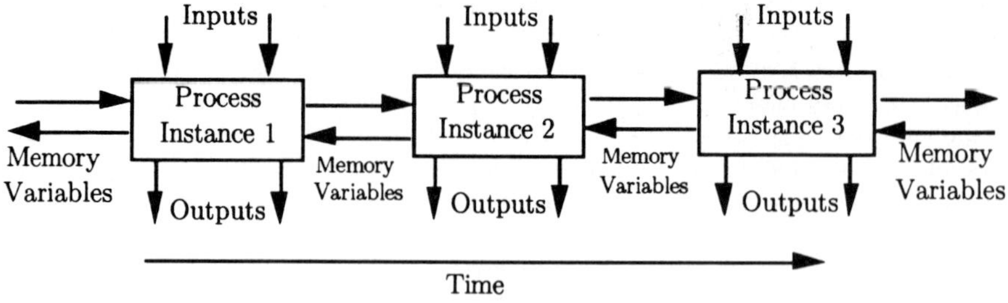

Figure 2: Temporal Control Structure's process chain. Each process instance reasons over a homogeneous interval. Memory variables (oracles and histories) pass between adjacent intervals. Hindsight reasoning occurs when memory variables move from right to left; view updating occurs when memory variables move from left to right. (Adapted from [5, pg. 39])

4. REVISING THE PRESENT

Clinical data frequently are not known in the same temporal order in which the data were obtained. Thus, a laboratory result may become known only after later test results have been used to derive conclusions. Just as new information may cause a reinterpretation of past conclusions (Section 3), the inclusion of newly acquired old data may invalidate present conclusions. Shahar has termed this feature *view updating* [6]. Using the same truth maintenance system and the propagation of memory variables, TCS re-evaluates present conclusions in light of new data from the past. Changes in memory variables move from the past to the present along the TCS process chain (Figure 2). In a similar manner, using a dependency graph of events, contexts, primitive data, and abstracted intervals, the RÉSUMÉ system by Shahar performs view updating when newly acquired past data invalidates current temporal abstractions. We describe RÉSUMÉ in more detail in Section 5.

Although previous inferences and current abstractions can be modified by old or new data, not all assertions can be retracted. For example, even though an action may have been based on an inference that no longer is valid, the action-fact cannot be withdrawn. Systems like TCS and RÉSUMÉ which permit revisions to past and present conclusions must support a temporal ontology which distinguishes between refutable and irrefutable temporal entities.

5. RELIVING THE FUTURE

Prediction, simulation, and envisioning are common methods for "living" in a future world. Because future outcomes are unknown, many alternative future worlds are possible. A diagram of branching future worlds which collapses at the ever-changing instance called "now" is a common topological structure. Programs which generate possible future states for later comparison embody a branching-future temporal structure. Information obtained at a later time is used to prune the unrealized alternative worlds – to select the future world that was realized. The ability to generate propositions about future states has many names: *foresight* is used within the temporal reasoning community [6] and *envisioning* is used within the qualitative reasoning community [7].

The RÉSUMÉ system supports foresight reasoning. RÉSUMÉ generates high-level abstractions from patient data using five temporal abstraction mechanisms (Figure 3) [6]. Like TCS, RÉSUMÉ maintains a dependency graph of events, contexts, primitive data, and abstracted intervals. RÉSUMÉ organizes abstractions around interpretation-context intervals – intervals of time during which a set of temporal definitions, assumptions, expectations, and derived abstractions are attached. Expected future states can be represented as interpretation-context intervals which appear in future time. RÉSUMÉ permits multiple interpretation-context intervals to exist concurrently, reflecting the possibility that differing interpretations are possible using different definitions or assumptions. When the future becomes the present, RÉSUMÉ uses its defeasible reasoning capability to refute or prune unrealized future states.

RÉSUMÉ can represent not only an ambiguous future, but also an ambiguous past and present. Each alternative past, present, or future is encapsulated in an interpretation-context interval which contains only those inferences and abstractions which are plausible using the definitions and assumptions contained within that context. Any new data, either by hindsight or foresight reasoning, can eliminate defeasible interpretation-context intervals. Irrefutable facts, such as therapeutic actions, are "global" and hence are not accessible for defeasible reasoning.

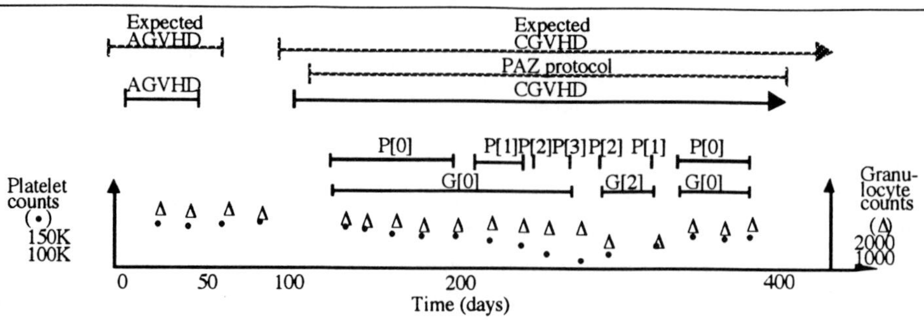

Figure 3: Temporal abstractions generated by RÉSUMÉ. (Adapted from [6, pg. 126])

6. CONCLUSION

In this short paper, we have examined only three medical expert systems which perform temporal reasoning. Many more examples have been described in the Artificial Intelligence in Medicine (AIM) literature [8]. With just these three examples, we have illustrated circular and branching temporal structures along with foresight and hindsight reasoning. The representation of temporal concepts and the reasoning methods required to manipulate these concepts show a rich diversity in their structure and their mechanisms. Creating new temporal models and more flexible temporal reasoning mechanisms remains an active area of research within the AIM community.

REFERENCES

[1] Rescher N, Urquhart A. *Temporal Logic*. Wien, Germany: Springer-Verlag, 1971.

[2] van Benthem J. *The Logic of Time*. Boston MA: D. Reidel, 1983.

[3] Fagan LM, Kunz JC, Feigenbaum EA, Osborn JJ. Extensions to the rule-based formalism for a monitoring task. In: Buchanan BG, Shortliffe EH, eds. *Rule-Based Expert Systems: the MYCIN Experiments of the Stanford Heuristic Programming Project*. Reading MA: Addison-Wesley, 1984: Chapter 22: 397–423.

[4] Fagan LM. *VM: Representing Time-Dependent Relations in a Medical Setting* [Dissertation]. Department of Computer Science, Stanford CA: Stanford University, 1980.

[5] Russ TA. Using hindsight in medical decision making. In: Kingsland LC, ed. *Proceedings Symposium on Computer Applications in Medical Care*. New York NY: IEEE Computer Society Press, 1989:38–44.

[6] Shahar Y, Musen MA. A temporal-abstraction system for patient monitoring. In: Frisse ME, ed. *Proceedings Symposium on Computer Applications in Medical Care*. New York NY: McGraw-Hill Inc., 1992:121–7.

[7] Kuipers B. Commonsense reasoning about causality: Deriving behavior from structure. In: Bobrow DG, ed. *Qualitative Reasoning About Physical Systems*. Cambridge MA: MIT Press, 1985: 169–204.

[8] Kahn MG. Modeling time in medical decision-support programs. Medical Decision Making 1991; *11*: 249–64.

Artificial Intelligence in Medecine
S. Andreassen et al. , Eds.
IOS Press, 1993

Criteria for the acceptance of decision-support systems by clinicians; lessons from ECG interpretation systems[1]

Jan H. van Bemmel

Dept of Medical Informatics, Faculty of Medicine and Health Sciences,
Erasmus University Rotterdam, The Netherlands

Abstract

An analysis is made of the reasons why clinical support systems in health care (e.g., imaging systems, laboratory systems) are in routine use whereas decision support systems have not been widely accepted. The conclusions of this review are illustrated by the results of a large evaluation study of systems for ECG interpretation.

1. INTRODUCTION

Decision-support systems are not well incorporated in medical practice. The possible reasons have been given by several authors [1-4]. To stimulate discussions, I have simply divided the field of clinical systems into two halves:
(a) the widely accepted *clinical support systems* (CSSs), and
(b) the not or only partly accepted *decision-support systems* (DSSs).

2. SYSTEMS

The road to successful and applicable medical DSSs is long and winding. Even for the early systems that are frequently cited in the literature, no widespread market has emerged.

Of the CSSs, imaging systems are undoubtedly a success story in medicine. And of no less importance: very early, industry became deeply involved in the R&D of imaging systems. Developers of DSSs do not always realize who will be the future users of their systems. This is especially true if systems are developed within a university environment, where the most direct goal is research.

CONCLUSION (1):

Some CSS, such as imaging systems, are very successful, offering data directly related to anatomy and function that the user needs for decision making. Although a prototype decision-support system might be successfully used at the center where it was developed, this is no guarantee that it can be transferred to other centers or industry.

3. EXPECTATIONS

Data interpretation can be depicted as part of the diagnostic-therapeutic loop, in which (1) observations (data), (2) decisions, and (3) therapies are circling. Where in this loop are support systems most needed?

---

[1] A more extensive version of this paper, giving proper credit to the literature, will be published in *Methods of Information in Medicine*.

In using imaging systems, the physician draws his diagnostic conclusions directly from the primary imaging data. A perfect example is 3-D reconstruction from CT slices, offering views that can compete with direct observations during surgery.

Other successful systems are seen in areas where the information stream is too large to be comprehended by the user: the data have to be reduced, transformed and presented in a comprehensible way. Such systems are, e.g., seen in operating theaters, intensive care units and laboratories. CSS handle data validation, administration, electronic transport via networks, and computer-storage. Decision support is mainly used for data validation and data reliability and to reduce the number of errors in reports or false alarms.

CONCLUSION (2):

In the diagnostic-therapeutic loop, the most important place for support systems is the first stage: data acquisition and presentation. Support systems are in demand when they offer: (1) medical data that cannot be obtained otherwise, (2) overviews necessary for decision making, (3) support of administration, documentation, and transportation, (4) handling of large data streams in routine environments. Decision support algorithms are primarily used to enhance data reliability.

4. USERS

In a study by De Dombal [5], three different support methods for inexperienced staff were mutually compared: structured data collection forms, real-time decision support, and computer-assisted teaching. A combination of forms and teaching gave equally good results as forms plus direct decision support. For example, De Dombal could show a large decrease in unnecessary interventions in perforation rates among patients with appendicitis.

Heckerling *et al.* investigated the *Iliad* system to generate diagnostic suggestions, and compared the results with the diagnoses of internists who diagnosed the cases before and after confrontation with *Iliad*'s verdicts [6]. Physicians were able to improve their diagnoses significantly for 28 of the 50 cases for which *Iliad* contained knowledge, but not so for the other 22 cases.

Feldman and Barnett [7] describe a strategy for evaluating the accuracy of *DXplain*'s differential diagnoses. In this study 46 test cases were obtained from a variety of sources. It appeared that the system agreed well with the consensus of experts, scoring for 27 of the 46 cases.

Van der Lei used data contained in a routine computer-based patient record system as input to a critiquing system for hypertension (*Hypercritic* [8]). It appeared that *Hypercritic* could compete with eight expert reviewers and that the computer-based patient record system contained sufficient data to be used as input for the expert system.

For several decades, computers have been in use in cardiology for the interpretation of the electrocardiogram (e.g., [9]). ECG decision support is fully integrated with data acquisition, and documentation and storage. ECG systems are in that way completely comparable with laboratory support systems, and deliver a fully interpreted final document, usually reviewed by the treating physician.

CONCLUSION (3):

Both experienced and inexperienced users of DSSs require that DSSs are fully integrated in their clinical practice and will use a DSS only if it increases the quality of care. In principle, DSSs may assist: (1) inexperienced users in complex decision making; (2) experienced users in enhancing the quality of their decisions; (3) users who require help in non-routine cases; (4) users who want to integrate the DSS in routine clinical practice.

5. VALIDATION

There are legal and ethical reasons why a medical system should not be introduced into clinical practice before it has been properly evaluated. Evaluation should cover all stages of the development process of a decision-support systems. An important point is that evaluation is a process to be continued after the introduction of a decision-support system into practice, as is done in post-marketing surveillance studies of drugs.

Only very few decision-support systems in medicine were as extensively assessed as ECG interpretation systems. Therefore, I give some details of the so-called CSE (Common Standards for quantitative Electrocardiography) study. [10,11]. The first part, dealing with the accuracy of waveform recognition, was completed in 1985 [10]. The second, on diagnostic interpretation, in 1990 [11].

In both stages there was the problem of defining an "Objective Reference". In the first stage a documented database was used, reviewed by 5 cardiologists [10]. In the second study, the diagnostic classifications of 10 ECG systems were compared with ECG-independent clinical evidence and with the group outcome of the interpretations by 8 cardiologists, with the help of 1,220 well-documented ECGs. The best systems had either an overall agreement with the clinical evidence of about 70%, and of about 80% when compared with the group of cardiologists.

Some interpretation systems appeared to be more accurate and stable than others. This resulted in major changes in the current systems and, in a few cases, even withdrawal of the system from further evaluation.

The second stage revealed that cardiologists (on average) perform no better than the best systems, and that a combination of diagnostic results from different systems is better than the diagnostic results from any individual system. The latter applies, however, also to the combined result of cardiologists.

CONCLUSION (4):

CSE underlined that a DSS can enhance the diagnostic performance of clinicians. The best interpretation systems reached a diagnostic accuracy approaching that of the best experts; a combination of the diagnostic results of experts and/or systems appeared to be better than either one of them. Evaluation of a medical DSS should be conducted in a multi-center study in which the principal investigators have no role in the collection of the patient material or the processing of the results. Standardization of terminology is a prerequisite for comparison of interpretation results.

6. CRITERIA FOR THE ACCEPTANCE OF DSSs

On the basis of the above review and considering many criteria for DSSs that are already given in the literature [1-4], I now formulate some criteria for the acceptance of clinical support systems (CSS) in general, and decision support systems (DSS) in particular:

1. *A CSS should support data acquisition*
   Clinical support systems are most successful at the first stage, i.e., when offering primary data for further decision making.

2. *A DSS may support data reliability*
   Decision-support systems are successful for enhancing primary data reliability, inconsistency, and completeness.
3. *A CSS does not require a DSS*
   Physicians are most often able to interpret the data offered by a clinical support system, based on their knowledge and experience, and do generally require no decision support.
4. *Local acceptance of DSS condition, no guarantee*
   The acceptance of a decision-support system at one location is a necessary condition, but no guarantee that it can be successfully transferred to other centers or adopted by industry.
5. *A DSS should be integrated with a CSS*
   A decision-support system should be integrated with a CSS to be successful, and be part of routine clinical practice. This should be considered as the most essential condition for the acceptance of DSSs in medicine.
6. *Assessment of DSS is condition*
   Physicians will accept decision-support systems only if they have proven to increase the quality of patient care.
7. *Independent evaluation of DSSs required*
   Validation of DSSs should be conducted in multi-center studies, in which the principal investigators have no principal role in the collection of patient material or in interpreting the results of the study.
8. *Standardization of terminology necessary*
   The assessment of decision-support systems requires standardization of terminology for the interpretation of the results.

7. REFERENCES

1. Miller RA, Masarie FE. The demise of the Greek oracle model for medical diagnosis systems. Meth Inform Med 1990;29;1-2.
2. Van Bemmel JH. Formalization of medical knowledge. Meth Inform Med 1986;25:191-3.
3. Wyatt J. Computer-based knowledge systems. Lancet 1991; 338:1431-6.
4. Heathfield HA, Wyatt J. Philosophies for the design and development of clinical decision-support systems. Meth Inform Med 1993;32:1-8.
5. De Dombal FT, Dallos V, McAdam WAF. Can computer aided teaching packages improve clinical care in patients with acute abdominal pain. BMJ 1991;302:149-57.
6. Heckerling PS, Elstein AS, Terzian CG, Kushner MS. The effect of incomplete knowledge on the diagnoses of a computer consultant system. Med Inf 1991;16:363-70.
7. Feldman MJ, Barnett GO. An approach to evaluating the accuracy of DXplain. Comput Meth Progr Biomed 1991;35:261-6.
8. Van der Lei J, Musen MA, van der Does E, Man in 't Veld A, van Bemmel JH. Review of physician decision making using data from computer-stored medical records. The Lancet 1991;338:1504-8.
9. Van Bemmel JH, Willems JL, eds. Special issue on CSE. Meth Inform Med 1990;29:259-423.
10. Willems JL, Arnaud P, van Bemmel JH, et al. Assessment of the performance of ECG computer programs with the use of a reference data base. Circulation 1985;71:523-34.
11. Willems JL, Abreu-Lima C, Arnaud P, van Bemmel JH et al. The diagnostic performance of computer programs for the interpretation of electrocardiograms. New Engl J Med 1991;325:1767-73.

Model Based Reasoning

Artificial Intelligence in Medecine
S. Andreassen et al. , Eds.
IOS Press, 1993

A tool for pathophysiological knowledge acquisition

L. Ironi[a], A. Cattaneo[a,b] and M. Stefanelli[b]

[a] Istituto di Analisi Numerica del C.N.R., C.so C. Alberto 5, 27100 Pavia (Italy)

[b] Dipartimento di Informatica e Sistemistica, Università di Pavia, Via Abbiategrasso 209, 27100 Pavia (Italy)

Abstract

The explanation power of a medical knowledge based system (MKBS) can be highly enhanced by the availability of deep pathophysiological knowledge. This kind of knowledge is well represented through mathematical models whose formulation, either quantitative or qualitative, requires both domain specific and domain independent knowledge. This paper describes QCMF, a tool which makes easier the acquisition, through an interactive graphical interface, of the domain knowledge and embeds the needed methodological knowledge to formulate a qualitative pathophysiological model. Such a model is directly coded in QSIM and is simulated in order to predict the system behavior under the effects of a variety of pathogenetic mechanisms and therapeutical treatments. Moreover, different models of a given pathophysiological system are stored in a library so that they can be efficiently retrieved and exploited within a MKBS.

1. INTRODUCTION

A powerful way of representing deep pathophysiological knowledge consists in the formulation of a model which describes both structure and behavior of the underlying system. The structure description, *structure model*, identifies the variables of interest and the existence of relationships between them, while the *behavior model* states the equations linking the variables. The variables represent attributes of the modeled system, and an equation describes the fact that a change of a variable produces a change in another variable. Therefore, a model of a system, which can reflect either normal or abnormal behavior of that system, allows to represent genuine biomedical theories as proposed in medical literature: a pathophysiological condition can be interpreted as the effect of some perturbations occurring on some system variables.

Within this context, a pathophysiological model is given by a behavior model of a structure associated with an initial state which describes the perturbations acting on the system.

A good pathophysiological knowledge allows the expert to model the structure of a system but it is not enough to reason about its behavior. To this end, a good knowledge about the suitable representation formalism and the simulation algorithm is necessary. Thus, we are developing a tool which makes easier the acquisition, through a user-friendly graphical interface, of the specific domain knowledge and embeds all the necessary domain independent knowledge to formulate a model and to derive predictions about the behavior of the system under different perturbations. More precisely, this tool, called QCMF (Qualitative Compartmental Modeling Framework), includes knowledge of the theory of compartmental systems [1, 3] and of QSIM [10]. The compartmental modeling ontology is the most common formal description of the dynamics of chemical reactions and material transfer processes in biological systems. In this modeling framework, the structure of a system is viewed as a finite set of subsystems, called *compartments*, interacting by exchanging material; while the behavior is described by the behavior of each compartment, namely a set of ordinary differential equations (ODE) based on the mass balance law.

In QCMF, a qualitative formulation of the behavior model has been preferred to a quantitative one because of both the reduced number of assumptions in building the model and the qualitative attitude of reasoning shown by physicians. The choice of QSIM [10] among the several proposed approaches [2, 20] to qualitative modeling is due to the fact that it seems the most suitable formalism to represent the dynamics of processes whose behavior is described by ODEs [6, 9, 13, 16].

The tasks performed by QCMF are:

(1) acquisition of the domain knowledge, namely the structure model, information about functional relationships between variables and single or multiple perturbations which may act on the system;

(2) formulation of the behavior model by an automatic analysis of the given structure;

(3) automatic generation of the behavior model in the QSIM code;

(4) automatic generation of the initial state corresponding to the perturbation on the system in the QSIM code;

(5) simulation of the model.

Since also the interpretation of the simulation results requires a good knowledge of the simulation algorithm, a module which generates a causal explanation of the predicted behaviors has been designed and is presently under development.

In a previous work [6] we have shown how qualitative pathophysiological models can be properly exploited in a MKBS [17]. To this end, for any given physiological system, a library of models associated with general categories of diseases or therapeutical treatments should be available. Beside the other tasks, QCMF stores in a library the previously formulated models: in the library the different entities composing models are represented through frames, and the whole set of frames is hierarchically organized. A browsing facility is provided by QCMF for retrieving and visualizing to the user all the information stored in the library. This paper is organized as follows: after a brief introduction of QSIM and compartmental modeling, the next sections deal with an overview of QCMF.

2. QSIM DESCRIPTION

QSIM provides (1) a descriptive language, consisting of qualitative constraints that abstract the relationships in an ordinary differential equation, to represent the behavior model of a pathophysiological system, and (2) a simulation algorithm to infer, starting from an initial state of the system, a qualitative description of all of its possible behaviors.

A model is characterized by a set of variables, continously differentiable functions of time, linked by constraints describing the structural relations of the system. The numeric value of a variable at any time does not need to be explicitely known, but may be characterized in terms of its ordinal relations with a finite and totally ordered set, called *quantity space*, of landmark values: the value can be either a landmark or an open interval between two adjacent landmarks. The qualitative state of a variable over time is given by its qualitative value and its direction of change, that is the sign of its time derivative. Time is symbolically represented as a sequence of symbolic time-points whose existence is associated with significant events. Such events occur when a function crosses one of its landmark values or the time derivative of a function becomes equal to zero. All of the time-points are generated by the simulation process. An important feature of QSIM is that during the simulation it can find new critical points, and thus add further landmarks to the quantity space.

The constraint notation used in this approach has a clear correspondence with ordinary differential equations by making explicit all the functions and operators in the equation. Therefore, constraints expressing some arithmetic and derivative operators are defined. The functional relationships between variables are not explicitely specified but just described in terms of monotonicity regions, making it possible to represent states of incomplete knowledge. Table I summarizes the basic operators in QSIM.

The constraints are expressed as predicates, at two or three-places, rather than as functions, since it is not yet clear how to define rigorously the function's range. Let us notice that M^+ (M^-) expresses a relation of strict monotonicity on the whole domain. However, this definition can be extended so that functions whose domain is divided in increasing and decreasing monotonicity regions can be described. (For example a function which is monotonic increasing over an interval and which takes constant values outside that interval can be defined by the constraint $S^+(f,g)\ (f_1,g_1)\ (f_2,g_2) := M^+(f,g)$ on (f_1,f_2); $g(t)=g_1$ if $f(t)\leq f_1$; $g(t)=g_2$ if $f(t)\geq f_2$), and a concave upward shaped function can be described by $U^+(f,g)\ (a\ b) := M^-(f,g)$ if $f(t)<a$ and $M^+(f,g)$ if $f(t)>a$, and $g(f(t))=b$ if

$f(t) = a$). The relationship between the variables in a constraint can be further restricted by *corresponding values*, which are landmarks simultaneously assumed by their respective variables. Each corresponding values statement consists of a list of landmarks, each of them corresponding respectively to the variable in the constraint of which the corresponding value statement is part.

Table 1
Basic constraints in QSIM.

Operator	Arguments	Definition	True iff $\forall t \in (a,b)$ it holds
ADD	f, g, h	$ADD(f, g, h)$	$f(t) + g(t) = h(t)$
$MULT$	f, g, h	$MULT(f, g, h)$	$f(t) \cdot g(t) = h(t)$
$MINUS$	f, g	$MINUS(f, g)$	$f(t) = -g(t)$
D/DT	f, g	$D/DT(f, g)$	$f'(t) = g(t)$
M^+	f, g	$M^+(f, g)$	$f(t) = H(g(t))$ and $H'(x) > 0$
M^-	f, g	$M^-(f, g)$	$f(t) = H(g(t))$ and $H'(x) < 0$
M_0^+	f, g	$M_0^+(f, g)$	$M^+(f, g)$ and $H(0) = 0$
M_0^-	f, g	$M_0^-(f, g)$	$M^-(f, g)$ and $H(0) = 0$

Given a set of constraints (QDEs) modeling a pathophysiological system F characterized by the set of variables $\{f_1, ..., f_m\}$ and an initial state, the simulation algorithm determines one or more qualitative behavior descriptions for the given variables. More precisely, it provides in output: (1) a tree of all possible behaviors whose nodes are qualitative state descriptions for F; (2) a sequence $\{t_0, t_1, ..., t_n\}$ representing the distinguished time-points of the system's behavior; (3) a totally ordered set of landmarks, possibly extending the original one, for each f_i; (4) the time course plot of each f_i.

The simulation proceeds by determining all of possible state transitions, then filtering out only combinations of transitions whose result is a state which fails to satisfy the constraints. Therefore, the predictions generated by QSIM include all real behaviors, but even spurious behaviors can be derived because of both the local nature of the criteria used for determining state changes and the qualitative level of descriptions. A great deal of current research in the qualitative simulation area deals with new methods to filter out spurious behaviors [5, 11, 12, 14, 15, 18, 19]. The common idea of all these methods is to add more knowledge and to make explicit some global properties of the system, such as, for example, the introduction of constraints expressing conservation laws which are implicitly embedded in a quantitative formulation.

3. COMPARTMENTAL MODELING

In the compartmental modeling framework, a system is represented as a finite set of subsystems, called *compartments*, interacting by exchanging material. A compartment is fundamentally an idealized store of a substance, homogeneously distributed: if a substance is present in a physiological system in several forms or locations and passes from one form or location to another one, then each form or location constitutes a separate compartment for the substance. It should be noted that different compartments can coexist in the same location of a biological system and that the compartments do not always correspond to physically identifiable components. Such modeling technique is applicable when the study concerns the flow of some substance through the system. The *structure* of a compartmental model, that is the system's decomposition and the network of interactions between compartments, is usually displayed by means of a compartmental diagram.

The decomposition of a system into compartments leads straightforward to a set of equations, based on the mass balance equation, which represents the *behavior* model of the system. Let's denote with the variable $x_i(t)$ the state variable of the system which represent the concentration or amount of substance in the i–th compartment which exchanges matter with other compartments at time t. The x_i rate of change is obtained by writing the equation:

$$\dot{x}_i = f_{i0} + \sum_{\substack{j=1 \\ j\neq i}}^{n} f_{ij}(x_j) - \sum_{\substack{j=1 \\ j\neq i}}^{n} f_{ji}(x_i) - f_{0i}(x_i) \qquad (1)$$

where $\dot{x}_i$ denotes the time derivative of x_i; f_{ij} and f_{ji} denote respectively the rates of mass transfer into the $i-th$ compartment from the $j-th$ compartment and into the $j-th$ compartment from the $i-th$ compartment. Both the variables f_{ij} and x_j take on non-negative values, that is:

$$x_i \geq 0 \;\; \forall i \quad , \quad f_{ij} \geq 0 \;\; \forall i, j, \;\; i \neq j \qquad (2)$$

In general, the flow of material depends on the quantity or concentration of material in the source compartment and may also be dependent on the quantity or concentration into some other compartments, that is: $f_{ij} = f_{ij}(x_j; x_l, x_m, ...)$ where x_l, x_m,.. denote the variables controlling f_{ij}. The dependence of f_{ij} on x_j and of f_{ji} on x_i can be either linear or non-linear. The nature of these functional dependencies will vary according to the system under investigation and be suggested either by the observation of the system or by the available pathophysiological knowledge. When the knowledge is complete enough to give an analytical expression for such dependencies, a quantitative formulation of the model can be given. In many circumstances, these dependencies can be expressed only through their monotonicity properties: in such a case a qualitative model is formulated.

The utility of a compartmental decomposition depends upon the applicability of the balance equation (1). The decomposition of a physiological system can be done at different levels of description: of course a finer description leads to a more complicated interaction network. How "coarse" or "fine" a description of the system is needed depends strictly on the purposes of model building.

4. THE ARCHITECTURE OF QCMF

QCMF offers a friendly environment that guides the user through the different steps of compartmental model-building: model formulation and generation, model simulation and result interpretation. The system, implemented in Lucid Common Lisp, is modular and each module allows the user to execute one of the above mentioned tasks. The user interacts with the system through a very straightforward graphical interface developed by extensively using the object-oriented programming facilities provided by the LispView Toolkit in the X Window System. From the point of view of the graphical interface, the generic window page is basically divided into three sub-windows (see next section). The bottom window is used for the dialogue with the user in the different phases. The central window is dedicated to the graphical input/output, namely for editing or showing structures and for presenting the simulation outcome. The right-hand window shows the functional buttons. Each button is associated with a different module corresponding to a specific phase of the analysis of a system. In more detail:

(1) GENERATE assists the user in the construction of a compartmental model and expresses it according to the QSIM formalism;

(2) SIMULATE receives in input the qualitative model and derives the possible behaviors of the system under different perturbations introduced by the user;

(3) EXPLAIN helps the user in the interpretation of the simulation outcome by giving a causal account of behavior and by highlighting the differences among behaviors;

(4) BROWSE is a module that retrieves and visualizes the information regarding the stored models by accessing the model library; this module allows the user to easily examine the assumptions made in building a model.

Figure 1 shows the conceptual structure underlying the organization of QCMF: it displays the main tasks executed by each module and the exchange of information that occurs between different modules and with the model library. Due to the methodological knowledge embedded in QCMF all steps are performed automatically except those that require the user to enter domain-dependent knowledge.

The two main issues concerning QCMF consist, on one side in representing pathophysiological knowledge through models, and on the other in dealing with the organization of this knowledge. The next two subsections illustrate the approach adopted by QCMF regarding these two issues.

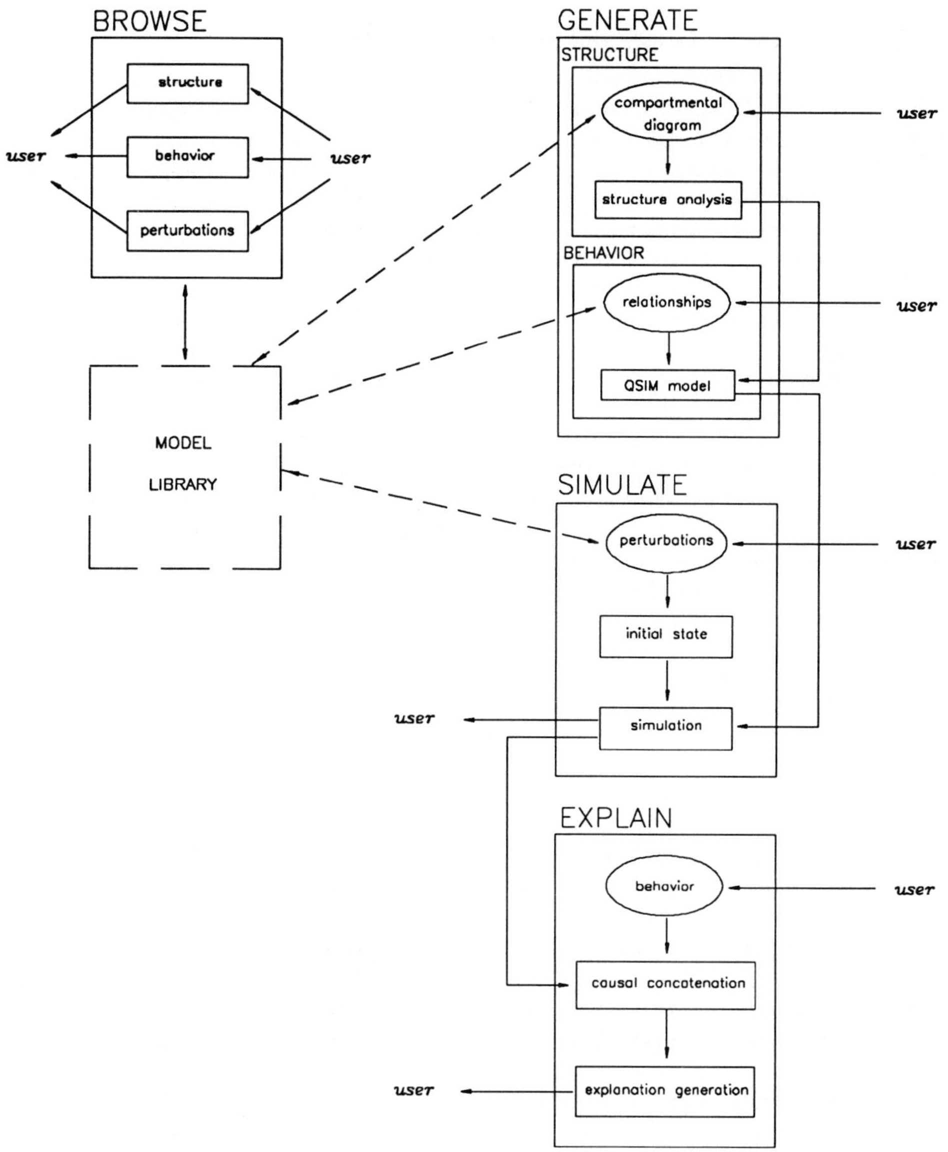

Figure 1. Conceptual structure of QCMF.

4.1. From pathophysiological knowledge to qualitative models

The following subsections describe exactly what information, representing the pathophysiological knowledge, the system expects in input from the user during the different model-building phases and how this information is exploited in formulating a model.

4.1.1. Model formulation and generation

Two different sub-modules, which are selected through a submenu of the GENERATE button, deal separately with structure and behavior model formulation and generation. The structure model consists of information gathered from the decomposition of the system into compartments, and about the network of exchanges between compartments and external environment.

The user can choose between entering the definition of a new structure or to retrieve and edit a previously defined structure.

In this phase the user is required to specify graphically through a compartmental diagram the components that identify the structure (i.e. compartments, flows, controls). This operation has been made simple by representing each type of component through an icon so that the user only has to click the corresponding menu-button option on entering a component or editing the structure. According to the selected component, further information must be provided by the user. Namely, it is required to specify:

- for a compartment: the name of the substance in it, and the position on the input/output graphical window;
- for a flow: the connections between compartments and the environment, i.e. which compartment the flow is leaving to reach another compartment or to the environment, and the compartment the flow is entering from another compartment or from the environment;
- for a control: the controlling variable and the controlled flow.

In view of the model-building process, QCMF associates a number to each compartment. This is useful in defining concisely the flows and the state variables in the model.

To make the input process easy, the flows and controls are drawn automatically. Particular attention has been given to the search of the optimal path in order to avoid the overlapping of components: this guarantees a clear view of the compartmental diagram.

Graphical editing facilities are available to the user in order to modify a structure: compartments can be moved to improve the layout of the compartmental diagram, in this case the compartment and the flows linked to it are erased and redrawn according to the new position; secondly, any component can be deleted choosing the *delete* option associated with the corresponding icon. If the user deletes a compartment the system renumbers the compartments and the flows are relabeled accordingly. The structure model, described by lists that contain all its specifications, can be stored and then retrieved; however, before saving a model the system performs an automatic debugging of the structure to verify that it complies to compartmental methodology.

When the compartmental diagram has been completed the system performs an analysis of the structure during which all the relevant variables are automatically identified: the numbering of the compartments allows to identify the state variables x_i, and their rate of change dx_i; the number i of the compartment the flow leaves from and the number j of the one in which the flow enters identifies the flow variables f_{ij}. Once the variables have been identified the system is capable of stating which variables are linked to one another, in fact each flow depends on the state variable of the compartment it leaves and from control variables, if any, while the rate of change of the state variables is described by the mass balance equations. The identification of the state variables each flow depends on is essential to the behavior sub-module because it allows the system to ask what kind of relationships there are between these variables.

The behavior sub-module has the function of writing down the differential equations related to a given compartmental structure and expressing them in QSIM code. To this end, the user is required to specify, on the basis of the pathophysiological knowledge available, what kind of functional relationship exists between variables. This operation is facilitated by a menu that presents the possible options in terms of monotonicity regions.

The generation of the QSIM code is invisible to the user and it begins as a first instantiation of the quantity spaces of the variables based on the inequalities (2) that will be updated with new landmark values according to the relationships chosen by the user. This updating is necessary because certain constraints (S+, S-, U+, U-) divide the domain of a variable and the corresponding codomain according to the different monotonicity regions. Therefore, when the user chooses one of these constraints the system has to introduce automatically the landmarks that characterize these regions into the corresponding quantity spaces.

The translation into QSIM of the relationships between variables is in most cases straightforward; however, since QSIM constraint operators are predicates at two or three places, the syntax does not allow to write down nested constraints in an explicit form. This is a drawback for the system that is compelled, when building complex expressions, to introduce intermediate variables with no physiological meaning. This is the case of controlled flows (i.e. multivalued functional dependencies between flow and state variables) which need to be expressed as sum or product of variables associated with single-valued functions.

After having derived the quantity space for each variable and translated the relationships between variables in QSIM code, the system, exploiting the structure analysis previously performed, generates automatically the QSIM code expressing the differential equations describing a pathophysiological system's dynamics (1). Moreover, QCMF singles out particular features of the structure in order to include in the model global properties, such as for example the mass conservation law in a closed structure, that are implicit in quantitative models but that would otherwise be lost in a qualitative formulation.

Once the behavior sub-module has generated the QSIM model, the user can store the code for later retrieval and move forward to the SIMULATE module.

4.1.2. Model simulation

When the behavior model generation has been completed or an already existing model retrieved, QCMF offers the chance of observing the possible behaviors of the modelled system.

QCMF allows the user to formulate two different kinds of scenario in defining the initial state. The first option simulates the effects of perturbations on the normal state of the system; the perturbations, representing a given pathophysiological situation, are entered by the user. The other option analyzes tracer kinetics supposing a tracer is given in input to the system. QCMF considers these two alternatives because they are of particular interest in the medical field.

In the first case, before perturbing the system QCMF identifies the normal value of each variable. The user is asked, whenever this operation may have different outcomes, to specify in which interval the normal value of state variables lies, but otherwise the operation is performed automatically. The user must then choose, through a menu, which variables are perturbed and whether their values increase or decrease. The options offered in the menu represent the variables that can be perturbed, i.e. state variables, constant flows and fractional transfer rate constants defining linear flows.

Once all the necessary information has been acquired the system generates the initial state function which describes the equilibrium state and the perturbed state by specifying, for both, the qualitative value of each variable and its rate of change.

The generation of the initial state function in the tracer kinetics option requires the user to state in which compartment the tracer enters and how the input occurs. The available choices regarding the kind of input are impulse and step signal.

In this second scenario, the variables represent the concentration and transfer of the tracer substance; therefore, all compartments are assumed to be empty before giving the tracer in input. If the input is described by an impulse QCMF derives the initial state by assuming the tracer is present only in the compartment the tracer enters. Instead the step signal may be considered as a constant flow of tracer into the selected compartment.

Once the initial state has been defined, the user can run a simulation by clicking the *simulate* option in the simulate menu or simply save the generated code.

4.2. Model library

Organizing efficiently the knowledge embedded in the stored models is an essential issue if the system is to allow, once the user has a clear view of a pathophysiological problem, to search and retrieve an appropriate model. QCMF tackles this issue by representing the pathophysiological knowledge and the related models through *frames*. In this representation the system organizes the knowledge in a manner similar to the user's reasoning process in building a model: first it identifies a system, then the possible structure and behavior models representing this system, and finally the initial states associated with a particular physiological model.

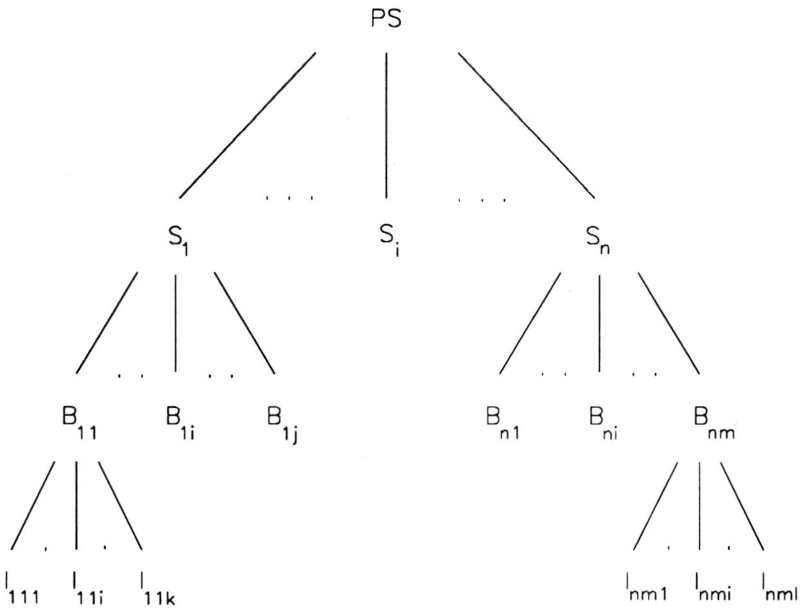

Figure 2. The tree structure of the model library.

All together the frames give rise to a tree structure (Figure 2) in which the nodes are given by the pathophysiological system frame (PS), the structure frames (S_i), the behavior frames (B_{ij}: the first index indicates which structure the behavior is associated with) and the initial state frames (I_{ijk}). Each frame contains:

- the name of the parent node;
- the names of all its children;
- the information given in input by the user regarding the frame.

This organization is useful on one side to QCMF to correctly access the model library, and on the other side to the user to easily examine the assumptions made in building the models. The latter of these operations is performed by the BROWSE module that allows the user to:

- visualize graphically a structure model;
- visualize all the functional relationships defined by the user in a given physiological model;
- visualize the assumptions underlying the initial state of a pathophysiological model.

5. AN EXAMPLE

This section describes a typical working session with QCMF at building and simulating a model. To this end, as an example, the glucose-insulin regulation system has been considered. When QCMF is invoked, an initialization window appears and the user is requested to enter a metabolic system which can be either selected among a list of previously defined systems through a menu or directly introduced (Figure 3). A corresponding pathophysiological frame is instantiated, and its slots, containing the names of structures, behaviors and initial states associated with it, are updated as soon as the related pieces of information are stored.

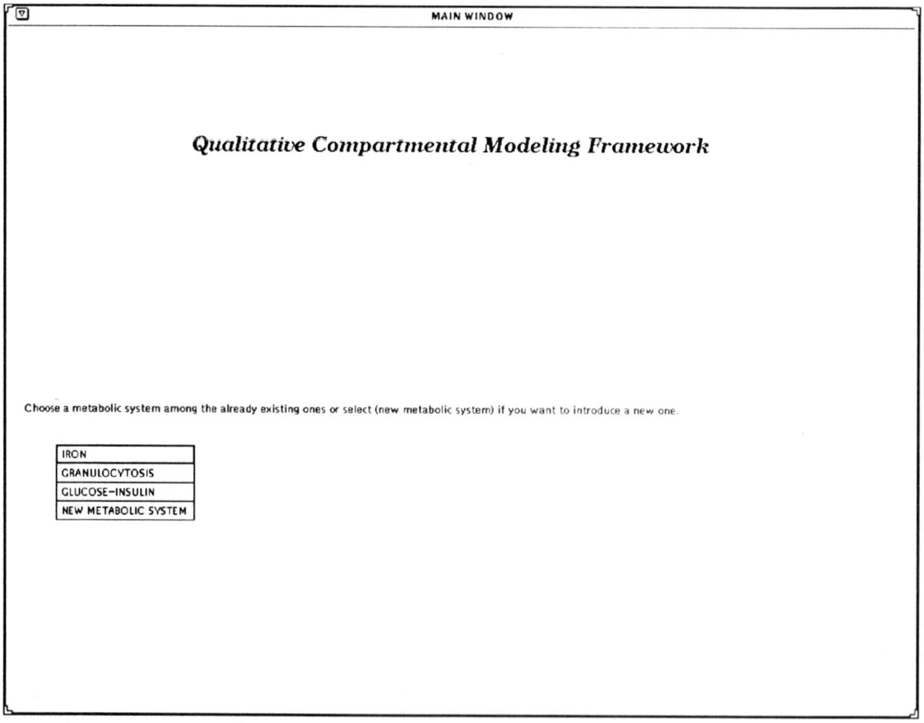

Figure 3. QCMF initialization window.

After the selection of the system, the working page window of QCMF appears. The user is then allowed to enter one of the model-reasoning phases. The GENERATE module makes the two sub-modules for generating a structure or behavior model accessible. Each of these sub-modules allows the user either to create a new structure or behavior model or to select a previously stored one.

When the structure module is selected, the icons representing the components of a compartmental diagram appears on the menu window.

Figure 4 shows a structure for the glucose-insulin regulation mechanism. This is the simplest structure describing such a mechanism: the system is decomposed into only two compartments containing respectively glucose and insulin. The two compartments exchange substance with the environment through input (production of glucose and insulin, respectively F10 and F20) and output flows (elimination of glucose and insulin, respectively F01, F02) but no substance is exchanged between them. The glucose elimination is due to the uptake renal excretion and the utilization by the central nervous system and red blood cells, as well as to the insulin-dependent glucose utilization by muscles and adipose tissues. The insulin production is controlled by the concentration of plasma glucose.

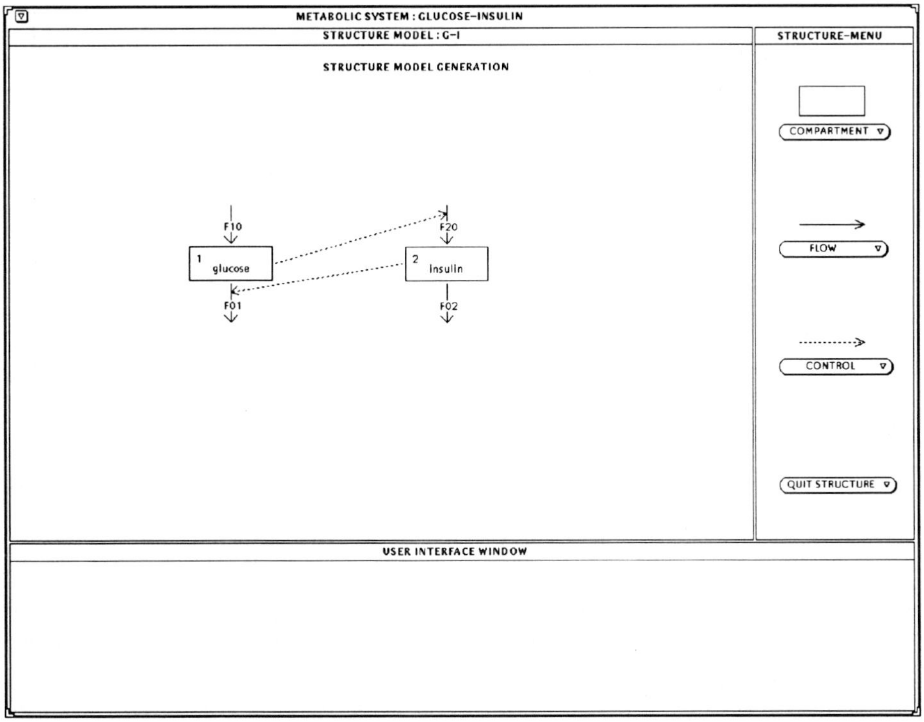

Figure 4. A structure model of the glucose-insulin regulation system.

After the structure has been entered, the user is allowed to build its associated behavior models. As shown in Figure 5, the variables and existing functional dependencies between variables are automatically identified by QCMF through the analysis of the structure, and the user is requested to select the kind of each relationship between the classes of functions listed in the menu. The listed classes of relationships allow the user to describe qualitatively a wide set of functional dependencies between variables in terms of their monotonicity properties.

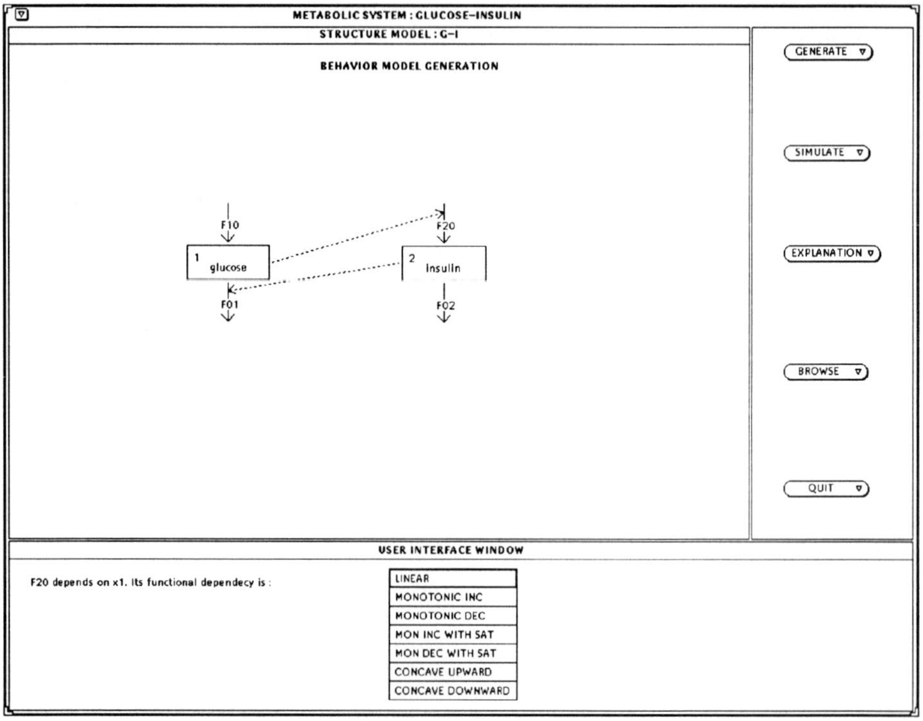

Figure 5. Relationships selection during the behavior model generation phase.

For the structure in Figure 4 a reasonable choice could be to assume the production of glucose $f10$ constantly equal to a normal value, and $f02$ to be a monotonic increasing function of $x2$. The flow $f20$ is controlled by $x1$, and it can be assumed that the production of insulin takes on a constant value (F20S) when the glucose is under a landmark value (X1S), beyond which it increases monotonically with the glucose and eventually reaches a saturation value (F20P) for $x1$=X1P. (In QSIM, this is well described by the constraint S^+). The landmarks X1S, X1P, F20S, F20P, which are given by the specific domain knowledge, are automatically entered into the respective quantity spaces for the variables $x1$ and $f20$, which have been firstly instantiated by exploiting the inequalities (2).

The multi-valued functional dependencies between flow and state variables (i.e. controlled flows) are expressed as sum or product of single-valued functions, according to the user's input. For example, the elimination of glucose $f01$, controlled by insulin, is both function of $x1$ and $x2$. In this case, it is reasonable to assume $f01(x1, x2) = gx1(x1) + gx2(x2)$, where $gx1 = M^{+}(x1)$ and $gx2 = S^{+}(x2)$, monotonic increasing in the interval $[0, x2^{*}]$ and then constant. This implies that the functions $gx1$, $gx2$, which actually are auxiliary variables, are added to the list of quantity spaces, and the quantity space of $x2$ is updated.

In addition to a quantity space for each variable, and to the translation into QSIM of the relationships between variables, QCMF derives automatically for each compartment the differential equation describing the dynamics of the contained substance.

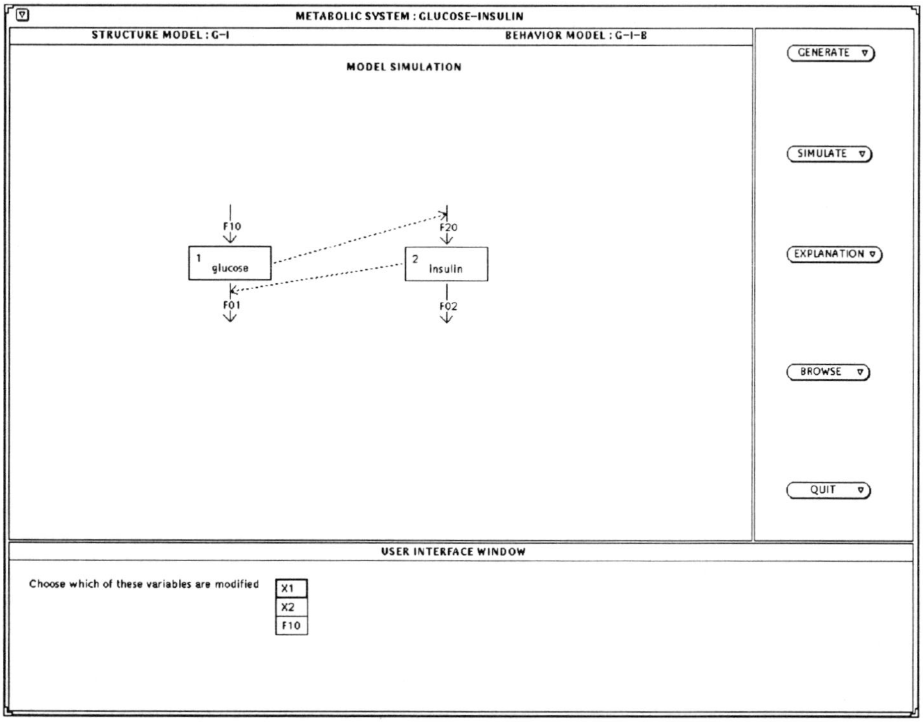

Figure 6. Selection of the perturbed variables.

Then, the user can access the SIMULATE module in order to simulate the glucose-insulin behavior model. In this case, the appropriate scenario is the perturbation of the normal state. QCMF automatically identifies which variables can be perturbed (Figure 6), and the user is asked to enter which variables are perturbed and if they are increased or decreased respect to the normal value. Then, QCMF automatically builds the initial state and invokes QSIM for simulating the model.

In Figure 7 one of the possible behaviors of the system obtained in response to an increased value of glucose is shown. At time t_0 the variable x_1 (glucose) has an increased value respect to the normal one (in correspondence to N). Then, the insulin production, which depends on x_1, assumes its maximum value (F20P), and consequently x_2 starts to increase. An increase of x_2 causes a higher glucose elimination, and then x_1 decreases till it reaches the landmark value X1P (displayed on the y-axis). When x_1 takes on the value X1P, the insulin production starts to decrease. The insulin (x_2) reaches its maximim value in t_1 and then decreases. Both x_1 and x_2 assume again the normal value in t_3.

This example does not consider any particular pathological situation but simply shows the dynamics of the system in a perturbed condition. Structural changes, for example the absence of the control by glucose of the insulin production, allows to model one type of diabetes.

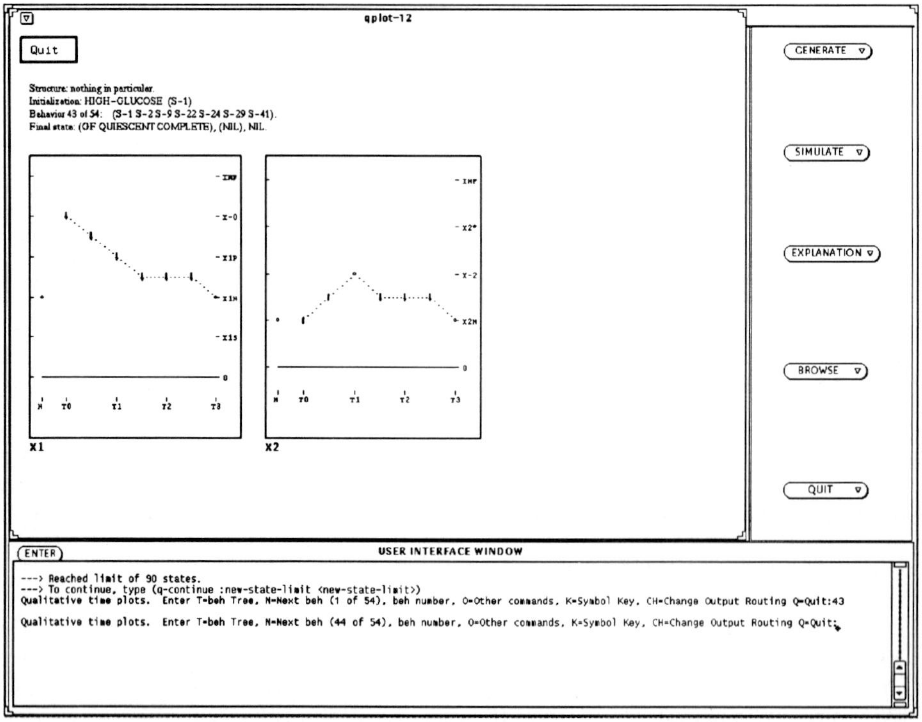

Figure 7. Simulation results of the effects of an increased glucose concentration.

6. CONCLUSION AND FUTURE WORK

System dynamics modeling is a powerful tool for reasoning about pathophysiological systems. Model-based reasoning goes through different steps, namely model formulation and generation, prediction and interpretation of the results. While the formulation and results interpretation phases require both the pathophysiological and methodological knowledge, the generation and simulation processes are strictly domain independent. The need of a large body of domain independent knowledge has been a serious deterrent for physicians from using system models in spite of their great utility. It is evident that a tool, like QCMF, which integrates the steps mentioned above should be of great help. In fact, such an integration allows sharing the domain knowledge and results obtained in each step, and moving automatically from one step to another.

As far as the possible uses of QCMF are concerned, two issues must be considered. First, QCMF has a practical value as a stand-alone system. The possibility to formulate and simulate, in an easy way, different qualitative models of a system allows the user to evaluate alternative hypotheses about functional relationships between variables on the basis of simulated behaviors which should reproduce behaviors either observed or reported in literature. This makes QCMF a powerful didactic tool for reasoning from the pathophysiological principles and for a deeper understanding of pathophysiological mechanisms. Second, it can be seen as a tool for both acquiring pathphysiological knowledge and building a library of models. Such a library should be integral part of the knowledge base of a MKBS and be properly exploited in the deductive inference of medical reasoning.

Although the current implementation makes QCMF already utilizable from the point of view of model building and simulation, some work has still to be done in order to make QCMF capable of generating explanations of the predicted behaviors. The generation of causal explanations of the behavior of a system is in itself an area of research in AI [4, 7, 8]. In our context, the problem of generating a causal explanation from an acausal description, as a QDE is, is restricted since the structure model is exploited as a causal graph where the effects of a change propagate following the paths in the structure topology. Of course, from the simulation point of view QCMF shows the same limitations of QSIM. But, a great deal of work is done both to reduce the generation of spurious behavior and to aggregate behaviors which do not differ significantly.

As far as the use of QCMF within a MKBS is concerned, future work will deal with the selection within the library of the appropriate models to test a set of hypotheses, and the formulation of a model of a complex system by assembling existing models of its components.

7. ACKNOWLEDGEMENTS

We especially thank B. Kuipers who provided the Common LISP implementation of QSIM. This work is part of the AIM project A2034, a General

Architecture for Medical Expert Systems II (GAMES II), which is supported by the European Community.

8. REFERENCES

1 G.L. Atkins. *Multicompartmental Models in Biological Systems.* Chapman and Hall, London, 1974.

2 D. G. Bobrow (ed.). *Qualitative Reasoning about Physical Systems.* North Holland, Amsterdam, 1984.

3 E. R. Carson, C. Cobelli and L. Finkenstein. *The Mathematical Modeling of Metabolic and Endocrine Systems.* Wiley, New York, 1983.

4 J. De Kleer, J.S. Brown. Theories of causal ordering. *Articial Intelligence*, 29 (1986) 33-61.

5 P. Fouchè, B.J. Kuipers. Reasoning about energy in qualitative simulation. *IEEE Transactions on Systems, Man and Cybernetics*, 22 (1992) 47-63.

6 L. Ironi, M. Stefanelli, and G. Lanzola. Qualitative models in medical diagnosis. *Artificial Intelligence in Medicine*, 2 (1990) 85–101.

7 Y. Iwasaki, H.A. Simon. Causality in device behavior. *Artificial Intelligence*, 29 (1986) 3-32.

8 Y. Iwaski, H.A. Simon. Theories of causal ordering: reply to De Kleer and Brown. *Artificial Intelligence*, 29 (1986) 63-72.

9 B. J. Kuipers, J.P. Kassirer. Causal reasoning in medicine: analysis of a protocol. *Cognitive Science*, 8 (1984) 363-385.

10 B. J. Kuipers. Qualitative simulation. *Artificial Intelligence*, 29 (1986) 280–338.

11 B.J. Kuipers B.J. Abstraction by time-scale in qualitative simulation. *Proceedings of the National Conference on Artificial Intelligence (AAAI-87).* Morgan Kaufmann, Los Altos, 621-625, 1987.

12 B.J. Kuipers, D. Bearlant. Using incomplete quantitative knowledge in qualitative reasoning. *Proceedings of the National Conference on Artificial Intelligence (AAAI-88).* Morgan Kaufmann, Los Altos, 324-329, 1988

13 B. J. Kuipers. Qualitative reasoning with causal models in diagnosis of complex systems. In: L.E. Widman, K.A. Loparo and N.R. Nielsen (eds.), *Artificial Intelligence, Simulation and Modeling.* Wiley, New York, 1989.

14 B.J. Kuipers, C.Chiu, D.T. Dalle Molle and D.R. Throop. Higher-order derivative constraints in qualitative simulation. *Artificial Intelligence*, 51 (1991) 343-380.

15 W.W. Lee, B.J. Kuipers. Non-intersection of trajectories in qualitative phase space: a global constraint for qualitative simulation. *Proceedings of the National Conference on Artificial Intelligence (AAAI-88)*, Morgan Kaufmann, Los Altos, 286-290, 1988.

16 E. Nicolosi, M.S. Leaning. Qualitative simulation of compartmental systems. In: C. Cobelli, L. Mariani (eds.), *Proc. 1st IFAC Symposium Modeling and Control in Biomedical Systems.* Pergamon, Oxford, 193-198, 1988.

17 M. Ramoni, M. Stefanelli, L. Magnani, and G. Barosi. An epistemological framework for medical knowledge based systems. *IEEE Transactions on Systems, Man, and Cybernetics*, 22, 6 (1992) 1361-1375.
18 Q. Shen, R.R. Leitch. Combining qualitative simulation and fuzzy sets. In: B. Faltings, P.Struss (eds.), *Recent Advances in Qualitative Physics*. MIT Press, 1991.
19 P. Struss. Global filters for qualitative behaviors. *Proceedings of the National Conference on Artificial Intelligence (AAAI-88)*, Morgan Kaufmann, Los Altos, 275-279, 1988.
20 D.S. Weld, J. De Kleer. *Readings in Qualitative Reasoning About Physical Systems*. Morgan Kaufmann, Los Altos, 1990.

Artificial Intelligence in Medecine
S. Andreassen et al. , Eds.
IOS Press, 1993

Knowledge-Based Interpretation of Magnetic Resonance Images : Detecting Multiple Sclerosis Lesions

M. Kamber[a,b], R. Shinghal[c], A.C. Evans[b,d], D.L. Collins[b], and G.S. Francis[d]

[a]School of Computing Science, Simon Fraser University, Burnaby, B.C. V5A 1S6, Canada

[b]NeuroImaging Laboratory, Montreal Neurological Institute, Montreal, Quebec H3A 2B4, Canada

[c]Department of Computer Science, Concordia University, Montreal, Quebec H3G 1M8, Canada

[d]Department of Neurology & Neurosurgery, McGill University, Montreal, Quebec H3A 2B4, Canada

Abstract

Magnetic Resonance (MR) imaging is a medical technique which permits the visualization of a variety of tumors, lesions, and abnormalities present within the soft biological tissues of the body. *Segmentation* of medical image data is the process of assigning anatomically-meaningful labels to each component of the image. This paper presents a method of knowledge-based interpretation of MR images of the head. In particular, the method is designed for the segmentation, or detection, of multiple sclerosis (MS) lesions of the brain. Knowledge of brain anatomy is represented in the form of a tissue probability model which provides *a priori* probabilities of brain tissue distribution per unit voxel in a standardized 3D 'brain space'. As 90-95% of MS lesions occur in white matter tissue [1], the model was used to confine the search for MS lesions to plausible white matter locations. Use of the model to segment multiple sclerosis lesions reduced the number of false positive lesions by 50-80% in comparison to non-model-based (i.e. purely data-driven) segmentation.

The performance of the statistical minimum distance and Bayesian classifiers (which both represent learned tissue classification rules as mathematical formulae) are compared to that of pruned and unpruned decision tree classifiers (which represent classification rules symbolically, as flow-chart-like tree structures). Although each classifier performed at about the same level of accuracy, the concise and symbolic representation of the rules generated by the pruned decision tree classifier may be preferred for its greater human interpretability.

1 INTRODUCTION

1.1 Problem definition

Magnetic Resonance Imaging (MRI) is a noninvasive medical technique employed to produce series of 2D cross-sectional images of the human body, permitting the detailed visualization of biological soft tissues. As a diagnostic tool, MRI is typically used qualitatively, with radiologists inspecting the acquired images for tumors, lesions, and other abnormalities present within internal anatomical structures. Although it can be applied to all parts of the body, MRI has been particularly useful for imaging the brain and spinal cord owing to its ability to discriminate between gray and white matter tissues, and fluid spaces.

Segmentation of medical images is the process of assigning a class label to each image pixel, where classes correspond to anatomical tissues, fluids, or structures. The segmentation of head MR data in routine clinical applications gives important quantitative information about anatomy in normal and diseased brain. An example of interest to this paper is the segmentation of multiple sclerosis lesions in MR images of the human brain. Multiple sclerosis (MS), a neurological disease affecting approximately 1 in 1000 persons [2], is characterized by lesions or 'damage' to the insulating myelin sheath surrounding nerve fibers of the brain and spinal cord. In MR images, these lesions appear as regions of hyperintensities, initially small and isolated, but becoming more extensive and connected as the disease progresses. Segmentation enables the quantitative measurement of MS lesion volumes and hence contributes to research in the study of the disease, the evaluation of drug treatments, and MS patient follow-up. Furthermore, segmentation allows the visualization of MS lesions in 3D, providing a means for studying how the locality of lesions affects the disease.

Manual segmentation of individual structures is tedious, time-consuming, and costly, with errors occurring owing to poor hand-eye coordination, low tissue contrast, and unclear tissue boundaries caused by *partial volumes* (where individual pixels contain more than one tissue type). Accurate automated segmentation of MR images is the first step towards promising quantitative applications of magnetic resonance imaging.

1.2 Justification of the use of artificial intelligence techniques

Magnetic resonance images contain noise and artifacts [3] which can cause regions of hyperintensity similar to that of MS lesions. Hence, techniques of automated segmentation which rely solely on image intensities (*data-driven* techniques) tend to produce a large number of *false positive* lesions (non-MS pixels incorrectly labeled as MS) even when images have been preprocessed to reduce impurities. Examples of data-driven methods include intensity thresholding and histogram analysis [4-5], edge-detection [6-7], region-growing [8-9], and multispectral feature-space classification [10-12]. When manually segmenting MS lesions, the physician will not base the hand-drawn outlines entirely on image intensities. Prior knowledge of anatomy and medical experience is also used in order to overcome noise, lack of tissue contrast, and artifacts in the image [9]. This is the premise behind model-based approaches to segmentation [13-15] which typically make use of knowledge such as the size and shape or relative location of anatomical structures in their classification. As 90-95% of MS lesions occur in white matter tissue [1], knowledge of whether a voxel (3D pixel) is in an area of the brain having a high probability of white matter tissue can be used in segmenting MS lesions. A tissue probability model [16] in a standardized 3D 'brain space' [17] was constructed based on MR brain image data obtained from twelve healthy volunteers, and gives the probabilities of each voxel belonging to each of the possible major healthy tissue types. Previous work in brain probability models can be found in von Keyserlingk's [18] probability density model for the presence of human 'sulci' (grooves separating the convolutions of the brain). This paper explores the use of our brain tissue probability model to guide the segmentation of MS lesions in MR image data. Model-based and non-model-based (i.e. purely data-driven) segmentation are compared.

This paper also presents a comparison of the performance of statistical and decision tree (pruned and unpruned) classifiers applied to MS lesion segmentation. Statistical classifiers, such as the minimum distance [12] and Bayesian [19] algorithms, represent learned classification rules as mathematical formulae. In decision tree algorithms [20], classification rules are represented as flow-chart-like tree structures where each internal node represents a test on a feature, each outgoing branch corresponds to a possible outcome of the test, and each leaf node represents a class. If both types of classifiers perform at the same level, then a decision tree classifier may be preferred for its symbolic rule representation.

2 EXPERIMENTAL METHODOLOGY

2.1 Image data sets used

Experiments were conducted on both real and simulated image data. Real MR brain image data were acquired with a Philips Gyroscan 1.5 Tesla superconducting magnet system from two patients diagnosed as having multiple sclerosis. A 2D Spin Echo sequence was used, with image acquisition parameters set at TR=1700 and TE=30/80ms. This sequence produced multispectral data, consisting of two channels (i.e. *dual-echos*), respectively reflecting the *T1-weighted* and *T2-weighted* tissue characteristic properties at each voxel. (For example, T1-weighted values help distinguish *c*erebro-*s*pinal *f*luid (CSF) from brain matter. T2-weighted values help differentiate MS lesions from brain matter. Use of these two tissue characteristics is important, as MS lesions may resemble CSF on single-echo data). Sixty-four non-overlapped dual-echo transverse slices were collected per patient at 2 mm intervals over the entire brain, and stored as 256 x 256 images with 1 mm square pixels. Each volume was transformed into the standardized brain space. Homomorphic filtering was applied to the images in order to reduce intensity variations for like tissues caused by the radiofrequency inhomogeneity artifact [21]. With the use of an edge-tracing routine, each lesion was manually outlined by an expert having an intra-observer variability of 3-5% in measurement of total MS lesion volume. The manual segmentation served as a 'gold standard' for quantifying the accuracy of the automated segmentation techniques, presuming that the human expert was always correct. In all experiments described below, classifier predictions which did not agree with the manual segmentation were regarded as incorrect.

The manual segmentation alone as a gold standard is insufficient owing to inter- and intra-observer variations in human decision-making, particularly when the images are of poor quality. Hence, segmentation was also performed on simulated image data where voxel class labels are known. Ten simulated brain MR image volumes depicting MS lesions were generated, each representing a different 'noise level', or variation in voxel intensity. In order to create the volumes, MR image data of a healthy brain were acquired, transformed into standardized space, and then segmented [16]. This resulted in a volume with voxels labeled according to the major cerebral tissues and fluid spaces. Using a mouse-controlled paint-edit function, MS lesions were added to the volume according to the size, shape, and location in which lesions can be found in real MR brain images of multiple sclerosis patients. A simulated 'noise-free' dual-echo MR volume was then created by replacing each voxel class label with the mean intensity value of its corresponding tissue and fluid spaces as determined from dual-echo images acquired in our laboratory [16]. The nine additional simulated volumes, were then generated by adding Gaussian noise with a mean of 0 and standard deviations in intensity of 5, 10, 15, 20, 30, 40, 60, 80, and 100 percent, respectively. Although we observed that the tissue intensity values in real-world image data typically vary from 4 to 20%, our aim was to study the accuracy of each classifier and the effectiveness of the model-based segmentation on data representing a wide range of noise.

2.2 Classification

This section give details concerning the implementation of each classifier. Owing to limited space, we are unable to present a description of the mathematics behind each method. For further theoretical details, the reader is directed towards the cited references. All algorithms were implemented in the 'C' programming language. Each of the classification algorithms is 'supervised' i.e. requires a training set of representative tissue samples in order to formulate classification rules. Associated with each tissue sample is an n-dimensional feature vector $X = (x_1, x_2, \ldots, x_n)$ depicting n measurements made on the tissue sample. Based on X, the sample is assigned to a tissue class.

In the minimum distance classifier implementation, an unknown sample is assigned the class to whose center (estimated by the mean class feature vector) it is the closest based on Euclidean distance.

In the Bayesian classifier implementation, classes were assumed to be equally likely since the prior probability distribution of MS lesions is not known.

The decision tree classifier uses an entropy function to measure the informativity of each attribute. A node is created to partition the training samples according to the values of the feature with the maximum information content ('test feature') [20]. To help keep trees at a manageable size by avoiding the growth of a branch for every possible test feature value, a single feature value, v, is selected to partition the training samples at a node into two branches (corresponding to the conditions $feature \leq v$ and $feature > v$) [22]. The tree grows as the test feature selection procedure is repeated recursively on each partition. A leaf is created when all samples of a partition belong to the same class, or when all samples of a partition have the same feature vector but are of different classes. In the former case, the leaf is labeled with the common class. In the latter case, the leaf is labeled with the class in majority among the partition samples [23].

When a decision tree is built, many of the branches will reflect noise caused by inaccurately measured or missing training data. Pruning methods identify and remove the least reliable branches, generally resulting in improved recognition rates [24]. The error-cost complexity pruning algorithm [25] was selected for pruned decision tree classification as it produces small and accurate trees [24].

2.3 Experiments

Model-based versus non-model-based segmentation. Knowledge of brain anatomy is encoded in the brain tissue probability model. Figure 1 shows a slice from the 80-slice model, illustrating probability masks for the major cerebral tissues and fluid spaces. These groups include gray matter tissue, white matter tissue, and CSF. Here, probabilities have been mapped to gray scale values. Low intensity voxels indicate areas of low tissue probability for the respective mask. High intensity voxels indicate voxels with high tissue type probability.

Non-model-based segmentation (using only the image intensity-based features described below) was compared to three methods of model-based segmentation in which the model was used, respectively, to :

1. *confine the search for MS lesions* to plausible white matter locations. All voxels having a white matter probability value (from the model) below the empirically-defined threshold of 50% were automatically labeled as non-MS. The features used were intensity-based, as described below.

2. *provide geometric features*, employing the probability values per voxel as features in addition to the intensity-based features below.

a)
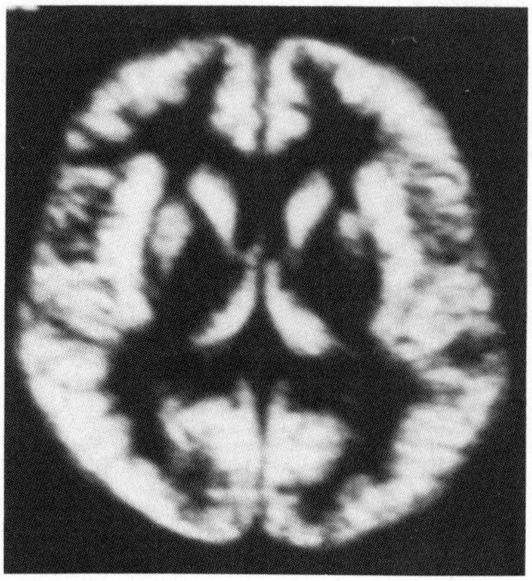
b)
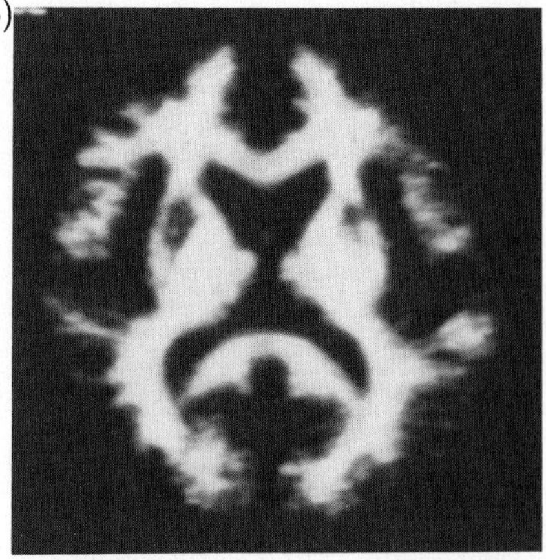
c)
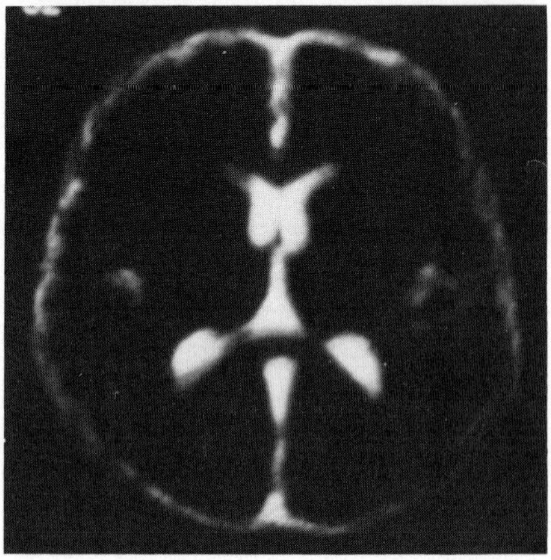

Figure 1: The tissue probability masks for *a*) gray matter, *b*) white matter, and *c*) CSF are mapped to gray scale values. These masks make up one slice of the 80-slice model.

3. *confine the search for MS lesions and provide geometric features* (i.e. a combination of model-based methods 1 and 2).

Comparison of classifiers. Segmentation was repeated on each image volume for each method with each classifier.

All experiments were conducted on a SUN Sparc 1 station with 24 Mbytes of memory. The intensity-based features employed were the dual-echo mean intensity and standard deviation about the mean from a window around each voxel. Each segmentation was repeated varying the window size (1, 3, 5 pixels) and dimension (2D or 3D). The training set consisted of 300 arbitrarily selected tissue samples. Volumes were segmented into MS and non-MS from above the eyeballs to just below the top of the brain (corresponding to the area covered in the tissue probability model). Because the percentage of MS lesions is small with respect to the entire volume, only the tissues within the brain were segmented.

3 RESULTS AND DISCUSSION

3.1 Model-based versus non-model-based segmentation

A segmentation example is given in Figure 2. Figures 2a and 2b correspond to the dual-echo images (respectively, T1-weighted and T2-weighted) obtained for a slice from one of the patient test volumes, transformed into standardized space. Figure 2c shows the non-model-based segmentation. Voxels classified as MS lesion are painted dark. Of the three model-based approaches, use of the model to confine the search for MS lesions to plausible white matter voxels was the most effective. Figure 2d shows the image segmentation obtained with this approach. In Figures 2c and 2d, the manual segmentation of MS lesions is displayed on top of the automated results. The use of the probability model to confine the MS lesion search space reduced the amount of false positive lesions by 50-80% (Figure 3). The elimination of false positive lesions is indicated with the 'F' pointers in Figure 2c and in their corresponding locations in Figure 2d. Although the use of the model has not eliminated all false positives (such as those at pointer 'E'), it has improved the segmentation of MS lesions considerably.

The overall accuracy of the non-model-based and model-based segmentation methods on each test volume are shown (here for the decision tree classifier) in Figure 4. Segmentation accuracy is computed as the recognition rate, i.e. the percentage of correct voxel tissue labelings (where the manual segmentation of the real image data, and known voxel class labels of the simulated image data served as gold standards). In comparison to non-model-based segmentation, the use of the model to confine the MS lesion search space improved accuracy by 3-5 percentage points for the real image data. For the simulated image data, the corresponding improvement was of around 5 percentage points when noise levels were 10-20 standard deviations, and 8-12 percentage points when noise levels were greater than or equal to 30 standard deviations. Accuracies of around 90% for non-model-based segmentation would seem to be quite high. However, as we have seen, close inspection of the non-model-based segmentation of Figure 2c reveals a large number of false positive lesions. The percentage of actual MS lesions is very small in relation to total brain size; it was observed to be 3.0-4.5% in our patients. Therefore, an accuracy of 90% is *not* considered acceptable when detecting MS lesions. The challenge lies in overcoming mis-classifications in the remaining 10%. Thus, an increase in accuracy of 3-12 percentage points (when the model is used to guide the MS lesion search) is considered to be a good improvement. Such a seemingly small increase has a large effect on the reduction of false position lesions, as shown by the 'F' pointers in Figures 2c and 2d.

The automated segmentation results obtained were more consistent than manual segmentation. The automated segmentation also identified true MS lesions that had been erroneously omitted in the manual segmentation, as is illustrated by the 'T' pointer of Figure 2d. Accurate and consistent segmentation of MS lesions is difficult to achieve manually, particularly when lesions are tiny, numerous, and spread over several thin (1 or 2 mm) slices. The model contains an overestimate of white matter tissue due to partial volumes. False positive lesions that were not eliminated with the use of the model are likely due to this discrepancy. The number of false positives should further decrease once errors in the white matter mask are corrected. The automated segmentation of an entire volume of 80 slices required roughly 15 minutes (including the time required for a user to produce a training set and to train the selected classifier). Manual segmentation of the same data by a human expert required approximately 4 hours.

a) b)

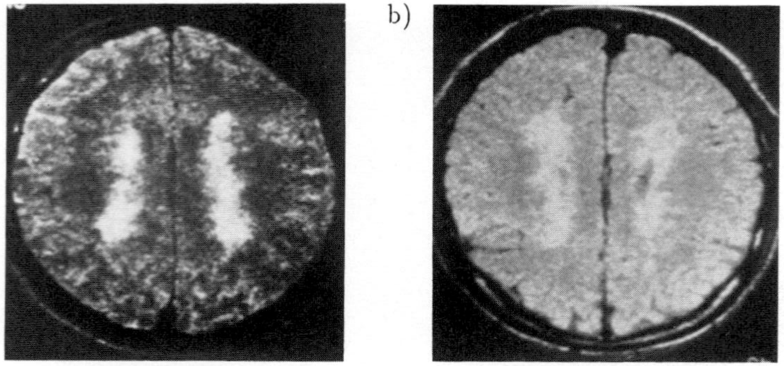

c) d)

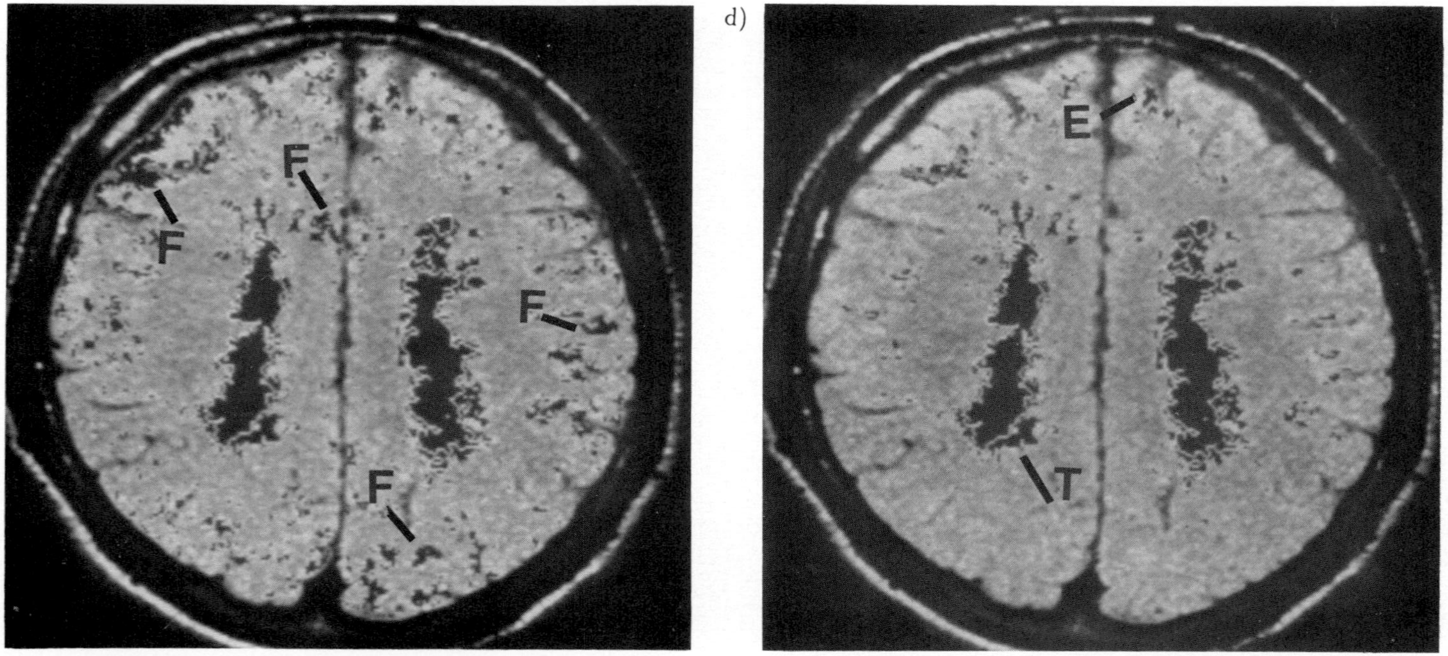

Figure 2: Segmentation of an image slice in standardized space: *a*) T1-weighted image *b*) T2-weighted image *c*) Non-model-based segmentation (purely data-driven) *d*) Model-based segmentation where the model was used to confine the search for MS lesions to voxels with high white matter probability. Voxels labeled as MS lesion by the automated segmentation are painted dark. Hand-drawn outlines of the MS lesions are displayed on top of the automated segmentation. Legend: T = true positive MS lesion, F = false positive MS lesion, E = errors not corrected with the model.

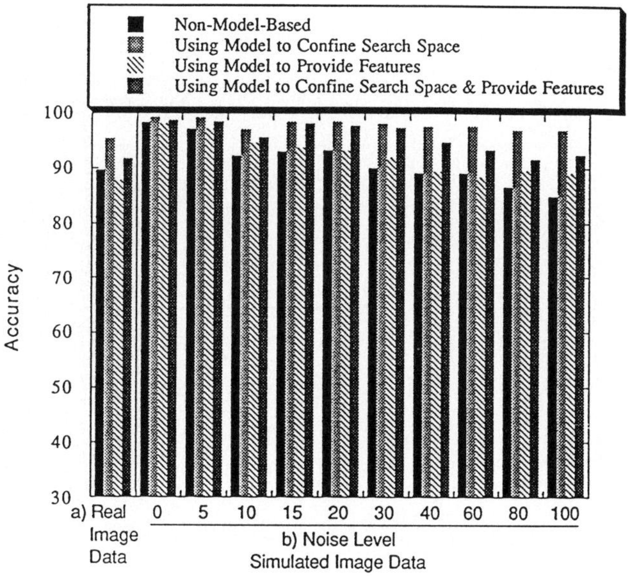

Figure 3: Non-model-based and model-based segmentation accuracy in *a*) real MR brain image data, and *b*) simulated MR brain image data.

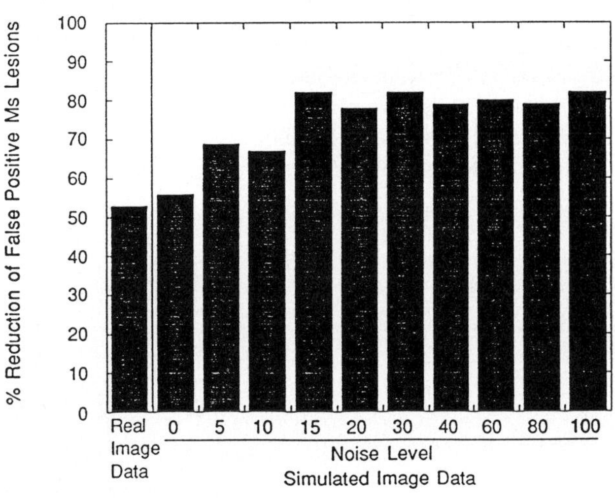

Figure 4: Percentage reduction of false positive lesions obtained when the model was used to confine the MS lesion search space to plausible white matter voxels. (A reduction of 100% means that all of the false positive lesions were eliminated).

3.2 Comparison of classifiers

The classifiers are compared in terms of accuracy (or recognition rate), training and recall times, and the interpretability of the derived classification rules. Figure 5 displays the overall accuracy of each classifier on the test image data (non-model-based). When classifying real image data, the level of accuracy of each classifier ranged from 89.0-92.5%. Pruning reduced the average number of decision tree leaves by 25-65%. Pruning improved decision tree classification by 1-3% in ten out of the twelve image test sets.

Figure 5: Accuracy of each classifier (non-model-based).

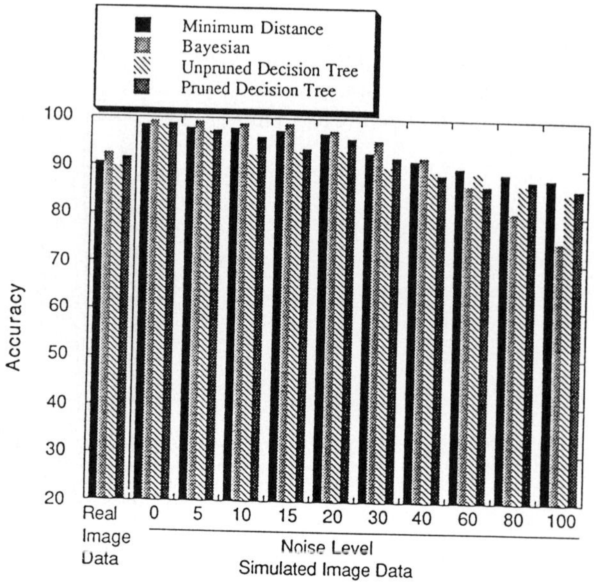

Figure 6: Training times of the statistical and decision tree classifiers (relative to the training time required by the Bayesian classifier on the noise-free simulated image data).

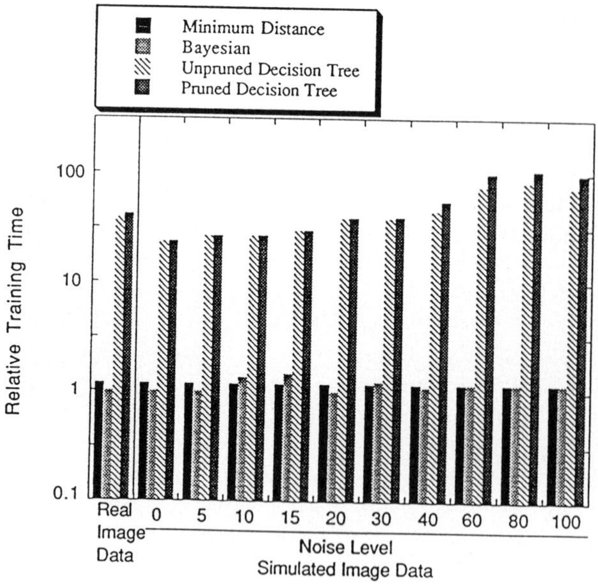

Training time is measured as the time required by a classifier to derive classification rules for recognizing tissue class labels of voxels in a given MR image. Figure 6 shows, for each image data set, the average classifier training time (relative to the training time required for Bayesian classification of the noise-free simulated image data). The statistical classifiers were faster in training than the decision tree algorithms. The average training times for the minimum distance, Bayesian, decision tree, and pruned decision tree classifiers on the real MR image data were, respectively, 0.020 CPU seconds, 0.017 CPU seconds, 0.649 CPU

Figure 7: Average recall time in CPU seconds (on a SUN Sparc 1) per slice for each classifier.

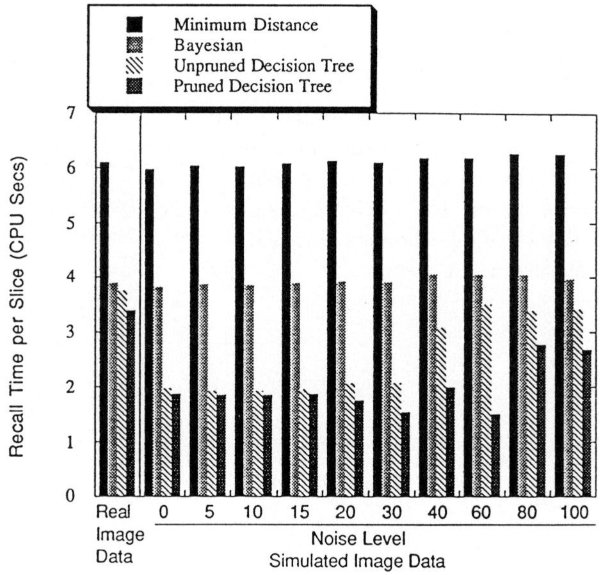

seconds, and 0.699 CPU seconds. Increasing levels of noise in the data caused the time required for the construction and pruning of decision trees to increase, yet did not affect the training times of the statistical classifiers. The higher the noise level in the data, the greater was the number of nodes in the decision trees.

Recall time is measured as the time required by a trained classifier to segment the brain region of an image slice (excluding the time required for feature extraction). The average recall time in CPU seconds per slice for each classifier on each image data set is shown in Figure 7. The decision tree classifiers were up to 4 CPU seconds faster in total recall time per slice than the minimum distance classifier, and up to 2 CPU seconds faster than the Bayesian classifier.

The statistical and decision tree classifiers differ in their representation of learned classification rules. To represent acquired knowledge of class descriptions, the minimum distance and Bayesian classifiers use mathematical formulae, whereas the decision tree classifiers use a symbolic representation. Although it can be difficult to access the human interpretability of learned classification rules, it was observed that the decision trees output by the unpruned decision tree classifier were barely intelligible. (The average unpruned decision tree was approximately ten levels deep). The pruned decision trees, however, were much smaller. An example of a pruned tree for the classification of MS lesion and non-MS is shown in Figure 8. Although a limited form of knowledge representation, the pruned decision tree is small enough to be easily understood. Since, on real MR image data, each classifier performed at about the same level of accuracy, the concise and symbolic representation of the rules generated by the pruned decision tree classifier may be preferred for its greater human interpretability.

Figure 8: Pruned decision tree for the classification of MS lesions. Although the input features were the dual-echo mean intensity and the standard deviation about the mean for a 3 x 3 x 3 window about each voxel, the classifier found only the dual-echo mean intensity features to be useful.

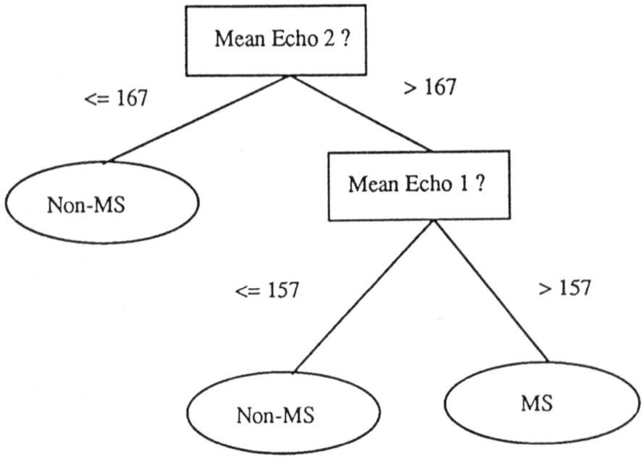

4 CONCLUSIONS

A knowledge-based approach was presented for the automated 3D segmentation of multiple sclerosis lesions in magnetic resonance images. *A priori* knowledge of brain anatomy was represented in the form of a brain tissue probability model which was used to limit the search for MS lesions to plausible white matter tissue locations. Although based on only twelve subjects, the model was useful in reducing the number of false positive lesions by 50-80% in comparison to non-model-based segmentation. The minimum distance and Bayesian classifiers, and the unpruned and pruned decision tree classifiers performed at about the same level of accuracy on real image data. Differences were observed regarding classifier training and recall times, and in the human interpretability of learned classification rules. The decision tree classifiers were the fastest at recall, yet were the slowest in training. Pruned decision tree learning may be preferred for its greater human interpretability. Future work involves the application of the probability model to the segmentation of healthy brain tissues, as well as to the segmentation of other types of lesions characterized by their location of occurrence. The model-based segmentation method was recently used to develop an MS lesion probability model [26]. Its usefulness in the segmentation of MS lesions is to be investigated. A brain atlas based on 300 normal brains is under development for use in the segmentation of finer gray and white matter structures [27]. Future plans include the investigation of methods for encoding the knowledge that clinicians use for lesion detection, and the development and application of unsupervised as well as hybrid learning systems [28-29].

5 ACKNOWLEDGEMENTS

We wish to thank Dr. D.L. Arnold, Mr. A. Gauvin, Mr. S. Hum, Dr. G. Partlow, Dr. T. Peters, Mr. A. Takahashi, Dr. Y. Zang, and the staff of the Brain Imaging Center at the Montreal Neurological

Institute. We also thank the Natural Sciences and Engineering Research Council of Canada, the Canadian Multiple Sclerosis Society, and the American Multiple Sclerosis Society.

6 REFERENCES

1. K.R. Maravilla. In D.D. Stark & W.G. Bradley (eds.), Magnetic Resonance Imaging, C.V. Mosby Company, St. Louis (1988) 344.
2. C. Martyn. In W.B. Matthews, A. Compston, I.V. Allen & C. Martyn (eds.), McAlpine's Multiple Sclerosis, Churchill Livingstone, New York, NY (1991) 3.
3. B.A. Porter, W. Hastrup, M.L. Richardson, G.E. Wesbey, D.O. Olson, L.D. Cromwell, & A.A. Moss. *RadioGraph.*, 7 (1987) 271.
4. K.O. Lim & A. Pfefferbaum. *J. Comp. Assist. Tomogr.*, 13 (1989) 588.
5. J.R. Mitchell, S.J. Karlik, D.H. Lee & A.Fenster. *Proc. SPIE Image Processing*, 1652 (1992) 99.
6. M. Bomans, K.-H. Hohne, U. Tiede & M. Reimer. *IEEE Trans. Med. Imag.*, 9 (1990) 177.
7. D.N. Kennedy, P.A. Filipek & V.S. Caviness Jr. *IEEE Trans. Med. Imag.*, 8 (1989) 1.
8. T.L. Jernigan, G.A. Press & J.R. Hesselink. *Arch. Neurol.*, 47 (1990) 27.
9. R.T. Fan, S.S. Trivedi, L.L. Fellingham & A. Gamboa-Aldeco. *Proc. SPIE Medical Imaging*, 767 (1987) 494.
10. G. Gerig, J. Martin, R. Kikinis, O. Kubler, M. Shenton & F.A. Jolesz. In A.C.F. Colchester & D.J. Hawkes (eds.), *Information Processing in Medical Imaging*, 511, Springer-Verlag, London, UK (1991) 175.
11. M. Ozkan, H.G. Sprenkels & B.M. Dawant. *Proc. Intl. Joint Conf. Neural Nets.*, 1 (1990) 429.
12. M.W. Vannier, R.L. Butterfield, D.L. Rickman, D.M. Jordan, W.A. Murphy & P.R. Biondetti. *CRC Crit. Reviews Biomed. Eng.*, 15 (1987) 117.
13. G.L. Vernazza, S.B. Serpico & S.G. Dellepiane. *IEEE Trans. Circuits & Syst.*, 34 (1987) 1399.
14. I. Kapouleas. *Comp. Meth. & Prog. in Biomed.*, 32 (1990) 17.
15. R. Dann, J. Hoford, S. Kovacic, M. Reivich & R. Bajcsy. *J. Comp. Assist. Tomogr.*, 13 (1989) 603.
16. M. Kamber, D.L. Collins, R. Shinghal, G.S. Francis & A.C. Evans. *Proc. Visualization Biomed. Computing*, 1808 (1992) 590.
17. J. Talairach & P. Tournoux. Co-Planar Stereotaxic Atlas of the Human Brain: 3-Dimensional Proportional System. Thieme Medical Publishers, New York, NY, 1988.
18. D.G. von Keyserlingk, K. Niemann & J. Wasel. *Acta Anat.*, 131 (1988) 127.
19. R.O. Duda & P.E. Hart. Pattern Classification and Scene Analysis, Wiley, New York, NY, 1973.
20. J. R. Quinlan. *Machine Learning*, 1 (1986) 81.
21. M.D. Levine. Vision in Man and Machine. McGraw-Hill, New York, NY, 1985.
22. J. R. Quinlan. *Intl. J. Man-Mach. Studies*, 27 (1987) 221.
23. J. R. Quinlan. In R.S. Michalski, J.G. Carbonell & T.M. Mitchell (eds.), Machine Learning: An Artificial Intelligence Approach II, Morgan Kaufmann, Los Altos, CA (1986) 149.
24. J. Mingers. *Machine Learning*, 4 (1989) 227.
25. L. Breiman, J. Friedman, R. Olshen & C. Stone. Classification and Regression Trees, Wadsworth, Monterrey, CA, 1984.
26. M. Kamber, D.L. Collins, S. Narayanan, E. Pioro, A.C. Evans & D.L. Arnold, *Proc. Soc. Magnetic Resonance in Med.*, (1993), in press.
27. A. C. Evans, D. L. Collins & B. Milner. *Soc. Neurosci. Abst.*, 18 (1992).
28. R.E. Stepp & R.S. Michalski. In R.S. Michalski, J.G. Carbonell & T.M. Mitchell (eds.), Machine Learning: An Artificial Intelligence Approach II, Morgan Kaufmann, Los Altos, CA (1986) 471.
29. J.W. Shavlik & G.G. Towell. *Connection Sci.*, 1 (1989) 233.

Artificial Intelligence in Medecine
S. Andreassen et al. , Eds.
IOS Press, 1993

Model Based Image Interpretation of Spiral CT Scans of the Abdomen

Englmeier K.-H.[1], Haubner M.[1], Fink B.K.[2], Fink U.[2]

[1] GSF-Institut für Medizinische Informatik und Systemforschung, Ingolstädter Landstr. 1, Neuherberg, 85758 Oberschleißheim, Germany

[2] Radiologische Klinik und Nephrologische Klinik des Klinikums Großhadern, Ludwig-Maximilians-Universität, Marchioninistr. 15, 81377 München, Germany

1. INTRODUCTION

The development of computer assisted imaging methods is one of the great advances in the medicine of the last years. Computer assisted imaging methods offer a lot of advantages in comparison to the conventional radiological technology:

By integration in a PACS image data are available in many places and at any time which may be the solution for the storage problem and makes the teamwork of clinicians and radiologists easier. Further computer assisted imaging methods offer a new presentation of anatomical and pathologic structures without superposition and with the possibility of post processing. In particular considerable are 3D-presentations which may be a good help in the preoperative planning and which may be an alternative to invasive methods as angiography.

This paper proposes a methology that enables an arbitrary Spiral-CT-scan of the abdomen to be automatically segmented and classified into bony structures, liver, kidneys and vessels. The image sequence is represented at a number of different scales (as in pyramid techniques) where a number of features are associated with each pixel al the particular scale (e.g. density, Hounsfield units, gradient magnitude).

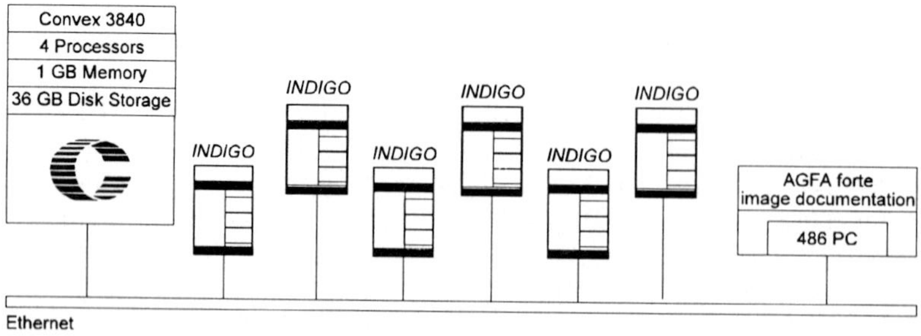

Fig. 1: Hardware environment

2. METHODS

2.1. Image acquisition

We examined 30 patients with renal tumors and 6 patients with stag horn calculi. All patients underwent surgery the day after the examination. The CT-scans were performed as spiral-CT-scans at a Siemens Somatom Plus. Based on slipring technology with continuous data acquisition over a multitude of 360° scans and continuous patient transport a volume of a maximum of 24 cm length can be scanned within 24 sec.

Patients with renal tumors were scanned with a table feed of 8 mm/sec, a slice thickness of 8 mm and an increment of 2 mm ca. 20 sec after a bolus injection of 150 ml non-ionic contrast medium. Bolus injection was done intravenously by an injector with a flow rate of 2 ml/sec.

Stag horn calculi were scanned dependent on their dimension with a table feed and a slice thickness of 4 mm or 2 mm and an increment of 2 mm or 1 mm before and 5 min after bolus injection of 100 ml contrast medium. Bolus injection was done by an injector with a flow rate of 1 ml/sec.

While the 24-sec spiral-CT-scan the patients were required not to move and to suspend respiration. All scans were taken at 165 mAs and 120 kV.

For the data calculation the algorithm implemented by Siemens was applied.

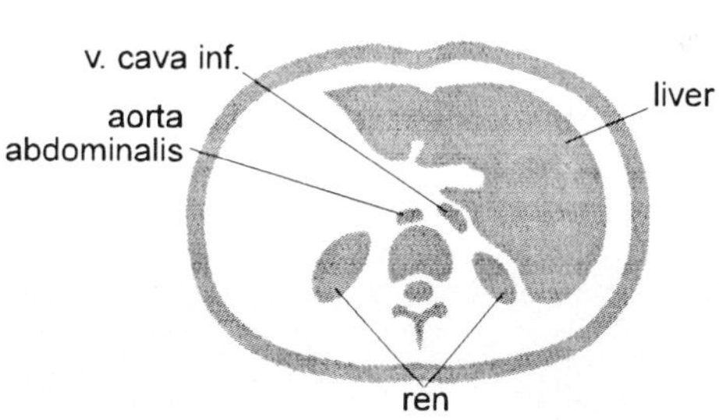

Fig. 2: Anatomical Model

2.2. Image processing and visualization

The stag horn calculi were reconstructed with the 3D-reconstruction program, which is implemented in Siemens software. The operating storage for these 3D-reconstructions contains a maximum of 64 slices. True to life reproductions were created in various projections. While the following endoscopic surgery - as a rule combined with ESWL (endoscopic shock wave lithotrypsy) - the 3D-model could be compared with the parts of the surgically removed calculus put together in order to control the completeness.

The process of this 3D-visualization as well as morphometry and density measurements are based on the process of segmentation and contour determination. To do this, the acquisitioned images were transferred to a parallel computer (CONVEX C3840) with 4 processors, 1 Gigabyte memory and 36 Gigabyte disc storage (Fig. 1). This supercomputing system is connected via Ethernet and network File System to a workstation cluster consisting of six Silicon Graphics IRIS-INDIGOS R 4000 with true color displays and z-buffers for surface and volume visualization. Using the Distributed Graphics Library (OPEN GL in the near future) both machine types can share the work load, each doing the task it is best suited for, resulting in a more balanced work load and better performance. The implemented software is embedded in a software system with the following specifications (see also 1):

- unique file format for CT, MRI, raw data of MRI, DR, DSA and scintigrams
- easy user interactions using file browsing and pull down menue techniques
- image processing utilities such as filtering, contour detection and segmentation
- image fusion techniques
- 3D-visualization techniques

In order to visualize the kidneys with their vessels, the segmentation of these anatomical structures is necessary. We developed an automatic segmentation method which reduces the number of user interactions. This method satisfies anatomical constraints to achieve structure identification and segmentation. These constraints of anatomical topology are described as follows: Both kidneys are localized side by side with the spinal column. Aorta abdominalis and vena cava inferior are in front of the spinal column. It is assumed that the crossection of both vessels is nearly elliptical (Fig. 2).

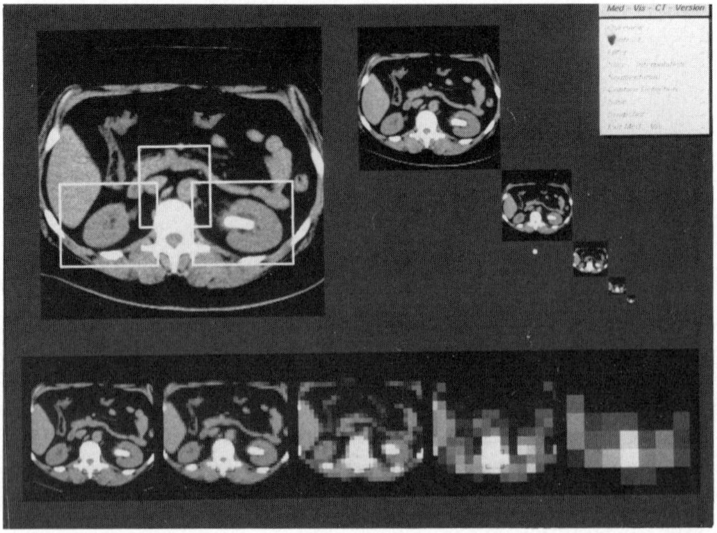

Fig. 3: Localization of the spinal column by the bright spot detection and the average image pyramids

In order to localize the region of the both kidneys, firstly the position of the spinal column is detected. The spinal column is a certain locality in the abdominal CT-image, which is noticeable brighter than the immediate surroundings. We exploit the advantage of the determination of this bright spot in the transversal CT, because the rectangular regions for the kidney segmentation are correctly localized beside the bright spot of the spinal column.

To detect the spinal column as a bright spot we use the average image pyramids. The algorithm of these pyramids has the characteristic of selecting a point, that is representative of a locally bright area at the image, if we combine the algorithm with a global maximum search (Fig. 3). The result of this process step is the position of the maximum density in the lowest resolution image of the image pyramid.

Following that three rectangular regions are created overlaying the localization of the kidneys and vessels. This procedure minimizes the influence of disturbances of the segmentation process caused by structures of similar density (liver). Within the rectangular regions, which overlays the position of the kidneys, a threshold oriented process is applied to the high resolution part of the image pyramid. Based on the a priori knowledge, that the kidneys are displayed as connected singular region in the CT-image, noise and disturbances are eliminated by recursive object labelling (Fig. 4).

Stag horn calculi are characterized by high density values, which are similar to bony structures. Therefore we can use threshold algorithm to localize the stag horn calculi within the region of the kidney.

Based on the a priori knowledge of closed elliptical contours the developed algorithm detects the actual contours of aorta abdominalis and vena cava by means of structure adapted filters via maximizing the cross correlation function (7).

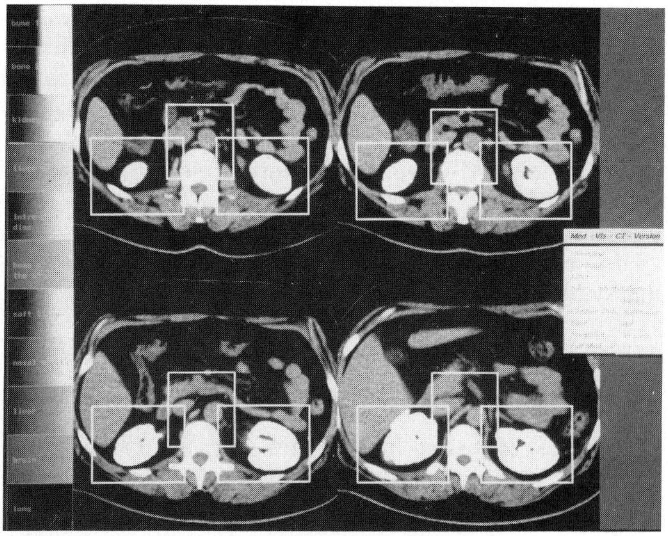

Fig. 4: Positioning of the raw rectangular regions and the result of the segmentation process overlayed in white color

3. RESULTS

In all 6 cases we created a 3D-model of stag horn calculus it could be proven as a true to life model of the surgically obtained concrement or the totality of its composed parts. For the surgeon this model proved to be an excellent possibility to control the complete removal of the stag horn calculus.

In all 30 cases of renal tumor the extension of the tumoral mass could be shown. In contrast to conventional CT-scans the data acquisition is performed with single breath-hold technique. In this way gaps or double imaged structures - in conventional CT-scans caused by inconstant respiration volumes - can be avoided. Multiplanar sections in each case improved the demonstration of spatial relation especially between kidney or tumor and liver or surrounding tissue. In a great number of cases the possibility of coronal imaging leads to a better delineation of the renal vessels. First results show, that the use of 3D-reconstruction and visualization in frontal, sagittal and oblique view might lead to a better staging of renal tumors.

4. DISCUSSION

The 3D-visualization of stag horn calculi is the only imaging method, which shows clearly the true 3D-topography, especially the extension of the calculus into the anterior or posterior calyces. This influences the surgical proceeding.

In the literature 3D-reconstruction is known especially from the visualization of bone structures (8,9). With conventional CT-scanning techniques a sufficient 3D-image of the kidneys mostly was not possible because of the inconstant levels of inspiration and due to this of the kidneys from scan to scan. This often caused omission of some anatomic levels or repeated scanning of others. With Spiral-CT-scanning in singlebreathold technique volumes can be scanned continuously without any gaps and little influence from patient motion. In this way one of the characterizing advantages of MRI in comparison to other imaging methods now with volume scanning is also available in CT-technique: The multiplanar imaging. In contrast to MRI-imaging this can be performed independently from breathing artefacts.

Another advantage is the short examination time because of the loss of inter scan times. This gives the chance of complete using of the bolus of contrast medium and may lead to a much better delineation of vessels.

A disadvantage of Spiral-CT may be the limitation of the available tube current at 165 mAs. This causes a decreased image quality in comparison to conventional CT-scans. With technical proceedings this may be improved in future.

One of the tasks of prime importance for the future seems to be the improvement of the image processing methods. The aim should be an image quality true to life as accurately as possible. Further the user interactions should be reduced and organized as easy as possible. In order to visualize the kidneys with artery and vein, the segmentation of these anatomical structures is necessary. Segmentation is normally described as the partitioning of an image into homogenous regions (characterized by grey values, textures) (3). Previous works on grey value based image segmentation can be considered to have taken two paths:

- edge based segmentation
- region based segmentation (2)

A lot of segmentation procedures (interactive or automatic) are described in the realm of CT and MRI image processing (3,4,5). We developed an automatic segmentation method which may reduce the user interactions and may lead to a better delineation of kidneys, tumor and vessels.

5. REFERENCES

1. **Englmeier K.-H., Fink U., Hilbertz T.:** Visualization of Multimodal Image Information in Medicine, Proc. of the Sixteenth Annual Symposium on Computer Applications in Medical Care, 8.-11.11.92, Baltimore, Eds.: M.E. Frisse, 25-29 (1992)
2. **Fu K.S., Mui J.K:** A survey on image segmentation. Patt.Recog.3: 3-16
3. **Griffin L D., Colchester A.C.F., Robinson G.P., Hawkes DJ.:** Structure sensitive scale and the hierarchical segmentation of grey-level imaging. Proc.of Visualization in Biomedical Computing, 13.-16.10.92, Chapel Hill, Ed. R.A.Robb, 24-32(1992)
4. **Schnemann T., Boman T., Tiede U., Höhne K-H.:** Interactive 3D-Segmentation of Tomographic Image Volumes, in: Mustererkennung '92, 14. DAGM-Symposium, Dresden, 14.-16.9.1992, ed.: S.Fuchs, R.Hofmann, 73-80 (1992)
5. **Vernazza G., Serpico S.B., Dellepiane S.G.:** A knowledge based system for biomedical image processing and recognition, IEEE transactions on circuits and systems, CAS-34 (11): 1399-1416 (1987)
6. **Blanford R.P., Tanimoto S.L.:** Bright-Spot Detection in Pyramids, Computer Vision, Graphics and Image Processing 43, 133-149 (1988)
7. **Englmeier K.-H., Hecker R., Hötzinger H., Pöppl S.J, Thiel H.:** Reconstruction and pseudo-3-dimensional presentation of the Uterus from Automatic Segmented Transversal Ultrasound Slices - a Fundamental Precondition for optimizing the individually Adjusted Therapy Planning in Case of Carcinoma of the Body of the Uterus, Proc. CAR '85, eds.: H.U.Lemke, M.L.Rhodes, C.C.Jaffe and R.Felix, Springer Verlag, Berlin, 358-370 (1985)
8. **Burk D.L.Jr., Mears D.C., Kennedy W.H., Cooperstein L.A., Herbert D.L.:** Three-dimensional computed tomography of acetabular fractures. Radiology 155(1985)183
9. **Pate D., Resnick D., Andre M., Sartoris D.J., Kursunoglu S., Bielecki D., Dev P., Vassiliadis A.:** Perspective: three-dimensional imaging of the musculosceletal system. AJR 147 545 (1986)

Artificial Intelligence in Medecine
S. Andreassen et al. , Eds.
IOS Press, 1993

Applying Qualitative Reasoning to Commonsense Physiology *

Inés Arana and Jim Hunter

Department of Computing Science, University of Aberdeen, Aberdeen AB9 2UE, Scotland, UK. *e-mail:*{arana, jhunter}@csd.abdn.ac.uk

Abstract

This paper describes ongoing basic research in the context of reasoning about naive physiology. A qualitative representation of commonsense physiology at various levels of abstraction and detail and high levels of interrelationships is described. This representation is then used to derive the behaviour of a physiological process from the behaviour of its subprocesses and the relationships between them. The model is then perturbed (possibly representing pathophysiology) and a method to derive the effect of such a perturbation by propagating it throughout the model is presented.

1. INTRODUCTION

During the last few years, considerable effort has been devoted to representing medical knowledge (eg. see [2]). Following some of the ideas described in the *Naive Physics Manifesto* [3], we believe that representations of commonsense knowledge are important,should be general and should reflect the way in which the domain perceived, i.e. be as close as possible to the models used by experts. A representation of commonsense† physiology should therefore be broad (represent the whole domain) and dense (reflect the complexity of the domain).

Qualitative models seem especially suitable for representing and reasoning about medicine, not only because numerical medical knowledge is frequently unavailable (unknown) but also because clinicians widely use symbolic knowledge when solving medical problems. Although these kinds of model have been successfully used to represent some particular physiological mechanism (eg. [4]), there has been little effort towards modeling commonsense physiology in a broader (more general) sense.

Qualitative representations often consist of a set of parameters and a set of differential equations. Although these seem appropiate for representing man-made physical systems, they often appear inappropiate when representing complex biological systems in general and human physiology in particular, as their level of description is often too detailed. For example, Kuipers' model of the water

*This paper is based on the work reported in [1].

†Or at least what could be considered commonsense by a clinician.

balance mechanism in the human body [5] consists of a set of parameters and a set of constraints between them, without representing structure (eg. the kidney is composed of nephrons) or the physiological processes involved (eg. urination). We believe representations of commonsense physiology need higher (less detailed) levels of description, as part of the knowledge is compiled.

We have therefore built a general representation of 'naive physiology' and are developing a system which displays commonsense abilities to reason with it. In particular, we are interested in the dynamics of medicine. Doctors frequently think about changes in terms of processes. They also use several levels of abstraction (generalised concepts obtained by extracting the common features of some specific concepts) and detail (extent to which a concept is described) depending on the problem they face. We have therefore taken a process-oriented representation and have described the various levels of abstraction and detail that doctors use in real life. Our notion of process is similar to the one used in QPT [6], although we represent time explicitly in the process description and we do not use 'histories'.

This representation is first used to reason about the behaviour of a complex physiological process as a combination of the behaviours of its subprocesses and the temporal relationships between them. Faults can then be introduced into the model in order to reason about their effects.

Several years ago, Smith [7] considered some of the ideas described in this paper although little work was done due to the inadequacy (as he saw it) of the representational techniques available at that time.

Other work was been done in modeling physiology. Abel [8] encodes knowledge of the physiology of acid-base electrolite disorders at various levels of detail, although only part of this knowledge is represented explicitly in the model. KBPMS [9], is a simple model of the respiratory system in which physiology is represented explicitly, but it lacks a coherent notion of important physiological processes such as *diffusion* and the representation of temporal aspects is limited to a simple ordering of processes.

The remainder of this paper is organised as follows: the representation we have developed is described in section 2; section 3 illustrates the reasoning task; some implementation details are given in section 4.

2. MODELING NAIVE PHYSIOLOGY

We have built a rich multi-functional knowledge base of commonsense medicine - a general purpose knowledge base not tailored to any specific use. As we want to cover a large, complex domain, the knowledge base is large, with many interrelationships. Although we cannot cover all of physiology, we want our system to be general enough to demonstrate the applicability of our ideas. We have therefore modeled five of the main systems in the human body: cardiovascular, respiratory, digestive, urinary and metabolic. We expect these systems to be sufficiently representative and that the addition of an extra system (eg. the reproductive system) will involve only minor changes to our representation.

Porter et al. [10] describe a similar approach to representing complex biological systems (botany in their case) at both the structural and physiological levels. Temporal descriptions are more complex in our representation.

2.1. The Knowledge Base

To represent the medical knowledge we have applied the following rule: do not represent anything which can be easily derived from the knowledge contained in the knowledge base; instead, give the necessary rules to derive it. For example, the *body parts* which are involved in a compound process can be expressed as *the union* of the *body parts* used in the subprocesses. It is therefore not necessary to ennumerate explicitly the body parts of a complex process but just to express this general rule. This philosophy of representation gives generality and eases changes in the system, as changes will be propagated. Both upwards and downwards inheritance are employed.

We need to represent the human body from two different points of view:

- **Anatomical objects - body parts:** We represent the body as a set of interrelated, inactive objects (body parts). We have built a highly structured description of human anatomy at various levels of abstraction and detail. At each level of abstraction, we have decomposed anatomical objects into their component parts and then decomposed these components into subcomponents, etc. until we have reached a detailed enough representation. Figure 1 shows an example of the representation at two levels of abstraction and at two levels of detail. A body part belongs to a class of anatomical objects from which it inherits properties. For example, the left side of the heart belongs to the class *side of heart*. It is therefore composed of an atrium (left atrium), a ventricle (left ventricle), an atrio-ventricular valve (bicuspid valve) and a semilunar valve (aortic valve); there is a *connected via valve* relationship involving the atrium, the ventricle and the atrio-ventricular valve.

  Conceptually a body part descriptor consists of:

  - *Name*: Eg. heart
  - *Components*: relationships to the parts which form the object. Eg. the heart is composed of the left side of the heart and the right side of the heart.
  - *Supercomponents*: relationship to the items the object is part of. Eg. the heart is part of the cardiovascular system.
  - *Structural relationships*: describe the structural relationships an object has with other objects. Eg. the heart is connected to the vascular system.
  - *Type of anatomical object*: specifies how the body part can be seen at an abstract level. Eg. a ventricle can be seen as a container.

  Other information can also be represented if necessary.

  At this level, the "no function in structure" principle [11] is applied, as the use a component is going to have is not specified. Figure 2 shows an example of the representation of anatomical objects.

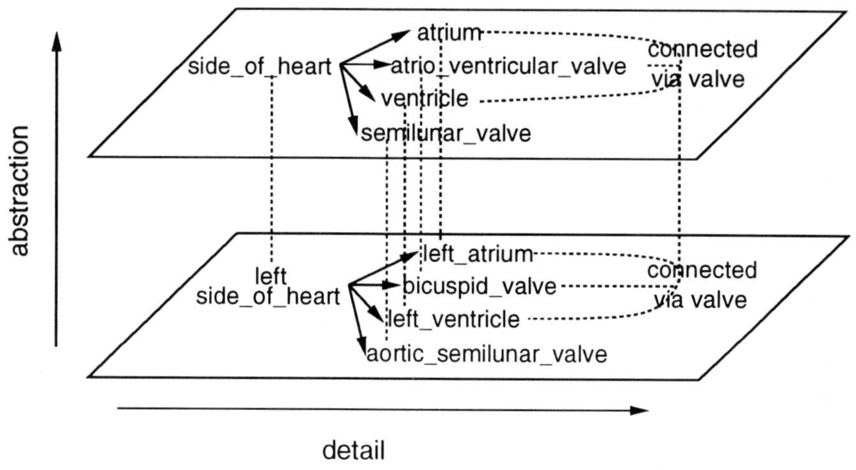

Figure 1: Decomposition of a structural component at two levels of abstraction.

Objects may contain materials, which are the elements that processes act on to produce an effect. Examples of materials are water, air, food, urine, blood, etc. We differentiate between a material abstraction and a material instance.

- **A material abstraction** is a general description of that material. It includes general information about the properties and behaviour of the material.
- **A material instance** is a particular *occurrence* of that material, which is contained in a *body part* or location. It is this relationship of containment in a location which defines the material instance. In other words, a material instance is uniquely identified by its location. A material instance can have properties in addition to those inherited from the material abstraction. This way of describing materials contained in locations is similar to the way in which liquids are conceived by Hayes [12].

For example, consider the material *blood.* This is an abstract concept which has properties such as being liquid, being red if oxygenated and blue otherwise, being able to contain substances in it, etc. A *blood instance* is, for example, the blood in the ventricle. This *blood instance* is defined through the relationship *being contained in* the ventricle. The relationship of containment can have properties like the quantity being contained, whether is oxygenated (which will vary depending, for example, on the particular ventricle), etc.

Object:	left_side_of_heart	Object:	left_ventricle
Components:	left_ventricle	Part_of:	left_side_of_heart
	bicuspid_valve	Valve_connected:	aorta via aortic_valve
	left_atrium		left_atrium via bicuspid_valve
	atrio_ventricular_valve	Type of object:	ventricle
Part_of:	heart		
Connected_to:	aorta		
	pulmonary_vein		
Type of object:	side_of_heart		

Figure 2: An example of representation of anatomical objects.

- **Physiological objects - processes:** We describe the processes which take place in the human body, together with their relationships and interactions. That is, we represent the body from a dynamic point of view. We have built a description of the human body at the level of the processes which take place in it at various levels of abstraction and detail. We use the concept *abstract process* (eg. transport of material from a source to a destination) to describe the general features and behaviour of a class of processes and *actual process* (eg. transport of food from the mouth to the stomach) to describe instances of *abstract processes*. This idea is based on the work on 'prime models' [13]. We have decomposed processes into their component subprocesses and the (temporal) relationships which hold between them.
  Conceptually, processes are described as follows:
  - *Name*: the name of the process. Eg. breakdown of food.
  - *Preconditions*: the conditions necessary to activate the process. Eg. some food in the gastrointestinal tract.
  - *Subprocesses*: processes which make up the process. Eg. mechanical breakdown of food and chemical breakdown of food.
  - *Superprocesses*: processes of which the process is a subprocess. Eg. digestion.
  - *Duration*: the time for which the process is normally active. Eg. some hours.
  - *Process nature*: a process can be either continuous or discrete. Eg. urine formation is a continuous process whereas urination is a discrete process.
  - *Temporal relationships to other processes*: Eg. breakdown of food is parallel to (occurs at the same time as) transport of food.
  - *Organs*: organs the process uses. Eg. gastrointestinal tract and blood stream.
  - *Materials*: materials the process uses. Eg food, saliva, bile.

- *Type of process*: how the process is seen at an abstract level. Eg. breakdown of food is a 'breakdown of material' process.

Other information can also be represented if necessary (for example, other kinds of relationships between processes). Figure 3 is an example of a process representation.

One of the most important relationships between processes is temporal. As the function of a process is dependent on its temporal relationships to other processes, we need a very rich set of such relationships. We are using and extension of Allen's representation of time [14] and have therefore the relationships: parallel, overlaps, before, during, starts, finishes and meets and their inverses and some combinations of these relationships. For example starts-before can be defined as a disjunction of before, overlaps, contains and meets. We are also incorporating the notion of cyclic processes (eg. *pulmonary-ventilation* is a continuous process which consists of the subprocesses *inspiration* and *expiration* which follow one another in sequence).

Temporal relationships play a key role in the reasoning task and are considered from two different points of view:

- times at which two processes are active. Eg. *glomerular filtration* and *tubular reabsorption* are active at the same time and are therefore *parallel*.
- times at which two processes act on the same "material instance". Eg. *glomerular filtration precedes tubular reabsorption* regarding a particular "urine instance".

2.2. Functionality of the Knowledge Base

The following questions may be asked directly of the knowledge base without using the reasoning module[‡]:

- Is the statement S true? Eg. Is the statement 'the stomach is part of the gastrointestinal tract' true? Answer 'Yes'.
- What is X? Eg. 'What is digestion?' will receive the answer 'Digestion is a process'.
- What are the properties of X? Eg. 'What properties does blood have?' will receive the answer 'Blood is a liquid. It's colour is red if oxygenated. It's colour is blue if not oxygenated. It is composed of water, red blood cells, ...etc'.
- What is the value of property P of X? Eg. 'What are the preconditions of breakdown of food?' will receive the answer 'The preconditions of breakdown of food is/are: food in gastrointestinal tract'.
- Which are the X which satisfy Y? Eg. 'Which are subprocesses of digestion?' will receive the answer 'The subprocesses of digestion are: ingestion, transport of food, breakdown of food, absorption of food and excretion'.

[‡]Note, however, that our system does not provide a natural language interface (which is used above for clarity only).

Process:	breakdown_of_food
Preconditions:	food in gastrointestinal tract food contains nutrients
Subprocesses:	chemical_breakdown mechanical_breakdown
Subprocess_of:	digestion
Duration:	hours
Process_nature:	discrete
Parallel_to:	transport_of_food
Starts_before:	absorption
After:	ingestion
Before:	excretion
Organs:	gastrointestinal_tract portal_vein outside
Materials:	food nutrients
Type_of_process:	breakdown

Figure 3: An example of representation of dynamic objects.

- What is the relationship (if any) between X and Y? Eg.'What is the relationship between the left ventricle and the left atrium?' The answer to this question is 'The left ventricle has a relationship *connected-via-valve* with the left atrium'.
- What are the structural/temporal relationships of X? Eg. 'What are the structural relationships of breakdown of food?' The answer to this question is 'Breakdown of food is a subprocess of digestion. It is composed of two subprocesses: chemical breakdown and mechanical breakdown.'

A separate module, the reasoning module, deals with questions which require more complex inferences. Thus, complex questions like 'What is the behaviour of process X?' or 'What would happen if Y were modified?' have to be put to the reasoning module. There is no clear boundary between the reasoning and the knowledge representation modules. It could be argued that the whole reasoning module could be integrated into the knowledge base module thus providing it with more functionality.

3. REASONING ABOUT COMMONSENSE PHYSIOLOGY

We are interested in a bottom-up type of reasoning: given a low level description of behaviours (misbehaviours), reason about the behaviour (misbehaviour) which takes place at a higher (less detailed) level. This kind of reasoning is used in the theory of consolidation [15], where the behaviour of a component is obtained from the behaviour of its subcomponents. In our case, we want to obtain the behaviour of a complex process (composed of subprocesses) by combining the behaviours of its subprocesses. We therefore want to specify a set of "rules of composition of behaviour" which, given two behaviours, the temporal relationship between them and a set of preconditions return the behaviour obtained by combining the two initial behaviours.

Rules of composition of behaviour are described as follows:

- *First and second behaviours*: the behaviours which take part in the composition.
- *Preconditions*: conditions which have to be satisfied for the rule to be valid. These conditions refer to parameters used in the first and second behaviours.
- *Temporal relationships*: time relationships between the first and second behaviours which make the rule valid. These could be considered as "further preconditions".
- *New behaviour*: the result of composing the first and second behaviours given the conditions specified in the preconditions and temporal relationships sections.

Figure 4 shows some examples of rules of composition of behaviour. These rules may be used to answer the question 'what is the behaviour of process X?'. Together with some knowledge about faulty processes, they may be used to predict 'what would happen if' a fault were introduced; in other words, the effect of such a fault could be propagated throughout the model. Our research therefore falls into two parts: reasoning about the behaviour of a process and reasoning about the effects of introducing a fault in the model.

It is important to notice that the reasoning mechanism used should be valid in the context of the information available, but that its conclusions may be wrong if not enough information is known or if the modification introduced is not physically possible.

3.1. Reasoning about the Behaviour of a Process

We use two methods to obtain the behaviour of a process depending on whether the process under consideration is a leaf process (with no subprocesses) or a complex process (composed of subprocesses).

The behaviour of a leaf process is obtained by accessing the abstract process of which the leaf process is an instance, getting the behaviour of that abstract process and instantiating this behaviour with the parameters of the real process. For example, the leaf process *urine transport* is an instance of the abstract process *transport*. The behaviour of a *transport* process is to move a substance from one location to another location. Instantiating parameters, the behaviour of *urine transport* is to move the urine in the kidney to the bladder.

The behaviour of a complex process can be derived from the behaviour of its subprocesses and the relationships between them. Rules of composition of behaviour

```
Rule 1:
    Behaviour_1:
            filtration    of_substance X
                          from location_1
                          to location_2
                          through_filter F
    Behaviour_2:
            transport     of_substance Y
                          from location_3
                          to location_4
    Preconditions:
            location_2 = location_3
            location_1 <> location_4
            Y = filtrate(X, F)
    Temporal Relationships:
            before, meets, precedes ...
    New Behaviour:
            filtration    of_substance X
                          from location_1
                          to location_4
                          through_filter F
```

```
Rule 2:
    Behaviour_1:
            filtration    of_substance X
                          from location_1
                          to location_2
                          through_filter F
    Behaviour_2:
            expel         substance Y
                          from location_3
                          to location_4
    Preconditions:
            location_2 = location_3
            location_1 <> location_4
            Y = filtrate(X, F)
    Temporal Relationships:
            before, meets, precedes ...
    New Behaviour:
            filtration    of_substance X
                          from location_1
                          to location_4
                          through_filter F
```

Figure 4: An example of rules of composition of behaviour.

are used to combine the behaviours of the subprocesses of a complex process to obtain the behaviour of the latter.

For example, the *urinary* process is composed of the subprocesses *urine formation, urine transport* and *urination*. *Urine formation* is a *filtration process* (it filters blood in the renal capillaries transfering urine as filtrate to the renal pelvis using the renal membrane as the filter; *urine transport* is a *transport process* (it moves urine from the kidney to the bladder); *urination* is an *expel process* (it expels urine from the bladder to outside the body). Using the rules of composition shown in figure 4 we can derive that:

- the process composed of *urine formation* and *urine transport* has a *filter* behaviour: it filters blood in the renal capillaries transfering urine as filtrate to the bladder using the renal membrane as the filter.
- from the above point and the behaviour of *urination*, the behaviour of the *urinary* process can be derived as *filtering* blood in the renal capillaries,

transfering urine as filtrate to outside the body using the renal membrane as the filter.

Composition of behaviours often involves a task of generalisation:

- Sometimes, two given behaviours will not be immediately available for composition because of incompatibility in the values of their attributes. For example, to be able to apply the first rule in figure 4 to compose the behaviours of *urine formation* and *urine transport*, the value of the *to-location* of the former (the *renal pelvis*) should be the same as the value of the *from-location* of the later (the *kidney*). As the *renal pelvis* is part of the *kidney* the *to-location* of *urine formation* can be generalised to be the *kidney*.
- Some of the behaviour conditions have to be weakened. For example, the to-location of a filtration process will normally be directly connected to the filter. When composing *urine formation* and *urine transport* above the result is a filter process from the renal capillaries to the bladder using as filter the renal membrane. The renal pelvis and the ureter are between the filter and the to-location but do not play any role in the composed behaviour.

3.2. Reasoning about the Effect of Modifications

A modification can be introduced into the model by either changing a body part or by changing a process. What would happen if a modification is introduced in the model? This section describes the reasoning mechanism used to answer this question.

As we have explained in section 2.1, we describe processes at different levels of abstraction. We are incorporating knowledge about 'faulty processes' into the abstract process descriptions. We are also adding rules of composition of 'faulty behaviours' to our set of rules of composition of behaviour. For example, we have the process *transport* (of material from a source to a destination) and information on how this process functions when there is a blockage in the conduit from the source to the destination. This is then used to reason about the effect of a modification introduced in the model, when the following steps are taken: a) see which processes are directly affected by the modification, and reason about how it affects their behaviour; b) look for processes which are influenced by the first ones and see how their behaviour is affected; c) use the rules of composition of behaviour to deduce how the behaviour of complex processes which use the processes already considered is affected. Steps b) and c) can be repeated for more complex processes.

For example, the *urinary* process is composed of *urine formation*, *urine transport* and *urination*. A fault is introduced into the model - the ureter is blocked. The reasoning module checks the information it has about ureters and discovers that it is an organ and a conduit. Then it looks at the processes which use the ureter to see how the fault affects their behaviour. There is one such process, *urine transport*, which uses the ureter as a conduit to move urine from the kidney to the bladder. It then searches for the type of process of *urine transport* and sees that is a *transport* process. Now it looks at whether it has information about *transport* when the conduit is blocked. This says that if there is a blockage, the process *transport* cannot take place. It then instantiates this information to deduce that the process *urine transport* cannot take place (so the kidney has urine and the bladder is empty). It now looks for processes influenced by *urine transport*. There are two such processes, *urine formation* and *urination*. It now turns to investigate *urine formation*, which is a filter process. Following the same reasoning as above, but applied to a filtering process in which the destination contains urine, it will deduce that *urine formation* will not take place. It now turns to investigate the process of *urination*. It discovers that the effect of 'urine transport' is one of the preconditions of *urination*. As *urine transport* does not take place, neither does *urination*.

It is now time to look at the superprocess of *urine transport*, the *urinary* process. This process is composed of three subprocesses, so its behaviour can be deduced by composing the behaviour of its subprocesses, as explained in section 3.1. As none of its subprocesses can take place, the urinary process cannot take place either (it has an 'empty behaviour').

3.3. Summary

We have seen two ways of reasoning about processes:

- Reasoning about the behaviour of a process: this answers the question 'What is the behaviour of process X?'. If X is a leaf process, its behaviour is instantiated from the behaviour of its abstract class. Otherwise, if X is a complex process, its behaviour is obtained by combining the behaviours of its subprocesses.
- Reasoning about the effect of introducing a modification in the model: this answers the question 'What would happen if a modification X were introduced in the model?'. The answer to this question depends on the kind of modification made.

4. IMPLEMENTATION

We have chosen Abel [16], an extension of ADAM [17], as a system in which to implement our ideas. Abel is an object oriented database written in Prolog which provides a number of basic constructs which can be easily extended (using metaclasses). The user can then adapt these constructs to his/her own needs. We consider that a simple but user-extensible set of facilities provides us with enough flexibility to implement our system (as opposed to a complex system which provides many facilities - some of them not needed - but difficult to extend). We are running Abel on a Sparc workstation under SEPIA Prolog [18].

We currently have a working knowledge base which is able to answer the questions mentioned in section 2.2. It now contains over 1000 objects (around 200 body parts, 170 processes and 950 relationships) and more knowledge may be incorporated to it. We are now implementing the reasoning system.

5. SUMMARY

We have described a system capable of reasoning about naive physiology displaying commonsense abilities. This system involves a model of the human body at the physiological level and a reasoning mechanism which uses it. The reasoning system is focused on how the behaviour of a complex process can be obtained by combining the behaviours of its subprocesses and on how introducing faults in the model can affect the behaviour of processes. This system could be used in reasoning about the effect a failure of a process will have in the global process of keeping the body alive.

One of the limitations of this approach is that the reasoning mechanism may not work in cases where a fault in the system activates alternative physiological mechanisms which are not described in our model (eg. a problem in the stomach may cause vomiting). This paper describes work in progress.

ACKNOWLEDGEMENTS

One of us (IA) acknowledges the support of the Spanish "Ministerio de Educación y Ciencia" in the form of a F.P.I. grant.

REFERENCES

[1] I. Arana & J. Hunter, "Representing and Reasoning about Naive Physiology," in Proceedings of QR'92 - The Sixth International Workshop on Qualitative Reasoning about Physical Systems, Edinburgh, 1992, 139–154.

[2] C. Sarmiento, "Representing Knowledge in Medical Decision Support Systems," Artificial Intelligence in Medicine 4 (1992), 417.

[3] P. Hayes, "The Second Naive Physics Manifesto," Formal Theories of the Commonsense World.

[4] I. K. Kirby & J. R. W. Hunter, "Further Progress in Qualitative Modeling of Cardiac Electrophysiology," in Proceedings of the 5th International Workshop on Qualitative Reasoning, Austin, Texas, 1991.

[5] B. Kuipers, "Qualitative Simulation as Causal Explanation," IEEE Transactions on Systems, Man, and Cybernetics SMC-17 (1987), 432–444.

[6] K. D. Forbus, "Qualitative Process Theory," Artificial Intelligence 24 (1984), 85–168.

[7] B. Smith, "A Proposal for a Computational Model of Anatomical and Physiological Reasoning," A.I Memo 493, MIT, 1978.

[8] R. S. Patil, P. Szolovits & W. B. Schwartz, "Causal Understanding of Patient Illness in Medical Diagnosis," Proceedings of IJCAI-81, Yale University, Newhaven (1981).

[9] R. Kunstaetter, "Intelligent Physiologic Modeling," Massachusetts Institute of Technology Report MIT/LCS/TR-360, 1986.

[10] B. W. Porter, J. Lester, K. Murray, K. Pittman, A. Souther, L. Acker & T. Jones, "AI Research in the Context of a Multifunctional Knowledge Base: The Botany Knowledge Base Project," Technical Report AI88-88, Artificial Intelligent Laboratory, The University of Texas at Austin, 1988.

[11] J. de Kleer & J. S. Brown, "A Qualitative Physics Based on Confluences," Artificial Intelligence 24 (1984), 7–83.

[12] P. Hayes, "Naive Physics 1: Ontology for Liquids," Formal Theories of the Commonsense World.

[13] R. Hewett & B. Hayes-Roth, "Representing and Reasoning About Physical Systems Using Prime Models," Technical Report KSL 90-40, Knowledge Systems Laboratory, Department of Computer Science, Stanford University, 1990.

[14] J. F. Allen, "Maintaining Knowledge about Temporal Intervals," Communications of the ACM 26 (1983).

[15] T. Bylander & B. Chandrasekaran, "Understanding Behaviour Using Consolidation," in Proceedings of IJCAI-85, Morgan Kauffman, 1985, 450–454.

[16] O. Díaz García,, "Making Object-Oriented Databases more Knowledgeable," Ph.D. Thesis, University of Aberdeen, 1992.

[17] N. W. Paton, "A Prolog Implementation of an Object-Oriented Database," Ph.D. Thesis, University of Aberdeen, 1989.

[18] ICL/ECRC, "SEPIA 3.1 User Manual," Ref. SEP/UM/064, ICL/ECRC, 1991.

Artificial Intelligence in Medecine
S. Andreassen et al. , Eds.
IOS Press, 1993

Implementation of a learning procedure for multiple observations in a Diabetes Advisory System based on causal probabilistic networks

O. K. Hejlesen, S. Andreassen and S. K. Andersen

Department of Medical Informatics and Image Analysis, Institute of Electronic Systems, Aalborg University, Fr. Bajersvej 7 D, DK-9220 Aalborg, Denmark

Abstract

An extension of a causal probabilistic network, modelling the humane glucose metabolism, making it possible to estimate patient specific parameters from data from multiple days, is presented. The importance of preserving information on both the patient specific means and standard deviations of the parameters is described. The approach is illustrated by examples of the role of the patient specific insulin sensitivity.

1. INTRODUCTION

An effective control of blood glucose is considered one of the key elements in the treatment of insulin dependent diabetes mellitus (Dahl-Jørgensen 1985, 1986). To achieve this, computers have been used in different ways. Some approaches are based on rules or algorithms for insulin dose adjustment derived from expert knowledge (Chanoch et al. 1985, Schriffin 1985, Harvey and Carson 1986, Chao and Albisser 1989, Deutsch et al. 1989, 1990). Others have used predictions of blood glucose levels based on mathematical models of the carbohydrate metabolism (Swan 1982, Shimauchi et al. 1988, Berger and Rodbard 1989, Salzsieder et al. 1990), and some systems have used a combination of the two approaches (Schneider et al. 1988, Berger et al. 1990, Lehmann et al. 1991). None of these systems seem to have gained widespread use or acceptance.

The model based systems generally predict a specific blood glucose profile in response to a given regimen (food intake, insulin injections etc.). The information provided by such models does not include the uncertainties of the prediction, although this kind of information, reflecting the stability of the patients blood glucose, is important to the clinician giving advise on the patients insulin doses. A computer system implementing this feature, based on causal probabilistic networks (CPN's), has already been described (Andreassen et al. 1991, 1993, Hovorka et al. 1992). It uses blood glucose measurements from one day to estimate patient specific parameters and then uses these parameters to predict the blood glucose for a following day, making it possible to suggest an optimal insulin regimen. The present paper describes an extension of the system, making it possible to estimate the patient specific parameters based on experience from multiple days.

2. THE MODEL

The model implemented in the Diabetes Advisory System, DIAS, is based on published physiologic data on insulin absorption (Binder 1969, Kölendorf 1978, Lauritzen et al. 1982, Kraegen 1984, Binder et al. 1984, Hildebrandt et al. 1984, Owen 1986, Vaag et al. 1990), carbohydrate absorption from the gut (Boroujerdi et al. 1987, Boroujerdi et al. 1988, Benn et al. 1989), renal clearance of glucose (Ganong 1983, Benn et al. 1989) hepatic production of glucose (Rizza et al. 1981, Best et al. 1981, Gottesman 1982, Gottesman 1984), insulin dependent utilization of glucose (Rizza et al. 1981, Best et al. 1981, Gottesman 1982, Gottesman 1984, Bell et al. 1986) and insulin independent utilization of glucose (Gottesman et al. 1983).

The model is a time discrete, variable discrete and parameter discrete CPN, simulating probability distributions for the blood glucose concentration in a 24 hour period in 1 hour steps. The model is constructed using the HUGIN tool (Andersen et al. 1989), and tools developed by the authors (Andreassen 1992, Olesen and Andreassen 1993). When simulating this glucose profile, the input to the model is the type, timing and amount of insulin injections and the timing and amount of carbohydrate intake. As shown in the simplified figure 1 the model includes two adjustable parameters describing the sensitivity to insulin and the absorption speed of the NPH insulin.

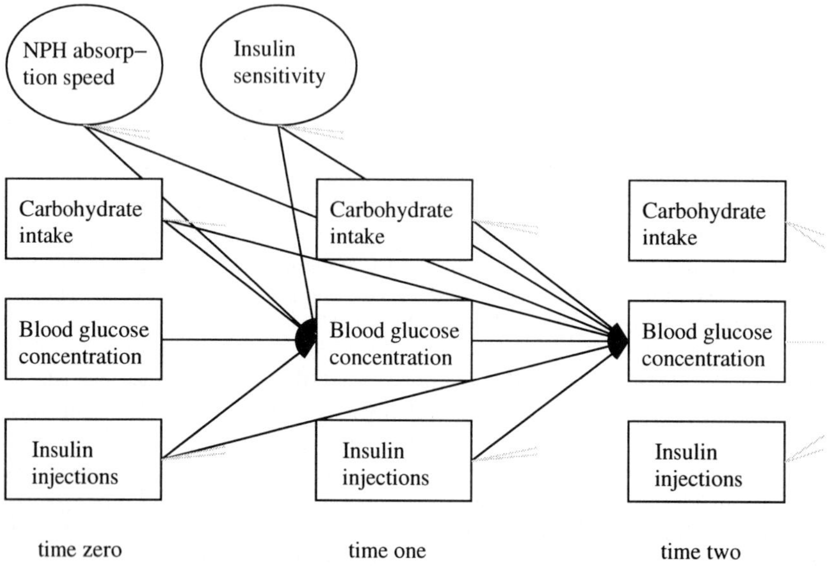

Figure 1. The three first time slices of the model in DIAS.

3. THE SYSTEM

In order to match the simulations to each individual patient, the system uses the two adjustable parameters, scaling the effect of the insulin on the glucose utilization (the insulin sensitivity), and scaling the absorption time for the intermediate acting NPH insulin (the NPH absorption speed).

The system is used in two phases. In phase I, the system is allowed to estimate the patient specific parameters on the basis of information on carbohydrate intake, insulin injections and measured blood glucose from a 24 hour learning period, called day 1. In phase II, the system estimates the expected distribution of the blood glucose for another 24 hour period, called day 2, on the basis of information on carbohydrate intake and insulin injections for day 2 plus the learned parameters from day 1. The first process is called retrieval of experience and the second is called dissemination of experience (Spiegelhalter and Lauritzen 1988).

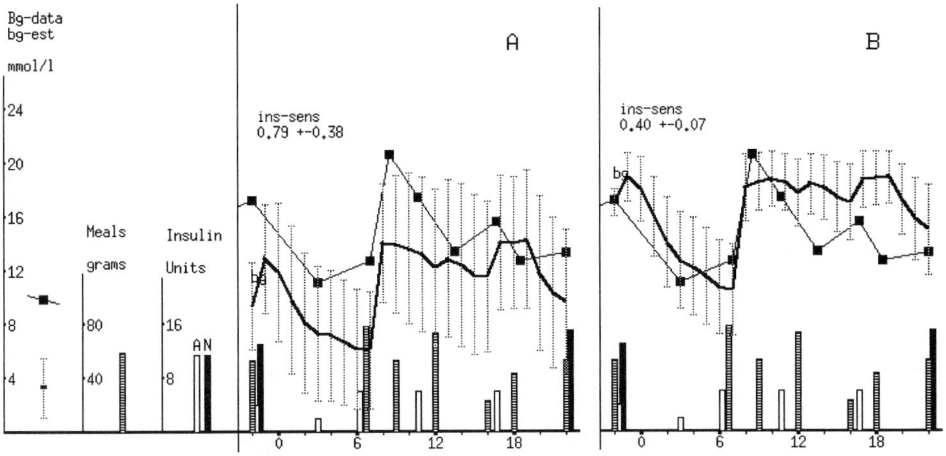

Figure 2. A) Prediction of blood glucose with a priori insulin sensitivity. Signatures for measured and predicted blood glucose (mean and sd), carbohydrate intake and Actrapid and NPH injections. B) Prediction of the blood glucose profile with the patient specific insulin sensitivity.

As an example, the effect of learning the insulin sensitivity is illustrated in figures 2A and 2B, where blood glucose measurements and predictions for the same day ('day 2') are shown. The simulation in figure 2A shows the probability distribution of the blood glucose, given a probability distribution of the insulin sensitivity equal to the diabetic population distribution used in DIAS as a priori knowledge, i.e. the system has not been given the opportunity to adapt to the particular patient. Figure 2B shows the blood glucose simulation on 'day 2' following a 'day 1' (not shown), where DIAS has been allowed to estimate the insulin sensitivity. It can be seen that the simulation in figure 2B after adapting the system to the patient is more precise and has a smaller standard deviation. The smaller standard deviation of the blood glucose is due to the fact that the learned insulin sensitivity has a smaller standard deviation than the a priori insulin sensitivity.

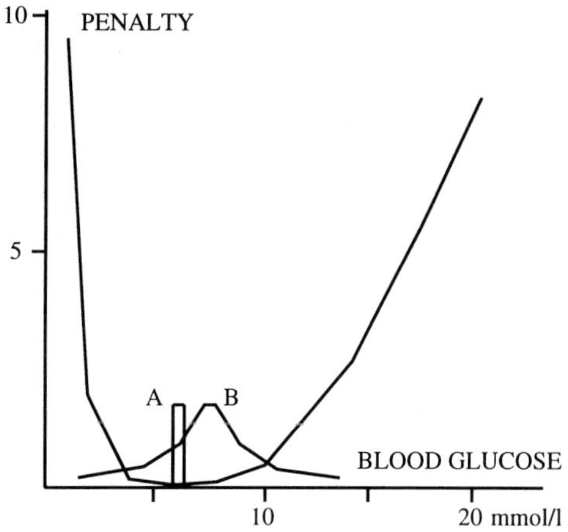

Figure 3. Finding the minimal penalty for A: zero standard deviation and B: standard deviation of 3 mmol/l.

The importance of estimating the standard deviation of the insulin sensitivity and thereby estimating the standard deviation of the predicted blood glucose should be discussed in combination with the automatic adjustment procedure for the insulin doses implemented in DIAS. The penalty function shown in figure 3 describes our suggested relation between the blood glucose level and the expected loss of life or life quality, and it has a resemblance to the M-value (Schlichtkrull et al. 1965). The function represents our subjective opinion on the detrimental effect of different blood glucose concentrations. Given the penalty function and a predicted probability distribution for the blood glucose in a 24 hour period, i.e. day 2, the penalty score, also called the risk, for the period can be calculated. This is done by integrating the product of the penalty function and the predicted blood glucose distribution for each time slice and then adding the risk for each time slice to give the total 24 hour expected risk or penalty score. The automatic adjustment of the insulin doses is then implemented as an iterative procedure of repeated simulations with different insulin doses to identify the insulin doses, which minimizes the total risk for day 2.

It should be noted that the penalty function rises more steeply for lower blood glucose than for higher, and that the system therefore in the adjusting procedure for smaller standard deviations of the blood glucose would aim at higher insulin doses, i.e. lower predicted blood glucose, than it would for larger standard deviations. This property seems to be in accordance with good medical practice. The reason for this behavior can be understood from a simple example with only one time slice, and assuming a normal distribution of the blood glucose. With a standard deviation of zero, it can be seen that the system would aim at a mean of 6 mmol/l in an adjust bringing the penalty down to zero (A in figure 3). If the standard deviation is larger, for example 3 mmol/l, the penalty would be larger too, and the minimal penalty is obtained with a mean blood glucose of approximately 7.5 mmol/l (B in figure 3). The mean is shifted up to keep a respectable distance to the steep left hand side of the penalty curve. Since a large standard deviation in the insulin sensitivity gives a large standard deviation in the predicted blood glucose, then a large standard deviation in the insulin sensitivity makes it advantageous to aim for a relatively high blood glucose.

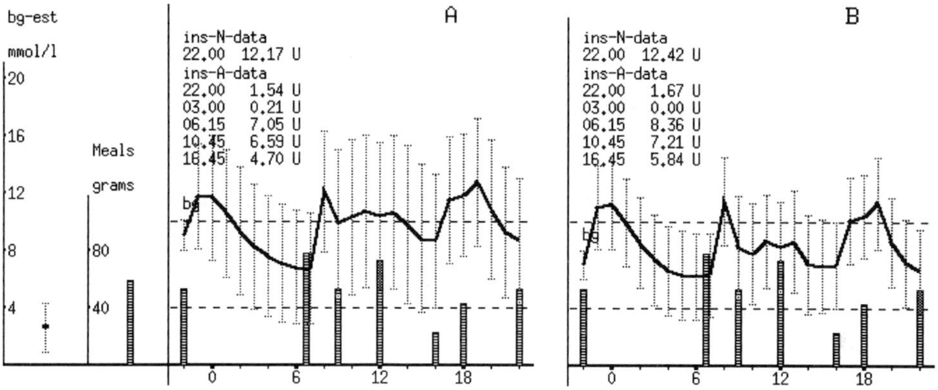

Figure 4. A) The result of an adjust of the insulin regimen for insulin sensitivity with normal mean and standard deviation of 34 %. B) The result of an adjust of the insulin regimen for insulin sensitivity with normal mean and zero standard deviation.

Figure 4A shows the result of an automatic adjustment of insulin doses for 'day 2'. The adjust was performed with a normal mean and a standard deviation of 34% on the insulin sensitivity. The average predicted blood glucose resulting from these "optimal" insulin doses is 9.74 mmol/l with a total insulin dose of 32.3 U. If the insulin sensitivity were known with certainty, i.e. a standard deviation of zero, then the optimal doses would give an average blood glucose of 8.3 mmol/l with a total insulin dose of 35.5 U, as shown in figure 4B. This illustrates that, when the insulin sensitivity is known better, then the system "dares" to be more aggressive in the insulin therapy, or in other words that a reliable estimation of the standard deviation is important.

4. THE PROBLEM

Often, measured blood glucose values (and data for meals and insulin regimen) from more than one day are available. A typical example is an ambulatory patient, seeing the doctor and bringing measured blood glucose for four days in the last month. We now want to consider how to learn from multiple days, and then simulate and adjust for one day based on parameters learned from multiple days. As mentioned in the previous section, the considerations should include means to preserve information on the variations of the parameters.

5. THE SOLUTION

One approach is to use estimated parameters from day 1 as a priori knowledge for learning from day 2, then using the learned parameters from day 2 as a priori for day 3 and so on. This strategy would be analogous to the previously described leaning of e.g. the insulin sensitivity from a single day, where the estimated insulin sensitivity is the product of the a priori distribution of the insulin sensitivity and the likelihood of the insulin sensitivity, given the data. The only difference would be that the likelihood would be the product of the likelihoods from the multiple days. Assuming normal distributions of the parameters, it can be seen that this approach would give estimated distributions converging against the patients means with zero standard deviation. This modelling of the means still leaves out the fact that there are day to day variations of the parameters, and, as already described, the result of an automatic adjust is depending, not only on the mean of a parameter, but also on the standard deviation. This means that the approach seems less suited to solve the problem.

In order to preserve information on both the means and standard deviations of the parameters, we have built a hierarchical model of the parameters. Others have built hierarchical models, where they use the different levels to model the population distribution in relation to the patient specific parameters (Bellazzi et al. 1991). The example with the insulin sensitivity will be used to illustrate our approach. Using a simplified CPN, figure 5 shows the relations between the a priori knowledge, the insulin sensitivity parameter and the observed blood glucose measurements in the case with only learning from day 1. It can be seen that the estimated insulin sensitivity to be used for simulations and adjusts are directly derived from the insulin sensitivity on day 1. In probabilistic terms, the estimated insulin sensitivity is the product of the a priori distribution of the insulin sensitivity and the likelihood of the insulin sensitivity, given the data. Assuming a normal distribution of the insulin sensitivity, we have formulated the model, shown simplified in figure 6, which has the desired property of preserving information on both mean and standard deviation. Here, the estimated insulin sensitivity is derived from the patient specific parameters, describing the mean and day to day standard deviation of the insulin sensitivity. The estimated insulin sensitivity to be used for simulations and adjustments are derived from the parameters, describing the mean and the day to day standard deviation. The price to pay for this approach is that, in contrast to the situation on figure 5, the estimated insulin sensitivity on figure 6 is forced to have a normal distribution. It should be noted that any parametric description could be used instead of the normal distribution.

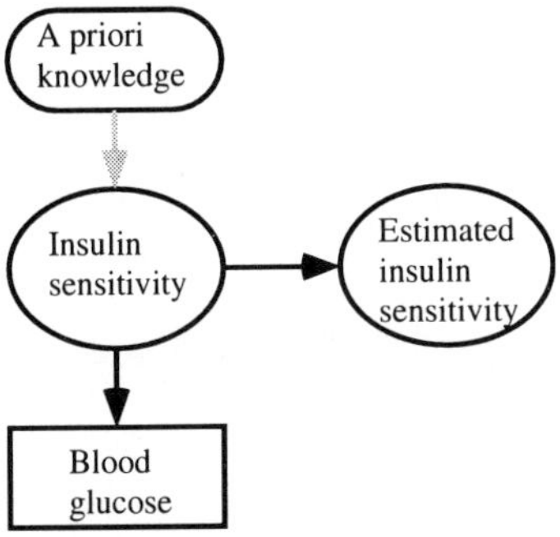

Figure 5. A CPN estimating insulin sensitivity from one day.

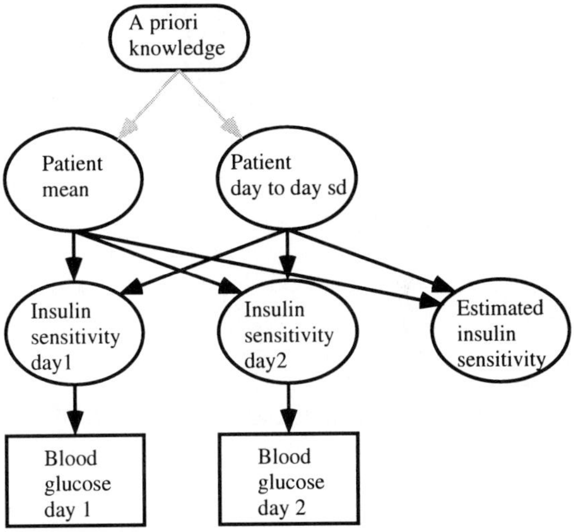

Figure 6. A CPN estimating the insulin sensitivity from multiple days. The patient mean and standard deviation (sd) are included.

6. AN EXAMPLE

In order to show the effect of learning from multiple days instead of one day, blood glucose measurements from one of the patients, who actually has been given insulin doses according to the advise provided by DIAS, is illustrated in figures 7, 8A and 8B. The system was asked to give advise for a 24 hour period, starting on March 22 at 9.00 am. The predicted insulin sensitivity and data for the preceding four days are indicated in figure 7, and a simulation for the 22th, based on the 21th, is shown in figure 8A. A simulation based on all four days from the 18th to the 21th is shown in figure 8B. It can be seen that the simulation based on all four days has a better fit to the actual data than the simulation based on one day. The RMS prediction errors are 3.3 mmol/l and 4.3 mmol/l, respectively.

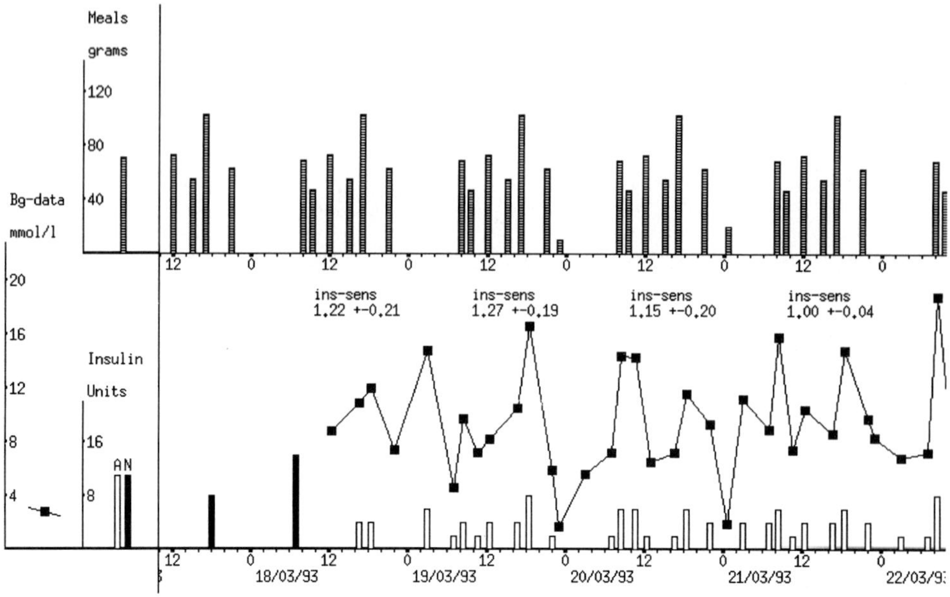

Figure 7. An example with estimated insulin sensitivities on March 18-21. The patient is hospitalized and shifted from NPH to regular insulin on March 18.

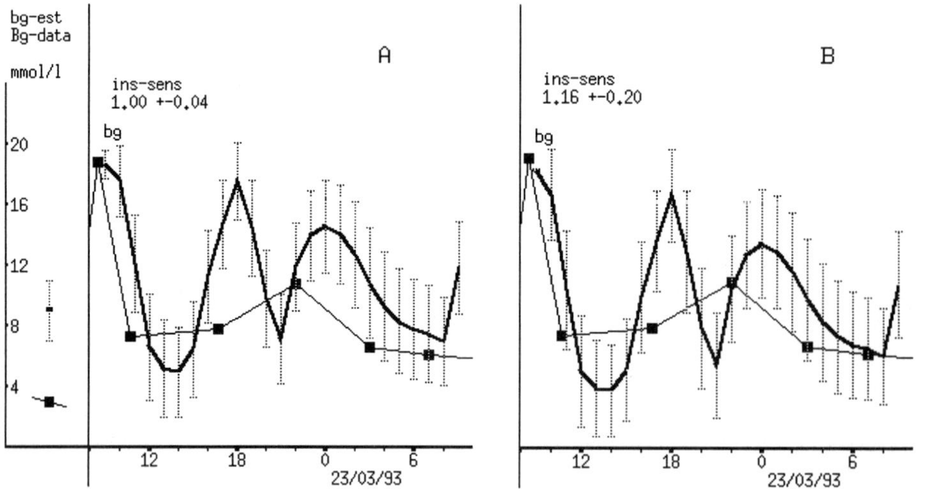

Figure 8. A) Simulation on March 22 based on estimated insulin sensitivity from one previous day. B) Simulation on March 22 based on estimated insulin sensitivity from four previous days.

7. MULTIPLE PARAMETERS

As shown in figure 1, the present version of DIAS has two adjustable parameters: the insulin sensitivity and the absorption speed of the NPH insulin. In order to handle more than one parameter without assuming independence between the parameters, the model has to handle the joint distributions of the parameters, i.e. to model the correlations between the individual parameters. The two-dimensional normally distributed parameters, implemented in DIAS, are shown simplified in the CPN formalism in figure 9.

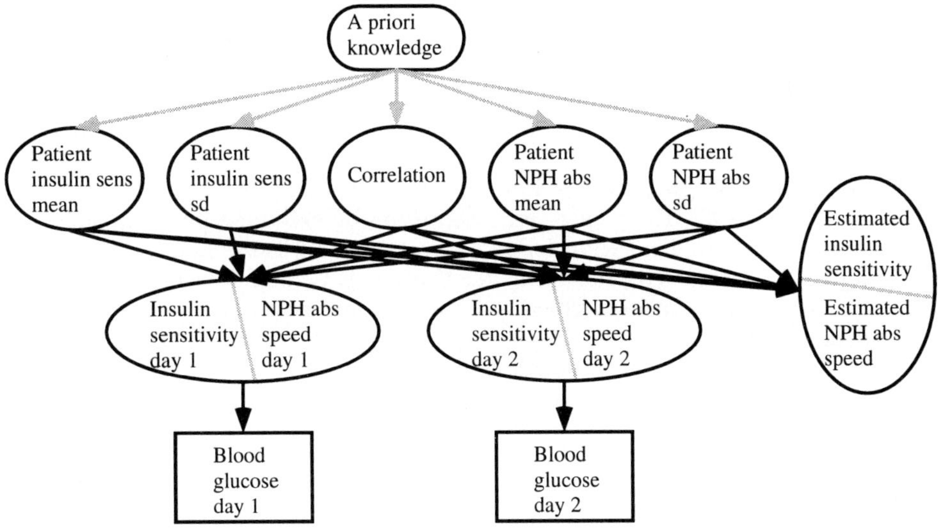

Figure 9. The principle of a CPN implementing estimates of multiple parameters from multiple days. Only two parameters and two days are shown.

8. DISCUSSION

The present paper has described an extension of the Diabetes Advisory System, DIAS, making it possible to estimate patient specific parameters from data from multiple days. The role of estimating the standard deviation of the parameters has been emphasized, using the insulin sensitivity as an example. A patient case has been used to illustrate the role of learning from multiple days and thereby minimizing the effect of the day to day variation of the parameters. For patients who for some reason or another are believed to have parameters drifting, we have plans for extending the approach by a mechanism for weighting the information in the multiple days. If the chosen parameters are regarded as independent, the need for handling the joint distributions disappears and the modelling of the correlation can be omitted. Preliminary investigations have lead us to believe that the correlation between the insulin sensitivity and the NPH absorption speed is relatively small compared to e.g. the correlation between the insulin absorption and the absorption of the carbohydrate from the guts, the latter being one of the strong candidates for an additional parameter in the model. Despite of the potential improvements to be considered in the future, we believe that the present implementation of the learning procedure from multiple days is an important contribution to the performance of DIAS, which is currently being tested clinically.

9. REFERENCES

Andersen, S.K., Olesen, K.G., Jensen, F.V., and Jensen, F. (1989). HUGIN - A shell for building Bayesian belief universes for expert systems. In: Proceedings of IJCAI 89 2, 1080-1085.

Andreassen, S., Hovorka, R., Benn, J. J., Olesen, K.G., and Carson, E.R. (1991). A model based approach to insulin adjustment. In: Lecture Notes in Medical Informatics (Proc. of AIME '91) 44, eds. Stefanelli, M., Hasman, A., Fieschi, M. and Talmon, J. pp. 239-249. Berlin: Springer-Verlag.

Andreassen, S. (1992). Knowledge representation by extended linear models. In: Deep Models for Medical Knowledge Engineering, ed. Keravnou, E. Elsevier.

Andreassen, S., Benn, J.J., Hovorka, R., Olesen, K.G. and Carson E.R. (1993). A probabilistic approach to glucose prediction and insulin dose adjustment - Description of a metabolic model and pilot evaluation study. Computer Methods and Programs in Biomedicine. In Press.

Bell, P.M., Firth, R.G., and Rizza, R.A. (1986). Effects of hyperglycemia on glucose production and utilization in humans. Measurement with [23H]-, [33H]-, and [614C] Glucose, Diabetes 35, 642-648.

Bellazzi, R., Berzuini, C, and Quaglini, S. (1991). Cytotoxic chemotherapy monitoring using stochastic simulation om graphical models. In: Lecture Notes in Medical Informatics (Proc. of AIME '91) 44, eds. Stefanelli, M., Hasman, A., Fieschi, M. and Talmon, J. pp. 227-238. Berlin: Springer-Verlag.

Benn, J.J., Bozzard, S.J., Kelley, D., Mitrakou, A., Aoki, T., Sorensen, J., Gerich, J., and Sonksen, P.H. (1989). Persistent abnormalities of the metabolism of an oral glucose load in insulin-treated type I diabetics, Metabolism 38, 1047-1055.

Berger, M.P. and Rodbard, D. (1989). Computer simulation of plasma insulin and glucose dynamics after subcutaneous insulin injection, Diabetes Care 12, 725-736.

Berger, M.P., Gelfand, R.A., and Miller, P.L. (1990). Combining statistical, rule-based and physiologic model-based methods to assist in the management of diabetes mellitus, Comput. Biomed. Res. 23, 346-357.

Best, J.D., Taborsky Jr., G.J., Halter, J.B., and Porte Jr., D. (1981). Glucose disposal is not proportional to plasma glucose level in man, Diabetes 30, 847-850.

Binder, C., Lauritzen, T., Faber O. and Pramming, S. (1984), Insulin pharmacokinetics, Diabetes Care 7, 188-199.

Boroujerdi, M.A., Williams, C.D., Carson, E.R., Piwernetz, K., Hepp K.D. and Sonksen, P.H. (1987). Simulation approach for planning insulin regimes. In: Int. Symp. on Advanced Models for Therapy of Insulin-dependent Diabetes,

eds. Brunetti, P., Waldhaust, W.K. pp. 41-46. New York: Raven Press.
Boroujerdi, M.A., Leaning, M.S., and Nicolosi, E. (1988). Knowledge-rich representations of carbohydrate metabolism for diabetic expert systems. In: Medical Informatics 88: Computers in Clinical Medicine pp. 89-96. London: British Medical Informatics Society.
Chanoch, L.H., Jovanovic, L., and Peterson, C.M. (1985). The evaluation of a pocket computer as an aid to insulin dose determination by patients, Diabetes Care 8, 172-176.
Chao, S.C. and Albisser, A.M. (1989). The diabetes simulator. In: Decision Support for Patient Management: Measurement, Modelling and Control, pp. 86-88. London: British Medical Informatics Society.
Deutsch, T., Boroujerdi, M.A., Carson, E.R., Harvey, F.E., Sonksen, P.H., Tamas, G., and Williams, C.D. (1989). The principles and prototyping of a knowledge-based diabetes management system, Comput. Methods Programs Biomed. 29, 75-88.
Deutsch, T., Carson, E.R., Harvey, F.E., Lehmann, E.D., Sonksen, P.H., Tamas G., Whitney G., and Williams, C.D. (1990). Computer-assisted diabetic management: a complex approach. Comput Methods Programs Biomed 32, 195-214.
Ganong W.F. (1983). Review of Medical Physiology, 11th ed., pp. 572-573. Los Altos: Lange.
Gottesman, I., Mandarino, L., Verdonk, C., Rizza, R., and Gerich, J. (1982). Insulin increases the maximum velocity for glucose uptake without altering the Michaelis constant in man, J. Clin. Invest. 70, 1310-1314.
Gottesman, I., Mandarino, L., and Gerich, J. (1983). Estimation and kinetic analysis of insulin-independent glucose uptake in human subjects, Am. J. Physiol. 244, E632-E635.
Gottesman, I., Mandarino, L. and Gerich, J. (1984). Use of glucose uptakeand glucose clearance for the evaluation of insulin action in vivo, Diabetes 33, 184-191.
Harvey, F.E. and Carson, E.R. (1986). Diabeta - an expert system for the management of diabetes. In: Objective Medical Decision-Making: Systems Approach in Disease, ed. Tsiftsis, D.D. pp. 166-174. Berlin: Springer-Verlag.
Hovorka, R., Andreassen, S., Benn, J.J., Olesen, K.G., and Carson, E. (1992). Causal probabilistic network modelling. An illustration of its role in the management of chronic diseases. IBM Systems Journal 31(4), 635-648.
Hildebrandt, P., Birch, K., Sestoft, L. and Vølund, AA. (1984). Dose-dependent subcutaneous absorption of porcine, bovine and human NPH insulin, Acta. Med. Scand. 215, 69-73.
Kolendorf, K., Aaby, P., Westergaard, S., and Deckert, T. (1978). Absorption, effectiveness and side effects of highly purified porcine NPH-insulin preparations (Leo), Eur. J. Clin. Pharmacol. 14, 117-124.
Kraegen, E.W. and Chisholm, D.J. (1984). Insulin reponses to varying profiles of subcutaneous insulin infusion: kinetic modelling studies, Diabetologia 26, 208-213.
Lauritzen, T., Pramming, S., Gale, E. A. M., Deckert, T. and Binder, C. (1982). Absorption of isophane (NPH) insulin and its clinical implications, British Medical Journal 285, 159-161.
Lehmann, E.D., Deutsch, T., Roudsari, A.V., Carson, E.R., Benn, J.J. and

Sonksen, P.H. (1991). A metabolic prototype to aid in the management of insulin treated diabetic patients, Diabetes Nutrition and Metabolism 4 Suppl. 1, 163-167.

Olesen, K.G. and Andreassen, S. (1993). Specification of models in large expert systems based on causal probabilistic networks. Artificial Intelligence in Medicine. In press.

Owen, D. R. (1986). Human Insulin - Clinical pharmacological studies in normal man. Lancaster U.K.: MTP Press Ltd.

Rizza, R.A., Mandarino, L.J. and Gerich, J.E. (1981). Dose-response characteristics for effects of insulin on production and utilization of glucose in man, Am. J. Physiol. 240, E630-E639.

Salzsieder, E., Albrecht, G., Fischer, U., Rutscher, A. and Thierbach, U. (1990). Computer-aided systems in the management of type I diabetes: the application of a model-based strategy, Computer Methods Programs Biomed 32, 215 - 224.

Schiffrin, A., Mihic, M., Leibel, B.S. and Albisser, M. (1985) .Computer assisted insulin dosage adjustment, Diabetes Care 8, 545-552.

Schlichtkrull, J., Munck, O. and Jersild, M. (1965). The M-value, an index of blood sugar control in diabetics, Acta Med. Scand. 177, 95-102.

Schneider, J., Piwernetz, K., Engelbrecht, R. and Renner, R. (1988). DIACONS - A consultation system to assist in the management of diabetes. In: Expert Systems and Decision Support in Medicine, eds. Reinhoff, O., Piccolo, U. and Schneider, B. pp. 44-49. Berlin: Springer-Verlag.

Swan, G.W. (1982). An optimal control model of diabetes mellitus, Bull. Math. Biol. 44, 793-808.

Shimauchi, T., Kugai, N., Nagata, N. and Takatani, O. (1988). Microcomputer-aided insulin dose determination in intensified conventional insulin therapy, IEEE Trans. Biomed.. Eng BME 35, 167-171.

Spiegelhalter, D. J. and Lauritzen, S. L. (1988). Updating probabilities in expert systems. Technical Report, MCR Biostatistics Unit, Cambridge .

Vaag, A., Damgaard Pedersen, K., Lauritzen, M., Hildebrandt, P. and Bech-Nielsen, H. (1990). Intramuscular versus subcutaneus injection of unmodified insulin: Consequences for blood glucose control in patients with type 1 diabetes mellitus, Diabetic Medicine 7, 335-342.

Vaag, A., Handberg, A., Lauritzen, M., Henriksen, J.E., Damgaard Pedersen, K. and Bech-Nielsen, H. (1990). Variation in absorption of NPH insulin due to intramuscular injection, Diabetes Care 13, 74-76.

Artificial Intelligence in Medecine
S. Andreassen et al. , Eds.
IOS Press, 1993

Reasoning with Causal Networks at Variable Depths

Pedro Barahona, Jorge Cruz and Susana Nascimento

Departamento de Informática, Universidade Nova de Lisboa, 2825 Monte da Caparica, Portugal

Abstract

In medical problem solving two main subproblems can be identified, namely the selection of possible hypotheses from some initial data, and the evaluation of these hypothesis, possibly taking into account some additional evidence. In a number of model-based systems, more superficial knowledge is used for generating diagnostic hypotheses, whereas deeper knowledge is used to assess them, but these systems are usually domain specific. In this paper we present a generic methodology for representing causal knowledge, which enables diagnostic reasoning to be made at the appropriate knowledge depth. In particular, to obtain candidate diagnoses from easily observable findings (superficial knowledge) and to assess them subsequently via less easily observable findings (e.g. signs and results from complementary tests, usually associated with deeper domain entities).

1. Introduction

In many medical tasks, namely in diagnosis, two main subproblems can be identified a) the selection of possible hypotheses (e.g. diagnoses), from some initial data (typically symptoms), and b) the evaluation of the merit of these hypothesis, possibly taking into account some additional evidence (e.g. results from complementary tests). Although this decomposition of the diagnostic task is quite consensual in such abstract terms, its exact formulation and implementation is, of course, largely dependent from the adopted representation of medical knowledge.

Despite their different implementation, most diagnostic systems can be regarded as containing some kind of causal network to represent medical (causal) knowledge, where direct arcs link causes to effects. Diagnostic reasoning with such networks is basically a set covering problem - to find diagnoses that, via the causal chains, justify the observed findings.

In the extreme case, diagnoses and manifestations are the only entities represented in the network. This simplified representation has the advantage of allowing relatively simple computation of candidate diagnoses, which has some similarities to the "intuition" that human experts use to guess candidate hypotheses. However, such simplification also imposes that the ranking of hypotheses can only be made via some numerical schema, e.g. assuming some minimality criteria (a set of diagnoses with less diagnoses is usually better than another set containing more diagnoses), or based on probabilities. In particular [PeRe91] use prior probabilities in diagnoses and a kind of conditional probabilities in the causal links to compute the posterior probability of the diagnoses. Nevertheless, the accuracy of these probabilities (or other numerical ranking schemes) at such high level of abstraction (i.e. where much, and possibly highly relevant, knowledge about pathophysiologic states is not represented) is quite difficult, if not impossible, to control, and the resulting ranking is open to debate. Incidently, the explanations provided by these networks are quite poor, given the fact that only superficial knowledge is represented in them.

Deeper knowledge can be represented in bayesean belief networks [Pear88], where the roots usually represent diagnoses, leafs represent observable findings and intermediate nodes represent pathophysiologic states [AnFO92]. Despite the possibility of representing pathophysiologic states, it seems that bayesean networks are not typically used to capture the typical behaviour of a physician performing diagnosis: formulate hypotheses based on the superficial knowledge (e.g. symptoms), and subsequently evaluate their merits taking into account deeper pathophysiological findings, usually requiring more demanding complementary tests.

Rather they seem to have been adopted mostly to rank hypothesis more accurately, with a sound probabilistic calculus. However, and although several algorithms have been proposed to efficiently compute posterior probabilities [LaSp88], the fact remains that they are still quite complex and only applicable to relatively small networks. Moreover, the above argument about the accuracy of the prior and conditional probabilities applies, possibly even strongly, to the rankings produced in bayesean belief networks.

The complementarity nature of superficial and deeper domain knowledge, has already been perceived in other systems such as ABEL [PaSS81] and CHECK [ToCo89], where several layers of increasing complexity where used: the most superficial to generate hypothesis and the deeper ones to assess and explain these hypotheses, at the light of evidence found about the entities which are solely represented in these deeper layers. The main problem with this approach seems to be its very specific nature - the above systems were developed for specific domains, and cannot be easily generalized for different domains.

In this paper we present a generic methodology for representing causal knowledge, which enables diagnostic reasoning to be made at the appropriate knowledge depth. In particular, to obtain candidate diagnosis from easily observable findings (superficial knowledge) and subsequently assess them via less easily observable findings (e.g. signs and results from complementary tests, usually associated with deeper domain entities).

The reasoning proposed in the paper has some similarities with that presented in [FoKr91], [FoKD92], where it is assumed that, if in the underlying domain theory, a diagnosis is known to possibly cause some observed finding, then it becomes a candidate diagnosis (or part of a more general diagnostic set). A logic of argumentation is then developed to rank the candidates, taken into account the strength of the arguments that can be generated from the domain theory and the existing evidence.

However this framework for formalizing diagnostic reasoning, being quite independent from the medical domain, can only capture a part of the diagnostic procedure. In particular, the sequencing of actions required to seek further evidence is largely ignored. Moreover, the ranking that can be obtained from counting arguments of a very qualitative nature {confirmed, eliminated, supported, opposed}, as proposed in [FoKr91] is very limited.

Our methodology can thus be regarded as providing a more precise qualification to the arguments used in the logic of argumentation, as well a generic formalism to produce such arguments from the exploitation of deeper layers of medical knowledge.

The structure of the paper is the following. In section 2 we describe the basic ontology of our knowledge representation (a causal network is described). In section 3, a set of operations are presented that abstract away the deeper knowledge from a causal network, to produce simpler and more superficial networks. Section 4 presents the arguments that can be derived from our causal networks, and a calculus for their aggregation. Section 5 presents a simple example, to illustrate the main features of our methodology. Finally, section 6 summarizes the main conclusions.

2. Causal Networks

A causal-functional model was originally developed [BaVe91] to represent medical knowledge, in particular anatomic and functional knowledge, making it suitable for causal reasoning. Its domain ontology contains two types of entities, structures and processes. Both these entities have a state that may change over time. Structures are used to represent anatomic entities such as organs and their parts, and processes are used to represent the changes that can take place in the states of the structures, or even in the state of other processes.

This paper is about causal reasoning with the causal functional model, and focuses on the decomposition of processes, and how such decomposition is used in causal reasoning. The temporal issues of such reasoning, addressed in [Bara93], are thus not considered. The decomposition of structures (and the functions they perform) into their components is also not addressed in the paper (see [Bara92]).

Domain knowledge in the causal-functional model, expressed by means of structures and processes, can be regarded as the specification of some kind of causal network. Different entities can be selected for these networks, according to the medical speciality, as well as the task in hand. By and large, in diagnosis these networks will be directed graphs, where the roots represent complex disorder states (the diagnostic set) and the leafs represent observable findings.

A major concern that led to the development of the causal-functional model, was the need to represent medical knowledge as deeply as necessary, since deep knowledge was assumed to be one of the solutions to overcome the brittleness of existing medical knowledge based systems. It is thus a major feature of the model that structures and processes can be represented at any adequate depth. In general, the deeper the knowledge represented, the larger and more complex are the corresponding networks. (Here the term depth can be regarded as denoting both the level of detail and the, closely related, observability of the medical phenomenae; not the fact that the behaviour of a system can be derived from its structure, given a deeper representation of functionality, e.g. by means of differential equations, or their equivalents in qualitative simulation [Kuip84].)

Figure 1 shows a (very simplified) fragment of a diagnostic network for the peripheral nerve system. Oval nodes represent the relevant state attributes of a structure, which can range over a finite set of values. Square nodes represent processes, relating the values of the attributes of their causes and effects.

Carpal tunnel and polineuropathy are complex organism conditions, which are considered as being not directly observed, but only diagnoseable. All the other structures can have their states observable, though with variable difficulty. Whereas symptoms such as painful hand are easily observed (they are usually prompted by the patient), signs and results from complementary tests are less easily observable (they require more or less complex test procedures) and can thus be considered deeper entities. Instead of explicitly representing test processes (and their visible results) associated with visible entities, we have simply associated labels to each oval node (except to diagnostic nodes), to denote their depth. Labels range over the integers, the most visible nodes having depth 0 (e.g. painful hand).

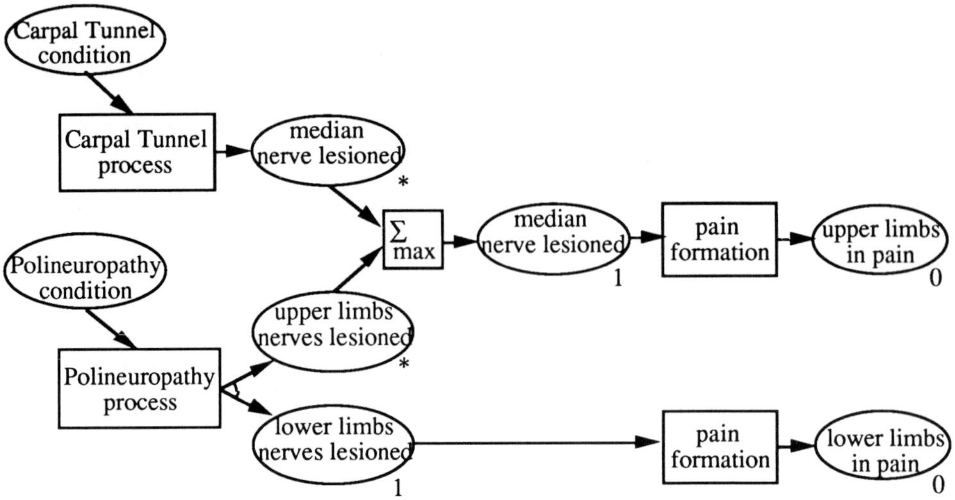

Figure 1. A simplified diagnostic network

As to the processes, they express more or less complex constraints relating the values of the attributes of process causes and effects. Generic processes may contain generic relations representing anatomic and functional knowledge (e.g. a lesioned nerve causes pain in the region it enervates). Since this paper is not concerned with such generic representation of medical knowledge, we assume that all the entities are already instantiated. Hence, the only constraints considered are the strength to which the causes are believed to cause the effects.

This belief can be represented in a variety of ways, more or less related to conditional probabilities. Because of the difficulty in obtaining accurate values for such probabilities (see discussion above), we will assume that the expert will provide some kind of qualitative measurement of the plausibility with which he/she believes in the cause-effect relationship (e.g. a severe lesion always causes a severe pain, or a severe lesion is more likely to cause a severe pain then a moderate pain, but still it can cause no pain at all).

When two or more processes affect the same node, then there is of course an interaction between the different values that each of the processes impose. Nevertheless, and because the plausibilities are assumed to express the effective causality, we represent explicitly each of the individual effects (with * in the figure) and collapse them into a single resulting node, via a special combination process, Σ_{max}. Assuming that abnormality overrides normality, the resulting node of such processes is considered to take the most abnormal value from all the individual inputs.

As will be seen in section 4, the plausibilities will eventually be quantified and used in some kind of probabilistic calculus. However, they are not used to compute posterior probabilities, given our assumption on the unreliability of the data which can be pragmatically be provided in real applications. Instead, they can be regarded as providing some quantifiable values for arguments about diagnostic hypotheses.

3. Network Abstraction

Because a deep causal network is supposed to represent the domain knowledge as completely as possible, reasoning about it can be quite complex, due to the number of nodes and links involved. In particular, the fast abduction of causes from observed findings in a way that "mimics" human intuition is hampered by such complexity.

This is thus the basic motivation for abstracting a deep causal network into a simpler one which, in the limit, only contains processes linking diagnostic nodes to findings of level 0 (e.g. symptoms). Such shallow networks simplify the abduction of diagnostic hypotheses. The original deeper networks should nonetheless remain available, namely to derive expected deeper findings abstracted away in the simplified network, or to explain findings not explainable in the abstracted network.

Instead of defining statically a set of layers of increased depth (and complexity) as done in ABEL[PaSS81] and CHECK [ToCo89] abstraction is performed in the causal-functional model by means of a set of abstraction rules, described below. To present these rules formally, we will use the notation

$$P :: c_1, \ldots, c_n \rightarrow e_1, \ldots, e_m \mid MC$$

to represent a process P, whose causes are attributes $c_1, \ldots, c_n$ of the states of different structures influencing the attributes $e_1, \ldots, e_m$ of the affected structures. MC denotes the matrix of conditional plausibilities discussed above (similar to conditional probabilities, but derived from a quantification of the causal strength believed by an expert).

3.1 Root Elimination

Rare diagnoses are usually not considered in the initial stages of the process of diagnosis. Therefore they can be assumed as not present by default, and abstracted away from the simplified causal network. Such elimination can be formalised as follows.

$$\frac{PSt :: c_1, \ldots, c_{i-1}, \mathbf{c_i}, c_{i+1}, \ldots, c_n \rightarrow e_1, \ldots, e_m \mid MC}{PSt' :: c_1, \ldots, c_{i-1}\ ,\ c_{i+1}, \ldots, c_n \rightarrow e_1, \ldots, e_m \mid MC'}$$

where $\mathbf{c_i}$ is a rare diagnosis. The resulting process has, of course, its matrix simplified, since there is one less cause. This simplification is performed by removing cause c from matrix MC. This function could be defined in several ways. Since we are assuming that the abstraction is due to the rarity of the diagnosis, we simply remove the lines from the input matrix where c_i is in a pathological state. For example, figure 2 shows the root elimination of c_2, a rare diagnosis, from process P.

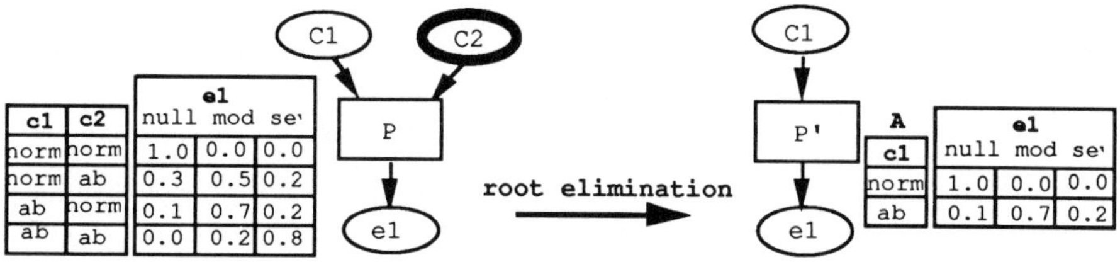

Figure 2. Root elimination

Notice that the abstracted network may be unable to explain certain situations explainable with the deeper network. For example, whereas a normal value of c_1 is not compatible with a moderate occurrence of e_1, which is obviously not the case with the initial network, where the effect is caused by the abnormal value of c_2 (the rare diagnosis).

3.2 Process Split

Spliting process P, through one of its effects e_j, turns this effect independent from the others and results in two processes, P_1 whose only effect is e_j, and P_2 with all the other effects of P. Formally,

$$\begin{array}{l} P{::}\ c_1,\ldots,\ c_n\ \to e_1,\ \ldots,\ e_{j-1},\ \mathbf{e_j},\ e_{j+1},\ \ldots,\ e_m\ |MC \\ \hline P_1{::}\ c_1,\ldots,\ c_n\ \to e_1,\ \ldots,\ e_{j-1},\ e_{j+1},\ ..,\ e_m|\ MC_1 \\ P_2{::}\ c_1,\ldots,\ c_n\ \to \mathbf{e_j}|\ MC_2 \end{array}$$

where the depth label of e_j is the highest (e.g. e_j is the highest depth) among the process other causes and effects. The plausibilities appearing in the matrices of P_1 and P_2 are the sum, over all values of the eliminated effects, of the corresponding plausibilities in the original matrix. In the example below, process P is split through e_2 (or through e_1, since there are only two effects).

	e 1 e 2			
c 1	null null	null sev	sev null	sev sev
norm	1.0	0.0	0.0	0.0
ab	0.0	0.3	0.3	0.4

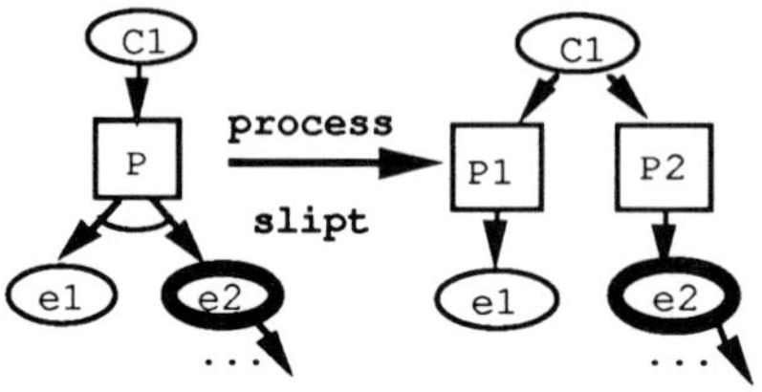

M 1	**e 1**	
c 1	null	sev
norm	1.0	0.0
ab	0.3	0.7

M 2	**e 2**	
c 1	null	sev
norm	1.0	0.0
ab	0.3	0.7

Figure 3. Process split

In contrast with the previous rule, the loss of information resulting from this rule, allows the abstract network to (wrongly) justify situations which are not justifiable in the complete network. For example, an abnormal value of c1 is compatible with e_1 and e_2 having both null values, which is certainly not the case with the initial network.

3.3 Process Aggregation

The purpose of process aggregation, through an entity e_j, is to eliminate this entity from the network and aggregate process P whose only effect is e_j (e.g. P may have resulted from a previous process split through e_j) with all those processes P_i that have e_j as one of their causes.

$$\begin{array}{l} P\ {::}\ c_1\ ,\ldots,\ c_n \qquad\qquad\qquad \to \mathbf{e_j}\ |\ MC \\ P_1{::}\ c_{11},\ldots,\ \mathbf{e_j},\ldots,\ c_{1k_1}\ \to e_{11},\ \ldots,\ e_{1j_1}\ |\ MC_1 \\ \ldots\ldots\ldots \\ P_s{::}\ c_{s1},\ldots,\ \mathbf{e_j},\ldots,\ c_{sk_s}\ \to e_{s1},\ \ldots,\ e_{sj_s}\ |\ MC_s \\ \hline P'_1{::}\ c_{11},\ldots,\ c_{1k_1},\ c_1\ ,\ldots,\ c_n\ \to e_{11},\ \ldots,\ e_{1j_1}\ |\ MC'_1 \\ \ldots\ldots\ldots \\ P'_s{::}\ c_{s1},\ldots,\ c_{sk_s},\ c_1\ ,\ldots,\ c_n \to e_{s1},\ \ldots,\ e_{sj_s}\ |\ MC'_s \end{array}$$

where $\mathbf{e_j}$ is the least visible among all the other entities involved in the rule, and matrices MC'_i are obtained by a generalization of the multiplication of the matrices through the common attribute e_j(it is indeed a matrix multiplication if e_j is the only cause of MC_i). An example is shown in Figure 4:

3.4 Process Elimination

This rule simply eliminates those processes which, through previous root eliminations lost all their causes. Formally

$$\begin{array}{l} P{::}\ \ \to e_1,\ \ldots,\ e_m\ |\ MC \\ \hline \end{array}$$

MP		ej
c	null	sev
null	1.0	0.0
sev	0.2	0.8

MP1			e1
c1	ej	null	sev
null	null	1.0	0.0
null	sev	0.4	0.6
sev	null	0.6	0.4
sev	sev	0.0	1.0

MP2		e2
ej	null	sev
null	0.8	0.2
sev	0.2	0.8

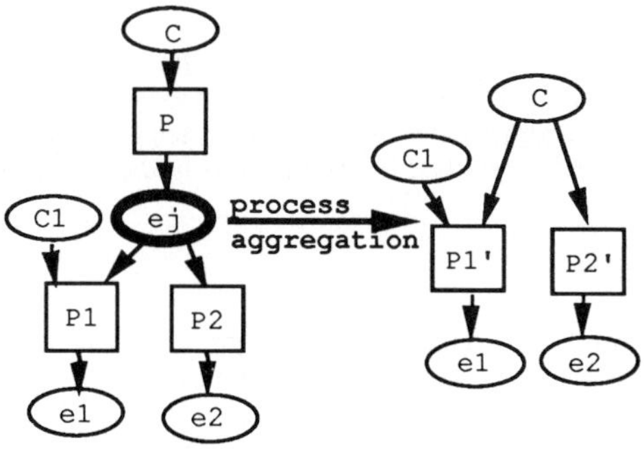

MP1'			e1
c1	c	null	sev
null	null	1.00	0.00
null	sev	0.52	0.48
sev	null	0.60	0.40
sev	sev	0.12	0.88

MP2		e2
c	null	sev
null	0.80	0.20
sev	0.32	0.68

Figure 4. Process aggregation

4. Causal Reasoning

With the causal network domain representation, causal reasoning can be regarded as deriving from the network adequate diagnoses which are compatible to the known findings, and is thus a composition of abduction and deduction. Abduction derives the antecedent from an implication, from the known consequent, and can be formalised as

$$\frac{A \rightarrow B \qquad B}{A}$$

If causality is paralleled to logical implication, then diagnosis A can be abducted from the observation of finding B. Of course the problem of abduction is that many diagnostic hypotheses can be generated from the same observed fact. Some of them can possibly be discarded by deduction, more precisely with the modus tolens rule below, specifying that an diagnostic hypothesis A which is expected to cause C, should be abandoned when this finding is not present.

$$\frac{A \rightarrow C \qquad \sim C}{\sim A}$$

There are several problems when considering the application of this kind of reasoning in medicine, namely in diagnosis. Firstly, the complexity of the computations required to abduct hypothesis depends on the complexity of the network. Secondly, a network with medical knowledge as complete as possible contains all relevant diagnoses, even those that are quite rare, and hence too many diagnostic hypothesis might be generated for further consideration. Thirdly, due to the uncertainty that pervades the medical domain, diagnostic hypotheses, as implausible as they might be, can hardly be discarded.

To cope with these problems, we have presented in the previous section a set of rules that enable focussing the problem by abstracting away less relevant information. The first problem, is basically handled by the Process Aggregation rule, that abstracts away deeper knowledge (which can nonetheless be retrieved for the evaluation of the hypotheses thus generated). The second problem is alleviated by the possibility of specifying rare diseases, and thus abstracts them away, even if only temporarily, from the network, via Root Elimination and Process Elimination rules.

To handle the third problem, we will use the process plausibilities to quantify the arguments that can be produced about diagnostic hypotheses, as proposed in [FoKD92]. In our notation, a diagnostic hypothesis can be represented by a set of triples O: < D, P >, one for each observed node O, where P is the process that most likely explains it and D are the inputs of this process.

4.1 Observed Evidence

Let us assume that an hypothesis contains a diagnostic node X in state s, denoted by X_s, which via process P, may cause an observable node O to be in one of 3 states O_1, O_2, and O_3, with causal plausibilities 0.2, 0.3 and 0.5, respectively. If O_3, the most likely outcome of X_s is observed, then the expectations about X_s are fulfilled, and the diagnostic task proceeds without penalizing hypothesis X_s. The observation of the most plausible outcome is therefore taken into account as an argument favouring X_s. On the other hand, if O_2 is observed then our expectations are somewhat contradicted, since O_2 is a less expected consequence of X_s. Nevertheless, this should not be considered as a complete contradiction (which would lead to discard hypothesis X_s by application of modus tollens), but rather make our expectations with respect to X_s to decrease somewhat. In a sense, this finding should be considered as an argument against X_s. The same rationale applies, *a fortiori*, if O_1 is observed.

The aggregation of evidence for and against the hypotheses can thus be made by specifying the plausibility π of an hypothesis, given the known evidence, and modify it as more arguments are obtained by the exploration of the causal network. The updating of the plausibility of an hypothesis H, once O is observed, can be made by adding a new triple O: < D, P > to H, with the corresponding value of π. The overall plausibility of the composed hypothesis H + O: < D, P > is assumed to be the minimum value of the individual π's of the composed hypothesis.

4.2 Process Decomposition

If O: < D, P >π is an explanation included in an hypothesis, and P is the result of the aggregation of processes P_1 and P_2, which has eliminated node I, and this node can be observed at a sensible cost (related to its depth), than more accurate arguments can be produced with respect to the hypothesis, by exploring this deeper knowledge. In general such exploitation is not necessary if π is equal to 1 (or some other sufficiently high value).

In particular, once the value I_v of I is observed, the expanded explanation is obtained by replacing the triple O: < D, P >π, by I_v: < D, P_1 >π_1 and O: < I_v, P_2> π_2, where π_1 and π_2 are computed as explained above.

5. Causal Reasoning Applied to an Example

At present we have not yet developed completely the diagnostic reasoning process, in the sense that we have not yet specified criteria to stop or proceed the application of the reasoning rules described in the previous section, and in case of proceeding, which of the available rules is applied to the hypothesis with higher plausibility. Hence, we will illustrate the reasoning process defined in the previous sections by mean of an example. Let the domain knowledge be represented by the deep causal network of Figure 5.

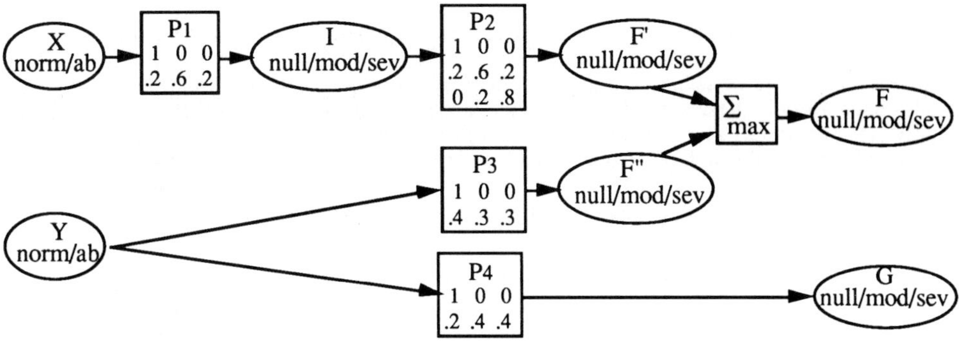

Figure 5. A deep causal network

Let us assume that F is observed. Assuming that Y is a rare disease, the full abstraction of the deep causal network results into the superficial network of Figure 6.

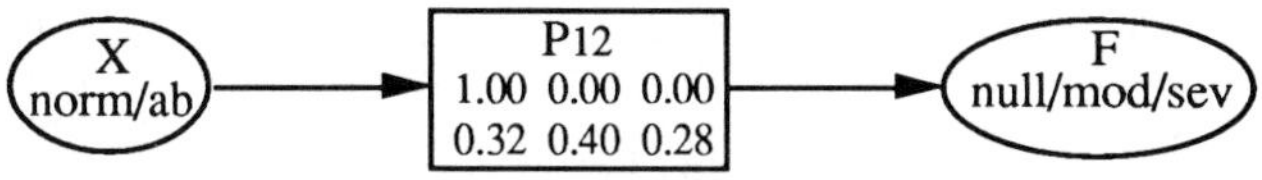

Figure 6. The superficial network

The system can now generate hypothesis X, which explains F. As explained in the previous section, the plausibility of an hypothesis H, given a certain observable fact F, in the context of a process P, is the ratio between the causal plausibility of F as an effect of process P, and that of the most expected effect. If F_{sev} is the observed value of F, the plausibility of it being produced by process P_{12} with inputs X_{norm} and X_{ab} is 0.0 and 0.28, respectively. Since the most likely outcomes X_{norm} and X_{ab} have causal plausibilities 1.0 and 0.40, the plausibility of these hypotheses are:

$$F_{sev} : < X_{norm} / P_{12} >_{0.00} \quad (0.00/1.00)$$
$$F_{sev} : < X_{ab} \; / P_{12} >_{0.70} \quad (0.28/0.40)$$

The first hypothesis is eliminated at this stage (as an explanation of F_{sev}) given its null plausibility. Moreover, there are reasons to suspect that X_{ab} is the actual cause of F_{sev}, given the fact that this is not the most likely outcome (reflected in the value of $\pi = 0.7$). We could thus proceed by investigating process P_{12} more deeply. Expanding it into the original processes P_1 and P_2 results into the network of Figure 7.

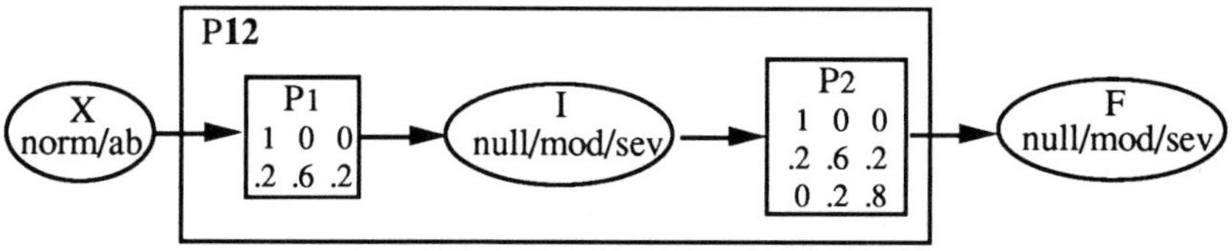

Figure 7. The intermediate network

Now this suggests observation of I. If I is sev, then our hypothesis is updated, since the plausibilities of I_{sev} being produced by X_{ab} and F_{sev} produced by I_{sev} are, respectively, 0.2/0.6 = 0.33 and 0.8/0.8 = 1.0. Our hypothesis thus becomes:

$$I_{sev}: < X_{ab} / P_1 >_{0.33} + F_{sev} : < I_{sev} / P_2 >_{1.0}$$

The low plausibility of the first component of the hypothesis, suggests that there might be other causes for I_{sev}, which seems to be the real cause of F_{sev}. We should then proceed by searching these other causes of I_{sev}, assuming that there might be rare diagnosis that could have been abstracted away in these simplified networks. Since there are no such diagnosis in our complete network, we would then terminate our search with the conclusion "X_{ab} is the best found diagnosis of I_{sev}, through process P_1, and I_{sev} is the likely cause of F_{sev} through process P_2".

If I_{null} is observed instead, the extended hypothesis would become:

$$I_{null}: < X_{ab} / P_1 >_{0.33} + F_{sev} : < I_{null} / P_2 >_{0.0}$$

This guarantees that the actual reason of F_{sev} is not I_{null}, and we should then find other reasons to explain F_{sev}. Moreover, we would also try to better justify I_{null}, since X_{ab} does not seem a plausible explanation. In this case, I_{null} is better explained with X_{norm}, via the same process P_1. We would then proceed with

$$I_{null}: < X_{norm} / P_1 >_{1.00} + F_{sev} : < I_{null} / P_2 >_{0.0}$$

If I_{mod} were observed instead, the same reasoning would lead us to hypothesis:

$$I_{mod}: < X_{ab} / P_1 >_{1.00} + F_{sev} : < I_{mod} / P_2 >_{0.33}$$

In both cases, the only way to better explain F_{sev} is to consider the rare diagnosis Y, previously abstracted away. The extended causal network would not only include Y, but also G, which has depth 0. This network corresponds to the initial deep network (see Figure 5).

Let us assume that G_{null} is observed. In this case, we have

$$G_{null} : < Y_{norm} / P_4 >_{1.00}$$
$$G_{null} : < Y_{ab} \ / P_4 >_{0.50}$$

Proceeding with the most plausible value of G, we have hypothesis

$$I_{mod}: < X_{ab} / P_1 >_{1.00} + F_{sev} : < I_{mod} / P_2 >_{0.33} + G_{null} : < Y_{norm} / P_4 >_{1.00}$$

We still have to improve our explanation for F_{sev}. Given our semantics of the Σ_{max} process, the plausibility of F_{sev} is the best of the plausibilities of F'_{sev} and F''_{sev}. But the explanation of F''_{sev}, i.e. F_{sev} from Y_{norm} via P_3, has plausibility 0, and so can not improve the explanation provided by F'_{sev} (F_{sev} from I_{mod} via P_2). The overall plausibility of the composed hypothesis is thus 0.33, the minimum of the individual plausibilities.

At this point, we would backtrack to try Y_{ab}, and form hypothesis

$$I_{mod}: < X_{ab} / P_1 >_{1.00} + F_{sev} : < I_{mod} / P_2 >_{0.33} + G_{null} : < Y_{ab} / P_4 >_{0.50}$$

Trying again to explain F_{sev} better, we realize that F_{sev} is indeed quite plausibly caused by Y_{ab}, via P_3, and the resulting plausibility $0.3/ 0.4 = 0.75$ overrides the previous explanation of F_{sev}. The composed hypothesis will thus become

$$I_{mod}: < X_{ab} / P_1 >_{1.00} + F_{sev} : < Y_{ab} / P_3 >_{0.75} + G_{null} : < Y_{ab} / P_4 >_{0.50}$$

Since there is no backtracking point the final explanation would be: "Y_{ab} is the most plausible diagnosis for both symptoms F_{sev} and G_{null}, given that I_{mod} was observed. X_{ab}, in turn, is the likely cause of I_{mod}".

6. Conclusion

In this paper we presented a scheme to causal reasoning with the causal functional network, developed earlier. Although this scheme borrows some notions from classical probability theory, it can be regarded as largely a scheme for abductive reasoning under some default assumptions.

The scheme presents a method to abstract simpler and "superficial" networks from more complex and complete causal networks, and to abstract properly identified rare diagnosis, to simplify the task of proposing diagnostic hypotheses. The evaluation of such hypotheses is done via the aggregation of arguments for and against these hypotheses, drawn from the plausibility assumed to the causal strength of the processes involved.

Being a preliminary first scheme proposed for causal reasoning with the causal-functional model, we believe that it can be subsequently improved, namely its weighting of arguments. The example presented, show that the present weighting scheme might be appropriate, at least for this toy problem. We are starting now to use it in more realistic applications, namely in electromiography (diagnosis of the peripheral neuro-muscular system). Results obtained from these experiences will clarify which improvements should be made to the scheme presented.

Acknowledgments

This research was carried out in the Artificial Intelligence Center of UNINOVA, and was supported by the Commission of the European Communities (Project ESTEEM A2010 from the AIM Programme), and JNICT, the Portuguese Council for Science and Technology (Project Rhesma, PMCT/C/TIT/861/90).

References

[AnFO92] S. Andreassen, B. Falck and K.G. Olesen, *Diagnostic Function of the Microhuman Prototype of the Expert System MUNIN*, Electroencephalography in Clinical Neurology, 1992.

[Bara92] P. Barahona, *A Causal-Functional Model for Medical Knowledge Representation*, in: Keravnou ed, Deep Models for Medical Knowledge Engineering. Elsevier, 1992.

[Bara93] P. Barahona, *Deep Causal and Temporal Reasoning for Decision Support on Drug Therapy*, Proceedings of MIE-93, Reichert A., Sadan B.A., Bengtsson S., Bryant J. and Piccolo U. (eds), April 1993.

[BaVe91] P. Barahona and M. Veloso, *A Framework for Causal Reasoning with a Functional Approach*, Proceedings of AIME-91, Lecture Notes in Medical Informatics, Springer-Verlag, June 1991.

[FoKD92] J. Fox, P. Krause and M. Dohnal, *A generic framework for uncertain reasoning*, Proceedings of the 8th Conference on Uncertainty in Artificial Intelligence, July 1992.

[FoKr91] J. Fox and P. Krause, *Symbolic Decision Theory and Autonomous Systems*, Uncertainty in Artificial Intelligence: Proceedings of the 7th Conference, D'Ambrosio B.D., Smets P. and Bonissone P.P. (eds), 1991.

[Kuip84] B. Kuipers, *Commonsense Reasoning about Causality: Deriving Behavior from Structure*, Artificial Intelligence 24, pp.169-203, 1984.

[LaSp88] S.L. Lauritzen and D.J. Spiegelhalter, *Local Computations with Probabilities on Graphical Structures and their Application to Expert Systems*, Journal of Royal Statistical Society, vol. B 50, pp. 157-224, 1988.

[PaSS81] R.S. Patil, P. Szolovits and W.B. Schwartz, *Causal Understanding of Patient Ilness in Medical Diagnosis*, in Procs. of Seventh International Joint Conference on Artificial Intelligence, 893-899, 1981.

[Pear88] J. Pearl, *Propabilistic Reasoning in Intelligent Systems: Networks of Plausible Inference,* Morgan Kaufmann, 1988.

[PeRe91] Y. Peng and J.A. Reggia, *Abductive Inference Models for Diagnostic Problem-Solving*, Springer-Verlag, 1991

[ToCo89] P. Torasso and L. Console, *Diagnostic Problem Solving: Combining Heuristic, Approximate and Causal Reasoning*, North Oxford Academic, 1989.

Artificial Intelligence in Medecine
S. Andreassen et al. , Eds.
IOS Press, 1993

Transformation of Compartmental Models into Sequences of Causal Probabilistic Networks

Ulrich G. Oppel*, Alexander Hierle*, Lydia Janke+, Wolfgang Moser+

*Mathematisches Institut, Universität München, Theresienstr. 39, D 80333 München, Germany. Email: ulrich.oppel@mathematik.uni—muenchen.d400.de

+GSF - Forschungszentrum für Umwelt und Gesundheit, Institut für Medizinische Informatik und Systemforschung, Ingolstädter Landstr. 1, D 85758 Oberschleißheim

Abstract: Some metabolic processes are described by compartmental models. They are characterized by a cyclic graph and a system of differential equations. We introduce a general method to transform such a system into a sequence of acyclic causal probabilistic networks (CPN). This method is based on the solution of the system of differential equations and a stochastification procedure. The result of this transformation is a more realistic model of the metabolic process which may be simulated and adapted to new evidence very easily using the shell HUGIN. In contrary to that, the adaption of the deterministic process of the compartmental model to new evidence in general is not possible. Furthermore, such a stochastified description of a metabolic process easily may be modified by adding additional nodes for additional effects to the CPN. We apply this method of transforming a compartmental model into a sequence of CPNs to a simple glucose - insulin model.

1. Introduction

Causal probabilistic networks are designed to describe biological, medical, social, economical, and technical systems which are subject to randomness and uncertainty. A causal probabilistic network (CPN) is a directed graph and a family of Markov kernels. The nodes of the graph represent random variables describing subsystems. The links connecting the nodes represent cause - effect relations which are quantified by conditional probabilities of events of the state space of a child node given states of the state spaces of the parent nodes; e.g. see Lauritzen et al. [6] and Pearl [8].

If the directed graph is acyclic and finite, the family of Markov kernels (given by the conditional probabilities) determines a probability measure $\mathbb{P}$ on the product of the state spaces of all nodes; this probability measure $\mathbb{P}$ is a directed Markov field which is completely determined by the given Markov kernels. If the directed graph is not acyclic, such a probability measure $\mathbb{P}$, representing the common distribution of all nodes, may not exist.

In medicine we encounter many very complex systems which are subject to randomness and uncertainty due to their complexity and inter- and intraindividual variation. To study these systems, it is necessary to simplify them extremely. Sometimes this is possible, sometimes it is necessary to complexify these oversimpifications afterwards again to obtain a better description of the system. Because of the randomness and uncertainty encountered everywhere, such a complexification necessarily includes a stochastification. Starting from a very simple compartmental model of a metabolic process we shall show how to stochastify such a model to obtain a more complex and operable CPN. Since the compartmental models and the CPNs obtained from them by stochastification usually contain cycles and since directed cycles are problematic, these directed cycles in the CPNs have to be transfered into sequences of repetitions of acyclic CPNs.

These sequences of CPNs have embedded Markov chains. The well known ergodic and periodic behavior of these Markov chains may be used to control, to motivate, and to exclude specific stochastifications. Here we cannot explain these procedures in more detail; it will be done in a forthcoming paper. However, here we can point out a remarkable effect of such a stochastification: *the (unrealistic) precision of a deterministic compartmental model usually does not allow to fit the model to new evidence, in contrary to that the (more realistic) imprecision of the stochastified model allows for such fitting.*

To understand this remarkable effect a little bit better, first let us explain the procedure of transforming a deterministic compartmental model into a stochastified model of a sequence of CPNs in general. A compartmental model is determined qualitatively by a (usually cyclic and not directed) graph and quantitatively by a system of differential equations. These differential equations determine the flow of masses between the compartments. Starting from the graph of the compartmental model we construct a sequence of properly connected acyclic graphs describing time slices of the metabolic process qualitatively. To describe the still deterministic metabolic process quantitatively, we solve the system of differential equations. For any finding at the beginning or at some other time point there is a unique trajectory determined by this finding and the system of differential equations. This trajectory is obtained by solving the system of differential equations iteratively starting from the time point and value of the finding and moving in the forward or backward direction of time. The deterministic process which is consistent with the finding and modeled by the system of differential equations is determined by this trajectory. The trajectory is uniquely determined by this one finding, another finding is not consistent with this model and the given finding, unless it lies on the trajectory. However, if we stochastify the model, this situation changes completely. To stochastify the model, we pass from the deterministic transitions (obtained from the system of differential equations) to properly designed stochastic transitions. Starting from the beginning we obtain a sequence of Markov kernels and , hence, an acyclic CPN. Into such a CPN according to the principles of Bayesian inference any kind of new evidence may be introduced, at any time points and in any order. The construction of such a CPN and the propagation of new evidence easily can be done using the well known shell HUGIN. Below we shall explain and demonstrate this procedure in more detail.

2. Compartmental models and CPNs.

The description of even a simple metabolic process in detail is immensely involved, comprising the anatomy of the organs, the physiology of organ function and transport processes, and long chains or numerous cycles of linked biochemical reactions. To make descriptions tractable abstractions and the description of diverse processes and phenomena in terms of a limited number of types of models are necessary.

A first and merely deterministic scheme of description of metabolic processes is concerned with masses of substances present at particular sites and mass flow rates between these sites. An example of such schemes of description are compartmental models for chemical reactions, transport processes (diffusion from one compartment to another, compartment washed by fluid, transport by fluid circulation), and parametrically controlled processes.

A compartment is an idealized store of a substance. If a substance is present in a biological system in several distinguishable forms or locations, then all the substance in a particular form and location is said to constitute a compartment. The function of the compartment is described by mass balance equations. The general form of the mass balance equation for a compartment i that interchanges matter with other compartments j then is the differential equation

$$dQ_i/dt = \sum_j R_{ij} - \sum_i R_{ji}$$

where Q_i is the quantity of substance in compartment i and R_{ij} is the rate of mass transfer from j to i and R_{ji} the rate of mass transfer from i to j. The exchange of mass between compartments takes place either by physical transport from one location to another or by chemical reactions. Both the rates of chemical reactions and of mass transfer in transport processes depend on the concentration which is in general not uniform. A compartment is characterized by the idealized concentration in a compartment. In such a compartmental model the rate of mass transfer from compartment j to compartment i is a deterministic function of the time t and the quantity Q_j in compartment j which may depend on some additional parameters of the model under consideration.

In the formulation of a compartmental model of chemical or mass transfer processes in a biological system, first the system is divided into relevant and convenient compartments. Then the mass balance equations for each compartment and its relations to linked compartments are established. Usually, these differential equations are of simple linear form in order to be able to solve these equations and to determine implicite parameters of the system of these coupled equations. A compartmental model is determined by the system of mass balance equations and a graph. The nodes of this graph are the compartments. The nodes of this graph are linked if the compartments which they represent are related by mass balance equations. Hence, the graph associated in such a way to a compartmental model describes this model qualitatively and the system of mass balance equations describes the model quantitatively. Such a point of view relates compartmenal models to CPNs. The system of mass balance equations in a compartmental model plays exactly the same role as the family of Markov kernels in a CPN. The Markov kernels of a CPN describe stochastic relations between the subsystems repesented by the nodes. Under certain conditions the system of mass balance equations has an eventually uniquely determined solution which describes deterministic flows of masses. Below we shall show how to stochastify compartmental models and how to transform them into CPNs. Since the graphs associated to compartmental models usually are not directed and contain cycles representing common feedback features of biological systems, we have to transform them into sequences of repetitions of a CPN with a directed graph. We shall obtain the family of Markov kernels of a sequence of CPNs associated to compartmental model by pr,operly stochastifying the deterministic relations of the compartmental model given by the system of mass balance equations. We shall demonstrate this for a well known example of a compartmental model for the glucose metabolism.

3. An example: glucose-insulin metabolism

The Bolie model for glucose-insulin interactions in mammals (see Bolie [3] and Carson et al. [5], p. 138 f.; see also Ackerman et. al. [1] and Braun [4], p. 178 ff.) is an example of a control system model which not only is based on simple mass balance consideratons, but also includes hypotheses as to control signal relationships between glucose and insulin. The model is a two compartment model and is described by the system of linear mass balance equations

$$dq_1/dt\ (t) = -\ p_1\ q_1(t) - p_2\ q_2(t) + \varphi(t) \qquad \text{(E1)}$$

$$dq_2/dt\ (t) = -\ p_3\ q_2(t) + p_4\ q_1(t) \qquad \text{(E2)}$$

and the initial values

$$q_1(0) = q_2(0) = 0$$

where $q_1 := Q_1 - Q_1^*$ and $q_2 := Q_2 - Q_2^*$ are the deviations of plasma glucose concentration Q_1 and insulin concentration Q_2 from their fasting levels Q_1^* and Q_2^*, respectively, $\varphi(t)$ is the impulsive intravenous injection of glucose, and p_1, p_2, p_3, p_4 are positive parameters that describe distribution and interactions of glucose and insulin (see Figur 1).

By considering plasma glucose the only measurable variable, the output is given by

$$y_1(t) = q_1(t)/V_p$$

where V_p is the plasma volume. The transfer function

$$H_{11}(s) := Y_1(s)/U(s) = (s+p_3)\ V_p^{-1}\ (s^2 + (p_1+p_3)s + p_1\ p_3 + p_2\ p_4$$

where $Y_1(s)$ and $U(s)$ are the Laplace transform of $y_1(t)$ and of the test input injection $\varphi(t)$, respectively. This model is unidentifiable, as there are five unknowns $(V_p, p_1, p_2, p_3, p_4)$ and four equations among them.

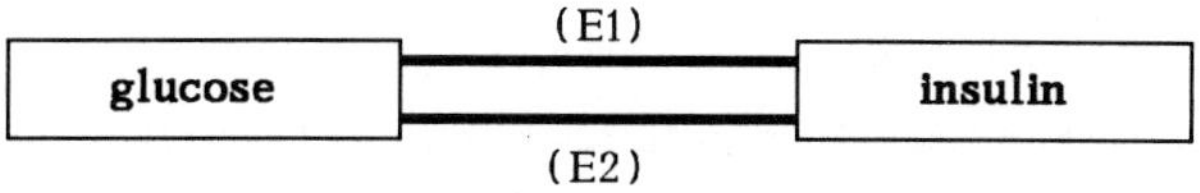

Figure 1: The graph of the two compartment model of the glucose insulin metabolism.

If the plasma concentration of insulin

$$y_2(t) = q_2(t)/V_p$$

is also measured, then a second transfer function is available, and hence, the 5 unknowns can be uniquely estimated from both plasma glucose and insulin data.

4. Stochastification of the example

In order to transform this compartmental model into a sequence of CPNs, first we solve the system of linear mass balance equations (E1) and (E2) for any initial values

$$q_1(t_o) = y_1 \quad \text{and} \quad q_2(t_o) = y_2 \ . \qquad \text{(E3)}$$

Furthermore, we shall solve the system (E1) and (E2) with (E3) for an arbitrary function $\varphi(t)$ which needs not describe an "impulsive intravenous injection" of glucose, but which might also describe some continuous process of supply of glucose.

One way of doing this is to differentiate (E1), we get

$$d^2 q_1/dt^2 = - p_1 \, dq_1/dt - p_2 \, dq_2/dt + d\varphi/dt \ .$$

Substituting (E2) we obtain that

$$d^2 q_1/dt^2 = - p_1 \, dq_1/dt + p_2 \, p_3 \, q_2 - p_2 \, p_4 \, q_1 + d\varphi/dt \, .$$

Solving (E1) for $p_2 \, q_2$ and substituting this, we arrive at the following nonhomogeneous linear differential equation of second order with constant coefficients:

$$d^2 q_1/dt^2 + (p_1 + p_3) \, dq_1/dt + (p_1 \, p_3 + p_2 \, p_4) \, q_1 = p_3 \, \varphi + d\varphi/dt \, . \qquad \text{(G1)}$$

The general solution of this equation is the sum of the general solution of the homogeneous equation

$$d^2 q_1/dt^2 + 2 \, \alpha \, dq_1/dt + \omega_0^2 \, q_1 = 0$$

$$\text{where} \quad \alpha := (p_1 + p_3)/2 \quad \text{and} \quad \omega_0^2 := p_1 \, p_3 + p_2 \, p_4$$

and a particular solution of the inhomogeneous equation

$$d^2 q_1/dt^2 + 2 \, \alpha \, dq_1/dt + \omega_0^2 \, q_1 = K$$

$$\text{where} \quad K := p_3 \, \varphi + d\varphi/dt.$$

Let us assume that $\omega^2 := \omega_0^2 - \alpha^2 > 0$. Then the characteristic polynomial of the homogeneous equation $\lambda^2 + 2 \, \alpha \, \lambda + \omega_0^2 = 0$ has the two roots $\lambda_1 := - \alpha + i \, \omega$ and $\lambda_2 := - \alpha - i \, \omega$ with $i^2 = - 1$ and $\omega > 0$. Hence, the general solution of the homogeneous equation is

$$h(t) := (\gamma_1 \cos(\omega t) + \gamma_2 \sin(\omega t)) \exp(-\alpha t) \quad \text{with } \gamma_i \in \mathbb{R},$$

where $h_1(t) := \cos(\omega t) \exp(-\alpha t)$ and $h_2(t) := \sin(\omega t) \exp(-\alpha t)$

is a fundamental system of solutions which has the following fundamental matrix

$$G(t) := \begin{pmatrix} \cos(\omega t) & \sin(\omega t) \\ -\omega \sin(\omega t) - \alpha \cos(\omega t) & \omega \cos(\omega t) - \alpha \sin(\omega t) \end{pmatrix} \exp(-\alpha t)$$

which has the Wronski determinant $W(t) = \omega \exp(-2\alpha t)$. Therefore, we obtain the following particular solution k of the inhomogeneous equation:

$$k(t) := -h_1(t) \int_t^t \sin(\omega t)/\omega \quad \exp(\alpha t)\, K(t)\, dt \; +$$

$$+ \; h_2(t) \int_{t_o}^t \cos(\omega t)/\omega \quad \exp(\alpha t)\, K(t)\, dt$$

The general solution of the inhomogeneous differential equation of second order is

$$q_1(t) := h(t) + k(t).$$

For any given initial values

$$q_1(t_o) = y_1 \quad \text{and} \quad q_2(t_o) = y_2$$

we obtain from (E1)

$$dq_1/dt\,(t_o) = -p_1 y_1 - p_2 y_2 + \varphi(t_o).$$

Hence, for any given t_o, y_1, and y_2 we can determine γ_1 and γ_2 of h(t), and therefore we get a unique solution of (G1) with $q_1(t_o) = y_1$; it depends on $\varphi(t)$, too; we denote it by $q_1(t;t_o,y_1,y_2;\varphi)$.

In order to solve the system (E1) and (E2) with the initial values (E3) we substitute the solution $q_1(t)$ of (G1), which we just obtained, into (E2) and solve it for $q_2(t)$ and the initial value $q_2(t_o) = y_2$. Fom (E2) we get the following inhomogeneous differential equation of first oder with constant coefficients

$$dq_2/dt\,(t) + p_3\, q_2(t) = p_4\, q_1(t;t_o,y_1,y_2;\varphi) \tag{G2}$$

We shall denote the solution $q_2(t)$ of (G2) with the property $q_2(t_o) = y_2$ by $q_2(t;t_o,y_1,y_2;\varphi)$. It has the following shape

$$q_2(t;t_o,y_1,y_2;\varphi) =$$

$$= \left(y_2 + \int_{t_o}^t p_4\, q_1(s;t_o,y_1,y_2;\varphi) \exp(p_3 (s-t_o))\, ds \right) \exp(-p_3(t-t_o)).$$

Our compartmental model has two compartments (representing the glucose concentration and the the insulin concentration); it is determined by the system of mass balance equations (E1) and (E2) which describe these concentrations as time goes by. Starting from this cyclic model, first we obtain a "deterministic" CPN which is a sequence of CPNs which we denote by $(\mathfrak{C}_n\colon n \in \mathbb{N})$. This is done by choosing a sequence of not necessarily equidistant time points t_n.

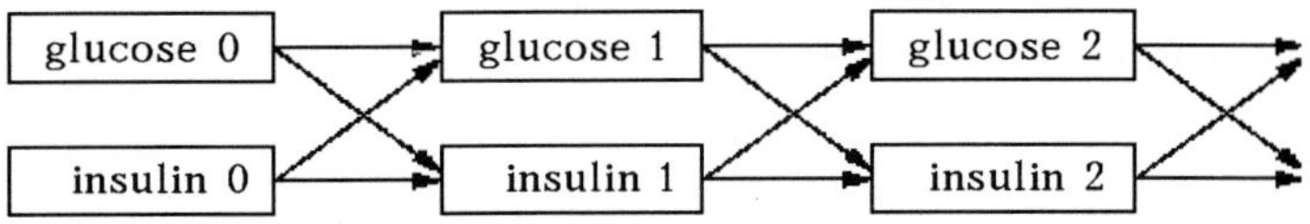

Figure 2: The graph of the glucose-insulin metabolism model of a sequence of CPNs obtained from the two compartmental model.

Each such CPN $\mathfrak{C}_n$ consists of two nodes "glucose n" and "insulin n" which describe the glucose and the insulin concentrations at time t_n, respectively. Let us now assume that the glucose supply in the time interval from t_{n-1} to t_n is given by a

supply function $\varphi_n(t)$

which is concentrated on this interval. (For example, if we know the supply function $\varphi(t)$ for all the time we can define $\varphi_n(t) := \varphi(t)$ for $t_{n-1} \leq t < t_n$ and $\varphi_n(t) := 0$ otherwise.) For each $n \geq 1$ and for "glucose n" and "insulin n" we can define "deterministic" Markov kernels

$$\mathfrak{G}_n: (S_{n-1,g} \times S_{n-1,i}) \times \mathfrak{S}_{n,g} \rightarrow [0,1] \quad \text{and} \quad \mathfrak{J}_n: (S_{n-1,g} \times S_{n-1,i}) \times \mathfrak{S}_{n,i} \rightarrow [0,1]$$

from the product $((S_{n-1,g} \times S_{n-1,i}) \times (\mathfrak{S}_{n-1,g} \otimes \mathfrak{S}_{n-1,i}))$ of the state spaces of "glucose n-1" and "insulin n-1" to the state space $(S_{n,g}, \mathfrak{S}_{n,g})$ of "glucose n" and $(S_{n,i}, \mathfrak{S}_{n,i})$ of "insulin n", respectively.

Let us assume that we know the state $y_{n-1,1}$ of the node "glucose n-1" and the state $y_{n-1,2}$ of the node "insulin n-1" at time t_{n-1}. Then we can calculate the solutions

$$q_1(t; t_{n-1}, y_{n-1,1}, y_{n-1,2}; \varphi_n) \text{ and } q_2(t; t_{n-1}, y_{n-1,1}, y_{n-1,2}; \varphi_n)$$

of the system

(E1) and (E2) with $\varphi_n(t)$ instead of $\varphi(t)$ (E1n) - (E2n)

and with the initial values

t_{n-1}, $y_{n-1,1}$, and $y_{n-1,2}$ instead of t_0, y_1, and y_2, (E3n)

respectively. From this we know what will be

the deviation of the glucose concentration $q_1(t_n; t_{n-1}, y_{n-1,1}, y_{n-1,2}; \varphi_n)$ and
the deviation of the insulin concentration $q_2(t_n; t_{n-1}, y_{n-1,1}, y_{n-1,2}; \varphi_n)$

at the time t_n with $t_{n-1} < t_n$ under the assumption that the process of

supply of glucose is given by $\varphi_n(t)$,
the deviation of the glucose concentration at time t_{n-1} was $y_{n-1,1}$, and
the deviation of the insulin concentration at time t_{n-1} was $y_{n-1,2}$.

Simply, we define

$$\mathfrak{G}_n(y_{n-1,1}, y_{n-1.2}; A) := \delta_{q_1(t_n; t_{n-1}, y_{n-1,1}, y_{n-1,2}; \varphi_n)}(A) \quad \text{and}$$

$$\mathfrak{J}_n(y_{n-1,1}, y_{n-1.2}; A) := \delta_{q_2(t_n; t_{n-1}, y_{n-1,1}, y_{n-1,2}; \varphi_n)}(A)$$

where δ_x is the normed Dirac measure in x; i.e. $\delta_x(A) := 1$ if $x \in A$ and $\delta_x(A) := 0$ if $x \notin A$ (see Figure 3).

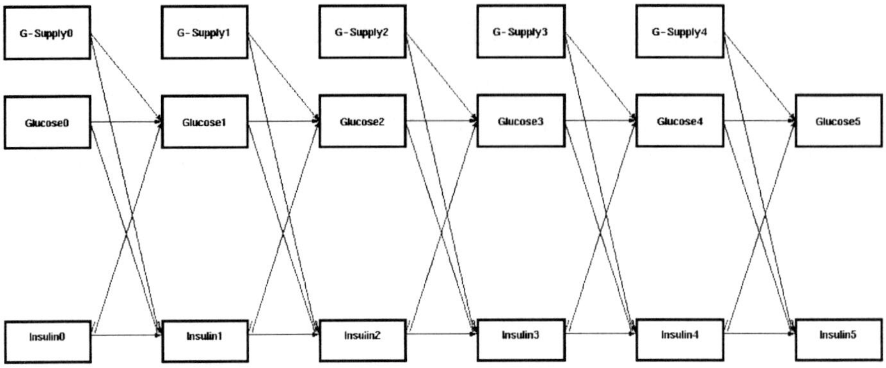

Figure 3: The glucose-insulin metabolism modeled as a sequence of CPNs with nodes added for glucose supply. This graph was constructed using the HUGIN shell. All windows are closed.

For the initial Markov kernels $\mathfrak{G}_0$ and $\mathfrak{I}_0$ we choose some Dirac measures or some other probability measures. If they are Dirac measures, the resulting Markov field is a completely deterministic process with all of its probability mass on a single trajectory which is uniquely determined by the initial values defined by the starting Dirac measures and furthermore iteratively by the solutions of the system of equations (E1n) and (E2n) with the initial values (E3n). If the initial Markov kernels are no Dirac measures, the resulting Markov field is a stochastic process with its probability mass distributed according to the starting distributions on the trajectories obtained from an initial value and from the associated solutions of (E1n), (E2n), and (E3n), i.e. it is a mixture of deterministic trajectories according to the initial distributions given by $\mathfrak{G}_0$ and $\mathfrak{I}_0$.

Because of the complexity of the metabolic processes indicated by glucose and insulin concentrations and because of inter- and intraindividual variations, such a deterministic or such a simple stochastic description of the metabolic process are inadequate. In a first approach towards a better stochastification of this process we stochastify the deterministic transition probabilities given by the deterministic Markov kernels $\mathfrak{G}_n$ and $\mathfrak{I}_n$. To do this, we take instead these Markov kernels the following "stochastic" Markov kernels

$$\mathcal{G}_n: (S_{n-1,g} \times S_{n-1,i}) \times \mathfrak{S}_{n,g} \rightarrow [0,1] \quad \text{and} \quad \mathcal{I}_n: (S_{n-1,g} \times S_{n-1,i}) \times \mathfrak{S}_{n,i} \rightarrow [0,1]$$

where for every $(y_{n-1,1}, y_{n-1.2}) \in (S_{n-1,g} \times S_{n-1,i})$ the functions

$$\mathcal{G}_n(y_{n-1,1}, y_{n-1.2}; \,.\,): \mathfrak{S}_{n,g} \rightarrow [0,1] \quad \text{and}$$

$$\mathfrak{I}_n(y_{n-1,1}, y_{n-1.2}; \,.\,): \mathfrak{S}_{n,i} \rightarrow [0,1] \quad \text{are}$$

real probability measures, and not degenerate one as $\delta_{q_1(t_n;t_{n-1},y_{n-1,1},y_{n-1,2};\varphi_n)}$ and $\delta_{q_2(t_1;t_0,y_{n-1,1},y_{n-1,2};\varphi_n)}$. Of course we have lots of possibilities to do this. For example, if the state spaces are the set of real numbers $\mathbb{R}$ with the Borel σ-algebra, we could take normal distributions or log-normal distributions with expectation $q_1(t_n,t_{n-1},y_{n-1,1},y_{n-1,2};\varphi_n)$ and $q_2(t_n;t_{n-1},y_{n-1,1},y_{n-1,2};\varphi_n)$ and variances $\sigma_1^2(t_n;t_{n-1},y_{n-1,1},y_{n-1,2};\varphi_n)$ and $\sigma_2^2(t_n;t_{n-1},y_{n-1,1},y_{n-1,2};\varphi_n)$, respectively. Of course, we also could choose other distributions with mean $q_1(t_n,t_{n-1},y_{n-1,1},y_{n-1,2};\varphi_n)$ and $q_2(t_n;t_{n-1},y_{n-1,1},y_{n-1,2};\varphi_n)$. The selection of these probability distributions depends on empirical or theoretical knowledge. It may also depend on the resulting Markov field associated to the chosen Markov kernels and its accordance with our knowledge of such a metabolic process.

5. Illustration of the results

Until now, all applications relying on exact methods have to be done using properly chosen discretizations of the state spaces. But because of existing continuity theorems about the construction of the Markov fields from the Markov kernels, this is no major problem; e.g. see Matthes et. al. [7].

The Markov kernels of the sequence of CPNs of the glucose-insulin metabolism were obtained from the iterative solutions of the system of the differential equations by stochastifying with normal distributions. Usually the parameters $p_1, \ldots, p_4$ have to be estimated for a specific patient from the response of his blood glucose level on a glucose injection. According to Ackerman [1] we simulated a non diabetic (that means $T_0 := 2\pi / \omega_0 < 4\,h$) with only slight damping (which means $\alpha \ll \omega_0$). We choose $p_1 = 0.0044$ 1/min, $p_2 = 0.04$ 1/min, $p_3 = 0.0045$ 1/min, and $p_4 = 0.03$ 1/min.

Figure 4 shows the development of the distributions of the glucose concentration and the insulin concentration under the assumptions of uniformly distributed initial concentration of glucose and insulin and of uniformly distributed glucose supply. (According to information theory, uniform distributions have maximal entropy and may be used to represent minimal knowledge.) The distributions of the glucose and insulin concentration converge very fast to "normal" distributions which are obviously the invariant distributions of glucose and insulin concentration.

Figure 5 shows the development of the distributions of the glucose and insulin concentrations under the quite different assumption of nonuniformly distributed initial glucose concentration, nonuniformly distributed initial insulin concentration, and uniformly distributed glucose supply. The system is starting with a relatively high level of glucose concentration (s 11) and a low level of insulin concentration (s2) which is a typical condition of a diabetic in the morning. After some initial fluctuation also here the distributions of the glucose concentration and the distributions of the insulin concentrations converge very fast to "normal" distributions which are obviously the invariant distributions of the system which are independent of the initial distributions. This shows the stability of the system.

Figure 6 shows the development of the distributions of the glucose and insulin concentrations under the assumption of nonuniformly distributed initial glucose concentration, nonuniformly distributed initial insulin concentration, and initially nonuniformly distributed glucose supply. In addition to that evidence is introduced in step 1 (normal glucose supply s1) and step 2 (high glucose supply s3, very low glucose concentration s2, and almost normal insulin concentration s5). Again after some initial fluctuation also here the distributions of the glucose concentration and the distributions of the insulin concentration converge very fast to "normal" distributions which are obviously the invariant distributions of the system which are independent of the initial distributions. This again shows the stability of the system. Furthermore the distributions of step 1 show a big change compared with the distributions of step 0 (the initial distributions) which "normally" is not expected within the system but is "enforced" here by the given evidence.

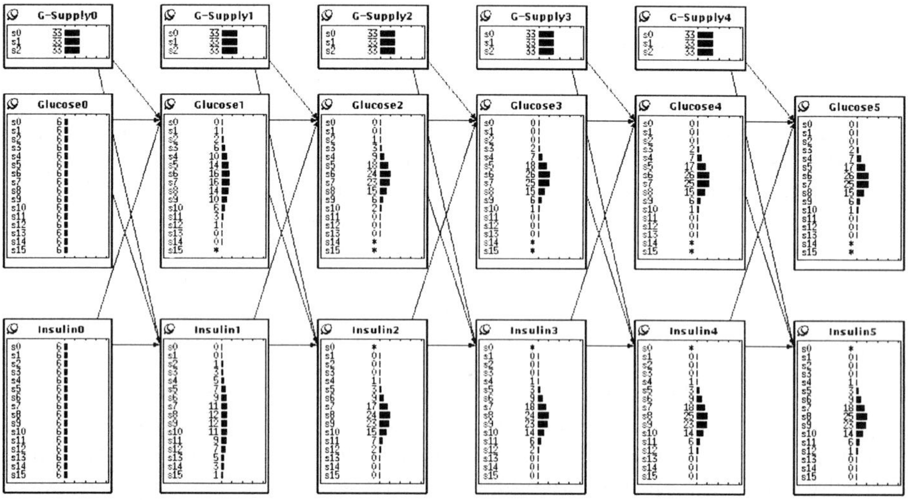

Figure 4: The sequence of CPNs of the glucose-insulin metabolism with six nodes for glucose concentration (Glucose; 16 states) and six nodes for insulin concentration (Insulin; 16 states) at six equidistant time points with five additional nodes for supply of glucose (G-Supply; 3 states). This CPN was constructed using the HUGIN shell. The windows of the nodes are open and displaying their distributions.

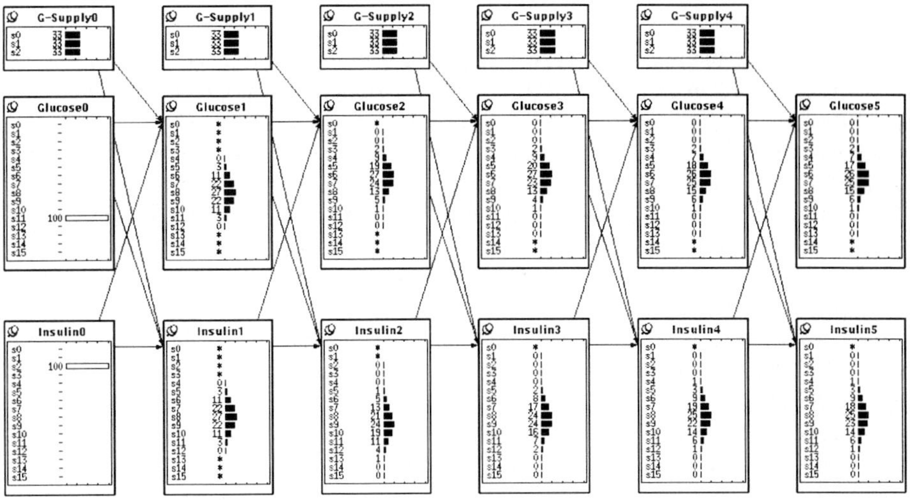

Figure 5: The development of the distributions of the glucose and insulin concentrations is shown under the quite different assumption of nonuniformly distributed initial glucose concentration, nonuniformly distributed initial insulin concentration, and uniformly distributed glucose supply. The system is starting with a relatively high level of glucose concentration (s 11) and a low level of insulin concentration (s2).

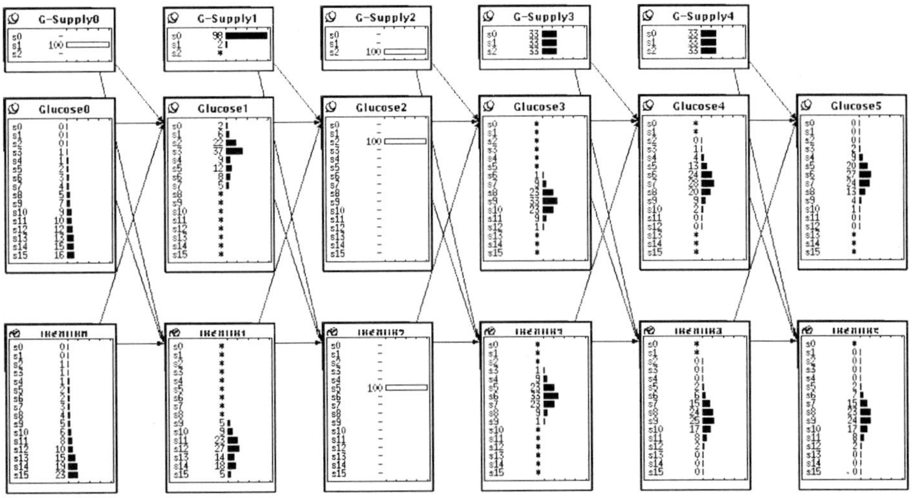

Figure 6: Here the development of the distributions of the glucose and insulin concentrations is shown under the assumption of nonuniformly distributed initial glucose concentration, nonuniformly distributed initial insulin concentration, and initially nonuniformly distributed glucose supply. In addition to that evidence is introduced in step 1 (normal glucose supply s1) and step 2 (high glucose supply s3, very low glucose concentration s2, and almost normal insulin concentration s5).

6. Conclusions

Compartmental models have been successfully used to get a better understanding of metabolic processes. This better understanding is provided by extreme simplification of very complex stochastic processes which leads to their description by a system of deterministic differential equations. One of the advantages of such a simplified deterministic description is to find solutions by determining the unknown parameters of the system. One of the disadvantages of such a deterministic description is the impossibility to fit the deterministic solution to experimental data, due to the stochastic nature of the metabolic processes. Another disadvantage of compartmental models is that they cannot be enlarged and complexified easily. Both these disadvantages may be dissolved by transforming these models into a sequence of CPNs. This transformation does not disregard the deep knowledge contained in the compartmental models, but makes use of it and leads to more complex and stochastic models which are more realistic and nevertheless easy to construct and to operate with the help of new techniques which are provided by the HUGIN shell.

Indeed, any deterministic model can be seen as a particular view of a more general stochastic model represented by a CPN. The dependencies in the deterministic compartmental model dissolve into a discrete time sequence of sets of conditional probabilities. The stochastified CPN allows to fit new knowledge derived from new data and promises to improve medical expert systems for prediction and control of complex systems.

References:

[1] Ackerman, E.; Gatewood, L.; Rosevear, J.; Mollnar, G.: Blood glucose regulation and diabetes. F. Heinmets (ed.): Concepts and Models in Biomathematics. Marcel Dekker: New York - Basel, 1969.

[2] Andreassen, S.; Hovorka, R.; Benn, J.; Olesen, K.G.; Carson, E.R.: A Model-Based Approach to Insulin Adjustment. In: Steffanelli, M,; Heisman, A,; Fieschi, M.; Talmon, J. (eds.): AIME 91, Proceedings of the Third Conference on Artificial Intelligence in Medicine, Maastricht, June 1991. Lecture Notes in Medical Informatics 44. Springer: Heidelberg, 1991.

[3] Bolie, V.W.: Coefficients of normal blood glucose regulation. J. Appl. Physiol., 16 (1979), 783-788.

[4] Braun, M.: Differential Equations and their Applications. Springer: New York etc., 1991.

[5] Carson, E.R.; Cobelli, C.; Finkelstein, L.: The Mathematical Modeling of Metabolic and Endocrine Systems. Model Formulation, Identification, and Validation. J. Wiley and Sons: New York, 1983.

[6] Lauritzen, S.L.; Spiegelhalter, D.: Local Computations with Probabilities on Graphical Structures and Their Application to Expert Systems. J. Roy. Stat. Soc. B, 50 (2) (1988), 157-224.

[7] Matthes, R.; Oppel, U.G.: Convergence of causal probabilistic networks. In: Bouchon-Meunier, B., Valverde, L.; Yager, R.R.(ed.): Intelligents systems with Uncertainty. Elsevier: to appear 1993.

[8] Pearl, J.: Probabilistic Reasoning in Intelligent Systems: Networks of Plausible Inference. Morgan Kaufmann: San Matteo, 1988.

Artificial Intelligence in Medecine
S. Andreassen et al. , Eds.
IOS Press, 1993

A Prototype Decision Support System for Diagnosing Polyneuropathies

Mikko Lipsanen[a], Steen Andreassen[b], Björn Falck[c] and Päivi Halonen[d]

[a]Dept. of Computer Sciences, Åbo Akademi, Lemminkäinengatan 14, SF-20520 Åbo, Finland

[b]Dept. of Medical Informatics and Image Analysis, Aalborg University, Fredrik Bajers Vej 7D, DK-9220 Aalborg, Denmark

[c]Dept. of Clinical Neurophysiology, University Hospital of Turku SF-20520 Turku, Finland

[d]Dept. of Neurology, University Hospital of Turku SF-20520 Turku, Finland

Abstract

We are developing a decision support system for the diagnosis of polyneuropathies. The system is based on a causal probabilistic network (CPN) which models the polyneuropathies, pathophysiological changes and symptoms. An evaluation of the system shows that the system is able to correctly diagnose a polyneuropathy and find its cause.

1. INTRODUCTION

Polyneuropathy is a generalized, widespread disorder of the peripheral nervous system, that affects all different types of nerves. Polyneuropathy is not a disease in its own right, usually it is a manifestation of a metabolic disorder or toxic effect on the peripheral nervous system. The most common reason for a polyneuropathy in the developed countries is diabetes. Other quite common reasons for polyneuropathy are uremia and chronic alcohol abuse. However, in many patients the etiology of the polyneuropathy is not so obvious and a thorough investigation is necessary to find the etiology. Currently more than 160 different causes for a polyneuropathy have been described. A number of polyneuropathies can be treated, such as B12 vitamin deficiency. Other polyneuropathies can be prevented, for instance polyneuropathies due to industrial lead exposure. On the other hand there are hereditary neuropathies in which the patient may need genetic counseling.

The diagnosis of a patient with a suspected polyneuropathy involves two stages. First the confirmation and characterization of the polyneuropathy. If the patient has a polyneuropathy, the next step is to find its etiology. The number of disorders that may cause a polyneuropathy is so high, that it is difficult, for even an experienced neurologist, to consider all appropriate etiologies and the laboratory examinations to detect these.

We have used the expert system shell HUGIN to build a causal probabilistic network (CPN) for representing our knowledge of polyneuropathies[1, 2]. The knowledge base is built using both expert knowledge and statistical information of different polyneuropathies and models the pathophysiological changes caused by different polyneuropathies. This project is an extension of a previous system called "MUNIN-the expert EMG assistant"[3, 4].

2. DOMAIN INFORMATION

The diagnosis of the polyneuropathy is based on (1) subjective symptoms, (2) clinical findings, (3) neurophysiological studies (EMG, quantitative sensory thresholds) and sometimes (4) histological findings. The suspicion of a polyneuropathy is raised by the subjective symptoms of the patient, usually numbness of the distal parts of the extremities, more the legs than the arm. There may be other symptoms, such as pain, cramps and decreased muscle strength. The clinical neurological examination will usually reveal decreased or absent tendon reflexes, decreased sensation of vibration and in more advanced cases decreased muscle strength and muscle atrophy. The neurophysiological studies can in most cases detect whether the patient has a polyneuropathy. With the EMG examination it is possible to determine the severity of the polyneuropathy. The EMG also characterizes the polyneuropathy, is the primary affection axonal damage or demyelination. In addition, the EMG examination will help to give an idea of the course of the polyneuropathy, is it acute or chronic.

When the polyneuropathy has been confirmed and characterized the next step is to find the etiology. The characterization will exclude some disorders and make a group of disorders more probable. To establish the etiology the clinician should do appropriate laboratory tests based on the likelihoods for different diseases, time, costs and whether the disease can be treated or not.

3. CPN FOR DIAGNOSING POLYNEUROPATHY

We have chosen a CPN to model our domain. With a CPN it is possible to model how different variables interact with each other[5]. When we get new information the state of the domain is changed by propagating the information throughout the network. We see how the information changed our other expectations in the model.

The CPN for diagnosing polyneuropathies is based on causal relations between diseases and pathophysiology and between pathophysiology and symptoms, clinical findings and neurophysiological findings[6, 7]. The causal relations are expressed with conditional probabilities between pairs of nodes in the network. The structure of the network shows the causal flow of information. The network consists of 146 nodes which have two to four states. In the network we use both continuous and discrete variables. The propagation time is under 2 seconds.

The CPN which links the diseases to the findings and symptoms is shown in Figure 1. The different layers in the network are (1) factors that affect disorders (time, dose, hereditary factors) (2) diseases which cause polyneuropathy, (3) polyneuropathies caused by the diseases, (4) severity of the polyneuropathies, (5) attributes used to describe the polyneuropathies (6) subjective symptoms, (7) clinical findings and (8) EMG findings.

Factors that affect diseases. This level contains facts that affect diseases which cause polyneuropathy. Such factors are time and dose for toxic exposure and heredity (Table 1).

Diseases which cause polyneuropathy. The prototype knows 12 diseases and in addition two disorders that cover the remaining polyneuropathies that have not yet been implemented: other axonal polyneuropathy and other demyelinating polyneuropathy. The diseases are given in Table 2.

Polyneuropathies caused by the diseases. Each of the disorders in Table 2 may cause a polyneuropathy, but not in every patient. The likelihood of a polyneuropathy differs from one patient to another. The probability of a polyneuropathy in a patient that has been treated with a drug called vincristine depends on the total dose of the drug he has received. On the other hand the time course of the neuropathy depends on how much time has passed since he received the treatment.

Attributes used to describe the polyneuropathies. The polyneuropathies are described in terms of (1) severity of the subjective symptoms, (2) severity of the clinical findings, (3) severity of the EMG findings, (4) overall severity, (5) time course, (6) pathology and (7) distribution (Table 3). Some of the polyneuropathies have quite typical features that characterize them.

Severity of the polyneuropathies. This attribute characterizes polyneuropathies severity. E.g. polyneuropathy caused by alcohol abuse is usually less severe than a polyneuropathy which is caused by Guillan-Barré syndrome.

Laboratory tests for diagnosing the causes. These tests include or exclude some causes for the polyneuropathy (Table 4).

Subjective symptoms. The only subjective symptoms that can be utilized in the prototype are paresthesia (numbness) in the legs and/or hands and cramps in the leg muscles (Table 5).

Clinical findings. The findings from the clinical examination that can be used are: vibration sensation in hands and legs, tendon reflexes and muscle atrophy (Table 6).

EMG findings. The findings from the EMG examination includes needle EMG from proximal and distal muscles in the upper and lower extremities. The muscles which are commonly investigated are m.deltoideus, m.interossius dorsalis 1, m.vastus lateralis and m.tibialis anterior. If these muscles have not been examined, findings from nearby muscles may be used instead. Both motor and sensory nerve conduction studies are used. The prototype motor nerves are n.medianus, n.peroneus, the sensory nerves are n.radialis and n.suralis. In the prototype findings from one side only are entered. Quantitative vibration threshold over the distal part of the first metatarsal bone is also included. The EMG findings are given in Table 7.

Figure 1. The polyneuropathy CPN in its a priori state.

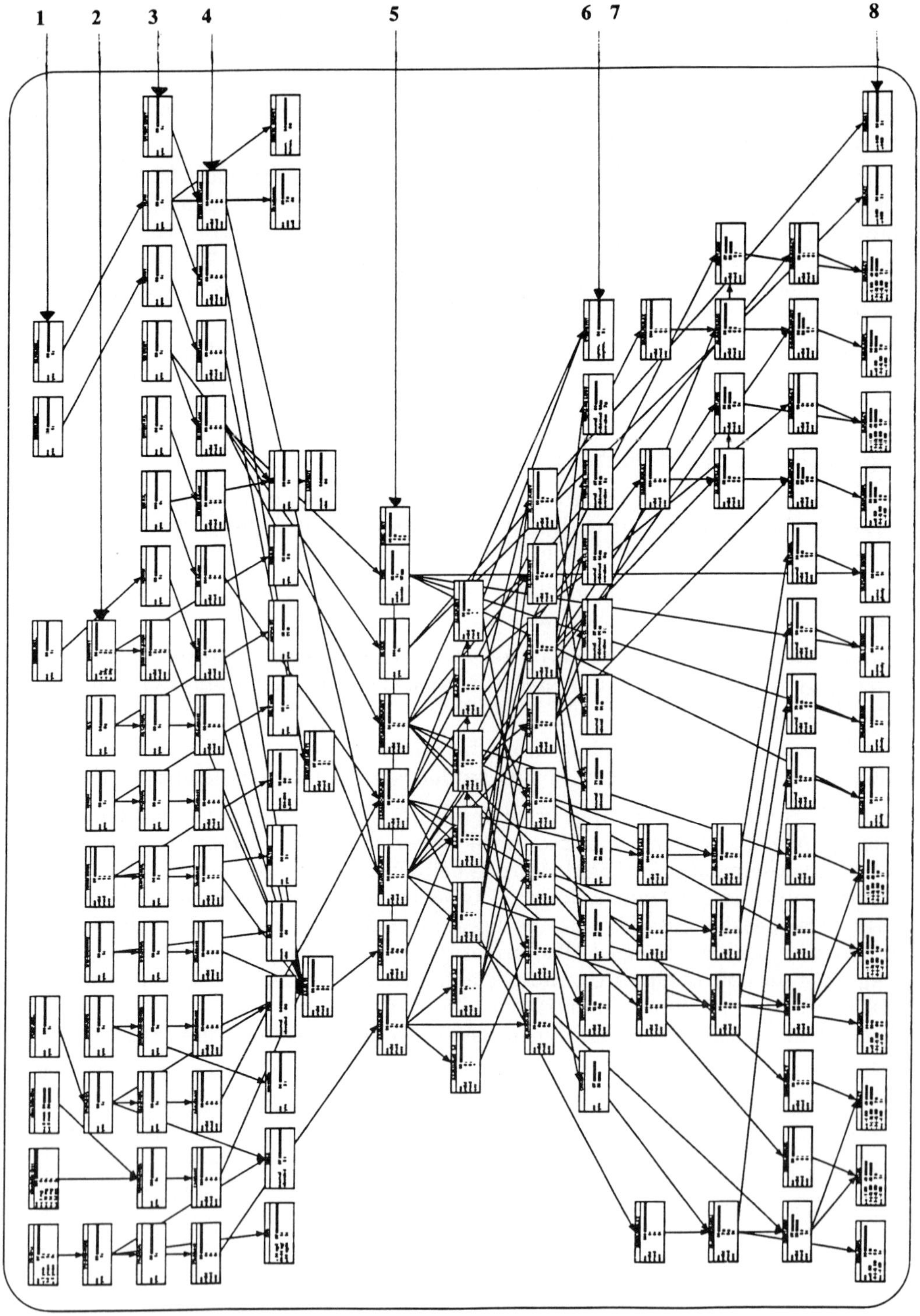

Table 1 Patient history

information	outcome
Lead exposure	no, < 1 year, 1-5 years, > 5 years
Treatment with vincristine	no, yes
Time since last treatment with vincristine	< 6 months, > 6 months
Total dose of vincristine	< 8 mg, 8-12 mg, 12-18 mg, > 18 mg
Family members with a similar disorder	no, yes
Occurrent of recurrent mononeuropathies	no, one, two or more
Insulin treatment	no, yes

Table 2 The disorders causing polyneuropathy and the apriori probability of the disorder in the department of neurology.

Chronic alcoholism	6.00 %
Type 1 diabetes (insulin dependent)	5.00 %
Chronic renal insufficiency	3.00 %
Guillan-Barré syndrome (polyradiculitis)	2.00 %
Other axonal polyneuropathy	2.00 %
Hereditary liability to pressure neuropathies (HLPN)	1.49 %
Hereditary motor and sensory polyneuropathy type 2 (HMSN 2)	1.49 %
Acute intermittent porphyria	1.25 %
Other demyelinating polyneuropathy	1.00 %
B_{12}-vitamin deficiency	1.00 %
Polyarteritis nodosa	1.00 %
Hereditary motor and sensory polyneuropathy type 1 (HMSN 1)	1.00 %
Lead exposure	0.65 %
AIDS	0.60 %
Vincristine treatment	0.35 %

Table 3 Attributes used to describe the polyneuropathies.

Severity of symptoms	no, mild, moderate, severe
Clinical severity	no, mild, moderate, severe
Severity of EMG-findings	no, mild, moderate, severe
Distribution	distal findings more severe in the lower extremi-
ties	
	distal findings more severe in the upper extremi-
ties,	
	proximal, random
Pathology	axonal, demyelinating, mixed
Symmetry	no, yes
Block	no, yes
Time course	acute, chronic

Table 4 Laboratory findings and anamnestic information used to diagnose the disorders.

laboratory tests	outcome
serum creatine	normal, elevated
serum gamma GT	normal, elevated
serum lead	< 50 ug/ml, 50-90 ug/ml, > 90 ug/ml
serum delta amino levulinic acid (DALA)	normal, elevated
serum porphobilinogen	normal, elevated
spinal fluid protein	normal, elevated
antibodies against HTL-virus (AIDS)	normal, elevated
signs of vasculitis on biopsy	normal, positive
serum glucose	normal, vasculitis

Table 5 Subjective symptoms.

symptom	outcome
paresthesia in the lower extremities	no, yes
muscle cramps	no, yes

Table 6 Clinical findings.

finding	outcome
Achilles tendon reflex	normal, absent
Patella tendon reflex	normal, absent
Atrophy of m.extensor digitorum brevis	no, yes
Vibration sensation over medial malleolus	normal, mild to moderate abnormality severe abnormality

Table 7 EMG findings.

1. Needle EMG findings

muscle	outcome
m.deltoideus	normal, mild, moderate, severe neuropathy
m.interosseus	normal, mild, moderate, severe neuropathy
m.vastus lateralis	normal, mild, moderate, severe neuropathy
m.tibialis	normal, mild, moderate, severe neuropathy

Table 7. EMG findings.

2. Motor nerve conduction studies

n.peroneus, knee to ankle
n.medianus, elbow to wrist

finding	**outcome**
maximal motor conduction velocity (MCV)	>= -1sd, -1- -2sd, -2- -4sd, < -4sd
motor action potential amplitude (MAPAMPL)	>= -1sd, -1- -2sd, -2- -4sd, < -4sd
motor distal latency (DL)	>= -1sd, -1- -2sd, -2- -4sd, < -4sd

3. Sensory nerve conduction studies

n.suralis, calf to ankle
n.radialis, forearm to wrist

finding	**outcome**
maximal sensory conduction velocity (MCV)	>= -1sd, -1- -2sd, -2- -4sd, < -4sd
motor action potential amplitude (SAPAMPL)	>= -1sd, -1- -2sd, -2- -4sd, < -4sd

4. Quantitative sensory thresholds

finding	**outcome**
vibration threshold, 1 metatarsal bone:	normal (< 2 sd), mild-moderate abnormality (2-4 sd), severe abnormality (> 4 sd)

3.1 DIAGNOSING POLYNEUROPATHIES WITH THE CPN

In the beginning of diagnosis the CPN is in its *a priori* state. This initial state is calculated from the *a priori* probabilities and it should represent our expectations for occurrences of different diseases and their severity (Table 2). During the diagnosis different findings are entered in the network and these findings are then propagated throughout the network. After the propagation we get *posterior* probabilities for the unknown variables. Based on these probabilities we can make more tests and get new findings which in turn are entered in to the network and propagated throughout the network. This procedure continues until we reach a diagnosis or give up the diagnosing.

3.1.1 A PATIENT CASE

To demonstrate how the network can be used for diagnosing we will go through a patient case. We have a patient who complains numbness in the legs. In the clinical examinations we diagnose absent achilles tendon reflexes. We enter these findings in the network and get expectations for possible polyneuropathy's type (Table 8). We see that the network believes most that the patient has an axonal distal polyneuropathy. The polyneuropathy is also characterized as chronic and symmetric.

Table 8 The disorders causing polyneuropathy and their probability given findings paresthesia in the lower extremities and absent achilles tendon reflex.

Type	**no**	**mild**	**mod**	**sev**
Axonal Distal Lower Polyneuropathy	36 %	21 %	20 %	24 %
Axonal Motor Proximal Upper Polyneuropathy	98 %	1 %	0 %	1 %
Demyelinating Distal Polyneuropathy	82 %	9 %	5 %	4 %
Axonal Random Polyneuropathy	99 %	1 %	0 %	0 %
Demyelinating Random Polyneuropathy	98 %	1 %	0 %	0 %
Time course	**no**	**acute**		**chronic**
Time course	21 %	1 %		78 %
Symmetry		**symm.**		**asymm.**
Symmetry		98 %		2 %

Based on these results we refer the patient for an EMG consultation. The results of this consultation are given in Table 9.

Table 9 Findings from the EMG examination.

1. Needle EMG findings		
muscle	**outcome**	
m.deltoideus	normal	
m.interosseus	normal	
m.vastus lateralis	normal	
m.tibialis	mild neuropathy	
2. Motor nerve conduction studies	**n.peroneus, knee to ankle**	**n.medianus, elbow to wrist**
maximal motor conduction velocity (MCV)	-1- -2sd	-1- -2sd
motor action potential amplitude (MAPAMPL)	-2- -4sd	-2- -4sd
motor distal latency (DL)	-1- -2sd	-1- -2sd
3. Sensory nerve conduction studies	**n.suralis, calf to ankle**	**n.radialis, forearm to wrist**
maximal sensory conduction velocity (MCV)	-1- -2sd	-1- -2sd
motor action potential amplitude (SAPAMPL)	-2- -4sd	-2- -4sd
4. Quantitative sensory thresholds		
vibration threshold, 1 metatarsal bone:	mild-moderate abnormality (2-4 sd)	

Results from the EMG examination are propagated throughout the network. New probabilities for a possible polyneuropathy are given in Table 10. The network expects that the patient suffers from moderate distal axonal polyneuropathy which is more severe in the lower extremities.

Table 10 The disorders causing polyneuropathy and their probability given the findings paresthesia in the lower extremities, absent achilles tendon reflex and the EMG findings from Table 9.

Type	Moderate Axonal Distal Lower Polyneuropathy	99 %
Time course	Chronic	100 %
Symmetry	Symmetric	99 %
Possible causes		
Type 1 diabetes (insulin dependent)		28 %
Other axonal polyneuropathy		15 %
Chronic alcoholism		15 %
Chronic renal insufficiency		13 %
Hereditary motor and sensory polyneuropathy type 1 (HMSN 1)		11 %
Polyarteritis nodosa		6 %
B_{12}-vitamin deficiency		6 %
AIDS		4 %
Vincristine treatment		2 %

We find out that the patient has had vincristine treatment for 4 months. The total dose was 10mg. We propagate this finding to the network and get new probabilities for causes . These probabilities are shown in Table 12. We see that the network now strongly believes that the patient suffers from a polyneuropathy which is caused by a vincristine treatment.

Table 11 The disorders causing polyneuropathy and their probability given the same findings as in table 11 plus finding about vincristine treatment.

Vincristine treatment	87 %
Type 1 diabetes (insulin dependent)	6 %

The CPN can be used for diagnosing as can be seen from above. The CPN can also be used in forward manner thus leading predictions of pathophysiological changes and findings given specific diseases.

4. VALIDATION AND EVALUATION OF THE PROTOTYPE

The diagnostic function of the system was evaluated with four patients that were sected by a neurologist not involved in the project. The patients had been referred to the outpatient clinic at the department of neurology for a suspicion of polyneuropathy. The outcome of the study are given in Table 12.

Table 12

	Type of polyneuropathy		Etiology	
	Final conclusion	Prototype conclusion	Final conclusion	Prototype conclusion
patient 1	moderate demyelinating	severe demyelinating 100 %	HMSN1	HMSN1 48 % Other dem. polyn. 48 % Diabetes 4 %
patient 2	severe mixed	severe mixed	Guillan-Barré 90 % Diabetes 10 %	Guillan-Barré 95 % Other dem. polyn. or HMSN 1 35 % Diabetes 24 %
patient 3	mild demyelinating	mild demyelinating	HLPN	HLPN 34 % HMSN 1 12 %
patient 4	severe axonal	severe axonal	HMSN 2	Other ax. polyn. 27 % HMSN 2 20 %

The prototype was able to characterize the polyneuropathy correctly in all patients. The etiology of all patients was correct. Overall the diagnostic performance was good.

5. DISCUSSION

A prototype decision support system for the diagnosis of polyneuropathies has been constructed. The system covers 12 most commonly occurring polyneuropathies that account for around 95 % of all patients with polyneuropathies. This prototype still lacks a substantial number of disorders that cause polyneuropathies. However the polyneuropathies that have been included represent the major types of polyneuropathies. The lower part of the CPN does not need major additions or modifications. The missing disorders that cause polyneuropathies can easily be added to the system.

The system was evaluated with a small number of patients. The evaluation showed that the prototype arrived at a correct characterization and diagnosis in all the cases studied. At this stage our intent was only to evaluate whether the system could be built as a CPN. Our results indicate that a complete decision support system can be constructed using a causal probabilistic network.

The network is able to deal with uncertain, missing or erroneous data. Another major advantage of a CPN is that it is able to diagnose multiple simultaneous disorders. Because all the causal relations can explicitly be seen and changes in nodes only affect the neighboring nodes the debugging of the network is easy even for a network of this size.

One of the problems with CPN is that all the probabilities that are used in the network cannot be obtained from actual experimental or clinical studies. Some of the information related to polyneuropathies can, however be obtained from the literature. For instance there are numerous studies on the occurrence of polyneuropathies in patients treated with vincristine. Some of the knowledge stems from the practical experience of the experts participated in the construction of the system. We have found it easy to express different causal relations with conditional probabilities. The most difficult thing has been to get the structure of the network right.

Our experience is that a decision support system for diagnosing polyneuropathies can be built using a CPN. Our current prototype can easily be expanded into a complete system only by adding disorders that cause polyneuropathies.

6. REFERENCES

1 Andreassen S, Jensen FV och Olesen KG (1991): *Medical Expert Systems Based on Causal Probabilistic Networks.* Int J Biomed Comput, 28 1-30.

2 Andersen, SK, Olesen KG, Jensen FV, Jensen F (1989): *HUGIN a shell for building belief universes for expert systems.* Proceedings of the 11th International Joint Conference on Artificial Intelligence, 1080-1085.

3 Andreassen S, Woldbye M, Falck B (1987): *MUNIN - A causal probabilistic network for interpretation of electromyographic findings.* IJCAI, Milan, 366-372. Kaufman.

4 Andreassen S, Jensen FV, Andersen SK, Falck B, Kjærulff U, Woldbye M, Sørensen AR, Rosenfalck A, Jensen F (1989): *MUNIN - an expert EMG assistant.* In Computer- Aided Electromyography and Expert Systems, Elsevier Science Publishers.

5 Hovorka R, Andreassen S, Benn JJ, Olesen KG, Carson ER (1992): *Causal probabilistic network modelling - An illustration of its role in the management of chronic diseases.* IBM Systems Journal, 4 635-648.

6 Schwartz WB, Patil RS and Szolovits P (1987): *Artificial intelligence in medicine: where do we stand?* New England Journal of Medicine, 316, 685-688.

7 Wallis JW, Shortliffe EH (1982): *Explanatory Power for Medical Expert Systems: Studies in the Representation of Causal Relationships for Clinical Consultations.* Report No. STAN-CS-82-923 Stanford University.

Artificial Intelligence in Medecine
S. Andreassen et al. , Eds.
IOS Press, 1993

Expert Systems and Mathematical Simulation

L.M. Müller[a], A. Hasman[a,b], J.A. Blom[a,b]

[a]Eindhoven University of Technology, Department of Medical Electrical Engineering, P.O. Box 513, 5600 MB Eindhoven, The Netherlands

[b]University of Limburg, Department of Medical Informatics, P.O. Box 616, 6200 MD Maastricht, The Netherlands

Abstract

Real time expert systems can be helpful to the anesthetist, being in charge of monitoring signals coming from the patient during an operation. The large stream of data can be organized, validated and interpreted by such an intelligent system. A physical model of the patient which is able to simulate the signals that are measured at an actual patient, combined with actual anesthesia equipment, can provide the signals, originating from known faults, from which the knowledge which forms the core of the expert system can be derived. Instead of physical patient models and actual equipment, mathematical models can be used for this task. Mathematical models are more flexible and cheaper than physical models. Our approach, in which we combine knowledge based methods with mathematical simulation models is described in this paper. The medical problem domain will be artificial ventilation of a patient during anesthesia.

1. INTRODUCTION

At Eindhoven University, Department of Medical Electrical Engineering, one of the research projects is aimed at automating patient monitoring during anesthesia.

During surgery a number of signals is being measured, and the anesthetist uses these measurements to determine the state of the patient. Many of these signals, like heart rate, blood pressure and respiration, have to be measured continuously because they contain important information on the current state of the patient. A critical situation can often immediately be recognized by the anesthetist when looking at these signals. The anesthetist has to process a lot of information simultaneously and has to act immediately when one or more of the measured signals show that there is something wrong with the patient. This is a difficult task which requires continuous attention of the anesthetist. To make this task easier attempts are made to (partially) automate patient monitoring. Efforts in this direction at Eindhoven University have resulted in a blood pressure control system and an intelligent alarm system for automatic ventilation.

These systems have been developed with the real time expert system generation program SIMPLEXYS, which itself was developed at Eindhoven University by Blom [2]. SIMPLEXYS is a useful tool for building expert systems which are to be applied in environments where information from different sources has to be processed in real time. An example of such an environment is patient monitoring during anesthesia.

1.1 Patient monitoring during anesthesia

When a patient is anesthetized, elementary body functions often are suppressed. The muscles, for example, are being relaxed artificially during surgery to prevent uncontrolled movements of the patient, which hinder the surgeon in his work. But as a consequence of muscle relaxation the patient is not able to breathe by himself. The ventilation of the patient has then to be taken care of by a mechanical ventilator. Also the arterial blood pressure is lowered, which is done in order to reduce blood loss during surgery, to improve the view of the surgeon, to reduce the risk of infections and to support the healing process of the operation wounds. This blood pressure lowering process must also be controlled by the anesthetist.

The suppression of the patient's body functions is not without risks. It is the task of the anesthetist to monitor the patient by interpreting the available data. The anesthetist knows what the important features are, recognizes critical states immediately and takes actions to solve problems which come up. Processing the data is a difficult task since a signal changes often and its value will be valid for only a short time. Also there is a large amount of data, coming from different sources, and all this information has to be processed at the same time. Often the measurements are noisy and it is hard to say if some abnormal signal wave form is caused by an artifact or by the physical state of the patient. The data have to be validated: when there is some disturbance which causes measurement errors, the measured signal which is affected by the disturbance has to be classified as invalid and can not take part in determining the patient's status. When the anesthetist concludes that an abnormal signal is caused by some problem in the anesthesia equipment, and the signal values are critical, he has to find that problem and solve it.

Finally, not all data are equally important to the health of the patient. The anesthetist has to distinguish between matters of major and matters of minor importance when processing the data.

2. PROBLEM FORMULATION

In spite of the knowledge and experience that anesthetists possess, in the United States alone 2000 to 5000 anesthetic deaths occur yearly. A large percentage of these are caused by faults in the breathing circuit used during artificial ventilation of patients [11].

The breathing circuit consists of ventilator, tubes and connections, fresh gas supplies and carbon dioxide absorber, and is used to help the patient breathe when he is not able to breathe autonomously. It is a complicated system in which different errors and defects can occur. For instance, leaks can develop in the tubes, and as a consequence the patient will not get the set tidal volume of air, obstructions in the tubes can hinder the air flow in and out of the patient, an exhausted carbon dioxide absorber causes a too high CO_2 content of the inspiratory air and a stuck air flow regulation valve will cause mixing of inspiratory and expiratory air.

Over the years, scientists have investigated possibilities to assist the anesthetist during breathing circuit monitoring, and ways to identify and localize faults which can occur. Different formalisms are used such as neural networks [11] and expert systems [1, 4]. Van der Aa [1] developed a real time expert system in SIMPLEXYS which is able to identify and localize faults that occur within the circle breathing circuit, a widely used breathing circuit, and provide the anesthetist with intelligent, helpful messages. Van der Aa's work is the starting point of this project.

Van der Aa used the Gainesville Anesthesia Simulator (GAS) at the University of Florida, a physical patient model that is connected to a real ventilator. Three signals are measured at this model: expiratory air flow, inspiratory air pressure and CO_2 content of in- and expired air. These signals are also measured during operations because they contain information about the state of the patient and the breathing circuit. In the ventilator, all sorts of errors and defects were introduced in order to study their effects on the measured signals. The influence of the errors on the signal features was used by Van der Aa to induce the production rules of his intelligent alarms expert system by hand.

This method of determining the effects of errors on the signals is accurate and exhaustive, all kinds of errors are reckoned with and the final version of the resulting expert system was able to detect 88% of the mechanical malfunctions correctly, when tested on real signals from sheep [1]. 'Patient' related perturbations were also applied to the sheep, like a low set tidal volume or a low oxygen delivery, and the expert system could classify them all correctly. When two faults were introduced simultaneously, the expert system was able to detect at least one of them.

But this method is also very time-consuming and expensive. For each new type of breathing circuit, the entire process of introducing faults, examining signal features, creating expert system production rules and testing those rules has to start all over again.

3. GOAL OF THE PROJECT

The goal of our project is to find a formalism to build, in a relatively fast way, real time expert systems which can be used to monitor an anesthetized patient. Instead of a physical patient model and ventilator we will use mathematical models, which are a lot more flexible and a lot cheaper to build. We introduce faults into our model as well, and for the present we assume that all faults that occur are equipment related, so the patient related part of our model can be kept relatively small.

Using mathematical models together with knowledge based formalisms is successfully practiced by AI scientists over the past years [3, 5, 6, 7, 10]. Mathematical models can support knowledge based systems, that operate in a qualitative way, with extra quantitative knowledge. Mathematical models are relatively easy to develop, compared to physical models, and since they can be implemented in a computer they can communicate with existing knowledge based systems immediately.

But not only the construction of the model can be speeded up. Van der Aa forms his production rules by inducting them by hand, based on the measured signals. We will also automate this latter part of the process. To do this, several possibilities exist. We will compare some of them in this project. At this time, the two main methods we study are *machine learning by induction* and *system identification*. But first will be explained what exactly our models look like.

4. MATHEMATICAL SIMULATION MODELS

The mathematical models that we use must generate the same signals as the ones that are measured at a patient during the operation. It is of great importance that those signals are as valid as possible. The models are adaptive in order to be able to simulate different patients during different conditions. Errors and defects in the breathing system can be modeled by adjusting model parameters.

Our models consist of a list of equations, describing the relations between the different signals. The models also contain patient and equipment specific parameters which can be adjusted to describe different patients, different ventilators and occurring faults. An example of such a model, describing the relationship between air flow and air pressure, is given below:

$$Plung = ((Vlung - V0lung)/Clung, thorax)$$

$$Qin = \text{constant}$$

$$Qout = (Pmouth - Plung)/(Rairways + Rhoses)$$

$$Vlung(t) = \int Q(t)dt$$

During inspiration: $Pmouth = (Qin \cdot (Rairways + Rhoses)) + Plung$

During expiration: $Pmouth = \text{PEEP}$

In these formulas, P stands for pressures, V for volumes, $V0$ for zero pressure volumes, C for compliances, R for resistances, Q for flows and PEEP is the positive end expiratory pressure.

A model like this can be translated to a computer routine which can calculate a value for the signals at every point in time. We have used the mathematical modeling software package TUTSIM [9] to build a first prototype of a mathematical model. It is able to generate expiratory air flow, inspiratory air pressure and carbon dioxide content of the air. Defects and errors like leaks, obstructions and disconnections, can be introduced into the model by changing the model parameters.

A TUTSIM model consists of blocks. Each block represents an elementary mathematical operation like multiplication, addition or integration. Blocks have inputs and outputs, and the outputs of one block can be the inputs of another. In this way, equations can be translated into TUTSIM block models. The way in which the blocks are connected defines the order of calculation. From all blocks an output signal is available. The output of the blocks which we are interested in (the ones generating expiratory air flow, inspiratory air pressure and CO_2 concentration) can be displayed graphically or numerically.

TUTSIM can generate numeric output in ASCII format which can be processed by other computer programs. A schematic picture of our model is shown in figure 1. The model consists of a patient part and an equipment part. As we will assume, for the time being, that the patient himself does not change during the operation, all occurring errors are equipment related and as a consequence of this, the patient specific part of the model can be kept simple. It contains five parameters. The patient parameters remain constant, because we assume nothing happens to the patient's lungs during the operation.

The equipment part of the model is more complicated and contains equipment specific parameters (resistances and compliances of hoses, sizes of leaks, percentage of CO_2 in inspiratory air) and user specified parameters, which are set by the anesthetist (tidal volume, I:E ratio). Modeling faults in the system is done by changing these parameters.

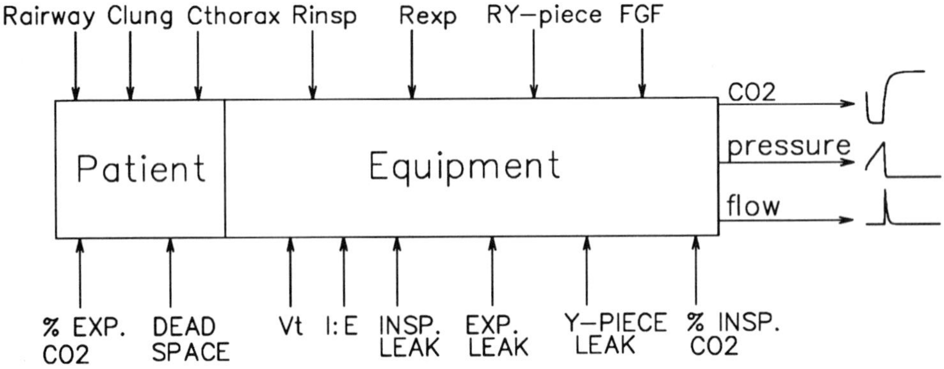

Figure 1. A model of the circle breathing circuit.

5. COOPERATION OF MODEL AND EXPERT SYSTEM

Now that we have described our models, we will explain in what ways we let them cooperate with the expert system. We will, for the present, study two ways of doing this: machine learning by induction and system identification. More methods are possible, like neural networks or causal nets, but those will be considered later on in the project.

5.1 Machine Learning by Induction

This method is similar to van der Aa's, in the sense that the production rules of the expert system are based immediately on the effects that faults have on the measured signals. Every respiration period a set of features is derived from each of these three signals (expiratory air flow, inspiratory air pressure, CO_2

content). Introducing a fault in the breathing circuit causes the signals and accordingly the extracted signal features to change. These effects on the signal features can be used to create the rules. This can be done by hand, like van der Aa did, but the process can be speeded up if it is automated.

This can be achieved using machine learning techniques. If we know which fault classes there are, and if we have a set of cases where for each member it is known to which fault class it belongs, a description for each fault class is generated in such a way that as many of the cases as possible can be classified correctly.

The method we apply is similar to that described by Bratko [3], the difference being that we use a quantitative model instead of a qualitative one. Each error or defect which can occur within the breathing circuit constitutes a fault class. The signal features of each fault class are probably affected by the fault, and the way they have changed compared to the situation in which no fault occurred. Examples of class features are: maximum pressure increased, flow time constant decreased, or inspired CO_2 concentration high.

The cases we have are different "patients", (different patients are modeled by varying the patient specific model parameters like lung- and thorax compliances and airway resistance), who are connected to a breathing circuit in which one of the errors occurs. Each case is described by the set of extracted signal features. We use an inductive machine learning algorithm which is similar to ID3 [8] and based on entropy reduction, and which is developed at the University of Limburg by Talmon [12]. This program produces a binary decision tree, in which the terminal nodes describe the different fault classes and the intermediate nodes have associated with them one signal feature and a numerical threshold value. If a case is being classified, the value which this case has for that signal feature is compared to the threshold value. Based on this comparison the case is further processed in one of the subtrees of the node, until a classification of the case is made.

The decision tree can be translated immediately into expert system production rules, or be used directly as the knowledge base of the expert system. An example of the creation of a decision tree is given below, but first the model that we used has to be validated. This is described in the next paragraph.

5.1.1 Validation of the Model

First, some of the signals were tried on Van der Aa's expert system, too see if it could recognize the introduced faults. In order to test this a 'patient' was created, with compliances of 0.22 l/mmHg and an airway resistance of 2.5 mmHg/l/sec. For this 'patient' the normal set of signals plus the eight faulty ones was created and fed to the expert system.

There is an important difference between the way the expert system recognizes faults and the way this is done by Talmon's program. The former looks at the signals with respect to the previous signals, as the latter looks at one signal at a time and judges them absolutely.

So to test the signals with the expert system, for each of the eight faults a series of signals, consisting of four normal periods followed by two faulty ones, was fed to the expert system. It proved that all three types of obstructions could be recognized correctly by the expert system. Also, a small leak in the inspiratory hose was recognized as a 'small leak in inspiratory or expiratory hose'. A small leak in the expiratory hose was however not recognized at all. This is caused by the fact that in case of a small expiratory leak the expired volume does not decrease enough to trigger the appropriate expert system rule.

A large expiratory leak is correctly recognized as a 'large leak at the ventilator side'. Van der Aa's expert system could see no difference between inspiratory and expiratory leaks. A large expiratory leak and a leak in the Y-piece are both judged 'obstruction in expiratory hose'. Although this seems rather strange, it can be easily explained by the fact that both types of leaks as well as the expiratory obstruction cause the flow time constant to rise, so the expert system confuses both types of errors. With higher values for the compliances the Y-piece leak was recognized correctly, because the time constant, which partially depends on the value of the lung and thorax compliances, was not affected much relatively, but the large expiratory leak was still judged by the expert system to be an expiratory obstruction.

5.1.2 An Example of Machine Learning

To test the possibility of machine learning in our domain, we applied it to a set consisting of 459 cases. We defined 51 'patients' by taking our TUTSIM model and varying the lung and thorax compliances and the airway resistance. We let the compliances range from 0.20 to 0.24 l/mmHg, with steps of 0.02 l/mmHg, and the resistance ranged from 1.0 to 2.6 mmHg/l/sec, with steps of 0.1 mmHg/l/sec. These values are realistic for a young male patient.

In this way, 51 different 'patients' were created. For each patient one of eight error conditions was introduced: small inspiratory leak, large inspiratory leak, small expiratory leak, large expiratory leak, leak in Y-piece, obstruction in inspiratory hose, obstruction in expiratory hose and obstruction in Y-piece. Apart from the fault situations, for each patient the normal situation was also modeled. So for each patient nine cases were created, resulting in 459 cases in total.

We had nine fault classes: the eight error situations plus the normal situation. In our data set each fault class contained 51 elements. Of each case it was known to which fault class it belonged. The three signals coming from each case were processed and nine features (maximum expired air flow, flow time constant, expired volume, minimum air pressure, maximum air pressure, pressure wave form slope, minimum CO_2 concentration, maximum CO_2 concentration and capnogram plateau time) were extracted from them. In Table 1 the resulting *confusion matrix* is shown. In the rows of this matrix for each fault class is displayed how many cases of a class are classified by the program in what fault class. The fault classes in which the cases are classified are displayed horizontally. From Table 1 we can see that leaks could be easily described. The small inspiratory leak is the only type of leak for which the program was not able to classify all cases correctly. Obstructions were more difficult to describe, and less than half of the 51 normal cases were classified correctly.

Table 1
Confusion matrix resulting from running machine learning program on 459 cases.

	small insp. leak	small exp. leak	large insp. leak	large exp. leak	Y-piece leak	insp. obst.	exp. obst.	Y-piece obst.	normal
s.i.l.	39				1				
s.e.l.		51							
l.i.l.			51						
l.e.l.				51					
Y-p.l.					51				
i.o.						12			
e.o.							21		
Y-p.o.								8	
norm.									23

The cause of the relatively weak performance of the program on obstruction cases could lie in the fact that the program bases its construction of classes on entropy reduction by choosing only one of the features. If two or more features cause an equal amount of entropy reduction the feature which is first in the list is chosen. Accidentally, the feature *expired volume* was each time chosen as the best feature, while other features could cause the same amount of entropy reduction. For recognizing leaks, the expired volume is one of the most important features and that is the reason why leaks are classified correctly in this case. To recognize obstructions other features like *maximum pressure* or *pressure wave form slope* are more significant. In the future, more experiments with varying orders of signal features and more cases, will be done.

5.2 System Identification

A second way to find the needed knowledge is the application of system identification methods. The models that we use consist of a set of mathematical equations, which contain parameters. Modeling an error is achieved by changing those model parameters in such a way that the models behavior is similar to that of the faulted system. When the model is set up in such a way that there is a direct mapping between model parameters and system parameters, a fault in the system, which is caused by a change in one or more of the system parameters, can be immediately modeled by making the same change to the corresponding model parameter(s). The other way around, if we can, given the output signals of the model, identify the parameter values of the model, we can identify the system parameters as well and based on this information we can conclude what kind of error has occurred within the system.

Determining values of the parameters of a set of equations, given the output, is known as system identification and several techniques exist to accomplish this. For example, a Kalman filter can be used, or a least squares estimator.

Fortunately, we have already a comprehensive description of our system, because that is exactly what our mathematical models are. Besides, some of the system parameters are constant and are not affected by any error. Information like this, for example patient specific information, like for instance the value of the dead space volume of the patient's lungs, are known in advance or easy to measure. Other parameters, which are more difficult to measure, like airway resistance or lung compliance, can be easily calculated from signal features like time constants. Model parameters which cannot be known in advance or calculated from the signal features, can be identified using a parameter estimation method. At this time we use a very simple signal parameter estimation technique based on interval reduction.

Besides parameter estimation techniques we can make use of some higher level, heuristic knowledge as well. An example of both will be given hereafter.

As a consequence the alarm expert system can be kept relatively simple: when via parameter estimation techniques it can be determined which part of the system is affected, we immediately know which part of the system behaves faulty. In fact, the expert system and the system identification part can be merged into one SIMPLEXYS program which contains procedural as well as heuristic knowledge.

5.2.1 An Example of System Identification

In figure 2, four production rules of the system identification expert system are shown in pseudo code. The first rule contains both types of knowledge: heuristic and procedural. The condition part tests if the time constant τ, which is extracted from the flow signal, has not changed since the last respiratory period. When this condition is satisfied, rule `adjust_Rs` is called, which adapts the parts of the model that represent leaks in the tubes. If τ has changed, new values for the compliances and resistances are calculated. With 'compliances' and 'resistances' we mean the values of patient specific airway compliances and resistances, lumped together with equipment specific hose compliances and resistances.

The heuristic knowledge consists of the fact that, if the time constant has not changed, the compliances and resistances have not changed either, so other model parameters have to be adjusted, and the procedural knowledge consists of the fact that resistance and compliance can be calculated from the derived signal features τ, minimum pressure and inspiratory flow, which is constant.

In the third and fourth rule new values for respectively the inspiratory and expiratory leak are calculated. This is done as follows: an interval for the value is chosen, initially this is the interval between 1 and 100. The size of the leak ranges from disconnection (1) to no leak (100). The right value is found by iteratively splitting the interval in halves and comparing the output of the model with the output of the system, choosing one of the two sub-intervals as the new interval. This goes on until a satisfactory value for the leak is found. To find the right value, multiple runs of the expert system are necessary. So when the model contains a lot of parameters for which the values will have to be searched like this, the expert system will slow down strongly and needs time to identify all parameters. When the model is extended, a more sophisticated parameter estimation technique will be needed in order to keep the expert system running in real time.

```
adjust: 'adjust the model'
if flow_time_constant = normal
then do adjust_Rs
else do
begin
  resistance := min_pressure/medium_insp_flow
  compliance := 2*(flow_time_constant/resistance)
end

adjust_Rs: 'adjust the additional resistances'
if max_pressure = normal
then do adjust_Rexp
else do adjust_Rinsp

adjust_Rinsp: 'adjust inspiratory leak resistance'
if max_pressure = low
then do
begin
  upper := Rinsp
  Rinsp := lower + ((Rinsp - lower) / 2)
end
else do
begin
  lower := Rinsp
  Rinsp := lower + ((upper - Rinsp) / 2)
end

adjust_Rexp: 'adjust expiratory leak resistance'
if expired_volume = low
then do
begin
  upper := Rexp;
  Rexp := lower + ((Rexp - lower) / 2);
end
else do
begin
  lower := Rexp;
  Rexp := lower + ((upper - Rexp) / 2);
end
```

Figure 2. Some production rules of the system identification expert system.

6. CONCLUSIONS AND FUTURE PLANS

With a mathematical model, consisting of a very simple model representation of the patient and a more complicated model of the breathing circuit, we are able to make reasonably realistic simulations of the expiratory air flow, the inspiratory air pressure and the capnogram of an artificially ventilated patient. Some of the faults that van der Aa could recognize with his expert system can be simulated by our model.

We validate our model by generating signals with it and testing those with the production rules of van der Aa. These production rules are validated and proven to be reliable [1] so they can serve as a good means of validation for our model. Right now, our model is able to generate leaks, obstructions and disconnections. Most of the introduced errors in our model can be recognized by van der Aa's expert system, but our model still has to be perfected and updated, in order to reach the same level of performance as a physical model of the breathing circuit.

At this time, we study two ways of communication between model and expert system: machine learning and system identification. The advantage of machine learning is the fact that the production rules can be found by induction and once they are found, they can be used immediately inside a real time expert system.

An advantage of the system identification method is that the model is a direct translation of the system components into model parameters so the resulting expert system rules become relatively simple. Both methods will be compared and tested thoroughly when the model is complete.

7. REFERENCES

[1] J.J. van der Aa: "Intelligent Alarms in Anesthesia - A Real Time Expert System Application", Ph.D. thesis, Department of Electrical Engineering, Eindhoven University of Technology, Eindhoven, the Netherlands, 1990.

[2] J.A. Blom: "The SIMPLEXYS Experiment - Real Time Expert Systems In Patient Monitoring", Ph.D. thesis, Department of Electrical Engineering, Eindhoven University of Technology, Eindhoven, the Netherlands, 1990.

[3] I. Bratko, I. Mozetic, N. Lavrac: "KARDIO - A Study in Deep and Qualitative Knowledge for Expert Systems", The MIT Press, Cambridge Massachusetts, London England, 1989.

[4] L.M. Fagan: "VM: Representing Time-Dependent Relations in a Medical Setting", Ph.D. dissertation, Department of Computer Science, Stanford University, Stanford CA, 1980.

[5] M. Hakman and T. Groth: "KBSIM: a System for Interactive Knowledge-Based Simulation", *Computer Methods and Programs in Biomedicine*, 34, pp. 91-113, 1991.

[6] M.G. Kahn, L.M. Fagan and L.B. Sheiner: "Combining Physiologic Models and Symbolic Methods to Interpret Time-Varying Patient Data", *Methods of Information in Medicine*, 30, pp. 167-178, 1991.

[7] E.D. Lehmann, T. Deutsch, A.V. Roudsari, E.R. Carson, J.J. Benn and P.H. Sonksen: "An Integrated Approach for the Computer-Assisted Treatment of Diabetic Patients on Insulin", *Medical Informatics*, vol. 17, no. 2, pp. 105-123, 1992.

[8] J.R. Quinlan: "Induction of Decision Trees", *Machine Learning 1*, pp. 81-106, 1986.

[9] W.E. Reynolds and J. Wolf: "TUTSIM, a Program for Engineering Design and Optimation by Simulation of Continuous Dynamic Systems", Meerman Automation, Neede, The Netherlands, v. 6.55, 1988.

[10] G.W. Rutledge, G.E. Thomsen, B.R. Farr, M.A. Tovar, J.X. Polaschek, I.A. Beinlich, L.B. Sheiner and L.M. Fagan: "The Design and Implementation of a Ventilator-Management Advisor", *Artificial Intelligence in Medicine*, 5, pp. 67-82, 1993.

[11] D.F. Sittig and J.A. Orr: "A Parallel Implementation of the Backward Error Propagation Neural Network Training Algorithm: Experiments in Event Identification", *Computers and Biomedical Research*, 25, pp. 547-561, 1992.

[12] J.L. Talmon: "A Multiclass Nonparametric Partitioning Algorithm", *Pattern Recognition Letters*, 4, pp. 31-38, 1986.

Strategies for Medical Reasoning

Artificial Intelligence in Medecine
S. Andreassen et al. , Eds.
IOS Press, 1993

Knowledge Based Systems and Techniques for the Health Sector

Pedro Barahona
UNINOVA
2825 Monte da Caparica
Portugal

Abstract

This paper reports on the EPISTOL project, set up to to provide a perspective on how are knowledge based systems systems going to be used in the health sector 5 to 10 years from now, and how should this expected use influence the planning of research and development work up to that period. The results of the project are aimed to aid the planning of future programmes concerned with research and development in health telematics, namely the fourth Framework Programme of the Comission of the European Communities.

1 Introduction

Due to the steady growing of health care services costs, pressures are being increasingly imposed on all the health care providers in order to decrease these costs, without jeopardising or even improving the quality of the services provided. Better management of resources is thus required, namely of the computers that are now found throughout the health sector, from large central hospitals and health centres down to the smallest private GP consultancy room. Computers that, in the present telematics age, are increasingly being connected through various kinds of networks.

Although computers in the health sector have been mostly used in administrative tasks (accountancy, statistics, etc), this pattern of use is likely to change in the near future. Medicine is growing in complexity at such a very fast pace, that the usual paper based channels for information and knowledge transfer (publications, reports, patient records) are not sufficient for the health care professionals. This has been a major motivation for the research and development of medical knowledge based systems and their underlying techniques - to provide support to the health care professionals so that the decisions they make might be better informed and take into account the medical knowledge embedded in these systems.

We have thus seen over the years a number of these systems and techniques being used in the medical field for a variety of purposes. The extent of their use is not as wide as originally expected and has not come about as fast as imagined. A steady growing use is taking place nonetheless, and they are being more and more integrated into other systems and routines and as such regarded as natural components of these systems or routines.

As part of the Telematics Programme of the Commission of the European Communities (CEC), the third Framework Programme the AIM '91 - '94 Programme is to some extent incorporating or addressing the area of knowledge based systems and techniques. About half of the 37 projects address this subject, a few of them as their main activity. The importance of this area was further acknowledged in the management of the current AIM Programme, where knowledge based systems were selected as one of the seven project lines in which the projects were grouped into for concertation purposes.

The EPISTOL project was therefore set up to clarify the impact, in the near future, of knowledge based systems and techniques for the health sector, in order to aid the planning of future programmes concerned with research and development (R&D)in health telematics, namely the fourth Framework Programme. More specifically, to provide a perspective on how are these systems and techniques going to be used in the health sector, 5 to 10 years from now, and how should this expected use influence the planning of R&D work up to that period.

2 Project Activities

The EPISTOL project started in the beginning of 1993 and was included, as a strategic study, in the accompanying measures of AIM '91 - '94, based on a contract between the CEC and UNINOVA. The activity was further supported by the MEDIS Institute, who also intends to use the results of the project in the planning of the future phases of the German MEDWIS Programme. The planning of this action encompassed a number of phases and events, shortly described in the next sections.

2.1 Core Group Meetings

A core group of specialists was appointed which consisted of six invited experts representing research, users, and industry plus the convenor from UNINOVA. Most of the members represented current AIM projects or have some other connection with the AIM programme. This group had a few two-days meetings, from January to April 1993, to discuss and create the basis of a Scenario Report of how it expects knowledge based systems and techniques to be used in the health sector 5-10 years from now.

The written scenario was meant to be visionary though based on as firm a ground as possible, and so it contains only little about the history of knowledge based systems and slightly more about the state of the art. Legal, ethical and regulatory aspects were not treated in this phase since no specialist of these areas was included in the group. The report is edited by the convenor with the approval from the core group experts.

2.2 Munich Workshop

The scenario report was presented at a three days working conference organised in Munich by the MEDIS Institute in 28-30 June 1993. The meeting was attended by the core goup, and by over 20 invited experts, who for some time have known the nature of the exercise. The experts representing research, industry, service providers, users, administration and the legal aspect were appointed by the core group after consultation with UNINOVA, MEDIS, and the AIM Office of the CEC.

During the morning sessions of this workshop the convenor presented the Scenario Report and each expert presented a short paper with his/her own vision of the future, as a supplement and/or comment to the scenario report. These presentations were further used as guidelines for the afternoon discussions, divided in 4 specialised working groups, each with a rapporteur and a specific topic but with multidisciplinary participants. The following topics were discussed:

1. How will knowledge based products change clinical practice;
2. How will knowledge based techniques be incorporated into commercial products;
3. Trends in knowledge based research that will enable its use in routine applications
4. Distributed knowledge and telematics in a changing health care environment.

The rapporteurs will produce written reports summarising these discussions. After the conference all participants may review their papers and submit a new version. The core group is also reviewing their scenario report in light of the new input and ideas, including the need for R&D work in the field. These approximately 25 papers will be collected by the coordinator in a draft document and be the basis for the next phase.

2.3 Brussels Seminar

An invitation will be distributed to as many relevant persons as possible to participate in a one day seminar, to be held in Brussels in the 19th of November 1993, chaired by the CEC. Anybody expressing interest in participating will receive the draft document and is requested to submit 1 - 2 pages of comments in advance of the seminar. These comments should include view points on the use of knowledge based systems and techniques in the health sector 5-10 years from now and the necessary R&D work leading up to this use.

At the seminar the core group presents the revised Scenario Report, the rapporteurs from the working groups of the Munich workshop present the groups' findings and a member of the core group presents an extract from the 20 plus papers from the same workshop. Finally two or three persons present overviews of the newly received papers from the participants. Following these 8 - 9 speeches a panel with the members of the core group will be the centre of a general debate for the rest of the day.

2.4 Deliverables

The major deliverable from this strategic study will be the publication of a book with a perspective on the future use of the knowledge based systems and techniques in the health sector and the nature and structure of the necessary R&D work in that field 2-5 years from now. This book, edited from the materials produced during the different stages of the study should be fed into the planning process of future AIM R&D actions. The book should be published by the beginning of 1994 (draft versions will be available earlier to the CEC).

3 Preliminary Conclusions

Although the study is not complete yet, a number of conclusions seem to have reached a large concensus among the study participants and are briefly outlined in this section. To begin with, the need for knowledge based systems and techniques as a means to effectively use the existing in computer infrastructure and provide better services, was indeed identified by the participating users (namely, medical doctors).

Future applications should nevertheless be well integrated into daily practices and routines. This requirement has a number of consequences, namely a) knowledge based systems should not be used in isolation but rather integrated with other software (e.g. communications, databases, signal and image processing, etc.), b) these systems should aim at providing global task support (e.g. to avoid the use of a system to support diagnosis, another for treatment, and still a different one for patient management).

¿From an industry point of view, the development of medical workstations that could integrate all these functionalities in a coherent environment should benefit from the expertise of different industrial sectors, namely those dealing with health care information systems software, medical electronic equipment, medical publishing, value added networking, and pharmaceutics. Knowledge based systems and techniques were identified in areas such as

Medical records: more powerful terminologies are required than those provided by current standards, integrated in shareable ontologies.

User interfaces: not only to improve the way in which information is presented (from graphical interfaces to multimedia) but also to deal with the problem of prompting the relevant information with the adequate timing (being context dependent, the solution of this problem has much to benefit from the use of knowledge based techniques).

Access to knowledge sources: for intelligent retrieval of information and knowledge from electronic supported textbooks and medical databases and knowledge bases.

Decision support: to support medical decisions in a variety of modes. In many cases decision support can be provided mostly in a watchdog mode, issuing warnings against "trivially" overlooked problems (most noticeably drugs interactions); in more difficult cases, knowledge based systems with more powerful inference capabilities are required, possibly to be used in a more interactive mode.

An interesting topic that was raised during the study, related to decision support and integration with routine practice, is the use of medical protocols and guidelines, which are being suggested or even imposed in many areas of the health sector, and for which electronic support is in demand. Superficially, protocols are categorical decision trees or flowcharts, and in that sense they virtually avoid the issue of dealing with uncertainty. Nevertheless, there are a number of problems with a "blind" following of protocols, since they do not cover all cases, and even in the covered cases still problems can arise (e.g. how mandatory is a guideline suggestion, should a protocol be abandoned given some unanticipated event or condition, interaction of conflicting protocols, etc.). As such, even protocol based care should benefit from the more advanced reasoning capabilities of knowledge based systems.

Annex

Participants in the Core Group Meetings

Pedro Barahona	UNINOVA	Portugal
F.T de Dombal	University of Leeds	United Kingdom
John Durinck	Philips	The Netherlands
Claude Florin	Hewlett - Packard Medical Product Group	Switzerland
Carlos Hernandez	Universitad Santiago de Compostela	Spain
Peter Hucklenbroich	GSF - MEDIS Institut	Germany
Mario Stefanelli	Universita di Pavia	Italia
Jens Christensen	AIM Office	Belgium
Jorge Cruz	UNINOVA	Portugal
Wolfgang Moser	GSF - MEDIS Institut	Germany
Susana Nascimento	UNINOVA	Portugal

Other Participants and Contributors to the Munich Workshop

Steen Andreassen	University of Aalborg	Denmark
Robert Baud	Hopital de Geneve	Switzerland
Enrico Coiera	Hewllett Packard Laboratories	United Kingdom
Luca Console	Universita di Torino	Italy
Wilhelm van Eimeren	GSF - MEDIS Institut	Germany
Rolf Engelbrecht	GSF - MEDIS Institut	Germany
John Fox	Imperial Cancer Research Fund	United Kingdom
Pierre Frutiger	Morges Hospital	Switzerland
Werner Horn	Austrian Res.Inst.for Artificial Intelligence	Austria
Johan van der Lei	Erasmus University	The Netherlands
Peter McNair	Hvidovre Hospital	Denmark
Hubert Mensch	Actir Sante	France
Francisco del Pozo	Universidad Politecnica de Madrid	Spain
Alan Rector	University of Manchester	United Kingdom
J.-L. Renaud-Salis	Fondation Bergonie	France
Anthony Rickards	Royal Brompton Hospital	United Kingdom
Paul Rubel	INSERM	France
B. de Schutter	Free University of Brussels	Belgium
Klaus Spitzer	University Heidelberg	Germany
Jürgen Stausberg	GSF - MEDIS Institut	Germany
Jan Talmon	University of Limburg	The Netherlands
Soren Vingtoft	Gentofte Hospital	Denmark
Thomas Wendler	Philips GmbH Forschungslaboratorien	Germany
Bob Wielinga	University of Amsterdam	The Netherlands
Jeremy Wyatt	Imperial Cancer Research Fund	United Kingdom
Isabelle de Zegher	BIM S.A.	Belgium

Artificial Intelligence in Medecine
S. Andreassen et al. , Eds.
IOS Press, 1993

A Knowledge-Based Advisor Supporting to Deal with Rare Diseases

Kindler H.*', Densow D.', Fliedner T. M.'

*) Institute for Applied Knowledge Processing, University of Ulm
Postfach 2060, D-89010 Ulm, kindler@dulfaw1a.bitnet

') Institute for Occupational Health, University of Ulm
WHO Collaborating Centre in Radiation Emergency Medical Preparedness and Assistance

This research was partially funded by the AIM Programme of the Commission of the European Communities as project number A2034 (GAMES II). The partners of this project are SAGO (Florence, Italy), Foundation of Research and Technology (Heraklion, Greece), Geneva University Hospital (Switzerland), University of Amsterdam (The Netherlands), University College of London (UK), the University of Pavia (Italy), and the University of Ulm (Germany)

Abstract

Ad hoc decision support is required for rare diseases. The construction of full-scale expert systems would be effective, but, too expensive. Co-operative problem-solving of a physician and a knowledge-based advisor combines their strengths efficiently. The architecture of a knowledge-based advisor is presented. The medical application domain is the acute radiation syndrome.

1. Introduction

Medical problems are often such complex that one single agent only is not efficiently capable to solve them autonomously. Thus, co-operative problem-solving involving the interaction of several agents is required to optimally manage the problems. In reality, a class of medical problems which necessarily must be solved and rarely occur can be identified. In general, these problems are composed out of many routine sub-problems and a minority of difficult, rare sub-problems. Both, training personnel or building expert systems is an expensive solution to provide the capability to master these problems. A third solution is the construction of a knowledge-based advisor which solves the rare sub problems, delegates the routine sub-problems to human agents, and composes the partial solutions to the overall solution. A common understanding of the problem management is required because several agents are involved.

2. The Domain of Application

The application domain is the medical management of the acute radiation syndrome (ARS). It is a rare disease. About 900 cases are known in the world including 150 Chernobyl cases, only.

A limited number of elder experts on the world knows how to manage the ARS. Today, young physicians rarely have the chance to gain experience in this medical management task. It would be rather expensive to train a larger fraction of them. On the other hand, it would be highly cost effective to develop an expert system to manage the acute radiation syndrome because coping with the management of an irradiated patient totally would require to model competence in surgery, dermatology, intensive care, internal medicine, haematology, and the specialists' knowledge about the acute radiation syndrome.

When the problem-solving behaviour of an expert who manages an acute radiation syndrome is examined it turns out that his problem-solving strategy is sequential diagnosis (Fliedner 81). The big task, the management of the ARS, is hierarchically decomposed into sub tasks which is done dynamically depending on the state of the individual patient.

These sub tasks are then solved in a sequential order. Many of the sub tasks are more or less routinely performed in a maximal care type hospital, e. g., creating an antibiogram, treating skin burns, and doing a bone marrow transplantation. Others are never performed in a normal hospital, e. g., dynamically developing the diagnostic and therapeutic strategy, determining the degree of the irradiation, taking into account the peculiarities of a bone marrow transplantation after accidental irradiation. Due to the multidisciplinarity this is co-operative problem-solving approach even when no knowledge-based advisor is involved.

As mentioned before, the most efficient way of problem-solving if several agents are involved will be to distribute each task to the agent who can perform it most efficiently. Since physicians especially have a lack in creating a management plan for the acute radiation syndrome the knowledge-based advisor must be able to advise the physician in charge. This key task and some small sub tasks which require relatively modest amounts of special knowledge about the acute radiation syndrome are not routinely solved by physicians. Whereas, they could be well done by the knowledge-based advisor which nevertheless must be able to explain and justify its propositions to the physician in charge. During the dynamic creation of the management plan it has to be decided continuously how to distribute the tasks to the physicians of the hospital. For instance, the treatment of skin burns is given to a dermatologist, a bone marrow transplantation is done by a haematologist, taking of blood samples can be done by a nurse.

3. The Architecture of a Knowledge-Based Advisor

3.1 Cognitive Problem-Solving Model and Blackboard Control Architecture

For co-operative problem-solving a basic plan common all agents involved has to be devised on how to best share the tasks among them. This plan must be developed by the knowledge-based advisor. Consequently, the knowledge-based advisor has to have strategic knowledge on tackling and decomposing the problem. This requires the explicit representation of strategic knowledge and virtual entities, i.e., the sub problems serving to control the reasoning.

The plan must be comprehensible to the human agents. Therefore, it must have a structure to which they are accustomed and the structural elements must be known. It is a well-known fact in cognitive science that humans solve large problems by hierarchically decomposing them into sub problems until means are found to solve the latter (Anderson 85). Experts managing the acute radiation syndrome apply the strategy of sequential diagnosis (Fliedner 81), which can be mapped to a cognitive problem-solving model (Kindler 91b). This strategy of sequential diagnosis is even more general (de Kleer 86). The select and test model (ST-model) has been derived from philosophy to cover all medical problem-solving processes (Ramoni 93). Current research has shown that this perfectly applies to sequential diagnosis, also.

The kernel of an advisor for a scenario as described above is knowledge on the problem-solving strategy. The advisor has to take the lead at the user's request and has to initiate the tackling of the problem. It therefore has to provide the competence to dynamically plan the problem-solving situation dependent on an abstract level. It must be able to decompose the problem into a hierarchy of cognitively relevant sub problems. The explicitly represented management plan has to be shared between all agents involved in the problem-solving process.

A blackboard control architecture (Hayes-Roth 85) is an appropriate mean to imitate human problem-solving behaviour by explicitly representing a dynamic problem-solving plan and controlling the problem-solving by the plan. A central focus decides which agent has to solve which task. This mimics the situation of an advisor supporting the physician in charge. Two blackboards contain the data in a blackboard control architecture.

The domain blackboard encompasses all domain data forming the description of a case suffering from the ARS. All of the objects on the control blackboard can be found which serve to represent the problem-solving plan. A plan is a dynamic hierarchy of tasks. It is dynamically created depending on the state of the domain blackboard. In case of a knowledge-based advisor for the ARS this is a task hierarchy representing a medical management plan developed according to the strategy of sequential diagnosis. The knowledge-sources are activated according to the state of processing of the task hierarchy on the control blackboard. After the solution of a task, the deduced information is stored on the domain blackboard. A knowledge source in general consists of production rules. Other inference methods like differential equation systems could be applied, too (Lanzola 90). Many of the tasks are communication tasks, e. g., the gathering of the laboratory results. The advisor has to know about a mapping of the sub problems to the agents. It must know which sub tasks can best be solved by which human agents or by itself, e. g., give the task to a surgeon, to a haematologist, or to a knowledge-source. It is marked for every type of task either by which knowledge source or by what human agent it shall be solved.

3.2 Human-Computer Interaction

For legal reasons the physician in charge has to take the full responsibility for the medical management. Therefore, the knowledge-based advisor must transparently share all its data and the developed problem-solving plan with the user. A patient chart gives a rapid overview about the state of the solution process. The immense information transfer capacity of man's visual sense can be utilised by applying graphical interfaces. In medicine the patient chart metaphor has been applied to provide an interface which is easy to use by a human user because he is already accustomed to it.

If several agents are involved in co-operative problem-solving it will be useful to provide one shared plan which is accessible to all of them. Reading the plan gives them information to perform their tasks adequately. Writing on the plan is necessary to relate their share of the problem-solving process to the others. On one of the cards the content of the control blackboard, i. e., the hierarchy of tasks, is visualised. This provides a good overview of the problem-solving process. Further cards illustrate the content of the domain blackboard. Blood cell concentrations as important signs to determine the most probable degree of the lesion of the haemopoietic system are displayed as time value plots. The other signs and symptoms are presented similarly. By this means the responsible physician, all the other personnel, and the knowledge-based advisor have a common access to all relevant data to manage the problem.

The communication between the humans and the knowledge-based advisor is done via forms (Lane 86). Due to the request for the laboratory results a set of questions for data of interest is constructed by rules and used to produce the layout of the form. This type of communication within organisations as a hospital is usual between humans, therefore, they are accustomed to it. Due to the graphical user interface, both, the human agents and the knowledge-based advisor have a representation at hand on which they can base their work.

3.3 Explanation

In medicine legal requirements and medical conventions force the physician in charge to take the personal responsibility of the medical management even when applying a technical aid like a knowledge-based advisor. The advisor must be able to explain and justify its deductions comprehensibly and give an overview of the problem-solving process. Therefore, answers must be provided to a set of "why" and "how" questions.

A justification-based truth maintenance system (JTMS) (Doyle 79) can record and withdraw the relations of the data given to the advisor and all the deductions derived by the strategic and domain rules and other knowledge-sources of the advisor. For each fact a deduction tree can be produced explaining how the fact was deduced.

A JTMS graph provides but poor explanation facilities. A better solution would be to map the JTMS graph on a hypertext graph (Nielsen 90). The textual form of a Horn clause with its instantiations is a hypertext node and the instantiating facts in the premises are the anchors leading to other hypertext nodes. The user can select by himself the detail of explanation. Equally for each task a deduction tree can be produced which explains why the task was executed. Thus, the possibility to give explanations is provided by recording the relations between deductions, facts, and tasks using a JTMS.

The justification form of a rule is a text that epistemologically justifies the deductive knowledge. For instance a quotation justifies that the medical measures have to be performed daily short after the irradiation if the haemopoietic lesions are of degree three. Supplementary physiological knowledge justifies why the initial increase of the granulocytes is a good indicator for the grading of haemopoietic lesions. The justifications of the knowledge can be provided in hypertext form, too.

4. Implementation

The demonstrator has been implemented on a Sparc 10 and on KEE 4.0, which provides basic routines for the user interface, a truth maintenance system, a production rule interpreter, and an object-oriented representation of the domain and inference ontology. The truth maintenance system provides the information to give explanations and justifications. However, the implementation still requires additional work.

5. Conclusion

We are on the way to implement a knowledge-based advisor that meets the following goals:

- responsible application complying with legal restrictions,
- efficient construction,
- easy maintenance,
- automatic documentation as a beneficial side-effect,
- support the human agents only when necessary, and
- efficient combination of man's skills and the expertise of the advisor.

A first demonstrator has been implemented as described above. It has not formally been evaluated yet. But, comments of experts in managing the acute radiation syndrome (WHO 93), both involved and not involved in the development of the system were positive. A database of case histories of the acute radiation syndrome is under completion (Kindler 93). It will be used to evaluate the competence of the system. The ergonomics and the interfacing with the users will be tested with medical staff.

We presume that in future only knowledge-based systems solving problems in co-operation with humans as outlined above will be successful. The effort to model the competence of humans will decrease in comparison with classical expert systems. On the contrary, the effort for modelling the communication between the agents is expected to increase.

6. Literature

[1] Anderson J. R.: "Cognitive Psychology and its Implications", W. H. Freeman and Company, New York, 1985

[2] Carroll J. M., McKendree J.: "Interface Design Issues for Advice-Giving Expert Systems", Communications of the ACM, 30, 1987

[3] Clancey W. J.: "Model Construction Operators", Artificial Intelligence, vol. 53, North Holland, 1992

[4] de Kleer J.: "An Assumption Based TMS", Artificial Intelligence, vol. 32, North Holland, 1986

[5] de Kleer J., Williams B. C.: "Diagnosing Multiple Faults", Artificial Intelligence, vol. 24, North Holland, 1987

[6] Doyle: "A Truth Maintenance System", Artificial Intelligence, vol. 12, North Holland, 1979

[7] Engelmore R., Morgan T. (eds.): "Blackboard Systems", Addison-Wesley, Wokingham, 1988

[8] Fischer G.: "Communication Requirements for Co-Operative Problem-Solving Systems", Information Systems, 15, 1990

[9] Fliedner T. M.: "Strategien zur strahlenschutzmedizinischen, ambulanten Versorgung von "Betroffenen" bei kerntechnischen Unfällen", Thieme, Stuttgart, 1981

[10] Greif I. (Ed.): "Computer Supported Co-operative Work: A Book of Readings.", Morgan-Kaufmann, San Mateo, 1988

[11] Hayes-Roth B.: "A Blackboard Architecture for Control", Artificial Intelligence, vol. 26, North Holland, 1985

[12] Hayes-Roth B., Hewett M.: "BB1: An Implementation of the Blackboard Control Architecture", in Engelmore R. S., Morgan A. J. (eds.): "Blackboard Systems", Addison-Wesley, Wokingham, 1988

[13] Kindler H., Densow D., Fliedner T. M.: "Better Justifiability and Less Rules by Using Deep Knowledge", Proceedings of the 10th MIE 91, Vienna, Springer, Heidelberg, 1991

[14] Kindler H., Densow D., Fliedner T. M.: "RADES - Medical Assistance System for the Management of Irradiated Persons", Proceedings of the 2nd DEXA 91, Berlin, Springer, Vienna, 1991

[15] Kindler H., Densow D., Fliedner T. M.: "How to Provide Computerised Decision Aid for Rare Diseases", Proceedings of the 11th MIE 93, Jerusalem, Freund, London, 1993

[16] Lane C. D., Walton J. D., Shortliffe E. H.: "Graphical Access to Medical Expert Systems: II. Design of an Interface for Physicians", Methods of Information in Medicine, vol. 25, Schattauer, 1986

[17] Lanzola G., Stefanelli M., Barosi G., Magnani L.: "NEOANEMIA: A Knowledge-Based System Emulating Diagnostic Reasoning", Computers and Biomedical Research 23, 1990

[18] Nielsen J.: "Through Hypertext", Communications of the ACM 33, 1990

[19] Ramoni M., Stefanelli M., Magnani L., Borosi G.: "An Epistemological Framework for Medical Knowledge-Based Systems", IEEE Transactions on Systems, Man, and Cybernetics, to appear 1993

[20] Swartout W. R.: "XPLAIN: A System for Creating and Explaining Expert Consulting Systems", Artificial Intelligence, vol. 21, 1983

[21] WHO-Report PEP/93.2: "Fourth Coordination Meeting of WHO Collaborating Centres in Radiation Emergency Medical Perparedness and Assistance", 1993

Artificial Intelligence in Medecine
S. Andreassen et al. , Eds.
IOS Press, 1993

On higher-level operational facets of diagnostic expert systems

M. Popper

National Centre for Health Promotion, Bratislava, Slovakia

Abstract

Macro-operations, as conveyors of strategy-directed diagnostic reasoning, are considered: they, as identifiable task-specific prescriptions, are to extend the expressiveness of knowledge representation and surpass the limitations of universal inferential operations.

1. INTRODUCTION

Both, expressiveness of knowledge representation and efficiency of its exploitation underlain expert system (ES) performance. While methods and technologies of knowledge representation has been evolving significantly in past years, it is not so with efficacy of their procedural - *operational* - counterparts. Some of the issues concerning operational facets of inference engine regarding strategy-directed diagnostic reasoning are sketched in this contribution. Noting the role and limitations of universal inferential operations the position of task-specific inference macro-operations are advocated. They are regarded as carriers of higherlevel operational means to increase the ES capabilities for providing more competent (diagnostic) performance.

2. HIGH-LEVEL OPERATIONS FOR REASONING STRATEGIES

Let us have an illustrating assertion: IF the patient's *findings suggest diffuse interstitial lung disease*, AND his/her *lung X-ray patterns* are one from the following: *(usually symmetric, diffuse, stable in localisation) ground-glass (granular), nodular, reticular, reticulonodular, honeycombing, bilateral hilar lymphadenopathy, larger confluent nodules,* AND his/her *tbc test is negative,* AND (though not necessarily) *erythema nodosum and positive Kveim's test have been detected,* AND at least one from the following is manifesting: *increased immunoglobulin or SACE level, hypercalcemia, hypercalciuria, lymphocytes in BAL more than 20%, positive Ga 67 lung scan,* AND *biopsy findings of sarcoid granulomas in lung or other lymphatic node are positive,* THEN his/her disease should be *sarcoidosis.*

The illustration, regardless whether it is fully acceptable for concerned professionals, has some important features to be noted. In it *only biological phenomena (substances) are referred to*. However, without their *complex (anatomic, physiologic, etiopathogenic, hierarchical, causal) relations* to other ones, free from explicit articulation of the *significance, credibility, attainability, differentiating power* of particular findings, their individual roles under diverse circumstances, etc. The relation of *logical equivalence* between the consequent and some items in the antecedent (as in our case) is ignored. *Neither regulations, nor constraints,* if any, are provided to comply with medical technologies in patient investigation. As *no particular inference control* is provided or implied by such an assertion, it itself does not indicate, at least not explicitly, the progression of its evaluation under various circumstances.

Irrespective of diverse ways the assertion is activated, the goal is to confirm or rule out its consequent: *sarcoidosis* - as a kind of *diffuse interstitial lung disease* (DILD). A physician does not judge such an assertion *in isolation*, a wider panorama is regarded. In our case at least the *context* of DILDs. In his/her mental model a general strategy to consider preferably easily attainable data with differentiating potential and the significant differentiating role of lung X-ray might be provided. Obviously, this influences the subsequent assessment process. If under given settings (s)he focuses the DILDs of known etiology, then patient interrogation related to e.g. his/her working environment and conditions, drug consumption, etc. takes place. Otherwise or succeedingly, positive X-ray findings are searched for (a subtask of own rights). While all positive findings listed in assertion may evidence any DILD, the bilateral hilar lymphadenopathy particularly strongly suggests sarcoidosis. For pursuing this disease, the assertion implicitly gives some hints. When no evidence for etiology occurs or the related line of reasoning does not yield an acceptable result, then other inference directions take their role. For example, if meaningful, consideration of colagenoses. This then shifts the attention to findings evidencing rheumatic diseases. Their absence, ruling out colagenoses, may switch next to another direction of reasoning - alveolitides. Consequently, the laboratory tests, siderophages in sputum, etc. are going to be examined. And so on, and so forth.

Evidently the sketched (partial) reasoning strategy does not follow directly from our assertion. Regardless of selected approaches, for ES inferencing also other provisions have to be furnished: proper *descriptions* and *prescriptions* [4]. The latter is our central issue: *operational prescriptions* as higher-level macro-operations standing for the low-level universal ones being dissolved in the inference procedures.

3. THE ROLE OF MACRO-OPERATIONS

In production rules - commonly representing assertions - the symbols standing for *terms* are related by operators of logic to form a propositionally evaluated expression. The evaluation implicitly follows rules of formal logic, usually yielding an exhaustive process regarding all its components in the provided sequence. Certainly, this approach frequently does not satisfy the real needs, especially regarding efficient cognitive manoeuvres.

For strategy-directed diagnostic reasoning underlain by explicitly expressed medical knowledge, considerations regarding well articulated, aggregated, organized, associated, hierarchical knowledge representation - observing mutual interrelations of biological substances - must be carefully regarded. Besides, case or event based efficient techniques and strategies being employed in course of diagnostic reasoning should be reflected as well. The corresponding inference operations and their control regimes, if they are to comply with natural knowledge employment, have to observe the demands for competent and efficient reasoning strategies and techniques having clear conceptual connection to the task-level operations. The too low-level computation-universal customary means for knowledge representation and their operational employment yields limitations in this respect. More complex well structured and organized specific operational units are needed for that. *Macro-operations*, as operational complements of specific declarative knowledge, highlighting real traits of tasks, with them associated relevant knowledge bodies, and their exploitation at the level complying appropriately with characteristic features of particular domains, may do. They should be dedicated to become problem, task, or case specific [1].

A macro-operation is not necessarily based only on formal logic. Diverse tasks can relay on various other productive symbolic knowledge representation (analytic expressions, bitmaps, sets, lists, etc.) associated with powerful computations providing efficient task-specific functions. (See e.g. [2],[5].)

Analyzing types of domain problems one can often see existence of knowledge organizations allowing *selection of small, highly relevant bodies of knowledge and recognize types of arguments which underpin actions and conclusions.* Consequently, one may reveal respective prescriptions and their interrelations to form macro-operations and strategies permitting their event or case driven invocations.

A structured sequence of operations related by a specific goal and referring to a subset of rules and/or subnet of frames (kind of a *description*) can be seen as an identifiable macro-operation. It actually signifies sort of instructions regarding particular employment of substance knowledge - a *prescription*. It might be regarded as a *scheme or pattern of reasoning* generating competent behaviour. Prescriptions, as operational units, in some context or situation might be triggered under diverse circumstances (e.g. based on available, lacking, or conflicting data, active defaults, content of the inference control infrastructure). With psychological feel one may talk about associating knowledge states with mental operators: *under particular conditions an individual descriptive piece of knowledge can invoke a distinctive task-specific macro-operation and, vice versa, a prescription, aside of its potential to invoke other related macro-operations, can appeal a description.* Facilitated by well conceptualized relations among task-specific macro-operations (type-type, type-subtype, dynamical precedence, etc.), the prescriptions might provide much potential for competent knowledge exploitation on task or case level properly and timely to derive needed conclusions effectively.

A situation-specific *line of reasoning* relevant to a task *links to a goal justified structural constituents as triggering cues, domain concepts, actions, and conclusions* [3]. In pursuing reasoning activities the lines of reasoning or their parts are chained: one feeds into another and, if necessary, they retract. Regardless of the particular knowledge used, the sequence of structural components reflect pattern-directed macro-operations. It is of advantage when they are *generic* as the patterns are not necessarily tight to any task specific knowledge. *Quantified, indirect, wild-card term references, and combination thereof in proper control structures enable their efficient implementation.*

4. SOME ILLUSTRATIONS AND CONCLUDIONG REMARKS

The *lines and patterns of reasoning* are to be perceived as conceptualized task-specific macro-operations. The inference workings can be then perceived as the process of constructing and comparing situation-specific models of processes for some diagnostic purpose based on macro-operations as the kinds described in the following.

For evoking a diagnostic hypothesis patient data are to be gathered, assembled, and organized in concordance with *networks of concepts and their relations.* A generic pattern, say a *conceiver,* may serve for creating particular views and select proper strategies, respecting constraints, options, discriminations, preferences, etc. The facts associated with patient present illness (history, physical examination) are collected in such a way. When a significant portion of patient data is either accumulated or changed, say a *discoverer* can be triggered to propose a kind of hypothesis for verification. Our illustrating assertion may be invoked by discovering in patient data evidence for DILDs (e.g. some combination of stress dyspnea, dry cough, crepitus, etc.). Prior triggering the discoverer, another macro-operation, let us call it *anticipator,* may take its role. Invoked by the process of information gathering it is to recognize a partially completed task related schema, a description, to fill up the gaps in it. Its potential is to invite directly or indirectly other contributing operations, e.g. assessment of lung X-ray. Recognizing unattainable, disregarded, confusing, or inconsistent facts, when provisions for that are given, might be the task of a *locator* which then triggers respective prescriptions for resolving the consequences, e.g. a *back-tracker* to retract the current sequence of reasoning and to shift it in a different direction. Even partially confirmed individual diagnoses may cause invoking a *pursuer* to refine the attained results, or an *endorser* to assess their credibility. Not seldom an adequate end-result can be developed only with a global assessing perspective, knowing or considering various matters concurrently. An *integrator,* recognizing available facts, inferred results, and their mutual complex relations, may then set up a global result (see [4] for illustration).

The sketched reasoning templates illustrate a potential to accommodate provisions for generic combination of a problem, knowledge representation, inference strategies, and explanation, each observant to the users' needs. As such, they can have an important role in knowledge acquisition as well. Diagnostic ESs aspiring to be attentive for solving realistic diagnostic problems are evidencing the necessity for inventing higher level (in contrast with low-level) inference operations. From this perspective, it was our aim to point out the significance and potential of the discussed operational patterns we consider vital for complementing declarative knowledge.

6. REFERENCES

1 D.C. Brown and B. Chandrasekaran, Design Problem Solving, Morgan Kaufmann Publ., California, 1989.

2 R.A. Miller and F.E. Masarie, Jr.: The Quick Medical Reference Relation Function: Description and Evaluation of a Simple Efficient "Multiple Diagnoses" Algorithm. In K.C. Lun et al.(eds.): MEDINFO'92, North-Holland, Amsterdam, (1992) 512.

3 Narayan S.M. et al.: Lines and Patterns of Reasoning: New Units of Analysis for Clinical Decision Making. Ibid., 426.

4 Popper M.: From Low-Level to High-Level Operations in Expert Systems. To appear in Proc. of DEXA'93 Conference, Springer-Verlag, Heidelberg, 1993.

5 Rotterdam E. et al.: Resolution of Constraint Inconsistency with the Aim to Provide Support in Anaesthesia. To appear in Proc. of DEXA'93 Conference, Springer-Verlag, Heidelberg, 1993.

Artificial Intelligence in Medecine
S. Andreassen et al. , Eds.
IOS Press, 1993

A framework for computer assisted medical decision making

B. Petkoff

RG Expert Systems, SysTA Biomed, Wielandstr. 28a, 4970 Bad Oeynhausen

Abstract

The promise of computers in medicine, including their role in decision support, can only be fulfilled if the overall effectiveness of the system is not constrained by a lack of coordination between the members of a group all sharing the same goal, namely patient care. Cooperative medical decision making involves a continuous process, assessing the validity of data, information and knowledge acquired and inferred by the colleagues, that is, a shared knowledge space must be transparent. The ACCORD methodology provides an interpretation framework for the mapping of domain facts - constituting the world model of the expert - onto conceptual models, which can be expressed in formal representations. The Maccord framework allows a stepwise and inarbitrary reconstruction of the problem solving competence of medical experts as a prerequisite for an appropriate architecture of both medical knowledge bases and the "reasoning device".

1. The need for a methodology of medical decision making

The use of computers in medical decision making has been a research area since the 1950s and the analytical approach of the Bayes´ Rule and Bayesian statistics towards the problem of medical diagnosis. By the late 1970s, programs that used symbolic "artificial intelligence" (AI) methods to give advice were becoming known as "expert systems" (XPS). Although the synergism of the statistical perspective and the heuristic approach is now well recognised and effectively implemented, there is increasing reason to doubt that systems based on this approach will ever yield wide acceptance, due to the dynamic quality of medical decision making. Modelling this dynamic nature adequately requires a constant iterative process consisting of stepwise decisions from one diagnostic or therapeutic category down to the next one, rather than an ad-hoc topological classification. In addition to this paradigmatic shift in the modelling of decision making, the notion of the stand-alone consulting program must be overcome, because the promise of computers in medicine, including their role in decision support, can only arrive within the next decade if the overall effectiveness of the system is not constrained by a lack of coordination between the individual members of the group sharing the same goal - patient care. This is the reason behind the need for a new metaphor and the emergence of a new line of research by the use of computers in medical decision making -*Computer Supported Cooperative Work* (CSCW). Three factors distinguish the MACCORD & CSCW metaphor from previous systems for medical decision making.

1.1. Articulating cooperative work

The commonly accepted view of what constitutes hospital organisation still relies heavily on cooperative efforts, involving a number of medical tasks in order to establish the diagnosis. Physicians are under pressure to act quickly, and meeting this challenge is very difficult without computer-based decision support. Such systems have to comply with the requirements of the working environment, usually calling for a hierarchical chain of decisions rather than a recommendation according to the final pathological classification.

1.2. Sharing an information space

Cooperative medical decision making involves a continuous process, assessing the validity of the knowledge acquired and inferred by the colleagues, i.e. a shared knowledge space must be transparent. Thus a computer-based system supporting cooperative work involving decision making should enhance the ability of cooperating colleagues to interrelate their partial and parochial domain knowledge and facilitate the expression and communication of alternative perspectives on a given problem. This requires a representation of the problem domain as a whole, as well as a representation, in some form, of the mappings between perspectives onto that problem domain. An important dichotomy between modelling activities in the field of medical decision support systems is often neglected. One may model the domain (concepts and relations of the universe of discourse) and/or the problem solver (acting in specific situations of interest). What is really needed is a methodology, providing an interpretation framework for the building of conceptual models of the universe of discourse. We use the term "conceptual model" to denote an abstract description of the problem solving process(es) and the different categories of knowledge employed therein. The conceptual model allows the mapping of the world model of the experts onto the representation language of the knowledge engineers.

1.3. Impact of AI - approaches

Over the past years a great deal of AI research has been directed towards the development of knowledge based systems (expert systems) for problem solving in complex domains. Several research groups have tried to formulate practical advice in "standard" textbooks and/or more advanced conceptualisations: generic task concept [1-2], KADS methodology [3-4] etc., but there is still no means for bridging the large conceptual gap between domain concepts and representational formalisms, which renders knowledge engineering an art rather than a science.

In the case of a medical domain this modelling requires an in depth epistemological analysis of the medical reasoning process which is not supported by any common approach. This analysis has to include the identification, formalisation and representation of the relevant concepts, notions and phenomena of the domain and their interrelations. These models of expertise have to comprise knowledge of various categories and at different levels of abstraction, according to the cognitively and epistemologically different problem solving activities, in order to enable effective communication between medical experts and knowledge engineers during the knowledge acquisition process.

We claim that the *ACCORD* conceptual models offer a methodological framework for interpreting unstructured data allowing the choice of appropriate formal representation by reconstructing the expert´s knowledge [8-10]:

- as a prescriptive tool it offers epistemologically motivated structuring and processing principles;
- as a descriptive tool it allows the meaningful reconstruction and correlation of different medical domains or different medical tasks - like diagnosis & therapy.

2. METHODOLOGY FOR MEDICAL KNOWLEDGE BASED SYSTEMS

The ACCORD metamodel has two major sources: the Experiential Learning Model (ELM), developed and elaborated by [5] and the epistemological studies of the structuralist philosophers [6-7]. ACCORD now tries to integrate both approaches into what can be called a "methodology of knowledge based systems" [8-10]. Developing a medical knowledge based system using the MACCORD model means reconstructing the problem solving behaviour of the medical expert in terms of empirical, hypothetical, theoretical or experimental models at various levels of abstraction, and the transitions between these [11-14]. There is another important point to be made about the goal of MACCORD : most "medical expert systems" and, even worse, many reconstruction´s of medical reasoning which serve as a theoretical foundation of, say, knowledge acquisition tools, do not address the clinical decision problem. With the term "clinical decision problem" we denote the problem of *deciding which action* (be it diagnostic or therapeutic) *is to be taken next in order to maximize the benefit for the patient*. This consideration is the heart of medical reasoning, the justification of any action taken or left in a medical context. Thus it is inappropriate that many medical kbs only attempt to *order* (diagnostic/ therapeutic) *alternatives by "plausibility"* based on *given* data. The question underlying any consultation of a medical xps is not "what is patient X´s illness?" but "what should I do next in order to obtain more specific information and to initiate a rational therapy?". Since procedures ("experimental models") and their meta-criteria, together with the kinds of information/knowledge they can provide, are represented explicitly, MACCORD enables knowledge bases to be "built around" the clinical decision problem.

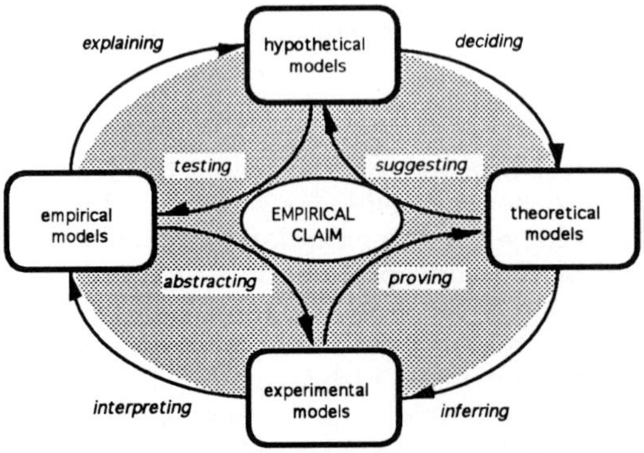

Figure 1. ACCORD:the abductive-deductive cycle

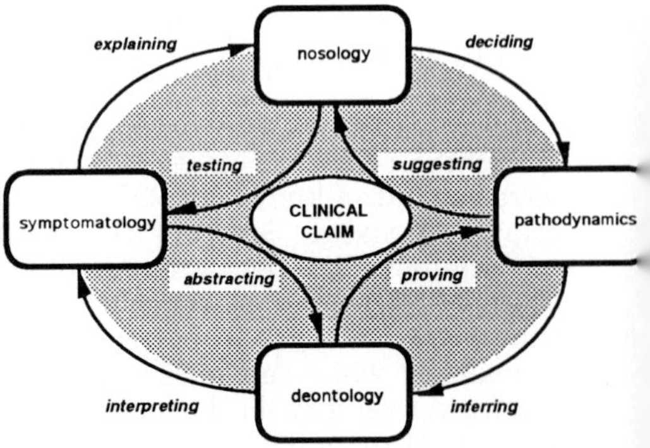

Figure 3. MACCORD

As one tries to apply the evolving concepts to a domain as complex as medicine one inevitably becomes confronted with the notion of conceptual levels. One reason for this is that very often meta-considerations or meta-decisions have to be taken into account. For instance, compared to the decision in favour of a certain form of therapy, the decision to treat the patient at all is a meta-decision. Another argument for conceptual levels is the idea that when reasoning reaches an impassé this has to be resolved at a somewhat "higher" level.

Furthermore, problem solving activities under different circumstances (scarce resources, time constraints, limited availability of data) tend to utilise knowledge located on levels that vary according to categories such as "heuristic vs. deterministic", "causal vs. associative" or "shallow vs. deep" models.

All levels (strategic, tactical, operative) have the form of abductive-deductive cycles, extended by backward leading transitions and are linked via (empirical, hypothetical, theoretical, experimental) columns.

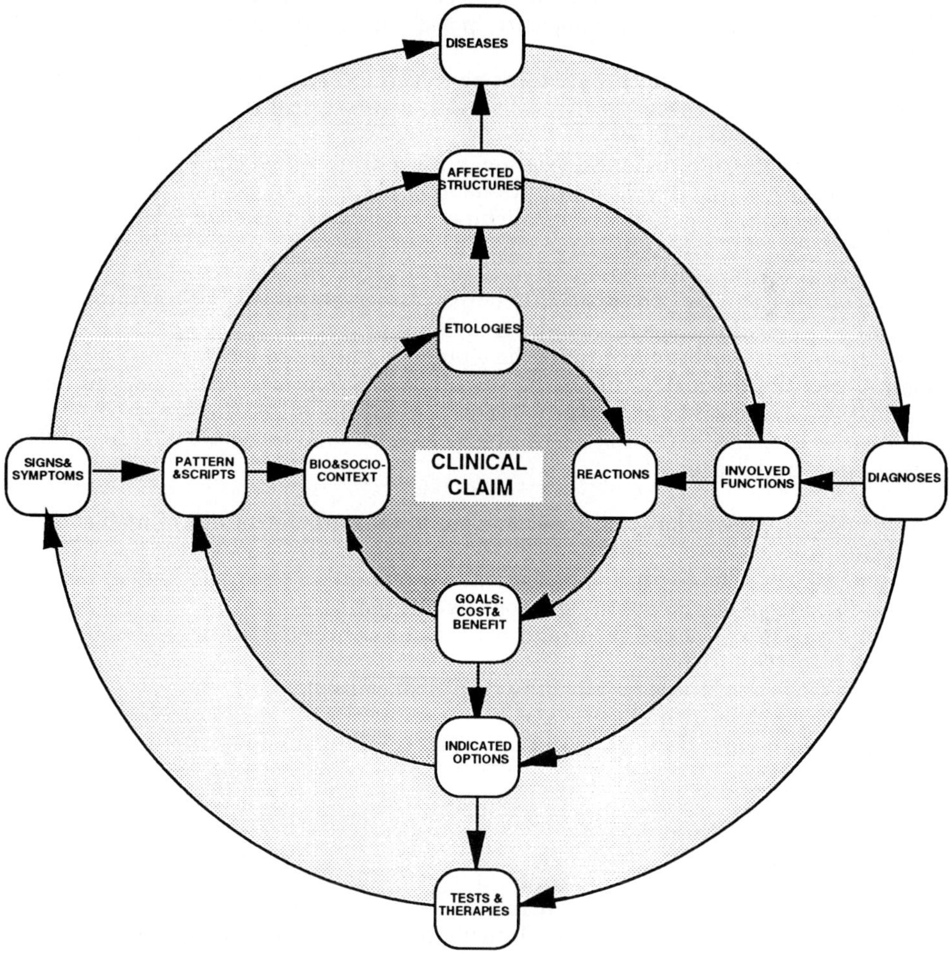

Figure 3. Diagnostic-therapeutical reasoning in the ACCORD model

The *strategic* level deals with knowledge of the environment in which problem solving takes place. With regard to medicine this may be the constitutional or situative factors of the patient (expositions, psychic and social situation), seasonal or epidemiological circumstances and the like, moreover the "never changing" anatomical and etiological categories, but also the (meta-)criteria for the evaluation of procedural methods (specificity, sensitivity, invasiveness, risk...) and the patient´s health status (comfort, abilities, development potential).

The knowledge provided by medical *specialtiies* is mainly found at the *tactical* level: pathognomonic constellations of findings and principal signs, specific knowledge concerning the etiological nature of disorders at various anatomical sites, detailed pathophysiological knowledge(...).

Knowledge organised at the lowest, the *operative*, level is most concrete: the raw, uninterpreted observations, specific hypotheses as well as diagnoses or particular tests and therapies are found at the operative level. To a degree, the operative level amounts to what constitutes expertise in a domain.

Similar to the intuitive introduction of levels, one may circumscribe the meaning of the columns that develop from opposite "poles" on the circumference of the circle by juxtaposing several levels:

The *empirical* column simply contains everything that is (or has been) observable. Signs, symptoms or values (concrete) as well as historical facts or epidemiological constellations (abstract).

The *hypothetical* column is the location of structures which can be *assumed* on the basis of observations. Such assumptions may concern anatomical localisations of varying precision (such as *hepatobiliary system* and *ductus choledochus*) or etiological classes (such as *infectious disease* and *inborn metabolic disturbance*).

Theoretical concepts can be found in the *theoretical* column. In clinical medicine, what we mean by theoretical concepts are mainly physiological or pathophysiological notions describing functional properties of the human body.

The *experimental* column contains the elements which render medicine an actional science oriented towards influencing the signs & symptoms of the patient. These are tests & therapies, procedural classes (such as *substitution, provocation, determination*) that are subject to meta-criteria such as *sensitivity, specificity, invasiveness* and the like.

It is relatively easy to locate the various subfields and disciplines of medicine. For example:

- anatomical knowledge can to a large extent be found in the hypothetical models at the tactical level: localisations, sites of predilection...
- pathophysiology provides the theoretical terms defining pathophysiological states and their interrelations
- epidemiology constitutes much of the empirical context
- the link between principal signs and suspected localisations / possible causes is the main content of standard textbooks on differential diagnosis
- ...

3. MACCORD & CSCW

The *MACCORD methodology* is an interpretation framework for the mapping of domain structures onto conceptual models able to be expressed in formal representations of a transparent knowledge space, as a basis for cooperative medical decision making - thus a step nearer to implementational constructs. From a technical point of view, a CSCW system has to be developed for the integration of multimedia documents and interfaces on the basis of integrated patient files.

The concept has to be supported by a knowledge based control system addressing staff members involved in examination schedules. Gaps within and contradictions of findings must be identified and further examinations then suggested. The advice is to be backed by multimedia support information concerning the execution of diagnostic steps. Incorporating a database of pertinent medical records, the diagnosis shall furthermore be assisted by case based reasoning. A knowledge based critique module of diagnoses can be attuned as an example of local diagnosis support systems. The knowledge based system can be applied as an on line-tutoring or decision support system.

We are technically ready to realise this vision, typically referred to as *"open systems"*. Open systems support an architectural framework that delivers *portatbility, scalability and interoperability*, giving us choice in selecting hardware platforms and standard ways for computing resources to communicate in heterogeneous computing environments. The UNIX operating system and OSI communications standards are well known technologies that fit the open systems framework, but not officially part of this framework are also RISC-based workstations and midrange server which run UNIX , relational database systems and graphical user interfaces. A convention typically used to denote very high level of computing performance is the term "on-line transaction processing". Workstation and server hardware technology has reached the needed level of performance, but some of the software components are critical: database management software, network management software, and transaction processing software. Although some of these components are at more advanced stages than others, they are still in early stages of maturity for open systems that need to support large "on-line transaction processing" environments.

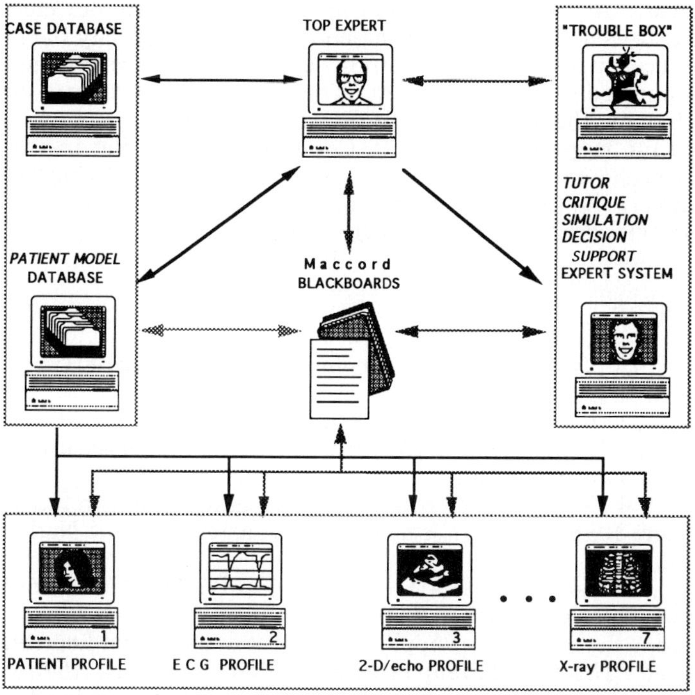

Figure 4. The structure of Maccord & CSCW in cardiology

Nevertheless there are advanced software-tools which could be used for the main parts of the Maccord&CSCW System, interacting via a blackboard-like formalism :
- database - containing patient data (*ORACLE, SYBASE*);
- knowledge base - containing knowledge about the entire diversity of medical reasoning, described in formal Maccord terminology (*NexpertObject*);
- hypermedia interface - exploiting thoroughly the possibilities of multimedia techniques both for user input and output (*Open Interface*).

According to the *"Knowledge-Sharing Effort"*-Project [15] we feel justified in stating that the problematic aspects of knowledge acquisition, representation and maintenance, the development of modular, extendible, flexible and explainable CSCW systems for medical domains can only be addressed with reasonable hope of success if an appropriate conceptual structure of the system has been gained.

4. CONCLUSIONS

In order to build a new generation of medical decision support systems, the large conceptual gap between the mental models of human experts and formal representations in programming languages / shell systems has to be bridged. The Maccord framework allows: realistic modelling of adequate support in cooperative diagnoses; efficient integration of human and technical performances; embedding of locally delimited expert systems; integration of easily understandable multimedia explanations via stepwise and inarbitrary reconstruction of the problem solving competence of medical experts as a prerequisite for an appropriate architecture of both medical data & knowledge bases and the "reasoning device".

The use of rigorous mathematical and logical methods within this framework can produce important theoretical and practical results. This is because the distributed knowledge base of ACCORD takes into consideration the complex character of the cognition process as a multi-level phenomenon and tries to satisfy the requirements of the formal reconstruction of intelligent behaviour with an architecture facilitating Computer Supported Cooperative Work. The appropriate structure for knowledge bases provided by the general ACCORD framework plays a very important heuristic role for Hypermedia Human Computer Interaction in the knowledge acquisition, storage and utilisation process, since existing AI programming tools efficiently support the ACCORD paradigm for problem solving and can be adopted for the building of "second generation" expert systems.

5. REFERENCES

1 Chandrasekaran B., Towards a Taxonomy of Problem Solving Types, AI Magazine, 4, 1, 1983
2 Bylander T., Chandrasekaran B., Generic Tasks for Knowledge-Based Reasoning: The "Right" Level of Abstraction for Knowledge Acquisition, International Journal of Man-Machine Studies, 26, 1, 1987.
3 J. Breuker et al., Model-Driven Knowledge Acquisition: Interpretation Models, Esprit Project 1098, Memo 87, University of Amsterdam, The Netherlands, 1987.
4 Wielinga B., Breuker J., KADS-II, Esprit Project P5248, Memo, University of Amsterdam, The Netherlands, 1990.
5 Kolb D.A., Fry R., Towards an Applied Theory of Experiential Learning, in: Cooper C. (ed.) Theories of group processes, Wiley, New York, 1975.
6 Sneed J.D., The Logical Structure of Mathematical Physics (rev. ed.), Reidel, Dordrecht, 1979.
7 W. Balzer , C.U. Moulines, J.D. Sneed, An Architectonic for Science - The Structuralist Program, D. Reidel Publishing Company, Dordrecht/ Boston/ Lancaster / Tokyo, 1987.
8 Petkoff B., Ein kybernetisches Modell der wissenschaftlichen Forschung, proc. 7th Int. Cong. on Logic, Methodology and Philosophy of Science, Salzburg, 1983.
9 Petkoff B., Artificial Intelligence and Computer Simulation of Scientific Discovery, proc. Artificial Intelligence - Methodology, Systems, Applications (AIMSA), Varna, W. Bibel & B. Petkoff (eds.), North-Holland, 1984.
10 Petkoff B., ACCORD - a Metamodel for IInd Generation Expert Systems, proc. 3rd International Conference Artificial Intelligence - Methodology, Systems, Applications (AIMSA), Amsterdam, North-Holland, 1988.

11 Kraus D., Petkoff B., Mannebach H., Maccord: Reconstructing Medical Problem Solving Competence, proc. Third European Conference on Artificial Intelligence in Medicine (AIME), Maastricht, Springer, 1991.
12 Mannebach H., Petkoff B., Kraus D., Maccord: Towards an Understanding of the Structure of Medical Knowledge, proc. AAAI Spring Symposium on Artifical Intelligence in Medicine, Stanford University, California, 1992
13 Petkoff B., Kraus D.,Computer Assisted Medical Decision Making, proc. 11th European Meeting on Cybernetics and System Research (EMCSR), Vienna, World Scientific Publishing Company, 1992.
14 Kraus D., Petkoff B., Mannebach H., Kirkby S., Reconstructing Medical Problem Solving Competence: MACCORD, Methods of Information in Medicine, Schatauer Verlagsgesellschaft, 1993
15 Neches R. et al. (1991): Enabling Thechnology for Knowledge Sharing, AI Magasine, FALL 91

Artificial Intelligence in Medecine
S. Andreassen et al. , Eds.
IOS Press, 1993

CLINICAL APPLICATION OF A GENERAL METHOD FOR DECISION - SUPPORT SYSTEMS

Mark Leaning[1], Peter Samuel[2],Tony Austin[1], Taher Hassan[1], Michael Modell[3], David Patterson[4] and Robert Rubens[5]

1. Clinical Operational Research Unit, University College London. 2. Concurrent Computer Corporation Ltd. 3. Department of Primary Health Care, Whittington Hospital, London. 4. Cardiac Department, Whittington Hospital, London. 5 ICRF Clinical Oncology Unit, Guy's Hospital, London.

ABSTRACT

The GAMES method for medical knowledge based decision support system construction is based on a select-and-test model of a medical decision making task. This paper reports the approach to clinical validation of the model which has been undertaken by applying it to a range of diagnostic and treatment planning tasks in asthma, cancer and intensive care. The potential applicability of the select-and-test model to patient monitoring is also discussed.

Keywords: artificial intelligence; medicine; knowledge-based systems; decision support systems; asthma; cancer; intensive care.

INTRODUCTION

The potential advantages of a general method for the development of medical knowledge based decision support systems are well understood: it should allow the development of common software tools for building different systems; greater rigour and system reliability achieved by following a standard tested approach; reusability of knowledge-bases in different applications. In addition, such methods provide a deeper understanding of medical knowledge and decision making. However, in order to justify the term "general" there is a need to establish the validity and applicability of a methodology across the range of medical domains in both clinical and scientific terms. These considerations apply over and above the issues of evaluating individual decision-support systems. This paper focuses on the clinical validation of a high level knowledge model (or "epistemological" model) which underlies the method for medical knowledge based system construction being developed as part of the CEC AIM GAMES-II project. The model is the select-and-test model (the "ST-model") of a generic medical decision making task (Ramoni et al., 1992).

[1]Correspondence: Dr Mark S Leaning, Clinical Operational Research Unit, Department of Statistical Science, University College London, Gower Street, London WC1E 6BT. Tel: (+44)-71-380-7835. Fax: (+44)-71-383-4703. Email: mark@uk.ac.ucl.coru.

DECISION MAKING TASKS IN PATIENT MANAGEMENT AND THE ST-MODEL

The patient management process is considered to comprise 3 basic decision-making tasks as shown in Fig. 1. The arrows show the usual sequences of tasks, although multiple tasks may be active simultaneously, for example in the management of a critically-ill patient. Each task generates a set of decisions, referred to as hypotheses, corresponding to diagnoses, treatment plans and monitoring outcomes.

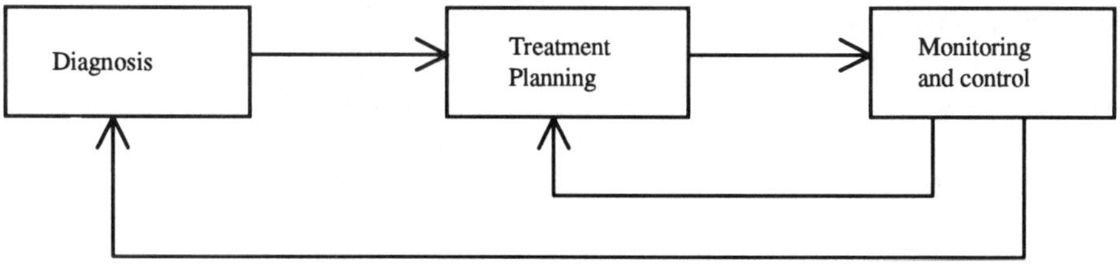

Figure 1. Basic Decision Making Tasks in the Patient Management Process

In GAMES, the aim is to represent each of the basic decision making tasks with the same underlying inference model - the ST-model in Fig. 2. The operation of the ST-model is as follows (for more detailed discussion refer to Ramoni et al, 1992). The decision making process begins with the abstraction of a schema from the currently available data. The schema is an organisation of the data, or subsets of the data, which may also contain qualitative and temporal abstractions. The schema triggers an abductive inference selecting those hypotheses which are consistent with the schema and data. Each hypothesis may have additional expected findings which can be deduced in order to guide the collection of more data. These data once collected will confirm or eliminate hypotheses through an inductive inference step.

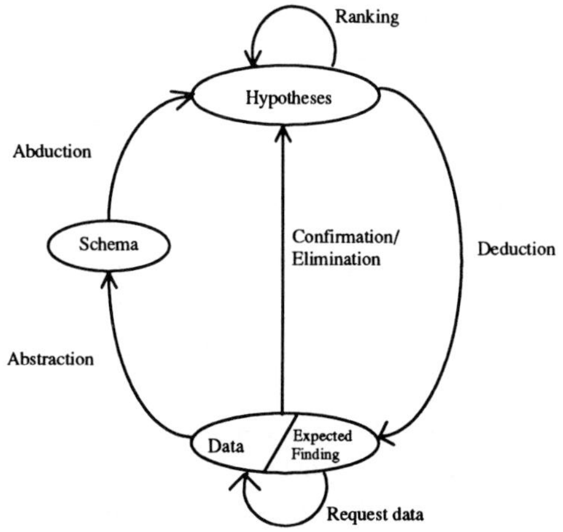

Figure 2. The Select-and-Test Model for a Decision Making Task

The ST-model is a high level knowledge, or epistemological model. It is not concerned with which formalisms are to be used for representation of factual knowledge (ontologies) or for implementing inference steps. In the following sections, we review the applications of the ST-model to a range of medical areas and decision tasks. This is achieved by filling-in the general model of Fig. 2 with classes of data, schemas and hypotheses relevant to each problem area. It is important to note that in the different applications of the ST-model it is only the contents of the ellipses (the ontologies) which change. The inference steps remain the same.

ST-MODELS FOR SINGLE TASKS

The simplest application of ST-models is to single decision tasks. Figure 3 shows the ST-model instantiated for the diagnosis of asthma. Here, the hypotheses are diagnoses of asthma and related respiratory disorders.

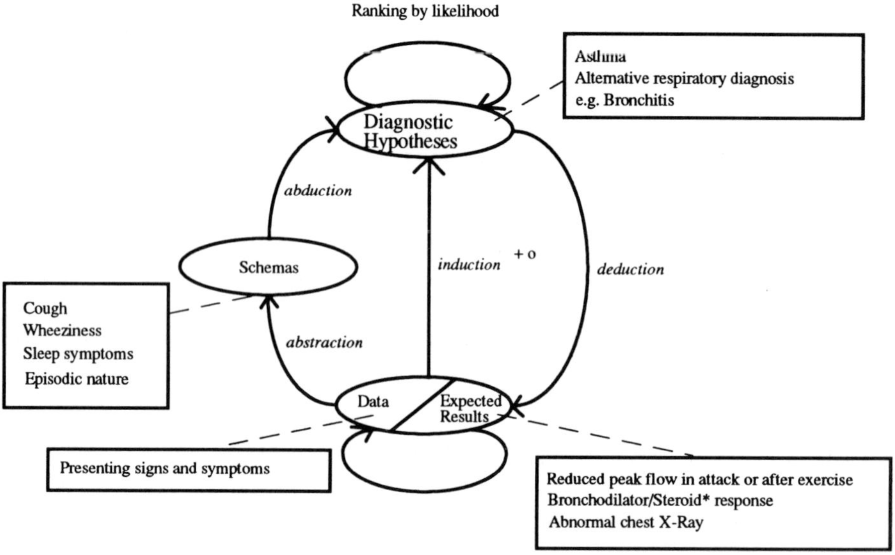

* Results from bronchodilators or steroid treatment

+ Reduced peak flow measurement reversible by bronchodilators or steroids will increase likelihood of asthma diagnosis

o Abnormal chest X-Ray increases likelihood of alternative diagnoses.

Figure 3. ST-Model for Diagnosis of Asthma

Figure 4 shows the model applied to planning chemotherapy for advanced cancer. Here, the hypotheses are treatment plans including its intentions and details of the regimens. An initial set of possible chemotherapy regimens is abducted from a schema containing the tumour type and the spread of the disease. The deduction and induction steps are concerned with eliminating regimens containing potentially contraindicated drugs. Once that has been completed the balance between expected response and toxic side effects needs to be made for each regimen before a decision is made. The final decision in this case will also need to consider patient's wishes. The behaviour of the model emulates that of an episodic skeletal plan refinement algorithm (Musen et al, 1992), gradually decomposing abstract plans into more detailed ones.

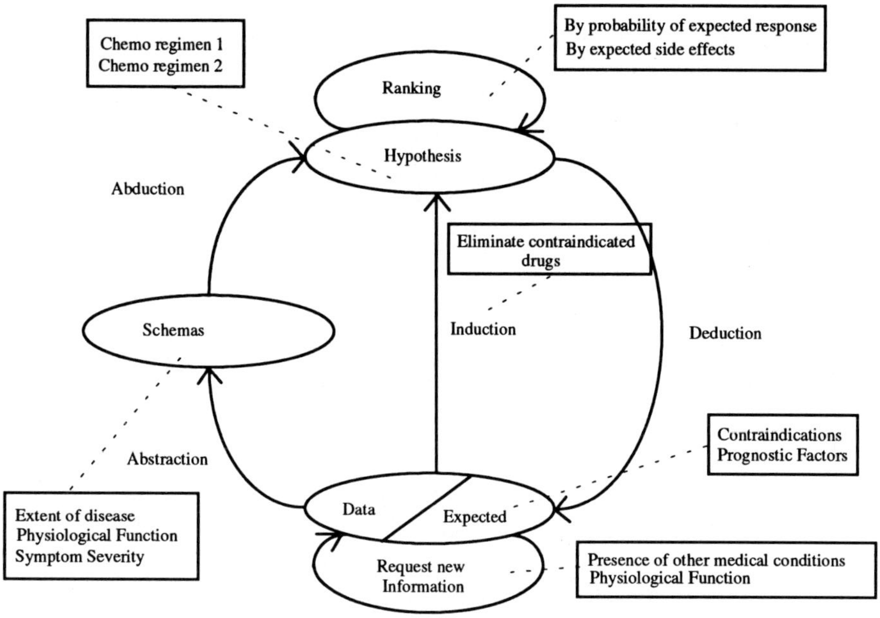

Figure 4. ST-Model for Treatment Planning of Palliative Chemotherapy in Advanced Cancer

INTERACTIONS BETWEEN ST-MODELS IN SEQUENTIAL AND ITERATIVE DECISION MAKING

Different ST-models for diagnosis, treatment planning and monitoring (Fig. 1) can be coupled to provide an overall knowledge model for patient management. In moving from task to task, the knowledge roles of different entities changes. For example, diagnoses are mapped to hypotheses in the diagnostic task but are regarded as data items in treatment planning. On the GAMES project, examples of sequentially connected ST-models have been developed for acute radiation syndrome, nosocomial infection, liver transplantation and shock (Fig. 5). However, there are many situations, ranging from chronic disease management to the unstable patient in intensive care, where there is constant iteration or feedback between medical decision tasks. At the overall level in Fig. 1 these are easy to depict. When showing the coupling between ST-models the interactions are more complex.

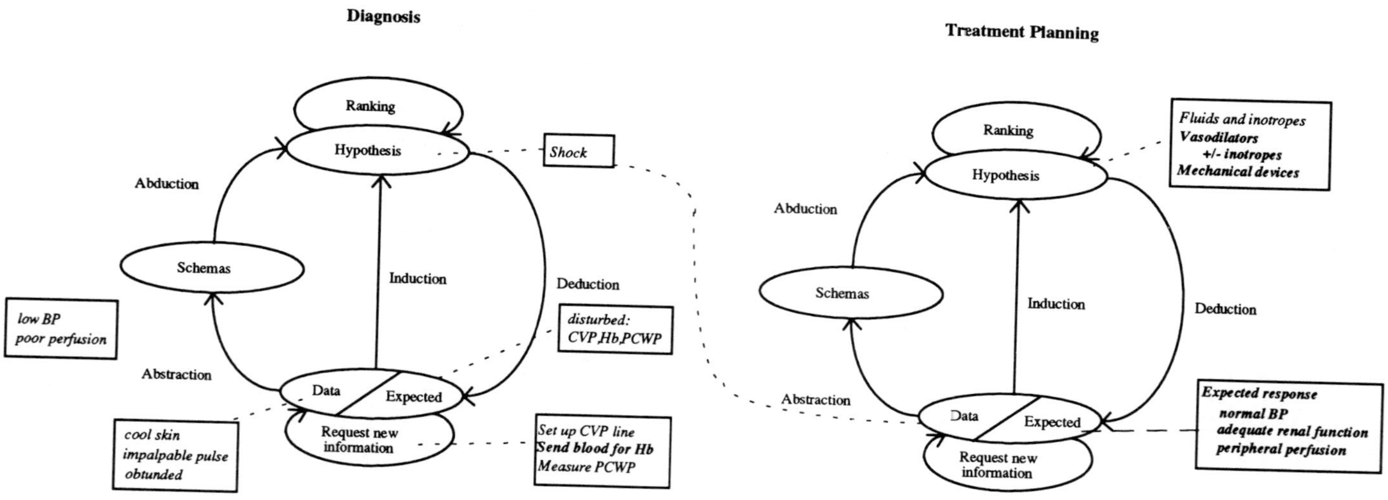

Figure 5. First Stage of Diagnosing Shock, Requesting Data and Initial Treatment Planning
Initial diagnosis of shock includes cardiac, septic, anaphylactic and haemorrhagic shock.

DISCUSSION

In addition to the medical areas described above, the ST-model has also been applied to graft versus host disease, liver transplantation, nosocomial infection, diabetes, asthma and neonatal icterus. The results indicate that the ST-model should have substantial face validity as a knowledge model for diagnostic and treatment planning tasks across a wide area of medicine, and is useful as a knowledge acquisition tool. As part of this work, detailed ontologies for findings, diagnoses and treatments in the various areas have also been developed. We have encountered areas where there is a case for additional basic tasks - for example, prognosis and prioritisation of potential patients for organ transplantation. We believe the ST-model should have validity for the monitoring task in which a comparison is made between the goals/expectation of treatment and outcome - if it is possible to identify the appropriate hypotheses for outcome. This reflects a general difficulty of defining and measuring outcomes in clinical care (Hopkins, 1992). It is also arguable that monitoring is a composite task involving assessment (equivalent to diagnosis) and prediction as well as comparison and control. The validity and applicability of the ST-model for the monitoring task is thus less well established.

The models presented here and in Leaning and Samuel (1992) are currently being implemented in M-KAT, a knowledge acquisition tool developed in the University of Pavia (Lanzola and Stefanelli, 1992). M-KAT is based on the ST-model and has an automatic facility for running ST-models at any stage in their development. It is written in KEE (Trademark, Intellicorp). M-KAT represents hypotheses, abstractions and findings classes as hierarchies, with abstraction, abduction and other inference knowledge implemented as rules. Meta-level rules control the overall inference process according to Fig. 2. In addition, the GAMES-II project is developing graphical editors for ontologies at the University of Amsterdam.

The clinicians on the project have found that the ST-model and other aspects of the GAMES method have provided them with a framework that provides insight into medical decision making in everyday clinical practice. This is a benefit independent of the eventual construction of decision support systems.

ACKNOWLEDGEMENTS

The Clinical Operational Research Unit is also funded by the UK Department of Health .

This paper reflects the views of its authors but draws upon the work of many colleagues, particularly that of Mario Stefanelli and his group to whom we are indebted. The work has been undertaken as part of the CEC AIM GAMES-II project (A2034) and we acknowledge the contributions of our partners: SAGO (Italy), University of Amsterdam (Holland), University of Pavia (Italy), Forth (Greece), Geneva University Hospital (Switzerland), University of Ulm (Germany). We particularly acknowledge the medical panel without whom this work would not have been possible.

REFERENCES

Hopkins A. Measuring the quality of medical care. *Royal College of Physicians*, 1990.

Lanzola G and Stefanelli M. A specialized framework for medical knowledge based systems. *Computers and Biomedical Research* 1992, 25: 351-365.

Leaning MS and Samuel P (Eds.). Identification of exemplar medical problems areas for evaluation of GAMES. *CEC GAMES-II Project (A2034)*, Deliverable 11, December 1992.

Musen M, Tu SW and Shahar Y. A problem-solving model for protocol-based care: from e-ONCOCIN to EON. In *Medinfo 92* 1992, 519-525.

Ramoni M, Stefanelli M, Barosi G and Magnani L. An epistemological framework for medical knowledge based systems. *IEEE Transactions on Systems, Man and Cybernetics* 1992, 2 1361-1375.

Artificial Intelligence in Medecine
S. Andreassen et al. , Eds.
IOS Press, 1993

Employment of Dr.Watson Type Systems (Dr.WTS) in medicine on the example of supporting decision making by a physician of the Regional Children Reanimation Consultative Centre.

S.I. Goldberg[a], E.K. Tsibulkin[b], A.O. Makhanek[a] and L.D. Meshalkin[c]

[a]Physiology Institute, Ural Branch of Russian Academy of Sciences
30 Popov Street, Yekaterinburg, 620014, Russia

[b]Emergency Pediatrics Chair, Sanct-Petersburg Pediatrics Institute
2 Litovsky Prospect, Sanct-Petersburg, Russia

[c]Mathematical Statistics Chair, Department of Applied Mathematics and Cybernetics, Moscow State University, Lenin's Hills, Moscow, Russia

Abstract.
A new class of computer intellectual systems for assisting high-skilled specialists is offered. Its destructive feature is an increased attention to stimulation methods of a specialist's intellectual activity. Characteristics of the class are demonstrated on the example of DINAR-2.2 system supporting decision making by the physician- reanimatologist on duty of the Regional Children Reanimation Consultative Centre (RCC).

1. INTRODUCTION

In spite of considerable successes achieved by artificial intelligence systems (AI) in medicine there is a common opinion that large intellectual and financial investments into this sphere have not been followed by an adequate effect, in practical application of machine intelligence.

Here, some ways of raising the efficiency of AI-systems are offered. And we fully agree with the administrative measures proposed by E. Shortliffe [1], with the ideas of Miller and Maserie [2] on maximum interactive style of the programs being developed and with necessity of rigorous scientific evaluation studies on systems [3]. However, we believe it expedient to consider one more direction proceeding from the fact that direct proposal of intellectual conclusions is not always acceptable for the specialist. Quite often even the best of the systems directly proposing decisions are used in an unreal scale of time, but as teaching, testing or a posteriori consulting ones.

At the same time, sometimes even an indirect intellectual aid, stimulating a specialist may prove to be very useful for him. Even such a famous specialist as Mr.Holmes willingly used to take services of a less skilled amateur-detective Dr.Watson and more often than of another famous deduction master - his brother Microft. Inspired by the example of relationship between Dr.Watson and Mr.Holmes. We tried to construct a new specific class of AI-systems. The systems, which like Dr.Watson document assist, provide for convenience in the work and, which is most important, stimulate the intellectual activity of the specialist, we shall call "Dr.Watson type systems" (Dr.WTS) [4].

The present report mainly deals with the description of their basic features (from our point of view) on the example of the latest version - DINAR-2.2, constructed along these lines the system of supporting decision making by a duty physician-consultant of the Regional Children Reanimation Consultative Centre. Its main task is to consult physicians of remote centres in diagnostics therapy and tactical actions for a severely ill infant [5].

2. METHODS

Turning to the description of Dr.WTS's characteristics, let us note that a part of them is peculiar not only to Dr.WTS, but for the successful practical functioning, as our experience shows, there is a necessity of fulfilling all the conditions mentioned below: "subordination", "integrability", "fullnes", and "stimulation".

2.1. Subordination

The priority of a specialist's opinion over the program conclusions is absolute and included in Dr.WTS - work technology. So in DINAR-2 the program offers quite a few successive conclusions: diagnosis assessment of state severity degree, state dynamics assessment, therapy effect assessment, tactics, treatment and so on. On each stage the physician can select his own decision and namely this is taken into account in all the following conclusions of the computer. That is more the physician knows that only his opinions stay in the computer's memory. Besides a somewhat small obligatory dialogue with a program, the physician himself selects the profundity of working out separate themes, employments of those or other additional functions of the system, trust degree to the information about a patient, being obtained from the local physician, qualification assessment of the consulted physician.

2.2. Integrability

This is the "carporability" of a system in an available world of informational technologies. This requirement becomes obligatory for all AI-systems, moreover it is necessary for Dr.WTS. So in DINAR there are an information-reference subsystem, a subsystem of forming analytical forms and forms of account, an electronic recording block. DINAR is joined to an independent system of acquisition and analysis of infant mortality.

2.3. Fullness

This is keeping all the aspects of a specialist's activity provided with informational and intellectual support. From the first versions of DINAR the scope of tasks being decided was put above decision accuracy of a separate task. One of the most important factors of "vitality" and broad inculcation of DINAR is that all intellectual tasks are decided with a program as it were "by side" while filling the effectively constructed electronic case history.

2.4. Stimulation

This is the most specific characteristic of Dr.WTS. It is directed to prompt a specialist to be more attentive and critical to his actions or to try to decide tasks beyond the limits of standard actions. For these purposes DINAR-2.2 uses the following means and methods:

(a) Psychological ones, for example a physician is offered to predict an effect of therapy he administered. Correlation of the prediction with the real course of the disease is the base for a game series, playing an important role for the whole system of DINAR-2.2.

(b) Methodological ones DINAR tries with the help of a full-length scheme of a successive decision making to work out a doctor's systemic approach in treatment of the concrete patient. A central part of DINAR is the formalized system of a patient's state severity assessment with consideration (besides physiological parameters assessment) of the current therapy, state dynamics, therapy efficacy.

(c) Visualization of information. An active use of charts and pictograms. In DINAR-2.2 development of a pathological process is reproduced in the form of "flower growth"and the collected clinical information about the patient's current state - in the form of a "specifically painted circle".

(d) Contecstual reference information.

(e) Offering alternative variants of decisions by the program.

The choice of adequate stimulation methods occurs through the understanding of common nature of errors which arise in a specialist. Quite often such errors are not limited to insuficient knowledge or a lack of logical mentality. So a physician during the process of information acquisition is often under the influence of some hypothesis and sees only "convenient" signs for him. In DINAR-2 a special mathematical apparatus is worked out for decision making in conditions of in such a way distorted information [6].

The principal idea of the method lies in a work with a great difference of information about a patient having been in the RCC from that of the real situation. It's supposed that the given distortion may be caused by four reasons:

- Inattentiveness or incompetence of the local physicians;
- Divergence of notions and terms in the RCC and among local physicians;
- The desire to present the patient's state milder or more severe than it is in reality;
- The desire to follow one's initially selected hypothesis, i.e. the physician sees only what he wants to.

Taking this into account, information about the patient is described as a fuzzy set. Information being suspected by the system DINAR for inaccuracy of the answer is specified with the help of assigning leading questions deciphering terms, breaking up complex notions into more simple ones. If a distortion of the state severity or a bent for a selected hypothesis is suspected then an algorithm of the DINAR goes on asking while the obtained decision **g** isn't steady with purposeful changing the information. So that

$$\mathbf{g(i^*)=g(D(I^*))} \quad \text{and} \quad \mathbf{g(i^*)=g(G(I^*))}$$

where **G(I*)** is maximally corrupted information aside of the initially established diagnosis, **D(I*)** is maximally corrupted information of the patient's state severity. Value and direction of a maximally possible data corruption are being changed in the process of the algorithm's work, and depend on co-ordination of the transmitted information.

3. CONCLUSIONS

Application of the stimulation methods from our point of view is very effective, but delicate as well. Lack of measure in the use of these methods may give a reverse effect. Especially dangerous is obliging a specialist to use these or other methods. Precisely a convenience and "imperceptibility" of Dr.WTS are basic characteristics of the systems. When introducing new methods of stimulation and for DINAR assessment as a whole in the Yekaterinburg RCC there were conducted questionings of users of DINAR and carried out statistics of appeals to various functions of the system.

The system DINAR which uses many of the methods described above has been bought by 12 regions of Russia, and Reanimation Consultative Centres working with it embrace more than 5,000,000 children. However, the joint consideration of DINAR-2.1 and the developed project on mathematical statistics as Dr.WTS allowed to enrich both of the projects and served as a base for creating DINAR-2.2. We hope that for other projects such a view can turn out to be useful too.

4. REFERENCES

1 E.H. Shortliff, Knowledge-based systems in medicine. In: Medical Informatics Europe 1991, Vienna, Austria, 1991, p.270-4.

2 R.A. Miller and F.E. Maserie, The Demise of the "Greek Oracle". Model for Medical Diagnostic Systems. Meth. Info. Med., 1990, v.29, p.1-2.

3 K. Clarke, R. O'Moore, R. Smeets, J. Talmon, J. Brender, P. McNair, J. Grimson and B. Barber, A Methodology for Evaluation of Knowledge-Based Systems. In: Medical Informatics Europe 1991, Vienna, Austria, 1991, p.361-366.

4 S.I. Goldberg, L.D. Meshalkin, A New Class of AI-Systems (DrWT-Systems). In: Tekhnicheskaya Kibernetika, N.5, 1992, p.217-223.

5 S.I. Goldberg, V.E. Lomovskikh, A.O. Makhanek, M.S. Sklyar, Expert system "DINAR-2" - methodological basis for the pediatric emergency aid organization in a large region. In: Medical Informatics Europe 1991, Vienna, Austria, 1991, p.270-274.

6 S.I. Goldberg, A.O. Makhanek, I.D. Novikov, Control consultation expert systems. Basic Properties and a realization example. Vestnik VOIVT, VIMI, v.1, 1991, p.46-52 (in russian).

Strategies for Medical Reasoning - Applications

Artificial Intelligence in Medecine
S. Andreassen et al. , Eds.
IOS Press, 1993

GAZE: An Attentional Mechanism for the Extraction of Prominent Facial Features

R. Herpers, H. Kattner and G. Sommer*

GSF - Medis Institut
Institut für medizinische Informatik und Systemforschung
Ingolstädter Landstr. 1 D-85764 Oberschleißheim
Email: herpers@gsf.de

Abstract

In this paper a technical realization of an attentional mechanism extracting salient regions in face images is presented. Using the knowledge of the eye movement strategies of the human visual system the attentional mechanism localizes prominent regions in natural images. Elementary visual features are derived from high-resolution digitized images and represented in a so called topographical attention map. A top-down algorithm analyzes this map implemented as a multi-scale representation by searching the most salient features in each represented scale. The scale information is propagated from coarse scales to the next higher resolutions while the extent of the fixated region is adapted. After the extraction the selected and now locally limited regions are analyzed and interpreted. The proposed attentional mechanism is part of an image processing system identifying faces with dysmorphic signs. To improve the classification of a local analysis module, it is intended to examine these characteristic areas with specialized algorithms. This knowledge based approach shows that an artificial attention control system is capable of localizing the prominent facial areas (eyes, mouth, nose, etc.) in face images only based on elementary image features. The proposed algorithm can also be used to detect other attentive regions in any images based on appropriate features.

1. Introduction

Image processing algorithms whose realization do not include attentional influences have been shown to be computationally intractable [1]. The visual search task in the bottom-up case is NP-Complete in the size of the image, while the task-directed case has linear time complexity in the number of items in the display. These complexity considerations suggest that attentional mechanisms may be required to perform successfully an image analysis problem in real time.

Inspired by the eye movement strategies of the human visual system [2] the attentional mechanism selects prominent areas of the image to analyze only the information essential to a current task [3]. Irrelevant image regions are ignored and do not need to be processed further. Thus, image processing with attention control simplifies computation and reduces the amount of processing [4].

*Present address: Institut für Informatik, Lehrstuhl Kognitive Systeme, Universität Kiel, Preußerstr. 1-9, D-24105 Kiel

At the early stage of preattentive processing elementary features like motion, color, orientation, edge information and others are derived in the human visual system [5]. These features establish a preattentive representation, the so called "primal sketch" [6]. The control of the visual attention is based on this representation, which localizes spatial regions of interest in the order of their importance.

This paper presents a technical realization of an attentional mechanism simulating these physiological strategies. The approach is based on investigations of J. Tsotsos, who first developed "a prototype for data-driven visual attention" [7, 8]. Certain aspects of this model are not addressed in the presented paper, such as the inhibition of not relevant regions or the neural like modelling. Instead, emphasis is placed on a fast data-driven realization of an attentional mechanism localizing the prominent regions in face images. Our attentional mechanism will be used as an essential component in the building of a complete image processing system identifying faces with dysmorphic abnormalities [9].

The proposed model consists of a topographical attention map coded in a multi-scale representation and an algorithm propagating the selected regions from coarse scales to the next higher resolution. For the results presented in this paper, two of the elementary visual features, edge and brightness information, are derived to guide the selective attention. The potential of the attention scheme is proposed by using facial 512x512 digitized gray-level images of normal and dysmorphic children.

2. Methods

The proposed attentional mechanism consists of a set of hierarchical computations. Task-oriented image information is derived and coded in a topological attention map comparable to preattentive visual stimuli. This map is transformed to a multi-scale representation and in the following analyzed to detect attentive image regions. A localized area is adapted to the extent of the underlying visual object and is extracted. After a local analysis it is suspended from the following processing of the attentional mechanism and the next salient region can be computed.

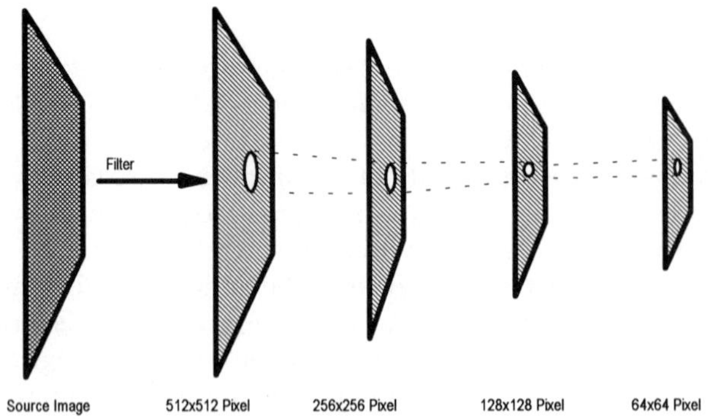

Fig. 1. Model of the multiscale representation. First, the original gray level image, the topological attention map in the highest resolution and 3 levels of an octave representation

2.1 Multi-scale representation

At the highest resolution, 512 x 512 pixel, the gray level image is transformed to a task-oriented image representation. The fast data-driven preattentive representation is given by the edge information provided by a 5 x 5 sobel filter, or alternatively by the brithtness information. The topological attention map is initialized with task-oriented weights which emphasize global image areas. For example, the image areas in the center are more important than the corners. The extracted image information is represented in the topological attention map by multiplication with a constant initialization. Multiresolution techniques are used to present the attention map in different scales [10]. We use a 5 x 5 gaussian convolution kernel to reduce the representation size (Fig. 1). The selection of an optimal scale representation is task-oriented and is one issue of this study. In a first approach tests were carried out using 4 or 5 octave pyramid levels and later 4 or less non octave levels of fixed size, because they enhance support of the detection of salient facial regions.

2.2 Adaptation of the extent

At the lowest resolution level of the attention map the actual, most attentive region is selected by a region based maximum search algorithm. The localized region is propagated through the entire hierarchy of the multi-resolution pyramid. The local extent of the underlying visual stimulus is adapted in a way that attentive visual objects will be detected completely. In each representation the region-growing is controlled by an algorithm which is determined by (1):

$$f(A) = 1 + \frac{A-1}{a\ (A-1)\ +\ b}; \qquad a, b > 0; \qquad (1)$$

where A is the area size and a, b are parameters determining the asymptotic properties of the region-growing algorithm [7,8].

In this study horizontal or vertical rectangles are used for matching attentive image regions (Fig. 2). During the adaptation process the edges of the calculated rectangle are expanded or reduced at each side of the rectangle.

2.3 Suspension of analyzed regions

At the highest resolution the detected regions are extracted and analyzed with specialized local algorithms [11]. After the analysis and local interpretation the focused regions are suspended from the following processing steps of the attentional mechanism. The intensity of the visual stimulus coded in the attention map is reduced to zero. We have examined two different procedures:

1) Constant reduction of the intensities in the whole detected area.
2) Gaussian like degradation beginning at the center of the extracted rectangle.

Schedular (2) produces a smooth alteration at the borders of the selected attentive region while the first one produces sharp changes. Very small attentive regions will suspend only corresponding small areas using the first proceeding. The second one can be tuned to suspend larger regions. We also investigated a temporal delay which gradually reduces the suspension. The temporal degradation enables a repeated detection of formerly suspended regions. Applying this procedure a dynamical artificial eye movement record is created during a continued processing of attentive image regions (Fig. 3).

3. Results and discussion

We have shown that an artificial attention mechanism based on elementary features is able to detect salient regions in face images. In this paper, only brightness and edge information is used as input to the presented mechanism. These two basic features are sufficient for the detection of prominent facial regions, although the use of other features is possible.

The selected regions (Fig. 2) as well as the computed scan path (Fig. 3), which resembles the eye movement strategies observed in the human visual system, show an appropriate accordance with the salient image areas.

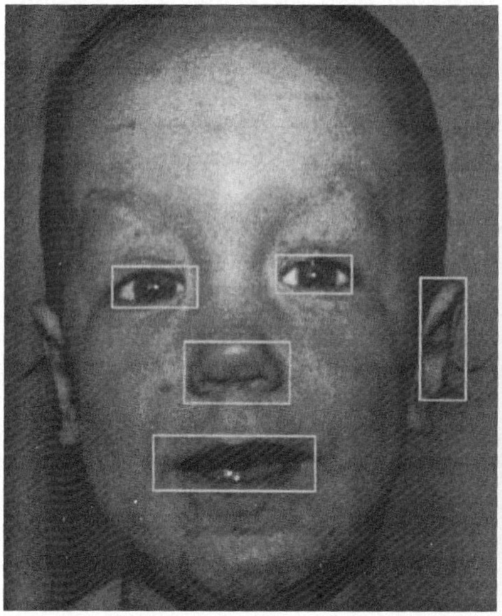

Fig. 2. Detection of characteristic facial regions

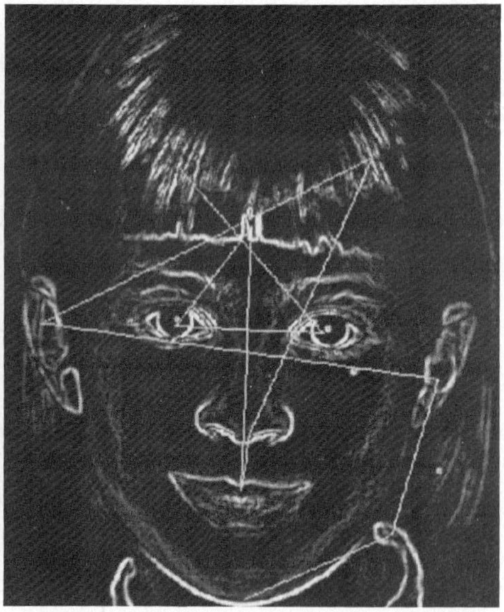

Fig. 3. Computer based attention record

The shown model is implemented in software on a SGI Indigo R4000 workstation and the measured performance in computing an attentional path with 20 steps lies between 7 and 10 seconds using high resolution, 8-bit, digitized, gray level images. The proposed algorithm is also tested on other real world images. The computed attentional mechanism localizes the salient areas in the natural scenes independent of the structure of the image data and the underlying task. There are no prerequisites to be taken like normalization or segmentation of the image data before the start of computation. The presented model can handle all sizes and arrangements of image objects within the processed data. The use of the model of processing hierarchies combined with a maximum search as against a neural based approach with inhibitory qualities enhances the performance of a sequential processing of the attentional mechanism.

Acknowledgements

We appreciate the support of Prof. Dr. S. Stengel-Rutkowski and Dr. C. Apacik, Institut für Soziale Pädiatrie und Jugendmedizin, Abteilung Genetik der Ludwig-Maximilian-Universität München, providing the images used in this study. We also thank Dr. W. Eckstein, Institut für Informatik IX der Technischen Universität München for helpful suggestions and stimulating discussions.

References

[1] J. K. Tsotsos, *The complexity of perceptual search task,* In: Proc. of the IJCAI, Detroit, pp. 1571-1577 (1989)

[2] A. L. Yarbus, *Eye Movements and Vision,* New York: Plenum Press (1967)

[3] C. Koch and S. Ullman, *Shifts in selective visual attention: Towards the underlying neural circuity,* Human Neurobiol. Vol. 4, pp. 279-283 (1985)

[4] B. Olshausen, C. Anderson and D. v. Essen, *A neural model of visual attention and invariant pattern recognition,* Tec. Rep CNS Memo 18, Caltech Pasadena (1992)

[5] A. Treisman, *Preattentive processing in vision,* CVGIP Vol. 31, pp. 156-177 (1985)

[6] D. Marr, *Vision,* W. H. Freeman, San Francisco (1982)

[7] S. M. Culhane and J. K. Tsotsos, *A prototype for data-driven visual attention,* In G. Sandini (ed.) Computer Vision ECCV´92, Springer-Verlag, pp. 551-560 (1992)

[8] J. K. Tsotsos, *Localizing stimuli in a sensory field using an inhibitory attentional beam* Tec.-Rep. M5s 1A4, University of Toronto, Dep. of Comp. Sc., Canada (1991)

[9] R. Herpers, H. Rodax and G. Sommer, *A neural network identifies faces with morphological syndromes,* In this proceedings (1993)

[10] P. J. Burt, *Multiresolution techniques for image representation, analysis and smart transmission,* SPIE Conf. 1199, pp. 1-14 (1989)

[11] M. Michaelis and G. Sommer, *Characterization of key-points in images,* accepted by Int. Symp. on Subst. Ident. Techn. ´93, Innsbruck (1993)

Artificial Intelligence in Medecine
S. Andreassen et al. , Eds.
IOS Press, 1993

PHARMNEPH: COMPUTER-SYSTEM FOR DRUG DOSAGE ADJUSTMENT IN RENAL FAILURE

Frieder Keller, Klaus Erdmann, Michael Giehl, David Czock.

Free University of Berlin, Steglitz Medical Complex, Medical Department, Hindenburgdamm 30, W-1000 (12200) Berlin 45, Germany. FON 030 798 3339, FAX 030 798 4141

Abstract

Drug dosage must be adjusted to kidney function to avoid toxic overdosage in patients with impaired renal function. These clinical demands must be attained within a hospital information system. The PHARMNEPH system is part of such a project. It is based on published pharmacokinetic knowledge standardized by nonparametric meta-analysis. A bayesian parameter estimate from population derived kinetics and sparce individual data will be implemented. Algorithms for a dosage calculation will be provided combining individual bayesian parameters with pharmacodynamic characteristics of each drug.

1. PRESENT DILEMMA

The kidneys are - next to the liver - the main route of drug elimination. It was the alarming experience with drug treatment in the 1970ies that severe adverse reactions occured mainly in patients with impaired renal function. The dosage of renally excreted drugs must be reduced if renal function is compromised [1]. It was the opposite extreme in the 1980ies that drug dosage was reduced too much to adjust for renal impairment. This had the detrimental consequence that the antiinfective treatment was subtherapeutic in many intensive care patients. It should be the aim of the 1990ies to avoid both overdosage and underdosage by a computer-assisted drug dosage adjustment.

Clinical pharmacokinetics of the last 20 years has elucidated how the elimination in nearly all commonly used drugs specifically depends on renal function [2]. This knowledge must be placed at the clinicians immediate disposal.

2. PREPARATORY WORK

We documented the published pharmacokinetic parameters of 1200 drugs in a 4 MB database with 980 primary citations of the literature (Figure 1). The documented parameters are the dominant elimination half life (T½), the volume of distribution (Vd), total drug clearance (CL), plasma protein binding (PB%) for normal renal function and anuria, respectively, along with the fraction eliminated by the renal route (fren) and the fraction (fR) eliminated by extracorporal procedures (hemodialysis, hemofiltration, hemoperfusion, plasmapheresis, peritoneal dialysis).

Evaluation of these 10.000 data revealed that the parameters of two thirds of all documented drugs depend on renal function. These documented population-derived pharmacokinetic parameters can be made accessible to be utilized for a computer-assisted dosage adjustment in renal failure. Such a utilization procedure is derived from Bayes' theorem. The probability (P) of a data set is the product of the probabilities of each point. These probabilities can be derived from Gaussian normal distribution and the standard deviation of parameters (SD).

$$P = \Pi [exp(-½([y - y(x)] / SD)^2)(dy)]$$

To maximize (P), the negative logarithm is minimized [3]. Thus, the probability (P) combines population derived knowledge on pharmacokinetic parameters (Kpop) with individual drug level measurements (Cind).

$$MIN = \Sigma([Kpop - Kind] / SDp)^2 + \Sigma([Cpop - Cind] / SDc)^2$$

This objective function is minimized to find out from a priori konowledge the a posteriori probability of individual parameters (Kind).

3. FUTURE PROJECT

Along with the factual knowledge, also procedural knowledge will be implemented into the database PHARMNEPH. The multitude of rough data published on each drug will be subjected to a statistical meta-analysis using the nonparametric median to generating the central parameter for the knowledge based drug information system. The most robust central value for a specific pharmacokinetic parameter (T½, Vd, Cl) is obtained by the nonparametric median with the 95 percent confidence interval [4]. In clinical practice the individual pharmacokinetics can rarely be calculated by standard pharmacostatistic programs. For this case the sparse clinical data (e.g. one single drug level) will be combined with the meta-analytically generated central parameter by the bayesian algorithm for an individual parameter estimate.

From these parameters an individual dosage proposal can be calculated according to explicitely stated therapeutic peak and trough levels. The decision on the appropriateness of dosage will be improved by graphic representation of the different drug level curves derived from usual dosage and from individual parameters [5]. Which concentration sould be considered therapeutic in renal failure patients, must be decided by an optimization algorithm which is based on the specific pharmacodynamics of efficacy and toxicity of each drug. Such a pharmacodynamic optimization procedure will be combined with pharmacokinetic algorithms for calculating dosage adjustments. In general, the pharmacodynamic effect (E) can be described by the Hill equation depending on the maximal effect (Emax), the concentration at half maximal effect (CE50) and the variable drug concentration (C).

$$E = (Emax\ C^h) / (CE50^h + C^h)$$

The more the Hill coefficient (h) exceeds 1.0 the more curved will be the function of that sigmoid Emax-model. For an effect with a CE50 much higher than drug concentration (CE50 >> C) pharmacodynamics will depend on drug concentration according to a power function as presumed for the aminoglycosides or cyclophosphamide.

$$E = (Emax / CE50)\ C^h$$

For the condition (CE50 << C) the effect will exhibit saturated zero order kinetics (E = Emax) according to the classical receptor-occupancy theory.

Whether the proposed dosage adjustments are therapeutic, ineffective or toxic, will be evaluated in prospective clinical studies with intensive care and renal failure patients.

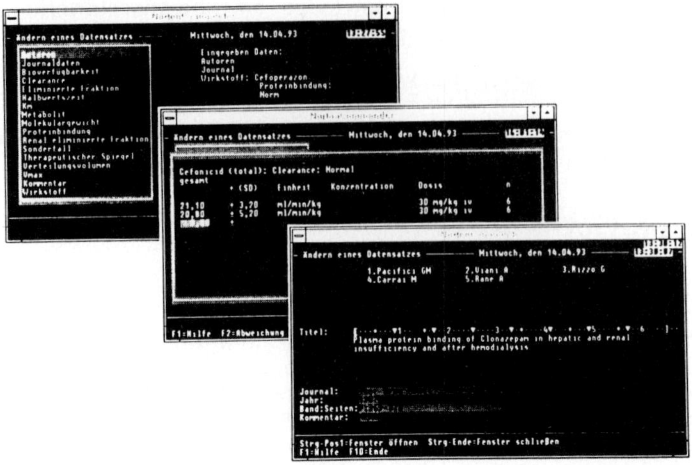

Figure 1: Database PHARMNEPH with pharmacokinetic parameters in normal renal function and anuria.

4. GENERAL PERSPECTIVE

Drug dosage in renal failure is only the special application of a general drug information system [6]. This system will be the task for both clinical practice and medical informatics in the next future. The main function to be implemented is to combine usual text word indexing with a standardized syntax [7]. Such a system should exemplarily be developed in a university hospital as part of a hospital information system, where at present pharmacy use amounts to only 6 percent of the retrieval activities [8].

The main functions of that system will encompass information about usual dosage, various indications, adverse reactions, interactions, pharmacokinetics, and changes of this knowledge in disease states (e.g. renal failure). This drug information must be connected with clinical patient data such as symptoms, body weight or serum creatinine to find out the right drug and the right dosage for an individual patient [9].

5. REFERENCES

1 Dettli L. Drug dosage and renal disease. Clin Pharmacol Therap 1974, 166: 274 - 279

2 Seyffart G. Drug Dosage in Renal Failure. Kluwer, Dordrecht 1991: 1 - 650

3 Lu DR, Mao F. An interactive program for pharmacokinetic modeling. J Pharm Sci 1993, 82: 537 - 542
4 Keller F, Erdmann K, Giehl M, Buettner P. Nonparametric meta-analysis of published data on kidney-function dependence of pharmacokinetic parameters for the aminoglycoside netilmicin. Clin Pharmacokinet 1993 (in press)
5 Lenert LA, Lurie J, Sheiner LB, Coleman R, Klostermann H, Blaschke TF. Advanced computer programs for drug dosing that combine pharmacokinetic and symbolic modeling of patients. Comp Biomed Res 1992, 25: 29 - 42
6 Prokosch U, Kamm S, Wieczorek D, Dudeck J. Knowledge representation in pharmacology: a possible application area for the Arden syntax? AMIA 1992: 243 - 247
7 Hersh WR, Hickam DH. A comparison of retrieval effectiveness for three methods of indexing medical literature. Am J Med Sci 1992, 303: 292 - 300
8 Bleich HL, Beckley RF, Horowitz GL, Jackson JD, Moody ES, Franklin C, Goodman SR, McKay MW, Pope RA, Walden T, Bloom SM, Slack WV. Clinical computing in a teaching hospital. N Engl J Med 1985, 312: 756 - 764
9 Langton K. The PREOP system. SCAM Proc 1991

Artificial Intelligence in Medecine
S. Andreassen et al. , Eds.
IOS Press, 1993

Building a Medical Knowledge Base: Tricks Facilitating the Simulation of the Expert´s Reasoning

Bernhard Puppe, University of Würzburg, Medizinische Klinik und Lehrstuhl für Informatik VI,
Am Hubland 12, 97218 Gerbrunn, Germany

Abstract: Detailed representation of intermediate pathophysiological concepts allows step-by-step diagnostic thinking which, starting from broad pathophysiologic terms, incrementally sharpens the focus of the working hypothesis and finally arrives at a specific diagosis. Rather than driving the diagnostic work-up with a single reasoning strategy, we let several - mainly forward-chained flow charts and hypothesize-and-test - compete in determining its course, i.e. the sequence of diagnostic tests.

1. Introduction

Since the early days of artificial intelligence in medicine, its researchers and developers did not only try to make their systems perform at the expert´s level, but also to get there in a way similar to the doctor´s mind. How he reasons has long been introspectively analyzed by preeminent physicians, but it was only by experimental research (Ellstein-78), (Kassirer-78) that the issue was investigated in depth and clarified to a point where system builders could start simulating the process in their programs (Shortliffe-76), (Pauker-76), (Kulikowski-82), (Miller-82). However, just as the overall impact of automated medical decision making on practical medicine has been only limited so far, so have the results of simulating the doctors´s line of reasoning. With regard to the latter, we will describe 2 principles which proved to be useful for our own evolving consultation system.

Beginning 10 years ago with a small system designed for the differential diagosis of thoracic pain (Puppe/Bernhard-85), we are now working on an intelligent tutorial system for diagnosis in general internal medicine which is already fairly competent in differentiating the various anemias. Since we plan using our system in medical student education, particular attention is being paid to model step by step the logic of informed medical decision making. Selectiveness in ordering laboratory studies instead of a "shotgun" approach is equally important as correct diagnosis for our work.

D3, the shell we use for building our knowledge base and which is applicable to any tasks that can be conceived of as classification problems (Puppe/Frank-87), facilitates simulation of medical reasoning by providing a broad array of mechanisms and sufficient control so that all important clinical reasoning strategies can be easily implemented in the program.

We begin our discussion with the description of a medical case and its computed solution to illustrate the main messages of this article. Since at present, our knowledge base is strongest in anemia, the example given is drawn from this domain. Full understanding and appreciation of the material would be enhanced by some hematologic knowledge, but the essentials should be readily understandable to anybody interested.

2. A Case of Pernicious Anemia and its Automatic Resolution

The following case - presenting a 62-year-old woman complaining of increasing fatigue and weight loss - is drawn from a textbook (Classen-91) and insignificantly adapted for our purpose. Suspecting some form of anemia, the systems immediately suggests a complete blood count that provides the following results: Hemoglobin 5.6 g/dL, hemotocrit 15.7 %, red blood cell count 1.4 million/µl, leucocyte count 3800/µl and thrombocyte count 90 000/µl blood.

After digesting this initial information, the systems presents its conclusions in 3 sections or windows: Secured or "established" diagnoses, diagnostic hypotheses and suggested further investigations. In our example, the secured diagnoses include anemia, tricytopenia/pancytopenia and, based on computation of the red blood cell indices, macrocytic and hyperchromic anemia. The diagostic hypotheses at this point are "macrocytic anemia/etiolgy unknown" and "megaloblastic changes of the peripheral blood", both derived from the already secured diagnoses.

The suggested investigations comprise routine tests necessary for any case of anemia, augmented by special tests selected on the basis of the information already gained and conclusions drawn therefrom.

The ordered reticulocyte count, reported to be 2.1%, is interpreted to be low in the face of severe anemia, spurring 2 additional entries to the list of secured diagnoses: "reduced erythropoiesis" and "hypoproliferative anemia". In addition, 2 new hypotheses - "myelodysplastic syndrome" and "aplastic anemia" - are invoked.

After finishing the straightforward routine work-up, the system switches to the selective mode of test-indication and suggests a white blood cell differential. This study is simultaneously indicated by the established diagnosis "tricytopenia/pancytopenia" (forward indication) and several hypotheses (backward-indication), all of which would profit from the results, i.e. could be refined. Indeed, by revealing marked neutrophil hypersegmentation, the test proves the suspected "megaloblastic changes of the peripheral blood", pushing this condition up from its former status of a hypothesis to a diagnosis.

Being established, this new diagnosis immediately generates a new hypothesis, "megaloblastic hematopoiesis", which in turn triggers a hypothesize-and-test cyle by indicating a bone marrow aspiration, this test being simultaneously asked for by "tricytopenia" (established diagnosis, indicates by forward reasoning) and "macrocytic anemia of unknown etiology" (hypothesis, indicates by backward reasoning).

The bone marrow aspiration results are interpreted to be positive for megaloblastic changes, allowing the system to add 2 more diagnoses (strictly speaking: patholphysiologic conditions) to its list of already accumulated conclusions: "megaloblastic hematopoiesis" (again a progression from hypothesis to accepted diagnosis) and, since the patient is anemic, "megaloblastic anemia". The latter gives birth to 2 new hypotheses: "megaloblastic anemia/etiology unknown" and "pernicious anemia", both of them crying immediately for a serum folate and vitamin B12 concentration. So did, by the way, the earlier hypothesis "macrocytic anemia/etiology unknown", which in the meantime has been replaced by the more specific hypothesis "megaloblastic anemia/etiology unknown".

The reported low vitamin B12 and normal folate serum levels together justify the conclusion of "vitamin B12 deficiency anemia". The new diagnosis - in a way the reader has already become familiar with - now generates, in an attempt to discover its cause, the hypothesis "vitamin B12 deficiency anemia/etiology unknown", which surplants its less specific predessesor-hypothesis "megaloblastic anemia/etiology unknown". "Pernicious anemia", of course, remains an active hypothesis (though with a higher index of suspicion). Both hypotheses now jointly suggest the decisive Schilling test whose pathognomonic results prove the major diagnosis of our case: pernicious anemia.

Though the diagnostic process has not yet arrived at its end point, we interrupt its description because the logic governing the system´s diagnostic behavior should have become sufficiently clear.

3. Detailed Representation of Intermediate Pathophysiologic Conditions

The described work-up of the case illustrates the detailed degree to which we represent what might be called "intermediate pathophysiologic conditions", insofar as they stand between the symptoms and signs presenting at the start of a diagnostic work-up and the specific diagnoses at its end. As a principle, we represent all pathoconditions which play a meaningful role in medical reasoning (Puppe/Bernhard-88). This decision entails a multiplication of represented conditions as compared to restricting representation to specific diagnoses. Furthermore, the terminolgy of the "intermediate terrain" in less standardized than that of specific diagnoses. However, we still believe that full representation should be a fundamental part of any consultation system aspiring to speak the physicians´ language.Since the cognitive distance between the presenting findings and final diagnoses is often wider than can be spanned by a single association, it is only convenient to structure the space in between by multiple mental constructs each of which can serve as a platform for differential diagnosis. Not yet specific enough to serve as a basis for the formulation of a therapy, the intermediate concepts help keeping the diagnostic process focused and allow the final goal to be approached in a convenient fashion of multiple small steps.

Although clinical decision making appears to vary widely in this regard - depending upon the case and scope of the physician's experience and knowledge - the controlled step-by-step approach is widely recommended in academic teaching for its logical appeal and reliability, especially to medical students lacking the experience to directly associate correctly a set of initial findings with a diagnosis. Thus, the intended role of our system in student education also favors detailed representation of the "in-between states".

Though it might seem paradoxical, this approach facilitates knowledge representation: When working out the symptomatic profile of a diagnosis, the difficulty of correctly assigning "certainty factors" (Heckerman-92) to findings increases rapidly with the number of findings simultaneously to be considered. In addition, ignoring their interdependancy results in under- or overrating of evidence. Our aproach points a promising way out of this complexity dilemma: Sequentially aggregating lower-level findings to higher-level concepts effectively reduces the number of findings involved in each single step.

Practically speaking, the upper limit of the scope of a symptomatic profile is defined by the magnitude of the screen. This might be discarded as a technical argument that should not affect the fundamental design of a knowledge base. However, there is much more to it than that. Extensive representation of intermediate-level concepts tends to transform probabilistic into categorical reasoning (Szolovits-78) which is exactly at which the human mind excels, explaining the abundance of intermediate-state terminology in medical science.

4. Interaction and Competition of Multiple Reasoning Strategies

A major problem of modern medical practice is indiscriminate use of costly diagnostic tests. There is general consensus that more selective test-ordering could help save costs for the payer and discomfort and time for the patient. It is not least in this area, that medical consultation systems might contribute to the improvement of the present situation.

The main reasoning strategies employed in the diagnostic process include hypothesize-and-test (a form of backward reasoning), differential diagnosis and forward reasoning. Flow charts - elaborate schemes consisting of multiple branched chains of forward-connected actions - seem to be gaining ground in medical teaching as well as in practice. We referred to them as "standardized forward reasoning" in (Puppe/Bernhard-89) describing their role in medical decision making especially in comparison with the hypothesize-and-test approach.

The classification shell D3 (Puppe/Frank-87) provides powerful specific mechanisms for the simulation of all 3 reasoning strategies. As demonstrated in our example, the diagnostic course is jointly steered by forward reasoning and hypothesize-and-test: Secured "established" pathoconcepts usually forward-indicate tests for their further refinement, whereas diagnostic hypotheses trigger hypothesize-and-test cycles. D3's specific mechanism for differential diagnosis is not evoked because the job was done by other means, mainly by hypotheses of the type "pathoconcept X/Etiology unknown".

When the diagnostic step-by-step process has arrived at an intermediate pathoconcept X, the term "pathoconcept X/Etiology unknown" comprehensively summarizes the diagnostic task ahead, better, while more concise, than explicitly evoking all possible candidates as hypotheses. More important, together with its affiliated procedures, a "pathoconcept X/Etiology unknown" serves as a powerful agent to resolve the differential diagnosis involved. For this purpose, it contains a number of tests sequentially evoked until a result shows up that is either diagnostic or allows the formulation of a narrower differential diagnosis based on a more specific "pathoconcept X/Etiology unknown". Thus, in the case discussed, the hypothesis "macroctic anemia/etiology unknown" is surplanted by "megaloblastic anemia/etiology unknown", which in turn, in the light of new information gathered, is replaced by "vitamin B12 deficiency anemia/etiology unknown" which narrows the set of differential diagnoses further, selects the decisive test (Schilling) proving the final diagnosis, pernicious anemia, and thereby eliminates itself.

Thus, hypotheses of the type "pathoconcept X/Etiology unknown" resolve problems of differential diagnosis in an orderly fashion as recommended by flow charts. Within D3, they proved to be the most efficient method to implement flow-chart logic. From a technical point of view, it is remarkable that, though flow-charts are a form of forward reasoning, our implementation by the means of a "pathoconcept X/Etiology unknown" reasons backward.

In our system, forward and backward reasoning constantly compete for guidance of the diagnostic process. This might seem like a luxury when each one of them alone is able to steer a logic course. However, although the competition places additional demands on the shell's control structure, we believe that consultation systems can only profit from a redundancy of problem solving capability. D3 allows competition on a still higher lever: All strategies discussed so far in this paper operate within D3's heuristic reasoning mode (Clancey-85), which is complemented by a case-comparison mode and a third one based on a functional model of the domain. However, our knowledge base does not yet include the knowledge required to exploit the 2 latter modes, thereby restricting competition to reasoning strategies operating within the heuristic mode.

In the example, forward and backward reasoning recommend a similar sequence of laboratory studies because the knowledge expressed is almost identical. Nevertheless, standardized forward reasoning and hypothesize-and-test have their strengths and weaknesses that should be taken into account when designing the problem solving approach of a diagnostics system (Puppe/Bernhard-89). When competing reasoning strategies disagree as to what test should be selected next, the shell's control structure must decide which one deserves priority. In D3, forward-indicated test selection generally gets preference over hypothesize-and-test because forward-chained selection often represents standardized practice, whereas hypothesize-and-test tends to be more individualized.

Acknowledgement

The reseach reported in this paper was conducted within the frame of the German MEDWIS-project "Tutoring Systems" supported by the German Ministry of Research and Technology and GSF Research Center for Environment and Health.

References:

(Bamberger-91) Bamberger S., Gappa U., Goss K. et. al.: The Classification Expert System Shell D3; Manuel; Karlsruhe University, Logic Institute, 1991

(Classen-91) Classen M., Diehl V., Kochsiek L.; (editors): Innere Medizin; Verlag Urban und Schwarzenberg, p. 181, 1991

(Clancey-85) Clancey W.J.: Hueristic Classification; Artificial Intelligence 27; p. 289-350; 1985

(Elstein-78) Elstein A., Shulman L., Sprafka S.: Medical Problem Solving; Harvard University Press, 1978

(Heckerman-92) Heckerman D., Shortliffe E.H.: From Certainty Factors to Belief Networks; Artificial Intelligence in Medicine 4; p. 35-52; 1992

(Kassirer-78) Kassirer J., Gorry A.: Clinical Problem Solving: a Behavioral Analysis; Annals of Internal Medicine 89, 245-255, 1978

(Kulikowski-82) Kulikowski C., Weiss S.: Representation of Expert Knowledge for Consultation: the CASNET and EXPERT Projects, in (Szolovits-82), 1982

(Miller-82) Miller R., Pople H., Myers J.: INTERNIST1: an Experimental Computer-Based Diagnostic Consultant for General Internal Medicine; NEJM 307, No. 8, p. 468-476, 1982

(Pauker-76) Pauker S., Gorry G., Kassirer J., Schwartz W.: Towards the Simulation of Clinical Cognition: Taking the Present Illness by Computer; American Journal of Medicine 60, 981-996, 1976

(Puppe/Bernhard-85) An Intelligent Computer Program for Thoracic Pain Diagnosis; Klinische Wochenschrift 63, 511-517; 1985

(Puppe/Bernhard-88) Puppe B., Puppe F.: A Knowledge Representation Concept Facilitating Construction and Maintenance of Large Knowledge Bases; Methods of Information in Medicine 27, 10-16, 1988

(Puppe/Bernhard-89) Puppe B.: Potential and Limits of Artificial Intelligence in Medicine; 5th TOYOBO Biotechnology Foundation Symposium on Artificial Intelligence in Medicine, 182-202; 1989

(Puppe/Frank-87) Puppe F.: Diagnostic Problem Solving with Expert Systems (in German), Springer-Verlag, 1987

(Shortliffe-76) Shortliffe E.H.: Computer Based Medical Consultation: MYCIN; American Elsevier, 1976

(Szolovits-78) Szolovits P., Pauker.: Categorical and Probabilistic Reasoning in Medical Diagnosis; AI-Journal 11, 115-144, 1978

(Szolovits-82) Szolovits P. (editor): Artificial Intelligence in Medicine; AAAS Selected Symposium 51, 1982

Artificial Intelligence in Medecine
S. Andreassen et al. , Eds.
IOS Press, 1993

Computer-Assisted Medical Decision Support by Analysis and Visualization of Multimodal Images

K-H Englmeier[1], M Haubner[1], H Förterer[1], B K Fink[2], W Perzl[1], R Waltram[1]

[1] GSF-Institut für Medizinische Informatik und Systemforschung, Ingolstädter Landstr. 1, Neuherberg, 85758 Oberschleißheim, Germany

[2] Radiologische Klinik, Klinikum Großhadern der Ludwig-Maximilians-Universität, Marchioninistr. 15, 81377 München, Germany

ABSTRACT:

Radiologic and clinical practice can be enhanced by improved access to multimodal image informations. Analysis, visualisation, method characteristic image processing and image synthesis is needed not only for the interpretation of the images but also for performing effective consultations with clinical colleagues and computer supported therapy planning and control strategies. A distributed visualization system is presented which enables the fast display, threedimensional visualization and the modality oriented analysis of multimodal image informations. Based on a unique image format, modality specific evaluation procedures and two- or threedimensional processing tools of image analysis produce the input data for therapy planning programs. The easy use of this multimedia visualisation tool enables radiologists and clinicians to deal with their image data. The description of methods and procedures of the prototype, as well as typical examples of radiologic practice will demonstrate the efficiency of the presented system.

1. INTRODUCTION AND STATE OF THE ART

The development of medical imaging modalities was strongly influenced by the use of computer technologies in the last twenty years. Since the introduction of examinations of the function and blood flow of organs by the help of the methods of nuclear medicine as well as the application of synthetic imaging methods such as computed x-ray tomography (CT) and magnetic resonance tomography (MRI) the use of computer technologies has been absolutely necessary in the field of medical imaging. Digital archiving of ultrasound images (US), Digital Radiography (DR) and Subtraction Angiography (DSA) are filmless alternatives to the conventional methods.The digital archiving of the images of the above mentioned methods could be managed by a central picture archiving and communication system (PACS) if the imaging devices are connected to the local area network of the hospital.

Although the above mentioned digital imaging systems are used beyond the conventional radiological examinations in radiologic practice the digital visualisation, analysis and synthesis of the multimodal images is not solved efficiently. The following technical and ergonomical barriers seem to be the reasons for that information and processing gap between medical imaging and image analysis based treatment planning systems:

- low transmission speed of the hospital networks
- missing capacity and performance of workstations to analyze and visualize images in real time
- minimum standardization of interfaces and file formats of the imaging devices
- missing techniques for user friendly and efficient human computer interaction [1]

One solution of the efficient data transport via networks seems to be the separation of management data and image data [2]. The ImNet/2 image network (described in [2]) has been developed for the fast image communication. The measurement of its effective transfer rate results in a value of 140 Mb/s. Other developments are FDDI with a carrier frequency of 125 MHz [2] or UltraNet 1000 Network Hub which is capable of transferring 1 Gb/s [3].

The variety and manufacturer dependency of interfaces and file formats of the imaging devices can be minimized by the introduction of image file format standards such as ACR-NEMA [4] which is mainly used for CT- and MRI-images. As the ACR-NEMA file description offers also the possibility of storing DR, DSA, US and NUK images, the conversion of manufacturer dependent file formats of these modalities to the ACR-NEMA format results in a unique image structure in medicine.

A lot of specific analysis, interpretation and visualization tools have been developed since the late seventies in the realm of medical imaging[5][6][7]. Most of the image analysis and synthesis systems have been developed for experimental purposes and only a few of them are commercialized [7]. Therefore we started the development of a distributed visualisation and analysis system. The system is capable to deal with two- and threedimensional images, including all imaging modalities mentioned above. It enables the simultanneous display of various images, the imaging method oriented processing, as well as twodimensional image fusion techniques.

2. METHOD

The implemented software system is entirely written in "C" with the support of the Distributed Graphics Library. The basic principles of the software system are:

- unique file format for CT, MRI, raw data of MRI, DR, DSA and scintigrams
- easy user interactions using file browsing and pull down menu techniques
- image processing utilities such as filtering, contour detection and segmentation
- image fusion techniques

All images of the various sources can be converted to a unique image file format containing patient, acquisition and image information. The unique format is similar to the ACR-NEMA image standard[4]. Manufacturer dependent file formats as well as compressed image data are converted to this unique image format. The user interaction is reduced to mousedriven selections of items within the pull down menus and file browsers. Parameter values, filter masks, distances and regions of interest are defined by sliders or interactive modifications in the image overlay.

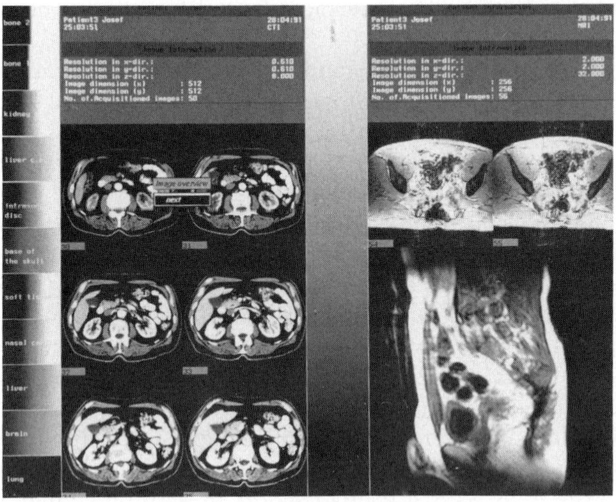

Fig. 1: In order to compare multimodal images the system enables the simultaneous display of multimodal images

2.1 Visualization

The visualization of the selected images of one patient is dependent on the image modality. The following display possibilities actually exists for CT and MRI:

- simultaneous display of multimodal images (s. fig. 1)
- Display of CT and MR images in cine mode using double buffering
- Image overview with zoom function
- Sequential image display combined with morphometric analysis (distances, areas, volumes) and interactive segmentation
- Use of 12 bit lookuptables and organ specific gray value windows in case of CT-presentation

Contrast modification is realized as an interactive tool by definition of the upper and lower threshold of the gray value window or in case of CT by selection of a fixed organ specific gray value window. Nevertheless fixed gray value windows have the advandage that they cannot be modified in an arbitrary manner by the user. This improves therapy control, because different CT-images are visualized under the same conditions.

DR and DSA images are visualized with a minimum resolution of 1024*1024 pixels and a gray value resolution of 10 bits. DR images with a resolution of 2368*1768 pixels are reduced in their size to monitor resolution. A magnifying glass enables the extraction of a part of the image and the presentation of this region in its original resolution. One important image preprocessing method of DR and DSA images is the following enhancement of edges:

$$g_r(x,y) = g_o(x,y) + k * (g_o(x,y) - g_{lp}(x,y))$$

$g_r(x,y)$	:=	resulting gray value;
$g_o(x,y)$	:=	orig. gray value;
k	:=	enhancement factor;
$g_{lp}(x,y)$	:=	low pass value;

The enhancement factor and the size of the low pass filter can be varied to change the degree of enhancement of lines and edges. The blurred version of the original image can be calculated by the convolution of the blurring filter mask with the original image. Another method is the digital subtraction of angiography images which enables the enhancement or reduction of the anatomical background of the visualized vessels (see fig. 2):

$$g_r(x,y) = g_c(x,y) - k * g_m(x,y)$$

$g_r(x,y)$	:=	resulting gray value;
$g_c(x,y)$	:=	contrast value;
$g_m(x,y)$	:=	subtraction mask;
k	:=	factor;

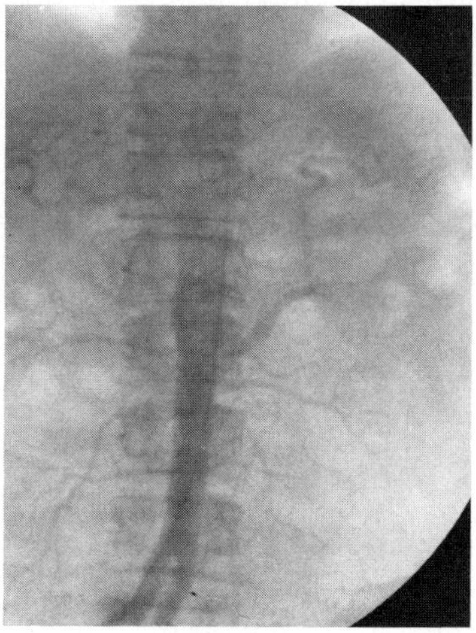

Fig. 2a: Digital Angiography: Original Image

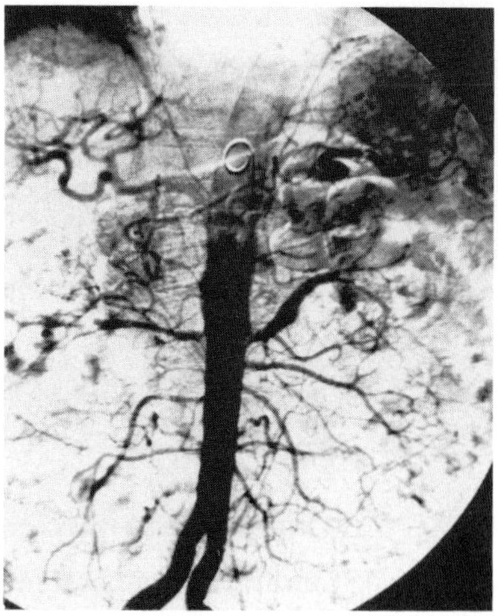

Fig. 2b: Subtraction result of fig.2a

2.2 Image Preprocessing and Analysis

The preprocessing and analysis of the multimodal image data actually includes the following methods:

- two- and threedimensional filters designed as Finite Impulse Response filters in the frequency domain
- gray value interpolation by the help of frequency dependent methods
- selective segmentation of regions of interest in CT images
- contour detection algorithms
- morphometry

Many filtering techniques focus on either space or frequency domains. In the following all of the implemented filters work exclusively in the frequency domain, because it allows a much simpler analysis of the image's noise and structure. The applied low-, high- and band pass filters as well as the band stop filters are designed as two- and threedimensional Finite Impulse Response filters of zero phase. As the extent of the unit sample response of these ideal filters is infinite, the nonrecursive approximation of the frequency response has to be established by the multiplication of the unit sample response with an appropriate window function[9][10]. The presented implementation of these well known filters in the twodimensional domain includes the extension to the threedimensional space. The application of the filters on medical images is realized as an interactive and easy method. The implemented filter system enables the reduction of noise, the enhancement of contours as well as the improved preprocessing of MRI raw data (noise removal) in the threedimensional domain in case of volume visualization. In case of CT-images these filtering method offers the advantage of non direction dependant slice image interpolation technique.

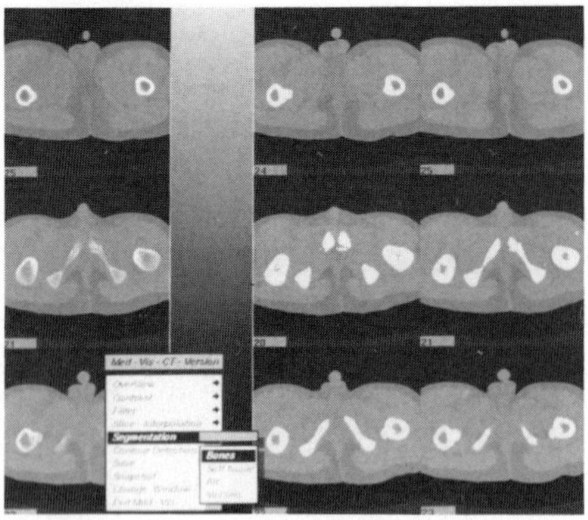

Fig. 3a: Automatic segmentation result of bony regions presented with the original CT-images

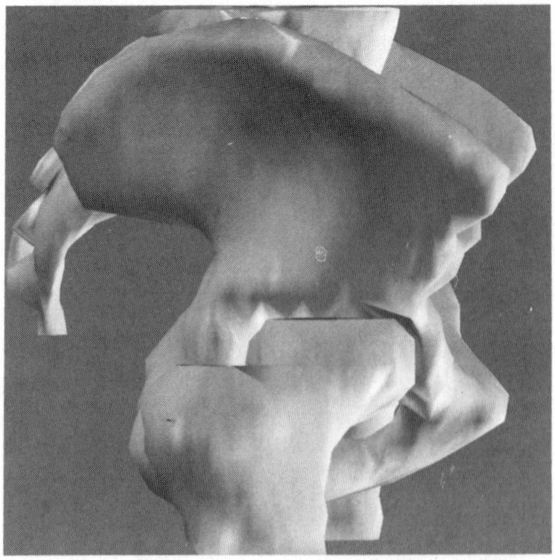

Fig. 3b: Surface oriented threedimensional presentation of the pelvis, the segmentation of which is presented in fig. 6a.

Automated segmentation and contour definition is one of the precondition of computer assisted therapy planning systems used in orthopedics or radiation treatment. The regions of bones and soft tissue can be detected automatically in case of CT-images: After the defintion of the body crossection the raw areas of the bony structures are detected by the application of a simple thresholding process. For these regions are overlayed with disturbances such as contour indentations as well as fused regions caused by the partial volume effect, an erosion and dilation process of these regions results in a partial elimination of the disturbances. The result of this segmentation process is the region of the interesting object, defined by the Houndsfield Units (fig. 3). After differentiating the binary images, a contour detection process stores the contour points on disk [13].

One method of postprocessing the detected contours is the threedimensional surface display. For this the contours are connected from one level to the next by the help of a hierarchical triangulation algorithm. The result of this calculation process is a data structure which enables the presentation of the surface as a wireframe or the colored presentation of opaque and transparent objects (fig. 6).

2.3 Registration and Fusion of Twodimensional Image Informations

The combination of lower resolution functional images from nuclear medicine with higher resolution anatomical information from CT or MRI has been reported in studies of the brain [14][15]. In order to improve anatomical localization of pathologic processes identified on the scintigram, a method was developed which enables the fusion of Digital Radiography with scintigrams in the diagnosis of spinal column injuries.

Based on the exact positioning of the patient for each image, three external or internal anatomical marker points have to be localized interactively by the user, after the images are displayed simultaneously. In order to match the low resolution image (source coordinate system) with the high resolution image (destination coordinate system) an image transformation matrix has to be calculated. The coefficients of this transformation matrix can be found by the method of least squares [16].

After the fusion of both images to one output image a true color display is used for the presentation of the matched image information. In order to remove unimportant background information in the scintigram a thresholding technique is applied. Following that the resulting hot spots in the scintigram are overlayed to the Digital Radiogram (s. fig. 4). An improvement of these overlay technique ist the calculation of transparent images. Therefore the scintigram is interpreted as an transparent object,which is overlayed to radiogram by the following formula which is mainly used in the realm of threedimensional computer graphics [17]:

$$R = t * D + (1 - t) * S$$

R: color of the final image
D: color of the DR image
S: color of the scinigram
t: transmission factor

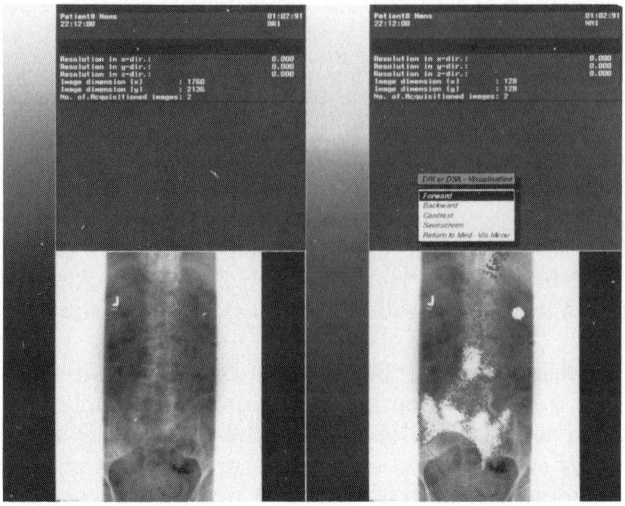

Fig. 4a: Interactive localisation of the positions of external and anatomical markers

Fig. 4b: Image fusion result of fig. 7a

3. CONCLUSION

Since the introduction of digital imaging modalities in medicine, analysis and visualization techniques are needed for the effective consultation of the radiologist with clinical collegues. The remote access to the multimodal image informatioons as well as the allocation of display and processing tools via networks enables this improved radiologic and therapeutic practice.

The userfriendly distributed prototype system displays and processes the images in a modality oriented manner. Based on a unique image file format, specific evaluation procedures produce the input data for therapy planning and surface rendering techniques. Future developments will extend the system by the following functions:

- communication with the radiologic information system (RIS)
- improvements of automated segmentation processes
- integration of volume rendering methods.

4. REFERENCES

[1] **Hendee W R:** Impact of Computer and Communication Technology on Radiology and Related Disciplines. In: Computer Assisted Radiology ´91. Lemke H U, Rhodes M L, Jaffe C C, Felix R (eds). Berlin: Springer, 1991: 249 - 255.

[2] **Meyer-Ebrecht D, Keizers A, Stut W J J, Vosseburger F:** Im Net/2 Transmits Images of 140 Mbit/s. In: Computer Assisted Radiology ´91. Lemke H U, Rhodes M L, Jaffe C C, Felix R (eds). Berlin: Springer, 1991: 482 - 487.

[3] **Tighe M:** Experiences installing an UltraNet on a Convex. In: 5th Annual CONVEX Use Group Worldwide Conference ´90. Dallas.

[4] **ACR-NEMA:** Digital Imaging and Communication. ACR-NEMA Standards Publication No 300-1985 (1986)

[5] **Tan A C, Richards S R Linney A D:** The MGI Workstation: An interactive System for 3D Medical Graphics Applications. In: Computer Assisted Radiology ´91. Lemke H U, Rhodes M L, Jaffe C C, Felix R (eds). Berlin: Springer, 1991: 705 - 710.

[6] **Dahm M, Glaser K, Jansen-Dittmer H, Keizers A, Krueger P, Meyer-Ebrecht D, Münker-Kaupp K, Rudolf H, Schilling C, Sieslack R, Winkler W, Wein B, Günther R:** Radiologists Start Designing their Digital Workplace: Prototyping with a Digital Image Workstation in the Radiology. In: Computer Assisted Radiology ´91. Lemke H U, Rhodes M L, Jaffe C C, Felix R (eds). Berlin: Springer, 1991: 699 - 704.

[7] **Robb R A:** 3-D Visiualization and Analysis of Biomedical Images Using ANALYZE. In: Computer Assisted Radiology ´91. Lemke H U, Rhodes M L, Jaffe C C, Felix R (eds). Berlin: Springer, 1991: 685 - 698.

[8] **Prokop M, Galanski M, Oestmann J W et. al.:** Storage phosphor versus screen film radiography: Effect of variety exposure parameters and unsharp mask filtering on the detectability of cortical bone defects. Radiology 1990, 177: 109 - 113.

[9] **Hecker R, Pöppl S J:** Structured Noise Removal by Using a High Flexible 2D FIR Digital Filter. In: IEEE Computer Society International Symposium on Medical Imaging and Image Interpretation '82. Silver Spring: IEEE Computer Society Press, 1982: 87 - 91.

[10] **Gonzalez R C, Wintz P:** Digital Image Processing. Reading: Addison-Wesley Publishing Company, 1987.

[11] **Watson A B:** The Cortex Transform: Rapid Computation of Simulated Neural Images. Computer Vision, Graphics and Image Processing 1987, 3: 311 - 327.

[12] **Achilles D:** Die Fourier-Transformation in der Signalverarbeitung. Berlin: Springer, 1985.

[13] **Englmeier K H, Wieber A, Pöppl S J, Hamburger C, Milachowski K A, Mittlmeier T:** Three-Dimensional Presentation of Human Organs in Medical Imaging and Therapy Planning. In: MEDINFO '89. Barber B Dexian C, Qin D, Wagner G (eds). Amsterdam: Norh Holland.1989: 403 - 408.

[14] **Schad L R, Boesecke R, Schlegel W, Hartmann G H, Sturm V, Strauss L G, Lorenz W J:** Three dimensional image correlation of CT, MR and PET studies in radiotherapy planning of brain tumours. J Comput Assist Tomogr 1987, 11: 948-954.

[15] **Pelizzari C A, Chen G T Y, Spelbring D R, Weichselbaum R R, Chen C-T:** Accurate three dimensional registration of CT, PET and/or MR images of the brain. J Comput Assist Tomogr 1989, 13: 20-26.

[16] **Hawkes D J, Robinson L, Crossmann J E, Sayman H B, Mistry R, Maisey M N, Spencer J D:** Registration and display of the combined bone scan and radiograph in the diagnosis and managment of wrist injuries. Eur J Nucl Med 1991, 18: 752-756.

[17] **Magnenat-Thalmann N, Thalmann D:** Image Synthesis, Theory and Practice.Tokyo: Springer Verlag, 1987.

Artificial Intelligence in Medecine
S. Andreassen et al. , Eds.
IOS Press, 1993

An evolutive alert system for diagnosis of nosocomial infections based on archiving distributed databases

E. SAFRAN[a], F. BORST[a], G. THURLER[a], D. PITTET[b], Ch. LOVIS[a], P. ROHNER[c], R. AUCKENTHALER[c] and J.-R. SCHERRER[a]

[a]Centre d'Informatique Hospitalière, [b]Division des Maladies Infectieuses and [c]Laboratoire central de Bactériologie, Hôpital Cantonal Universitaire, 24, rue Micheli-du-Crest, CH-1211 Geneva 14, Switzerland

Abstract

The GAMES European Community project deals with the general architecture of medical expert systems. Within the framework of this project, a methodology has been proposed, based on an epistemological model of reasoning of the hypothetico-deductive type. We applied this methodological approach to the design and the building of a system for diagnosing and predicting hospital-acquired infections, in the environment of DIOGENE, the Hospital Information System (HIS) of Geneva University.

Diagnostic rules were applied to DIOGENE databases, allowing the establishment of a daily list of selected patients with suspected infection: the process was applied to the data of 15 laboratories which are transferred everyday from the dedicated laboratory system to Archimed, an integrated archiving system.

Our goal was to test a sensitive diagnostic process, in a particularly well-suited HIS architecture. We tested this method for the diagnosis of pneumonia in the surgical intensive care unit: a list of patients with suspected infection was established daily on the basis of this process. Validation of the system was performed by applying the standard rules published by the Centers for Disease Control (CDC) of Atlanta for the diagnosis of nosocomial infections to all the patients of the care unit.

This highly sensitive system has a practical interest for the infection control staff for their reporting of nosocomial infections. In a high-risk unit, where all the patients' charts should be checked, the system allows to control only a small proportion of the patients, approximately one fifth with suspected infection, and therefore to save work time.

This strategy is made possible with the Geneva University HIS, firstly by a new open distributed architecture, and secondly, by the development of Archimed, a system for archiving distributed databases.

A computerized system for surveillance of nosocomial infections will play a major role for the quality of patient care and reduction of hospital costs, and furthermore, represents a commercial potential within the field of hospital information systems.

1. INTRODUCTION

Nosocomial or hospital-acquired infections represent an important problem in hospitals since they are a major cause of increased morbidity, mortality and costs. An infection control team has the responsibility to survey for nosocomial infections, in order to take adequate control measures. The need for computer systems as an aid to perform hospital-wide surveillance is well recognized; however, its feasability is entirely dependent on archiving and accessibility of reliable patients' data [1-6].

To design and build a system for surveillance of nosocomial infections, we applied the methodology for building knowledge-based systems developed within the framework of the GAMES project [7-11]. This methodology emphasizes the formulation of an epistemological model of reasoning: the Select and Test Model (ST-Model) has been proposed, with three main inference processes: *abduction* (from clinical evidence to hypotheses), *deduction* (from hypotheses to the request of additional data), and *induction* (confirming or eliminating a hypothesis) [7-11]. It corresponds to a hypothetico-deductive model of reasoning [12].

Since alerting systems are currently used as computer-assisted decision support [13-16], we have investigated the steps in the establishment of diagnosis which could be formalized as medical alerts. We used a pragmatic strategy of formalizing rules using data available in DIOGENE databases.

2. METHODS

2.1. Diagnostic tasks

We have identified two diagnostic tasks. The first task is patient-care oriented, and consists of detecting patients either infected, or at risk of developing infection, in order to take therapeutic or preventive measures. The second diagnostic task is audit-oriented: it is the reporting performed by the Hospital Infection Control Team using the rules published by the Centers for Disease Control of Atlanta, for the establishment of the statistics of nosocomial infections on a retrospective basis [17]. These rules serve also as standard criteria for validation of the system.

2.2. Application to nosocomial infection diagnosis

Steps required in medical practice for the establishment of nosocomial infection diagnosis were matched with the three main processes of the ST-Model, with special emphasis on the formulation of alerts for the Infection Control Team.

Abduction (from clinical evidence to hypotheses)

Structured data available in DIOGENE databases concerning hospitalized patients are laboratory, demographic and administrative data, and previous hospitalizations diagnoses and procedures [18]. Abductive rules were formalized, using available data, through queries applied to DIOGENE databases; a list of patients selected according to the chosen criteria was established daily and sent every morning as an alert directly to the Infection Control Team printer. High sensitivity of the diagnostic rules is a critical point for such a method, in order to ensure that the number of infected patients that may be missed is insignificant.

The method was tested in the surgical intensive care unit, for the diagnosis of pneumonia. The diagnostic process was mainly based on bronchio-alveolar material showing a significant presence of leukocytes upon direct examination; as shown in the paper by Lauwers (1990) [3], presence of leukocytes found upon direct examination is a useful sign for laboratory-based computerized monitoring of infection.

Validation of the method was performed by applying to all the patients in the unit the worldwide standard reference criteria for diagnosing nosocomial infections, published by the Centers for Disease Control (CDC) of Atlanta [17].

Deduction (from hypothesis to the request of additional data)

Complementary data for diagnosis (fever, chest X-ray criteria, ..) were obtained in the ward by the infection control nurse by checking the patients' charts, or requesting them from the personnel.

Induction (confirmation of hypothesis)

Final confirmation of the diagnosis was made by a physician.

2.3. The DIOGENE environment: an open distributed architecture and a system for archiving distributed databases

Applying diagnostic rules to the various distributed databases of DIOGENE, for selecting patients to be checked on the basis of specific criteria, has now been made possible, firstly by a new open distributed architecture, and secondly, by the present development of Archimed, a system for archiving distributed databases. In Archimed, all the patients' data are stored in their original raw form, allowing a user to formulate any combination of criteria for selecting patients [19].

3. RESULTS

Over an initial testing period of thirty days in the surgical intensive care unit, the number of daily patients ranged from 7 to 18, and the number of patients selected by the diagnostic rule varied between 1 and 6 per day; approximately half of the selected patients had pneumonia. The sensitivity of the method was very high, since over a total of 13 patients with pneumonia, 12 were detected by the alerting system; results are of course dependent on the chosen context of a unit with a high-risk of nosocomial infection where patients have their sputum routinely checked for bacteriological examination.

4. DISCUSSION

Computers play an important role in the surveillance of nosocomial infections; various systems have been built for selecting patients with key infection indicators [1,3,5] and models for identifying patients at risk of developing infection proposed [4]. However, their utility is greatly dependent on the presence, quality [1] and accessibility of data.

Archimed now stores both laboratory and demographic data, which is a particularly useful combination for surveillance of nosocomial infections [4,20]; it also stores laboratory requests, lists of patients' imaging exams, and links to some medical reports and imaging [18,19]. All data are stored in raw form and can be easily retrieved; this feature is the key to flexibility, allowing the rules to be changed for the selection of patients along with results of validation and requirements of the infection control staff.

Progress in data availability is dependent on the present development of dedicated applications for collecting clinical data, such as the archiving of medical reports and progress notes, or interactive laboratory requests.

With new data available, diagnostic rules may be refined, and the present project will help to identify the data of the medical chart that should be structured in priority, the ultimate goal of a system for the surveillance of nosocomial infections being to establish rules to detect high-risk patients, in order to prevent the occurrence of infections.

5. CONCLUSION

A system based on applying diagnostic rules to the database of the Geneva University HIS automatically helps to select a subset of patients who have to be checked for nosocomial infection. It has time-saving consequences for the work of the infection control nurses, and will have a major impact for the quality of patient care and reduction of hospital costs. The key element for building such a system is the presence of an archiving system of distributed databases, where all the patients' data are stored in raw form.

6. ACKNOWLEDGEMENTS

This work is part of the AIM (Advance Informatics in Medicine) Commission of the European Communities project A-2034 entitled "GAMES-II: A General Architecture for Medical Expert Systems", and was supported in part by the Swiss government OFES (Office fédéral de l'éducation et de la science), contract AI010.

The authors thank Ms. Hazel Morse for translation assistance.

7. REFERENCES

1 Evans R.S., Larsen R.A., Burke J.P., Gardner R.M., Meier F.A., Jacobson J.A., Conti M.T., Jacobson J.T. and Hulse R.K. : Computer surveillance of hospital-acquired infections and antibiotic use. JAMA 256: 1007-1011, 1986.

2 Schaffner W. : The global impact of hospital-acquired infections. In: Wenzel R.P. (ed.), Prevention and Control of Nosocomial Infections. Williams & Wilkins, Baltimore, 1987, pp. 13-18.

3 Wenzel R.P. and Streed S.A. : Surveillance and use of computers. J. Hosp. Infect. 13: 217-229, 1989.

4 Broderick A., Mori M., Nettleman M.D., Streed S.A. and Wenzel R.P. : Nosocomial infections: validation of surveillance and computer modeling to identify patients at risk. Am. J. Epidemiol. 131: 734-742, 1990.

5 Lauwers S., De Smet F., Van Zeebroeck A. and Van de Velde R. : Description of a computerized surveillance system for nosocomial infections used in a Belgian teaching hospital. 2nd International Conference of the Hospital Infection Society, London, 2-6 September 1990.

6 Pittet D. and Wenzel R.P. : Nosocomial bloodstream infections: secular trends in rates, mortality and contribution to total hospital deaths (in preparation).

7 Lanzola G., Stefanelli M., Barosi G. and Magnani L. : NEOANEMIA: a knowledge-based system emulating diagnostic reasoning. Comput. Biomed.

Res. 23: 560-582, 1990.
8 Stefanelli et al. The GAMES Team : GAMES: A general architecture for medical expert systems. In: Proc. of the Conference AIM-EUROFORUM, Sevilla, Spain, December 13-15, 1990.
9 Lanzola G. and Stefanelli M. : A knowledge acquisition tool for medical diagnostic knowledge-based systems. In: Stefanelli M., Hasman A., Fieschi M. and Talmon J. (eds.), AIME 91, Proc. of the Third Conference on Artificial Intelligence in Medicine, Maastricht, June 24-27, 1991. Springer-Verlag, Berlin, 1991, pp. 273-282.
10 Lanzola G. and Stefanelli M. : A specialized framework for medical diagnosis knowledge-based systems. Comput. Biomed. Res. 25: 351-365, 1992.
11 Stefanelli M., Bellazzi R., Berzuini C., Bugliesi M., Calzadilla J., Hunter J., Kolary P., Lanzola G., Leaning M., Mantas J., Moustakis V., Qualini S., Ramoni M., Ruggieri C. and Zambon F. : GAMES: A general architecture for medical expert systems. In: Noothoven van Goor J., Christensen J.P. (eds.), Advances in Medical Informatics, IOS Press, Amsterdam, 1992, pp. 133-140.
12 Fieschi M. : Intelligence Artificielle en Médecine. Masson, Paris, 1984, pp. 20-21.
13 Hripcsak G., Clayton P.D., Pryor T.A., Haug P., Wigertz O.B. and Van der Lei J. : The Arden syntax for Medical Logic Modules. In: Miller R.A. (ed.), Proc. of Fourteenth Annual Symposium on Computer Applications in Medical Care. IEEE Computer Society Press, New York, 1990, pp. 200-204.
14 Pryor T.A. : Development of decision support systems. Int. J. Clin. Monit. Comput. 7: 137-146, 1990.
15 Evans R.S., Pestotnik S.L., Classen D.C., Bass S.B., Menlove R.L., Gardner R.M. and Burke J.P. : Development of a computerized adverse drug event monitor. In: Clayton P.D. (ed.), Proc. of Fifteen Annual Symposium on Computer Application in Medical Care. McGraw Hill, Inc., New York, 1992, pp. 23-27.
16 Rind D.M., Safran C., Phillips R.S., Slack W.V., Calkins D.R., Delblanco T.L. and Bleich H.L.: The effect of computer-based reminders on the management of hospitalized patients with worsening renal function. In: Clayton P.D. (ed.), Proc. of Fifteen Annual Symposium on Computer Application in Medical Care. McGraw Hill, Inc., New York, 1992, pp. 28-32.
17 Gardner J.S., Jarvis W.R., Emori T.G., Horan T.C. and Hughes J.M. : CDC definitions for nosocomial infections. J. Infect. Control 16: 128-140, 1988.
18 Scherrer J.-R., Baud R., Hochstrasser D. and Ratib O. : "The DIOGENE Hospital Information System". M.D. Computing 7: 81-89, 1990.
19 Thurler G. : Archimed, Archivage - Interrogations - Statistiques. Internal Document, Centre d'Informatique Hospitalière, Hôpital Cantonal Universitaire de Genève, 1992.
20 Pittet D., Omahen J., Tarara D. and Wenzel R.P. : Current risk factors for nosocomial bloodstream infections in a tertiary health care center. 31st Interscience Conference on Antimicrobial Agents and Chemotherapy; Infections Diseases Society of America Meeting. Chicago, October 1991, A800.

Artificial Intelligence in Medecine
S. Andreassen et al. , Eds.
IOS Press, 1993

A knowledge-based system to classify and diagnose HIV-pneumonias

M. Fiore*, F. Sicurello*°, M. Viganò°, R. Pizzi°, S. Bandini°

*National Research Council, Institute of Advanced Biomedical Technologies, via Ampère 56, 20131, Milano.

°University of Milan, Department of Computer Science, via Comelico 39, 20135 Milano

Abstract

The paper describes an intelligent system for the automated diagnosis of HIV-pneumonias. The particular object-oriented approach adopted to set out the knowledge base allows to make use of the features of reusability and inheritance of objects, ensuring an easy and dynamical development of the knowledge base.

Classes and objects are implemented by means of frames, but another less specialized knowledge is codified by means of production rules. The system is able to identify diagnosis hypotheses and to suggest the suitable therapy.

Due to the possibility of displaying the inferential chains followed by the system, its didactical aspect is stressed.

1. INTRODUCTION

Complex problems with a number of variables, as for example the AIDS and its many collateral diseases, have raised the need for the physicians to have the available a computerized tool for decision making in order to define an appropriate diagnosis and therapy.

Patients who develop lung disease, particularly Pneumocystis Carinii pneumonia (PCP) , nearly always present clinically obvious immunosuppression. Often the patient's medical history is dominated by symptoms of the underlying immunosuppressive process, such as leukemia or lymphoma, or a disease for which immunosuppressive therapy is being given. In such patients, respiratory symptoms may be a consequence of the pre-existing disease and its treatment, or a new process; thus, the differential diagnosis contains a large number of processes, including a spectrum of opportunistic infections. Patients with human immunodeficiency virus (HIV) infection often have had nonspecific symptoms, such as fever, fatigue, and weigth loss for week to months prior to develope respiratory diseases or other disorders that categorize them as having a ARC (AIDS-Related Complex) or AIDS [1].

As regards the respiratory diseases, most patients present symptoms of PCP and Cytomegalovirus pneumonia, but pneumonia due to pyogenic bacteria has often been noted in particular caused by Pneumococcus and Haemophilus influenzae. Other agents responsible for infections are Branhamella catarrhalis, group B streptococci, S. aureus, Legionella, Mycoplasma pneumoniae and other Haemophilus species (see Fig. 1).

A differential diagnosis of such a number of pneumonias represents a difficult task for the physician, in which a decision support tool could be useful.

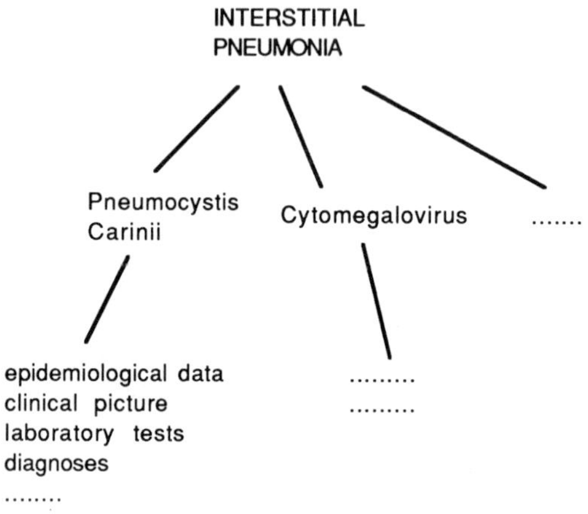

Fig. 1

Thus, we constructed a system able to perform a diagnostic and therapeutic evaluation of subjects affected by likely HIV-pneumonia, starting from a restricted number of data and lab tests, and to formulate diagnostic hypotheses in order to settle the most suitable therapy.

The physician can interact with the system, not only at the stage of the patients' data input, but even in the inference level: the system can give the physician the possibility to formulate diagnostic and therapeutic hypotheses and to check their correctness. This feature makes the system particularly suitable for didactical purposes as well as for decision support.

Special attention has been paid to the accomplishment of the user interface, which allows the physician to interact with the system in a simple way, overcoming the difficulties raised by the particular knowledge representation formalism. This allows the user to easily add new knowledge and modify the pre-existent one, in such a way to keep the system always up-to-date.

2. DESCRIPTION OF THE SYSTEM

To develope the knowledge-based system it is important to do an appropriate choice of the knowledge representation according to the features of the problem [2].

Thus, according to the features of our problem, we chose a knowledge representation which took into account the fact that the diseases of interest had common elements as regard the physiopathological states: epidemiological data, clinical features, lab tests, instrumental examinations.

Each state is characterized by the presence of data deriving from the lab and instrumental tests or from objective observation: the whole of this information settles the clinical evidence of every kind of pneumonia.

Therefore the peculiarity of a common description structure for any pathology suggests to adopt an object-oriented approach as the most natural one.

Several advantages have been claimed for this paradigm. Objects are modules which correspond directly to the types of object found in the domain of the application program. Fikes and Kehler [3] claim that this knowledge representation capture the way in which domain experts typically think about their knowledge. The structure of the domain about which the knowledge is modeled is directly reflected in the knowledge base. Thus corresponding to a class of entities in the domain there will be a class frame in the knowledge base, and for each individual entity in the domain, there will be an instance frame [4]. However the hierarchical structure of this knowledge representation has not only advantages from an representational point of view: the inference procedure that uses the taxonomic structure (inheritance) has its own advantages. Inheritance provides a natural way of dealing with default reasoning; through inheritance we can built new classes on the top of an existing less specialized hierarchy of classes, instead of redesigning everything from scratch [5].

We implemented classes and objects using frames, which, as a "data-structure for representing a stereotyped situation" [6], are particularly suitable to codify the kind of knowledge we are dealing with.

For example, let us consider the structure of Cytomegalovirus pneumonia as described by the card N° 1:

A) EPIDEMIOLOGICAL DATA
- it generally appears in association with different pneumonia, principally Pneumocystis Carinii (rarely it is the only etiological agent of pneumonia, likely in less than 5% of cases)
- it comes up almost always in patients with CD4<200/mmc

B) CLINICAL PICTURE
- it is generally associated with Cytamegalovirus infection in other sites (retina, liver, gastrointestinal tract, central nervous system, ...)
- symptoms (frequent, but not compulsory): fever, nonproductive cough, dyspnea , worsening of general conditions
- signs: cyanosis and tachypnea, lung findings often negative

C) LABORATORY TESTS
- chest X-RAY: diffuse bilateral interstitial infiltrates, rarely lumps and small cavities

D) DIAGNOSIS
- dimostration of evidence of Cytomegalovirus in blood, bronchoalveolar lavage, sputum, lung biopsy, urines
- exclusion of other kinds of interstitial pneumonia

Card N°1

Every frame has a name identifying the particular pneumonia and a set of four slots corresponding to the physiopathological states of the disease. Inside of the slots are stored data and lab tests related to the disease.

In this way, from the class INTERSTITIAL PNEUMONIA, the object Cytomegalovirus pneumonia is defined and is constituted by four slots which define the disease's attributes.

Every frame includes the particular slot AKO (a kind of) which contains information about what frames the analyzed frame is a specialization of [7]. In this way the inheritance mechanism is implemented, which describes the father frame and allows the analyzed frame to inherit the common data and attributes.

The pathology described by the card n° 1 is represented by the frame shown in the card n° 2:

```
frame(cytomegalovirus,[ako-[intestitial_pneumonia],
                  epidemiological_data-
                   [other_kinds_of_pneumonia-[yes],
                     CD4-[less_than_200/mmc]],
                   clinical_picture-
                  [symptoms-[fever,nonproductive_cough,dyspnea],
                     signs-[cyanosys_tachypnea],
                     lung_findings-[negative]],
                 laboratory_tests-[PO2-[lowering],
                            CD4-[less_than_200/mmc],
                              LDH-[growing]],
                   strumental_tests-
                   [chest_XRAY-[interstit_spread,no_lumps]]]).
```

Card N° 2

The domain knowledge is therefore represented by means of frames linked each other by means of relationships of specialization, generalization and causality.

Besides, another kind of knowledge is stored which is less specialized and concerned with more general medical aspects and which is used by the system during its diagnostic process. This kind of knowledge allows the system to perform generalization about the input data and is codified by means of production rules expressed in the following form: IF <condition> THEN <action>/<conclusion>, as for example:

```
IF       years(more_than_18) AND
           n_leucocytes(less_than_2500)
THEN     n_leucocytes(low).
```

A further classification is then performed, which relates concepts belonging to different classifications by means of inferences. When the data provided represent the solution's features, the process is direct when such features are, on the other hand, not provided in the form of data, it is possible to infer them by means of the data abstraction.

The inference structure of the system can be showed in Fig. n° 2

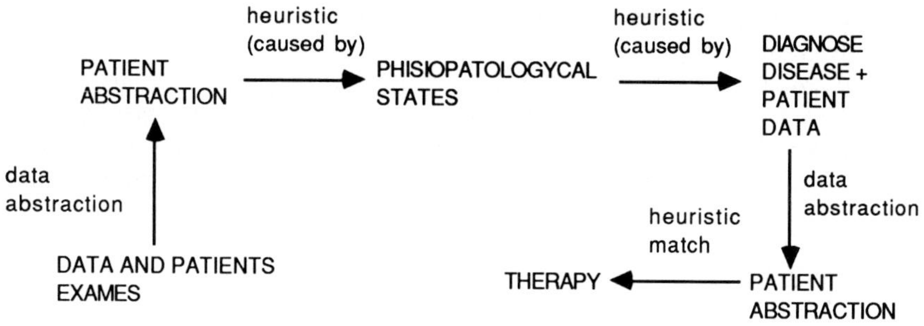

Fig. 2

Production rules are matched with the data related to the specific patient using data abstraction, allowing to identify some objects or symptoms as members of a known class of objects or diseases.

We have added the heuristic inference to this feature, which permits to perform the relationship between different concepts belonging to different entities and to establish a causal relationship between symptoms and diseases.

Besides, the uncertainty associated to rules and facts has led to allot a numeric weight to their importance in the diagnostic process. Such weight can take values between 0 and 100 and becomes negative when a reference datum in the system database cannot be found.

The system has been implemented on PC 386 using PROLOG II, whose main feature is an internal backword inference engine applied to the codified rules [8]. This logical-deductive process has been modified in order to adapt it to the frame formalism. The method we used to develop our system can be summarized as follows:

- -identification of a list of all possible solutions, data and intermediate categories;
- -identification of all the inference chains and classification of all the relationships between concepts;
- -building of the inference diagram which represents hierarchical relationships between classes and heuristic relationships;
- -transformation of the diagram into the PROLOG representation language, taking account of the suitable instructions for the frame codification and the necessary weights.

3. CONCLUSIONS

With the development of this system we hope to obtain some important results as regards AIDS pathology. The formalization of HIV pneumonia and therapies as object classes and with particular features is a step to find the agent which causes the disease and the suitable therapy.

Present knowledge about this disease is restricted but always growing and such an approach will allow an extension of the knowledge base, adding new knowledge to the system or modifying the existing one by means of new approaches and new discoveries.

We consider this aspect particularly important as we intend to implement in the future a mechanism which will allow to increment the knowledge base by means of new therapies suggested by physicians and complete with the reasons of the new choices. In this way the system will be able to suggest the most appropriate therapy, already chosen by the physician, every time a situation comes up, which will be suitable to the request features.

Last but not least is the didactical aspect of this system, which is linked to the feature of explaining the inferential chains followed by the system and the possibility for the physician to verify the correctness of diagnostic and therapeutic hypotheses.

A further step will be the translation of the system into an object-oriented language, in order to make it more portable and more suitable to the medical testing [9].

4. REFERENCES

1 M. A. Sande, P. A. Volberding, The medical management of AIDS. W. B. Saunders Company, 1988
2 Sicurello F., Lanzarone G. A., Taioli S., Pizzi R., Moroni M., Saracco A., D'Arminio Monforte A., Una base di dati e un nucleo di base di conoscenza sui fattori predittivi dello sviluppo di AIDS conclamata. Atti AIIM 89 Como, ottobre 1989:285-290.
3 R. Fikes, T. Kehler, The role of frame-based representation in reasoning. Communication of the ACM, 28,1985:904-920.
4 H. Reichgelt, Knowledge Representation: an AI perspective. Ablex Publishing Corporation,1991.
5 K. Parsaye, M. Chignell, S. Khoshafian, H. Wong, Intelligent Databases. John Wiley & Sons , 1989.
6 Minsky M., A framework for representing knowledge. In P. Winston (Ed.), The Psychology of Computer Vision, McGraw-Hill 1975.
7 Merritt D., Building Expert Systems in Prolog. Springer-Verlag, 1989.
8 Bratko I., Prolog programming for A.I.. Addison-Wesley, 1990.
9 Yourdon E., Coad P., Object Oriented Analysis. Yourdon Press Computing Series, 1991.

Artificial Intelligence in Medecine
S. Andreassen et al. , Eds.
IOS Press, 1993

How to appreciate expert principles for antibiotic prescription in a fuzzy context

B. Le Blanc, P. Morlat and G. Palmer

Département d'Informatique Médicale,
Université de Bordeaux 2, 33076 Bordeaux cedex, France

We describe the main functions of our expert system AntibES. This program is designed to help practitioners for prescribing antibiotics. We show the process of decision making in a fuzzy environment through a description of our decision engine. First, we use production rules for representation of expert principles. Then we make the comparison between these principles and context observations. Finally we produce a classification of decisions in a best choice way.

1. INTRODUCTION

By considering the prescription problem, we hope to answer to a large family of decision making problems in Medicine. The software has to choose most appropriated decisions in a large set of entities. This action completes the traditional diagnosis process. Our goal for decision making is a combination between Possibility Logic [1] and Social Choice Theory [2].

Our system, named AntibES (for Antibiotics Expert System), uses a fuzzy knowledge representation. The system is composed of two different engines : an inference one which prepares a short diagnosis [3], and a decision one for the decision process based on this diagnosis. In this presentation, we only consider the second one.

This engine is briefly presented in §2. The use of this system is discussed in §3. A short conclusion exposes the future of AntibES.

2. ANTIBES

Knowledge representation is an acute problem, in medicine as in other fields. The vague or uncertain form of considered informations is one particularity of the medical approach (a *possible* renal insufficiency, an *envisaged* infectious, ...).

The fuzzy set theory [4] is a good (and now classical) solution for representing fuzzy information. This theory is extended by the possibility logic [1] and gives a powerful frame for knowledge expression and manipulation. With this tool we are able to use continuous fuzzy notions, as discrete ones (cf. fig. 1) (see [5], [6] for instance).

On other hand, decision problem was most traditionally used in economic research (for instance the election of a candidate). But the interest into the choice of a candidate in an election context is close to the choice of a drug in a patient context. So we apply the Social Choice Theory [2] to our medical problem. To go beyond the K. Arrow's Impossibility Theorem several authors have proposed to improve the process of election by adding a ponderation to the vote.

Each elector gives a coefficient for each candidate. Coefficient of 1.0 means that the candidate is well recommended. A value between 1.0 and 0.0 expresses a more or less intensity of preference. Then, if we consider for each vote the set of candidates with these numerical intensities, we obtain a discrete fuzzy set.

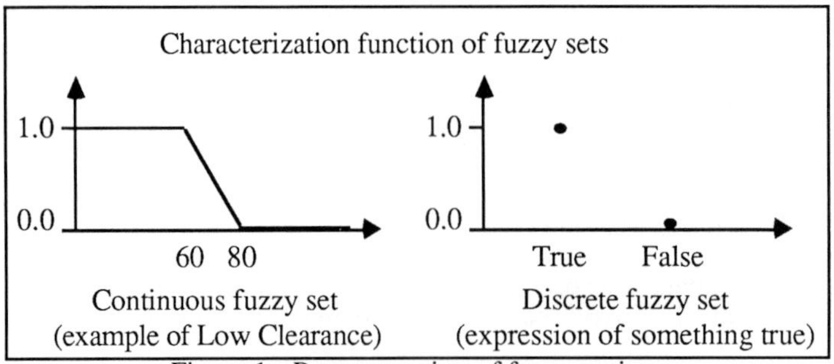

Figure 1 - Representation of fuzzy notions

2.1. Decision rule

Decision rules are the main knowledge of our ES. They look like traditional production rules. An hypothesis part exposes the context of application of the rule. The conclusion part is a little different from usual rules : it describes expert intention of prescription in front of the specific context of application. An element of conclusion is the association of a drug and a coefficient which characterizes the good choice degree of this drug in the appropriated principle.

In fact, each rule is a presentation of an individual vote. Decision making consists in the aggregation of all of these votes.

Figure 2 presents on left part an example of a decision rule, and on right part the interpretation of its conclusions in a discrete fuzzy set.

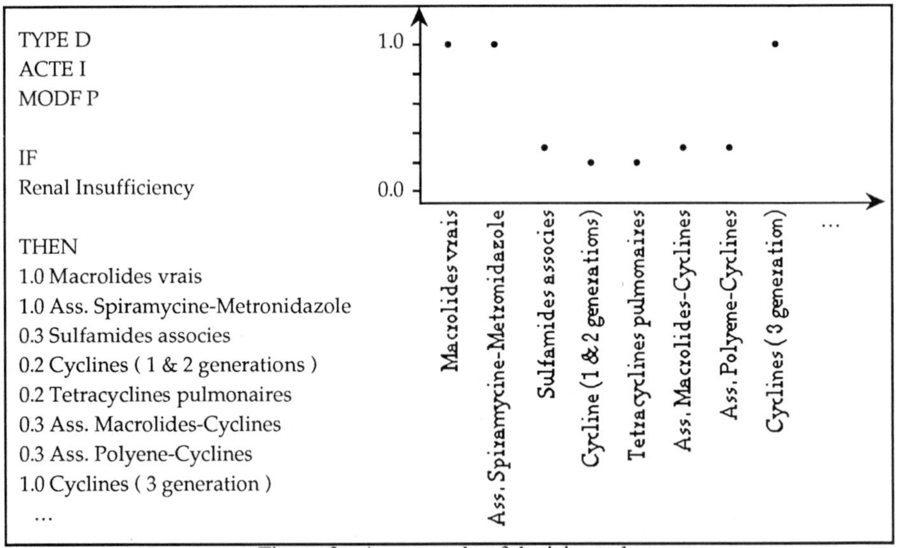

Figure 2 - An example of decision rule

2.2. Decision inference

The comparison between rule hypothesis (expert principle : Pri) and consultation situation (observation : Obs) is done by a possibilistic matching [3]. The measure of distance separating principle and observation is calculated with the Possibility and the Necessity measures. The result of this comparison is a couple of numbers (Poss(Pri:Obs) , Nec(Pri:Obs)).

Expert coefficients of each possible decision are not modified by the inference process, but the certitude in these coefficients may be decreased. We introduce a doubt in the conclusion by adding a new ponderation which expresses the uncertainty that the system has about the initial decision preference. If the observation exactly matches the expert principle then system infers an uncertainty level of 0.0. The more the distance between observation and principle increases, the more the doubt grows. A consistent difference between principle and observation infers a decision (with coefficients depending on the rule conclusion) with a total uncertainty.

Finally AntibES decision engine infers triplets : a decision and two coefficients, one for the expert certitude that the decision is correct and one other produced by the system which means the doubt in the suitability of the expert principle in the local consultation.

Figure 3 shows how to consider inferred decision as discrete fuzzy set.

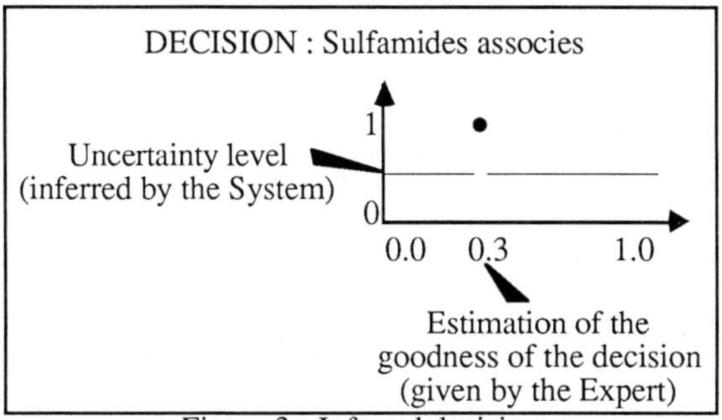

Figure 3 - Inferred decision

2.3. Decision making

The last step consists in sorting the inferred decisions. For this action the expert explains his definition of a "Good Decision" : what are good coefficients and bad ones for decision. For example, as shown in figure 4, a good decision has no uncertainty and a coefficient greater then 0.7 ; a bad decision has a coefficient smaller then 0.3.

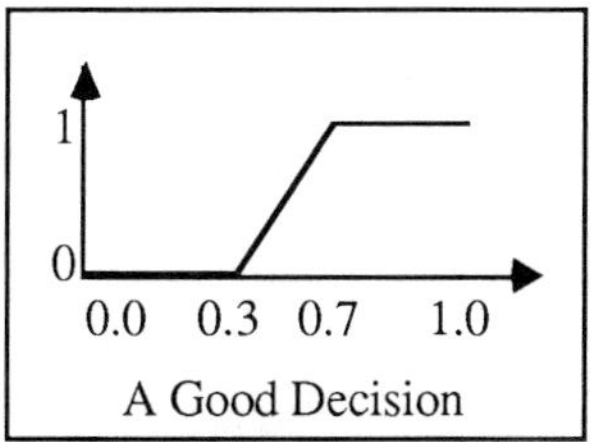

Figure 4 - Expert description of a "Good" Decision

Using the possibility theory, the system calculates the Poss and Nec measures of the distance between each inferred decision and the good decision. With these numbers (one couple P/N for each decision), it is easy to sort decisions in decreasing order.

The sorting process uses both possibility and necessity results. The scale of sorting is : best (P=1,N=1) ; then (P=1,N=n) ; then (P=1,N=0) ; then (P=p,N=0) and worse (P=0,N=0).

This action means that, for expert eyes, it is better to select a decision with a reasonable but not high coefficient (ex : 0.7) and a very small doubt (ex : 0.2) than a better decision (with coeff. of 0.8) with a great doubt (ex : 0.5).

Using the figure 4 profile of a good decision, this example leads to numeric results : P=1,N=0.8 (for the first decision which is favourite) and P=1,N=0.5 (for the second one).

3. DISCUSSION

The complete system consists of one Knowledge Base about antibiotic field and two engines (one for deduction, one for decision making). They are working together and are reusable for other kinds of application. The total KB has more than 500 rules (50 for deductions, others for decisions) and this system produces results in few seconds with a 386 classic PC.

Consultant chooses one infectious site and isolated or just suspected germs ; system asks for some informations about patient biological and clinical context. According to these informations, the deduction engine infers new knowledge about patient category (renal insufficiency, hepatic insufficiency, ...) not in a crisp classification but in a fuzzy adherence to categorical sets. This engine is able to appreciate distance separating real and complete insufficiency to patient case. Then the decision engine uses these distances to interpret expert prescriptions, in the way described above.

An explanation tool is added, rebuilding reasoning of decision engine. This module explains modifications of final decision coefficients. This explanation is considered as sufficient by practitioners for understanding system selections.

Correctness of results has been appreciated by several bacterial field specialists. They consider that system conclusions are correct and relevant ; but this is not a scientific validation of our system. A more global validation of AntibES will be done, including five different hospitals, and several real-life situations. Difficulty rests in the lack of expert decision unanimity in front of specific cases. System conclusion would be considered as another expert opinion and compared with still existing differences between expert advises.

4. CONCLUSION

The decision part of our AntibES system has been presented. This description hides several problems of decision making (concurrent decisions, equivalence rules, associations of decisions, mono or multi-criteria approach ...), with which we have been confronted. Our total decision support system needs more than this short summary to be completely exposed.

We developed the expert system with a modular approach. Engines and database are totally separated. Reasoning modules are completely reusable for other application, medical or not.

Future works consist in introduction of some new possibilities about dynamic constructions of decision associations. First, we must envisage a scientific study for AntibES validation.

References

1. D. Dubois and H. Prade, Possibility Theory : An approach to the Computerised Processing of Information, Plenum Press, New-York, 1988
2. K. Arrow, Social choice and individual values, Wiley, 1963
3. B. Le Blanc and G. Palmer, AntibES : an expert system for antibiotic prescription, Thirteenth International Conference on Expert Systems, vol. 1, pp 123-132, EC2, Avignon, May 1993
4. L. Zadeh, Fuzzy sets, Information and control, vol. 8, pp 338-353, 1965
5. K. Yoshida, S. Ikeda and E. Tazaki, Medical Application of Fuzzy Decision Making, Medinfo 92, vol.1, pp 461, North-Holland, 1992
6. MC. Jaulent, Application du filtrage flou à la classification des lésions de l'artère rénale, Les applications des ensembles flous, pp 91-98, EC2, Nîmes, Nov. 1992

Strategies for Medical Reasoning - ICU Applications

Artificial Intelligence in Medecine
S. Andreassen et al. , Eds.
IOS Press, 1993

ILE-VT: An Intelligent Learning Environment in Ventilator Therapy

Svein-Ivar Lillehaug

Institute of Community Medicine, University of Tromsø, N-9037 Tromsø, Norway

Abstract

Mechanical ventilation of the lungs is considered to be a complex field which takes several years of practice to achieve mastery. New practitioners in ventilator therapy are plunged from theory and didactic instruction directly into clinical work where training continues on real patients. This often results in sub-optimal therapy which might be dangerous for both the health and life of the patient. With the ventilator therapy patient recognised as one of the most expensive and resource demanding, a sub-optimal therapy also influences the health care economy. One way to improve the quality of ventilator therapy is by improving the ICU personnel's knowledge about, and skills in giving this kind of treatment.

This paper describes the conceptual architecture of ILE-VT, an intelligent learning environment in ventilator therapy. ILE-VT is based on cognitive apprenticeship and when used as an educational supplement provides advantages over traditional ventilator therapy education. The ILE-VT's conceptual architecture utilises and combines the advantages of several different approaches including critiquing and articulate expert systems, student modelling, knowledge-based simulation, and instructional planning.

1. INTRODUCTION

Ventilator therapy is a complex field where sub-optimal therapy might be dangerous for both the health and life of the patient. Furthermore, the discipline is considered to be very resource demanding in respect of personnel and totally costs. A 1984 survey [1] reported that between 15-20% of the USA's hospital budget, or almost 1% of the US gross national product, was spent on intensive care. This is important because ventilator therapy is the intensive care unit (ICU) treatment that takes the most resources. Thoner et. al. [2] describe ventilator therapy patients as the most expensive—five times as expensive as the average hospital patient. Through the eyes of the patient and the health care personnel, the therapy is optimal when the duration time is minimised while complications and harm are avoided. This view complies with the economic way of appraising the costs and benefits of the therapy, where the average costs of one patient is calculated by dividing the total cost of ventilator therapy by the number of patients discharged from the unit.

It is generally agreed that the quality of the therapy is not at an optimal level [3-5], and surveys discussing the cost-benefit relation in ventilator therapy [2,6] propose a restriction on who receives ventilator therapy in order to improve the relationship. From both a human and an economic perspective, a preferable alternative would be to raise the personnel's level of knowledge and skills within ventilator therapy. The proposal for a computer-based *intelligent learning environment in ventilator therapy* (ILE-VT) that addresses this preference is based on the following conclusions from [7]:

- The given ventilator therapy is, on average, not optimal. This can result in: longer therapy duration, unpleasantness and danger for the patient, less job-satisfaction for the personnel, and higher costs.
- The undesirable results of ventilator therapy can partially be explained by weaknesses in the current education on ventilator therapy.
- The undesirable situation should be addressed by improving the theoretical knowledge and practical skills of the personnel.
- Computer-based education is the least resource demanding way to implement the desired improvement.

2. EDUCATIONAL REQUIREMENTS

The shortcomings of traditional ventilator therapy education as given at the University Hospital in Tromsø (UHT), Norway, were identified through questionnaires and interviews with physicians and nurses taking their special education in intensive care medicine and anaesthesiology, and with those in charge of the education. As reported in [7] these can be summarised as follows:

- There are weaknesses in the supervisor's ability to explain cases/problems and their solutions.
- Feedback on student performance is missing or of varying quality.
- Students are rarely required to explain cases/problems encountered or their own solutions.
- Rarely occurring cases are seldom encountered for demonstration and further training experience.
- Supervisors are not available when needed, and when available, time limitations prevent the supervisor from demonstrating or giving detailed enough explanations.

The identified shortcomings represent a wide variety of problems all of which address the process of acquiring knowledge and skills through practical experience. In order to address the shortcomings, the ILE-VT is required to:

- identify relevant aspects of a case, suggest possible solutions, and solve sub-problems or the entire case. For all aspects, the ILE-VT must also be capable of explaining the reasoning.
- watch student behaviour when the student is dealing with a case and provide the student with feedback whenever appropriate — both positive and negative.
- encourage the student to explain the patient cases and his own actions, and further, to discuss the pros and cons about their own problem solving.
- provide a variety of relevant/realistic cases for demonstration/problem solving, including rarely occurring cases.
- be available on demand.

3. AN ADOPTION OF THE COGNITIVE APPRENTICESHIP MODEL

As Jelovsek et al. [8] claim, the quality and the educational outcome of an application for computer-based education in medicine is strongly dependent upon the incorporation of established principles from instructional theories. This claim is taken into consideration in the process of specifying the conceptual framework of the ILE-VT.

The practical parts of the UHT special education are oriented around the *role model*, where the student first follows and observes an experienced practitioner, then solves the problems together with the experienced practitioner, and then finally, takes over the problem solving with the experienced practitioner standing behind, but still being in control. Education within ventilator therapy has its parallel in instructional theory in what Brown and Collins [9-11] have proposed as the *cognitive apprenticeship* (CA) *model* for instruction of cognitive skills.

The CA model comprises three methods described in [9] as:

- *Situated modelling*: The teacher/coach promotes learning, first by making explicit their tacit knowledge or by modelling their strategies for students in authentic activity.
- *Coaching*: The teacher/coach supports the student's attempts at doing the task.
- *Fading*: The teacher/coach empowers the student to continue independently as support is gradually withdrawn.

Brown and Collins have used the CA model as the basis for computer-based tools for teaching cognitive processes such as writing and solving mathematics problems [10]. As opposed to the formal schooling curricula which usually focuses on domain-specific knowledge only, the CA model stresses the importance of teaching such domain-specific knowledge along with various kinds of strategic knowledge that indicate *when and how to apply the domain knowledge*. In this way the CA model addresses both the domain knowledge and its practical application in a given domain. Although the physicians claimed they had too little time to acquire the theoretical material, the shortcomings in the nurse and physician special education were identified in the situations which called for practical application of their theoretical knowledge. Thus, aspects of the CA model that stress the application of domain knowledge will be particularly useful in addressing the shortcomings of the special education in ventilator therapy.

The CA model has been adopted and further adapted by others for computational use. One example is SHERLOCK, a computer-coached practice environment for training troubleshooting on electronic equipment used to diagnose faulty devices in aircraft [12]. After less experienced technicians practiced on SHERLOCK for about twenty-five hours, they compared in their ability to troubleshoot test station failures with colleagues who had four more years of on-the-job experience [12]. Another project that has adopted the CA model is the SAFE project [13-14]. The main objective of SAFE is to design an Intelligent Simulation Learning Environment (ISLE) shell and an integrated set of authoring tools, SIMULATE, for constructing simulations that are embedded in an intelligent learning environment (ILE). Unlike the SHERLOCK project, however, which was aimed at a specific domain (electronic troubleshooting), targeted to technicians with some experience, and emphasised giving hints tailored to the students performance, the SAFE project makes no such assumptions. The intention is to specify a generic, domain independent architecture, with no presupposition about the student's experience. Thus, the final requirements are broadly specified. While developing the functional requirements for the ISLE architecture, van Berkum [15] has used a framework based on the CA model to specify the requirements of a generic system. The framework looks at CA from the perspectives of *content*, *methods*, *sequencing*, and *sociology*.

In summary, the ILE-VT is based on the CA model because:

- The CA model is a highly accepted and well established method for effective instruction of cognitive skills.
- The CA model corresponds to, and gives a formal framework for the education of nurses and physicians in ventilator therapy.
- The CA model is one out of a very few instructional models that has been implemented with success.

Using the CA framework proposed by van Berkum [15], forty-three functional requirements that cover the content, method, sequencing and sociology of the domain of ventilator therapy are given in [7]. Table 1 gives some examples. The ILE-VT built on these requirements has the potential to address more than just the shortcomings of today's ventilator therapy education. It can be used for introducing nursing and medical students to ventilator therapy, as a tool for other personnel involved in giving ventilator therapy, and it can be a life-long learning tool for those who have completed their special education. For the main category of users, nurses and physicians receiving their special education, it should be pointed out that the ILE-VT is intended for use as a supplement to the current education.

Table 1 Example ILE-VT functional requirements

Content:	
Req-01	The ILE-VT must be able to represent and communicate all different types of domain-specific knowledge as well as strategic knowledge within ventilator therapy.
Methods:	
Req-03	Learning with the ILE-VT should mainly proceed through treatment of simulated patient cases either chosen by the student or the ILE-VT.
Req-23	The ILE-VT must be able to remind the student of relevant prior knowledge.
Req-31	The ILE-VT must be able to store all relevant data of a session, and further, to let the student inspect this history through a browser.
Sequencing:	
Req-36	The ILE-VT must be able to select and present the student with problems and patient cases of increasing complexity suitable for the student's level of knowledge and skills.
Sociology:	
Req-43	The ILE-VT must maintain its coaching facilities, also in sessions where the roles are reversed.

4. THE ILE-VT CONCEPTUAL ARCHITECTURE

The ILE-VT's conceptual architecture, given in Figure 1, consists of six system components and a *Media Module* through which the user interacts with the ILE-VT.

The **Media Module** (MM) provides the user with facilities necessary to communicate with the ILE-VT. Central in the MM is a work station (WS) that is connected to a printer, and may be connected to a mechanical ventilator (MV). The student – ILE-VT interaction that deals with the setting and presentation of patient and ventilator parameters needs to reflect the real therapy situation. This can be handled by connecting the actual MV to the WS where the user can make the ventilator settings and read the patient parameters, or by having the ILE-VT simulate the MV's functionality and present an interface to the simulated MV on the WS. Either approach gives both advantages and disadvantages.

Using the actual MV obviously provides the student with the same interface as in a real therapy situation. On the other hand, the MV is unusable (without modifications from the manufacturer) for demonstrations or problem solving given by the ILE-VT as it's settings require physical "push, pull & turn" actions. The MV interface has another limitation as the student will have to select, with an option button, *which* parameters or trends to be displayed at any given time. On the WS monitor many parameters and trends can be displayed simultaneously using multiple windows. This has been shown to be advantageous from a pedagogical point of view [16]. Another advantage in using the WS monitor to present the MV interface, is that it is required for the other communication such as dialogues, messages and requests between the student and the ILE-VT. In addition, the WS is also needed for providing the student with facilities such as a scratchpad editor for note taking. For the benefit of simplifying the remainder of the discussions, it will be assumed that the ILE-VT simulates the MV functionality and the MV interface is presented to the student on the WS.

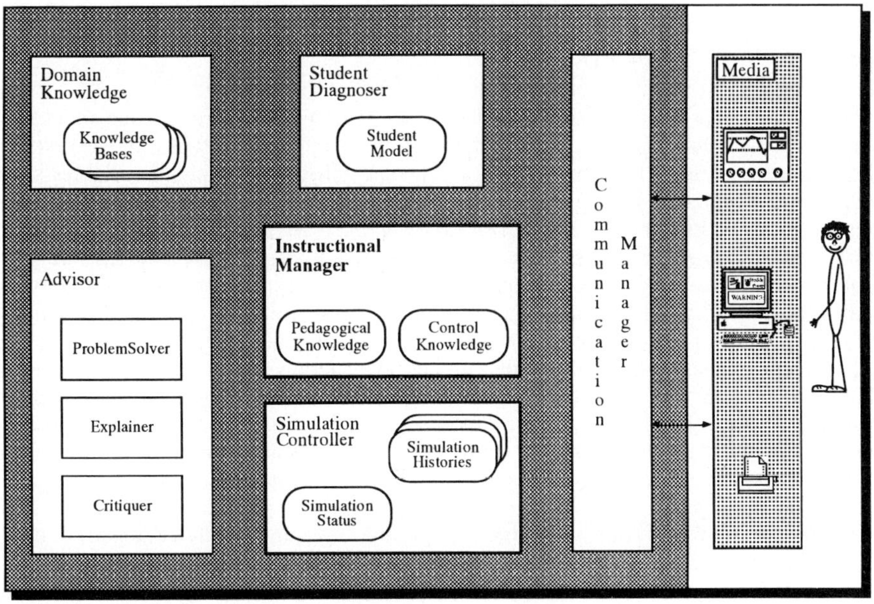

Figure 1. The ILE-VT conceptual architecture

The **Communications Manager** (CM) manages all interaction between the student (on the WS) and the ILE-VT. It translates the system's internal representation of what it wants to communicate into an understandable version for the student and vice versa. Central in this exchange of information is: the ILE-VT's output on the WS of the *simulated patient case* (visualised through continuously updated numerical, symbolical and trend parameters); an *interactive mechanical ventilator interface* through which the student manipulates and the ILE-VT displays and manipulates the different MV parameters; *display windows* in which the ILE-VT provides the student instructional support (e.g. an explanation window or critique window); and finally, *menus* from which the student can access different control actions (e.g., stop/start the simulation) and request instructional support (e.g., request an explanation or critique).

The **Domain Knowledge** (DK) represents the knowledge to be learned in forms that enable the other ILE-VT components to accomplish their tasks. In the ILE-VT, it is the problem solving of the ventilator therapy specialist that the student is to learn by interacting with the ILE-VT to solve patient cases while receiving instructional support. Thus, the domain knowledge must be organised and represented in formats that enable the following ILE-VT activities to take place:

- simulation of the patient case
- explanation of the patient case simulation
- monitoring of the patient case simulation
- explanation of specialist problem solving
- critique of specialist problem solving
- specialist problem solving of patient cases, with alternatives
- generating suitable next patient case
- critique of the student's problem solving performance
- evaluation of student's knowledge

- presentation of goal hierarchies
- monitoring of the student's performance
- providing the student with textual information, examples, demonstrations

The specialist's problem solving knowledge can be described as knowledge about how to initiate a patient to the ventilator, how to maintain the stable state obtained in the first phase, and to wean the patient from the ventilator. The specialist reasons about variables such as *general patient information* (e.g., age, sex, smoker/non-smoker, disease group (i.e. why the patient requires ventilator therapy)), *ventilator monitored parameters* (e.g. arterial gas tensions), *externally monitored parameters* (e.g., temperature), *visual parameters* (e.g., skin colour), *trends* (e.g., the change in oxygen intake over time), *complications* that arise (e.g. airway bleeding or accidental disconnection from the ventilator), and *current ventilator settings* (e.g., amount of oxygen delivered) to determine the next therapy action to be taken. In other words, the specialist has a model of ventilator therapy (developed through education and experience) that describes the relationship between all these variables and the adjustments that can be made to the ventilator. The representation of this model of ventilator therapy is complicated. For example, some of the variables are adjustable by the specialist through the ventilator (e.g., amount of oxygen delivered), while others are non-adjustable by the therapist (e.g., pulse rate), but are indirectly adjustable by the adjustment of several adjustable parameters. Thus, we constantly have dynamic activity ensured by this interrelationship of indirect adjustability. In addition to the challenge of determining the complex relationships between the variables, the choice of representation is complicated by the intended use for of the model. For example, in the ILE-VT, at least two types of ventilator therapy models are needed. One on which the simulation of the patient case can run (i.e., the runnable model) and explanations of the problem solving can be generated, and a second that represents the view of ventilator therapy that the student is to acquire (i.e., the learnable model).

White et al. [17] have shown that expert problem solving knowledge, to be learned through an ILE, is best represented as a series of models that capture the progression from novice to expert reasoning about a particular domain. These models can be arranged according to increasing complexity with problems to be solved classified according to the model level required for the correct solution, and explanations focused on the differences between a model and its predecessors. Applying this approach to modelling in the ILE-VT implies that the specialist's problem solving can be represented as a series of increasingly complex models of ventilator therapy. A model of ventilator therapy represents the knowledge required to identify relevant parameters, diagnosis the problem (taking those parameters into account), and plan the therapy action. Thus, the lowest level ventilator therapy model identifies a certain number of parameters as being important, and the diagnosis and therapy plan are based on those parameters. Then, each subsequent model will include more parameters, thus increasing the model's complexity. Correspondingly, patient cases, which are represented by a set of parameters and their initial values to be identified (i.e., the other parameters can be fixed at a reasonable setting), must be associated with the lowest model whose knowledge is required to solve the patient case.

The **Advisor Component** (AC) provides the ILE-VT with a set of support facilities that the instructional manager requires to provide the student with an effective learning environment. Essential in AC are operations on the specialist's problem solving knowledge, and a promotion of an understanding of the applied knowledge. The AC is responsible for the following ILE-VT activities:

- monitoring of the patient case simulation
- explanation of the patient case simulation
- explanation of specialist problem solving

- specialist problem solving of patient cases, with alternatives
- critique of specialist problem solving
- monitoring of the student's performance
- critique of the student's problem solving performance
- facilitating the presentation of textual information, examples, and demonstrations

To perform these tasks, the AC makes use of the **problem solver** (PS), the **explainer** (EX), and the **critiquer** (CQ). Specialist problem solving, performed by the PS, is required by the ILE-VT in several situations such as when the ILE-VT is demonstrating specialist performance, when the ILE-VT needs to provide the student with a hint or a solution to the current problem, and when the student asks a what-if question that requires specialist explanation. It is required indirectly when the CQ critiques the performance of the student or the ILE-VT. To perform problem solving, the PS works as a traditional expert system by using the domain knowledge to solve simulated patient cases. The problem solving also involves monitoring the on-going simulation to determine when an action must be taken (e.g., to watch for alarm states) and using the domain knowledge representation of specialist problem solving knowledge to determine what action.

The EX is responsible for making the knowledge more understandable for the student by using articulate expert system techniques to explain the therapy actions that the ILE-VT takes when demonstrating ventilator therapy, the different advice that it provides for the student when the student is practising ventilator therapy, and the answers given to a student's general question. It also supports the presentation of examples and textual information. In addition to providing these typical functionalities, the EX can provide the ILE-VT with an explanation of the simulation. This advantage is made possible by running the simulation on a knowledge-based representation (i.e., the runnable model) of specialist's problem solving.

The CQ is responsible for giving constructive criticism on a given hypothesis or problem solving performance. The problem solving performance can be on a single task, over a time interval, or over an entire patient case. Furthermore, the CQ makes use of EX's services when generating critiques of the student's or the ILE-VT's performance. The critique can either be a criticism that only discusses pros, cons and consequences of the criticised solution, or it can add a discussion of how the solution relates to alternative solutions.

The **Simulation Controller** (SC) is responsible for a *continuous simulation* of a given patient case. In the DK an instance of a patient case is defined through a set of variables, thus, a change in the patient's state can be described as a change in the value of one or several variables over time. It is also possible to force a change in the patient's state by changing the value of one or several of the variables which describe the patient's current state. This can be accomplished by running a qualitative knowledge representation of the patient case through a forward chaining mechanism that models ventilator therapy [18]. The SC uses a knowledge-based simulation to simulate a patient undergoing ventilator therapy. Ventilator therapy actions that can be performed on a patient are described in the DK's runnable model. The patient state's progression over time depends on the patient's history (described through current state and trends) and the student or the ILE-VT changes to the ventilator settings. To meet the requirement for a representation of time, the SC makes use of an internal clock which is also represented in the runnable model. It is this clock, together with the direct changes to the ventilator settings made by the student or the ILE-VT (through the PS), that drives the simulation. The direct adjustment to one ventilator parameter (or a combination) might in turn indirectly adjust other parameters thereby giving a continuous simulation. The internal clock also enables the simulation to be frozen at some point in time. This might be required in situations where the student is investigating some hypothesis and the student wants to absorb the information without the simulation running on, while the ILE-VT is providing the student with some information, or when the student wants to test out some alternative ventilator therapy action (e.g. changing a different parameter). Another advantage of the ILE-VT is obtained through it's sophisticated use of the time dimension. The use of alternative time modes (e.g., faster, slower, advance to next action required) enables the ILE-VT to avoid long periods where no therapy actions are required by speeding up the internal clock until a state where therapy actions are required again. Thus, patient cases that last a long time in reality can be presented in a reasonable time by the ILE-VT.

The SC has two knowledge bases, the *simulation status* (SSKB) and the *simulation histories* (SHKB), which store simulation states. A patient state is represented by its parameter values at a given time (i.e., the values have been updated as the simulation runs and therapy is given). The SSKB stores a sequence of patient states beginning with the initial state (defined in DK), and continuing through all the states that arise from both direct and indirect therapy actions. In addition, the set of actions that caused the patient state to change from the one state to the next state—the causes—are saved. Thus, the SSKB represents a progression of the patient's state over time, expressed as state1-actions-state2-actions, etc. The current state of the patient is the most recent state (according to time) represented in the SSKB. If the student wants to save a particular simulation state (e.g., indicated by selecting save the simulation state from a menu) then the SC can keep track of this by making a mark in the SSKB. Later, the simulation can be restarted from this point (e.g., the student wants to go back to a saved state and rerun the simulation performing different therapy actions) . Furthermore, the student can ask for an entire, or partial, simulation session to be stored for future use (e.g., to save an interesting case to rerun later with a supervisor, or to have more explanations given when the student has more time). The SC stores these sessions in the SHKB. The ILE-VT takes full advantage the potential of knowledge-based simulations (as opposed to CHRIS which does not [18]), and uses the causes represented in the SSKB to provide instructional support for the student. For example, the causes are used by the EX to give explanations about the simulation and the current patient state, and about why the changes in the patient state have occurred throughout the session, and by the student diagnoser to generate a diagnosis of the student's knowledge state.

The **Student Diagnoser** (SD) is responsible for developing and maintaining a *student model* which, at any given time, reflects an *adequate* model of the student's knowledge state and a history of the student – ILE-VT interaction. The student's knowledge state is described in terms of the ILE-VT's beliefs about what the student knows, does not know, might possible know, and what misconceptions are held. A *diagnosis* of the student's knowledge is based on the following:

- the student's performance (e.g., setting of ventilator parameters, inspection of trend variable, etc.)
- the student's requests for instructional support (e.g., answer to a question, an explanation, a critique, a hint, etc.)
- the student's answers to questions asked by the ILE-VT (e.g., to clarify whether the student holds a particular misconception, knows about a relationship, etc.)
- the information that has been given to the student (e.g., question answers, explanations, critiques, etc.)
- the particular domain knowledge that the student is to acquire (e.g., the specialist's solution for the particular patient case the student has been presented, the relationship between parameters that the student should learn to recognise, etc.)

The **Instructional Manager** (IM) coordinates the functions performed by the other ILE-VT components to continuously monitor the student's performance and determine when, how and exactly what instructional interaction is to take place. The IM is responsible for the following ILE-VT instructional activities:

- determination of what is to be taught/learned next (e.g., negotiating a learning goal)
- determination of the diversity and complexity of the ventilator therapy model for which the student is ready

- generation or selection of the next patient case (i.e., adapted to this student)
- determination of the most suitable time to interact with the student
- determination of whether to give an explanation, critique, example, hint or textual information
- generation of explanations, critiques, examples, hints and textual information at the appropriate level
- determination of when fading and scaffolding are required

The IM needs *pedagogical* and *control* knowledge that encode the ILE-VT's instructional strategies in a way that enables the IM to behave in a pedagogically valid manner. The pedagogical knowledge includes a pedagogical representation of what the student is to learn (e.g., it might be a conceptual organisation of ventilator therapy problem solving knowledge, or a hierarchical arrangement of patient cases), and represents the CA methods of modelling, fading, scaffolding, coaching, articulation, reflection, and exploration, and the additional strategy critiquing. The control knowledge represents where to obtain the functional support required to implement each of the strategies.

5. CONCLUSIONS

This paper has proposed an ILE that, when used as a supplement, provides advantages over traditional ventilator therapy education. First, the ILE-VT directly addresses the shortcomings in the current education reported in section 2 as it is always available with both often and rare cases. Demonstrations can be given with deep argumentation/explanation of both the changes in the patient's state and the performed therapy. Throughout student performance the ILE-VT has mechanisms to trigger student articulation and to provide the student with hints and constructive criticism.

By using the ILE-VT the student is provided with some additional advantages that are impossible to address through the current education. Through the ability to manipulate the time dimension the student can control the speed of the session. Patient cases requiring a long duration time can be completed during one session, while it is possible to spend more time on complicated problem situations than would have been possible (or natural) in a real setting. In addition, a session can also be frozen at the current state while the student is busy with other activities, or it can be stored for later inspections or reruns. Furthermore, the student can also step back to a particular state, thereby providing him with the possibility to test out alternative hypotheses. The ILE-VT also provides the student with an environment were he can exercise ventilator therapy without any danger for patients.

The ILE-VT also provides the speciality of ventilator therapy with an environment that provides life-long learning for the personnel. Other ways to use the ILE-VT are as a practical testbench for comparison of various therapy plans for an actual patient receiving ventilator therapy or as a theoretical testbench where benefits of new ventilator therapy techniques can be investigated. In the last case the ILE-VT contributes to optimising the discipline of ventilator therapy.

As an indirect consequence of these three categories of contributions, some extra benefits are incurred. First, the personnel will feel more self-confident in their jobs through an increase in their level of knowledge and skills. Second, an increase in the quality of the ventilator therapy implies less danger, fewer complications, less unpleasantness and shorter duration times for the ventilator patients. Finally, an increase in the quality of the ventilator therapy will also result in a better overall cost-benefit relation in ventilator therapy.

6. FUTURE RESEARCH

Shuell [19] describes a learning functions theory that summarises the current cognitive research on learning and education. This theory can also be used as a framework for evaluating the effectiveness of a computer-based learning environment. In [7] the ILE's conceptual architecture was evaluated according to it's support Shuell's twelve learning functions. The evaluation concluded that the ILE-VT's conceptual architecture is a highly acceptable architecture upon which future ILE-VT design decisions can be made. Thus, the next step is to refine the ILE-VT design and implement aspects of the system.

Being based upon an integration of several techniques such as critiquing and articulate expert systems, student modelling, knowledge-based simulation, and instructional planning, the future research on ILE-VT is provided with many challenges that will eventually be tested out in an implementation. In addition to tailoring and optimising these techniques for the ILE-VT, the domain of ventilator therapy will have to be considered from several perspectives. These include modelling of: patients receiving ventilator therapy (for the simulation); ventilator therapy performance by the specialist; problem solving in ventilator therapy as a series of increasingly complex models; and, the additional knowledge needed for textual information and examples.

Acknowledgements: The author would like to thank Thore Danielsen for supervising this masters research and Barbara Wasson for her helpful comments and discussions on this paper.

7. REFERENCES

1 Gardner, R.M. (1990). Patient-Monitoring Systems. Medical Informatics. In: E.H. Shortliffe, L.E. Perrault (Eds) Computer Applications in Health Care, 366-399. Amsterdam: Addison-Wesley.

2 Thoner, J., Sivertsen, O.M. (1982). Respiratorbehandling av kritisk syke pasienter. En kost/nytte-undersøkelse. *Tidsskr Nor Lægefor*, 102(25), 1291-1295. (In Norwegian)

3 Grossman, R., Hew, E., Aberman, A. (1983/1984). Assessment of the Ability to Manage Patients on Mechanical Ventilators using a Computer Model. *Acute Care* 10, 95-100.

4 Carson, E.R., Shamsolmaali, A., Summers, M.S., Leaning, M.S., Cramp, D.G. (1988). In: E.R. Carson et al. (Eds) Intelligent Instrumentation in Critical Care Medicine. *Advances in Biomedical Measurement,* 351- 358. New York: Plenum Press.

5 Summers, R., Carson, E.R., Cramp, D.G., Leaning, M.S. (1989). AIRS - An Artificial Intelligent Respirator System. In: C. Cobelli, L. Mariani (Eds) *IFAC Modelling and Control in Biomedical Systems*, 583-587.

6 Halvorsen, F.A., Ritland, S. (1991). Resultater av respiratorbehandling i en medisinsk intensivavdeling. *Tidsskr Nor Lægefor*, 111(2), 191-192. (In Norwegian)

7 Lillehaug, S-I. (1992). ILE-VT: Towards An Intelligent Learning Environment in Ventilator Therapy. *Cand. Scient. Thesis* (Master Thesis) in Computer Science, Department of Computer Science, University of Tromsø, Norway. Also available as Norwegian Telecom research report TF U 6/92.

8 Jelovsek, F. R., Catanzarite, V.A., Prince, R.D., Stull, R.E. (1989). Application of Teaching and Learning Principles to Computer-Aided Instruction. *M.D. Computing*, 6(5), 267-273.

9 Brown, J.S., Collins, A., Duguid, P. (1989). Situated cognition and the culture of learning. *Educational Research*, 18, 32-41.

10 Collins, A., Brown, J.S. (1988). The Computer as a Tool for Learning Through Reflection. In: H. Mandl, A.M. Lesgold (Eds) *Learning Issues for Intelligent Tutoring Systems*, 1-18. New York: Springer Verlag.

11 Collins, A., Brown, J.S., Newman, S.E. (1989). Cognitive Apprenticeship: Teaching Students the Crafts of Reading, Writing and Mathematics. In: L.B. Resnick (Ed) *Knowing, Learning and Instruction: Essays in Honor of Robert Glaser.* Lawrence Erlaum Associates.
12 Lajoie, S.P., Lesgold, A. (1988). Apprenticeship Training in the Workplace: Computer-Coached Practice Environment as a New Form of Apprenticeship. *Man-Mediated Learning*, 3, 7-28.
13 de Jong, T. (Ed) (1990). *The Safe Project: Computer Simulations in an Instructional Context.* DELTA-Project P7061, SAFE Report No. SIM/21.
14 Hijne, H., van Berkum, J. (1990). A Functional Architecture for Intelligent Simulation Learning Environments. *Paper presented at DELTA & Beyond*, 18-19 October, The Hague, The Netherlands).
15 van Berkum, J.J.A. (1991). Functional Requirements for an Intelligent Simulation Learning Environment: A Cognitive Apprenticeship Perspective. *DELTA-Project SAFE Report No. SIM/24B.*
16 Woolf, B., Blegen, D., Jansen, J.H., Verloop, A. (1987). Teaching a Complex Industrial Process. In. R.W. Lawler, M. Yazdani (Eds) *Artificial Intelligence and Education Volume One*, 413-427. Norwood, New Jersey: Ablex.
17 White, B.Y., Frederikson, J.R. (1990). Causal model Progressions as a Foundation for Intelligent Learning Environments. *Artificial Intelligence*, 42, 99-157.
18 Berger, R.A., Sonenberg, E.A., Zelcher, J. (1988). A Knowledge Based Simulation of Critical Incidents in Anaesthesia. Proceedings of the Australian Joint Intelligence Conference 1988, 203-217.
19 Shuell, T.J. (1992). Designing Instructional Computing Systems for Meaningful Learning. In: M. Jones, P. Winne (Eds) *Foundations and Frontiers of Adaptive Learning Environments*, New York: Springer-Verlag.

Artificial Intelligence in Medecine
S. Andreassen et al. , Eds.
IOS Press, 1993

Oxygen Status Model for the Ventilatory and Circulatory Contribution to Tissue Oxygenation

S. Andreassen[a], J. Egeberg[a], M.P. Schröter[a] and P.T. Andersen, M.D.[b]

[a] Department of Medical Informatics and Image Analysis, Institute for Electronic Systems. Aalborg University, Denmark

[b] Department of Intensive Care, Aalborg Sygehus, Aalborg, Denmark

Abstract

The paper presents an oxygen status model (OSM) for simulation of major respiratory and circulatory malfunctions and the effect of ventilatory or hemodynamic medical intervention. The OSM includes a model of a ventilator and the human respiratory and circulatory systems, implemented as a causal probabilistic network (CPN). The CPN representation makes OSM able to consider uncertainties during simulation. OSM was tested as a simulation tool on two fictive cardiovascular or ventilatory disease states. The results demonstrate the potential of the OSM with respect to simulation of disease states and their treatments.

1. INTRODUCTION

Critically ill patients often suffer from both respiratory and circulatory malfunction, which may cause an insufficient oxygen delivery to the tissues. In order to treat such a condition, the patients often will be ventilator-assisted and pharmacalogically manipulated with respect to the blood circulation. Yet, the treatment of patients in the intensive care unit is often a difficult task and some treatment strategies may have fatal consequences for the patient. This paper describes an expert system, the Oxygen Status Model (OSM) for simulating the effects of therapeutic intervention.

OSM is implemented as a Causal Probabilistic Network (CPN) modelling the human respiratory and circulatory systems and either a volume or pressure controlled ventilator. A CPN contains stochastic variables, linked by conditional probabilities. The CPN calculates the probability distributions of the stochastic variables.

OSM was tested as a simulation tool on two fictive disease states. The aim of the test was to simulate the characteristics of a patient with a cardiovascular disease and a patient with a ventilatory disease, as well as the effects of treatment.

2. STRUCTURE OF THE OSM

The OSM is divided into the five physiological blocks shown in Fig. 1. Each block contains a representation of the relevant physiology for its particular area.

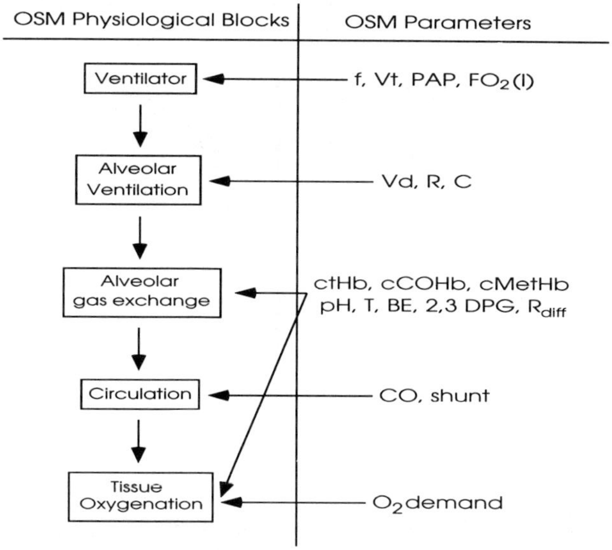

Fig. 1. The five physiological blocks of the OSM are given in the left column. OSM parameters (see text) are given in the right column.

The function of the *ventilator* is determined by the settings of the ventilator: The respiratory frequency (f) and the tidal volume (V_t) or the positive airway pressure (PAP), depending on whether the ventilator mode is volume or pressure control. We also include the inspired oxygen fraction ($FO_2(I)$) as a ventilator setting.

The resultant *alveolar ventilation* depends on dead space (V_d), airway resistance (R) and the mechanical compliance (C) of the lungs and thorax.

The *alveolar gas exchange* is the most complex part of the OSM, influenced by 8 parameters. Three parameters describe the composition of hemoglobin, the total hemoglobin concentration (ctHb), the concentration of carbonmonoxide hemoglobin (cCOHb) and the concentration of methemoglobin (cMetHb). Four parameters describe the oxygen affinity of hemoglobin: pH, temperature (T), base excess (BE) and 2,3 diphosphoglycerate (2,3 DPG). Finally, the alveolar diffusion resistance (R_{diff}) describes the diffusion resistance of oxygen between the alveoles and the pulmonary capillaries.

For the *circulation* the relevant parameters are cardiac output (CO) and veno-arterial shunt, typically a pulmonary shunt.

Sufficient *tissue oxygenation* depends on the amount of oxygen delivered by the circulatory system, but also on the tissues oxygen demand (O_2-demand). In addition the concentration of the various types of hemoglobin and the oxygen affinity of hemoglobin influence the oxygen partial pressures, and thereby the diffusion of oxygen from the capillaries to the oxygen consuming tissues.

The OSM is based on two status variables representing the oxygen status of the body. The status variables were chosen as the alveolar and

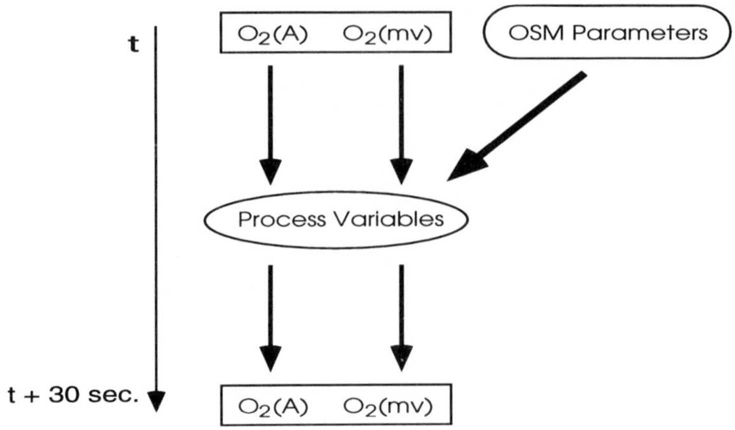

Fig. 2. The OSM is based on two status variables: oxygen stored in the alveoli (O_2(A)) and oxygen stored in the mixed venous blood (O_2(mv)). The system is parameterized such that the state of the system is determined by the 18 parameters listed in Fig. 1. These parameters influence the process variables, which in turn determine the changes of the status variables over a 30 sec time period.

mixed venous oxygen concentrations (O_2(A) and O_2(mv)), as they represent 87% of the total oxygen stored in the body (Nunn 1987).
The OSM allows changes in the status variables to be calculated over a number of 30 sec time slices (Fig. 2). Eventually, the status variables will reach an equilibrium, which reflects the current values of the parameters.

3. CAUSAL PROBABILISTIC NETWORK (CPN) REPRESENTATION

A causal probabilistic network consists of nodes and directed links (arrows). The nodes represent stochastic variables and the arrows represent conditional probabilities that allow the variables to influence each other (Andreassen *et al.* 1991, Pearl 1988). In the HUGIN shell used to construct this CPN (Andersen *et al.* 1989, Lauritzen and Spiegelhalter 1988) all stochastic variables are discrete and knowledge about the variables is expressed as discrete probability distributions over the states in each variable. In the OSM most of the variables are continuous. This is handled by sampling the continuous variables and treating the sampling points as states in a discrete stochastic variable.

In the OSM each of the parameters are represented as a node in the CPN, for example the temperature is represented as a node with 10 states, ranging from 32°C to 41°C. Each of the parameters has an a priori probability distribution associated with it. The a priori probability distribution reflects the probability distribution in the patient population. Other nodes represent sampled versions of the process and status variables.

The OSM has a total of 79 nodes in one time slice. A frequently occurring problem in CPN modelling of physiological systems is feedback, because most physiological systems have feedback mechanisms and feedback loops cannot be expressed in CPNs. In the OSM this was solved by dividing the model into time slices: variables in one time slice feedback to variables in the next, a strategy borrowed from a CPN model of glucose metabolism (Hovorka *et al.* 1992).

The choice of sampling points in the continuous variables is a somewhat tedious task that requires considerable care. If the variables are oversampled the computational load becomes unnecessarily large, and if the variables are undersampled the computational accuracy suffers (Andreassen 1992). However, one of the advantages of the representation of continuous variables as sampled (discrete) variables is that non-linear relations can be handled just as easily as linear relations. An example of a pronounced nonlinearity is the relation between oxygen partial pressure (pO_2) and oxygen saturation (sO_2). Under standard condition, i.e. normal pH, base excess ect., sO_2 is a function of pO_2:

$$sO_2 = f(pO_2) \tag{1}$$

This function can be implemented by reading the sampled values from the oxygen saturation curve (Fig. 3).

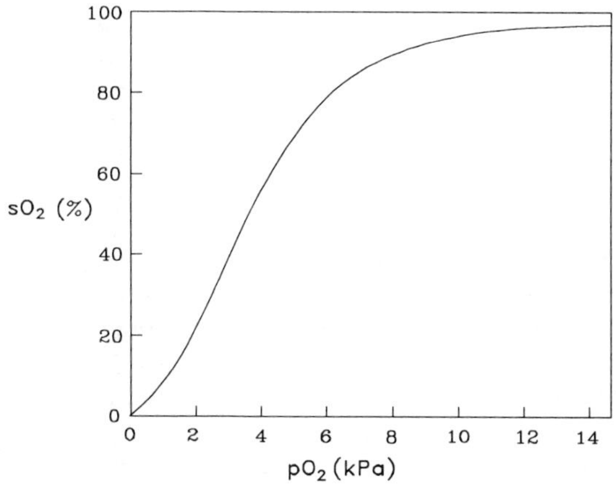

Fig. 3 The Oxygen Dissociation Curve (ODC) specifies the relation between oxygen pressure (pO_2) and oxygen saturation of hemoglobin (sO_2). The ODC is shown in its normal position.

This is an example where the variables are linked one to one. Typically the variables depend on two or more other variables, for example the alveolar oxygen ventilation, $VentO_2(A)$, depends on the alveolar ventilation of air, Vent(A), and the difference between inspired oxygen fraction $FO_2(I)$ and expired oxygen fraction $FO_2(E)$:

$$VentO_2(A) = Vent(A) \cdot (FO_2(I) - FO_2(E)) \qquad (2)$$

The conversion of equations of these types to conditional probabilities is made easier by using a tool designed for this purpose (Olesen and Andreassen 1993).

In this paper the OSM's ability to simulate patient status, given the values of the parameters will be explored. This type of reasoning is sometimes called causal or deductive reasoning, because the reasoning is performed in the direction of causality: from the parameters (causes) towards the effects (the status and process variables). However, a CPN can just as easily reason in the opposite direction, i.e. generate parameter estimates from measured variables, a type of reasoning that is sometimes called diagnostic or abductive reasoning. In practical use the applicability of the OSM depends on both types of reasoning, first patient specific parameter estimates are provided by diagnostic reasoning based on measured variables, and subsequently causal reasoning is used to derive the consequences of therapeutic interventions.

4. RESULTS

To illustrate the capability of the OSM in simulating the characteristics of the disease states and the effects of ventilatory and hemodynamic medical intervention, two fictive cases will be presented in the following paragraphs. The first case is a patient with a coronary thrombosis, causing myocardial infarction and low cardiac output. The second case is a patient with pneumonia, causing a high pulmonary shunt and a high oxygen diffusion resistance of the alveolar membrane.

4.1 Case 1:

The patient suffers a coronary thrombosis and myocardial infarction. He is not ventilator assisted. The respiratory system of the patient is normal and therefore shunt and diffusion resistance are initially assumed to be negligible. The initial data from the patient are summarized in Table I.

The myocardial infarction causes a decrease in cardiac output from 5 l/min to 1.9 l/min.

Fig. 4a shows the probability distributions for arterial and mixed venous pressures, saturations and concentrations, as the OSM predicts them. When CO equals 1.9 l/min, the OSM predicts a critically low $pO_2(mv)$, because the oxygen extraction in the tissues will increase, partially compensating for the low cardiac output. Treatment of low cardiac output could be inotrophic and vascular dilatatory drugs. If we assume that this treatment increases CO to 3.1 l/min, the OSM predicts the values shown in Fig. 4b.

Table I. Initial values for Case 1.

Respiratory frequency (f)	14 /min
Tidal volumen (V_t)	500 ml
Inspired oxygen fraction $FO_2(I)$	21 %
Hemoglobin concentration (Hb)	8 mmol/l
Base excess (BE)	0 mmol/l
Temperature (T)	37 °C
pH	7.40
Alveolar oxygen diffusion resistance	0 kPa/l/min

It shows that the increased CO does not affect the arterial pO_2 values, because the oxygenation of blood in the pulmonary capillaries is still optimal and no shunt is present. Instead, the increase in CO improves the mixed venous pO_2. From a clinical point of view the rise in mixed venous pO_2 accomplished by an increase of CO to 3.1 l/min is satisfactory. A further increase in CO by pharmacological manipulation would not be of major benefit to the patient. By simulation of the effects of circulatory manipulations, overmedication with vasoactive drugs might be avoided as many of the associated side effects of this treatment.

4.2 Case 2:

The patient suffers from pneumonia, causing a part of the lung to be a 100% shunt. In the remaining part of the lung, the alveolar diffusion barrier has increased (increased R_{diff}), due to inflammation and edema. This part of the lung does, however, not contribute to the shunt.

The patient is put into ventilator therapy due to hypoxia and exhaustion. Inspired oxygen fraction is 60%. Table II shows the initial values assumed for this patient.

Table II. Initial values for Case 2.

Respiratory frequency (f)	14 /min
Tidal volumen (V_t)	500 ml
Inspired oxygen fraction $FO_2(I)$	60 %
Hemoglobin concentration (Hb)	8 mmol/l
Base excess (BE)	0 mmol/l
Temperature (T)	37 °C
pH	7.40

In Table III, the column labelled Situation 1 shows the pulmonary capillary, arterial and mixed venous oxygen values, when both shunt and R_{diff} are high. The column shows critically low mixed venous oxygen values.

To improve the condition of the patient, PEEP (Positive End Expiratory Pressure) is instituted, causing a decrease in R_{diff}. Another effect of PEEP may be, that some alveoli which were shunted because of complete obliteration, are transformed into alveoli with high R_{diff}. The effect of PEEP is seen in Table III, Situations 2 and 3.

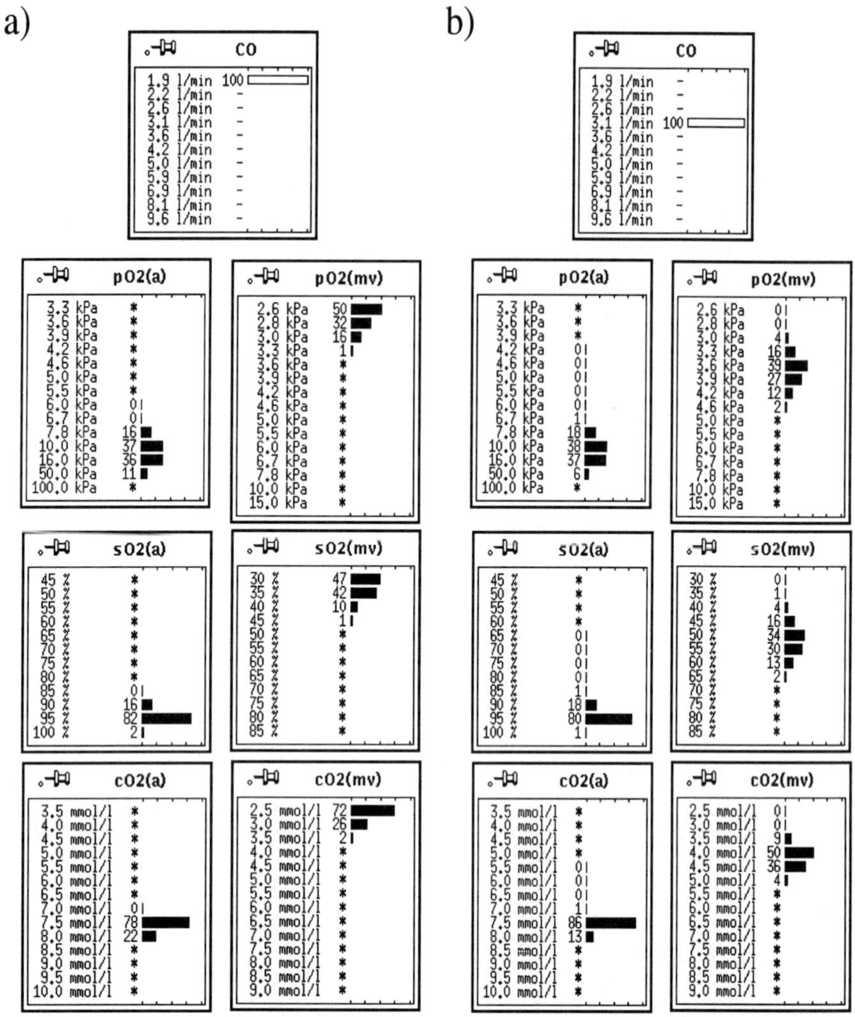

Fig. 4. The OSM is calculating the probability distributions of variables and parameteres. The leftmost numbers are the possible states. The length of the bars show the probability of the variable/parameter being in the respective states. The probabilities are also given in percent to the left of the bars. a) shows the oxygen status when cardiac output (CO) is 1.9 l/min, and b) shows the oxygen status when CO is raised to 3.1 l/min. pO_2, sO_2, and cO_2 refer to oxygen pressure, saturation and concentration, respectively. (a) denotes arterial and (mv) mixed venous.

In the column labelled Situation 2 the PEEP effect on R_{diff} is showing increased oxygen values. This is due to an increase in pulmonary capillary pO_2. In the column labelled Situation 3 the additional PEEP effect on shunt

Table III. The oxygen status when alveolar shunt and oxygen diffusion resistance of the alveolar membrane (R_{diff}) are high. The column labelled Situation 1 regards the initial values for a patient suffering from pneumonia causing increased shunt and R_{diff}. The column labelled Situation 2 shows the PEEP effect causing a decrease in R_{diff}. The column labelled Situation 3 shows the effect of decreased R_{diff} and decreased shunt. The figures are given as mean values ± standard deviations.

CASE 2		Situation 1	Situation 2	Situation 3
R_{diff}	kPa/l/min	153	101	101
shunt	%	50	50	30
$pO_2(c)$	kPa	7.3 ± 0.7	22.3 ± 14.7	21.1 ± 14.4
$pO_2(a)$	kPa	4.4 ± 0.3	4.7 ± 0.5	7.1 ± 3.4
$sO_2(a)$	%	63.1 ± 3.1	66.7 ± 5.6	82.8 ± 6.9
$cO_2(a)$	mmol/l	5.1 ± 0.2	5.4 ± 0.4	6.6 ± 0.5
$pO_2(mv)$	kPa	2.7 ± 0.1	2.8 ± 0.2	3.6 ± 0.5
$sO_2(mv)$	%	32.3 ± 2.9	35.4 ± 5.2	50.1 ± 7.9
$cO_2(mv)$	mmol/l	2.6 ± 0.2	2.8 ± 0.4	4.4 ± 0.6

is shown. The arterial and mixed venous oxygen values increases as shunt decreases. Simulating this disease state may help to derive the most beneficial therapeutic intervention by visualizing the result of manipulation of R_{diff} and pulmonary shunt.

5. DISCUSSION

We have presented an expert system (OSM) for simulating major ventilatory and circulatory malfunctions and the effects of ventilatory or hemodynamic medical intervention. The OSM was implemented as a CPN.

Two fictive disease states showed that the OSM simulated the diseases and treatments as would be clinically expected. However, to prove its clinical value, the OSM has to be tested on real patient data.

We are planing to carry out further testing by entering measurements from patients into the OSM. Propagation of these measurements in the CPN implementation of the OSM leads to revised (a posteriori) probability distributions for the OSM parameters. These revised probability distributions represent an estimate of the patient's current physiological status, based on the available measurements. After the probability distributions of the OSM parameters have been revised, the OSM can be used to predict the consequences of a range of therapeutic interventions.

Typically, there will not be enough measurements to generate accurate estimates for all parameters. Some of the parameters will have fairly wide a posteriori probability distributions. This residual uncertainty about the OSM parameters, expressed by the probability distributions, will in a consistant way be translated into a corresponding uncertainty about the predicted consequences of the therapeutic interventions. The performance of the OSM can be tested by comparing the predicted consequences to actual measurements performed after a therapeutic intervention.

The physiological models of alveolar gas exchange and circulation (Fig. 1) are essentially identical to the models implemented in the Oxygen Status Algorithm (OSA) (Siggaard-Andersen *et al.* 1990a, 1990b). The main difference is that the OSA implementation is based on a set of non-linear equations, while the OSM is based on a CPN implementation of essentially the same equations. We have added models of the ventilator and the alveolar ventilation, and a more detailed model of tissue oxygenation, in the expectation that the somewhat larger scope of the physiological modelling will increase the clinical applicability of the OSM. Further clinical testing will show whether or not this expectation is justified.

6. ACKNOWLEDGMENTS

We would like to thank the following for their advice and other contributions to this work: Lecturer Ron Summers, Ph.D., City University, London; Professor Ewart R. Carson, City University, London and Dr. Cliff Morgan, Royal Brompton National Heart & Lung Hospital, London.

7. REFERENCES

Andersen S.K., Olesen K.G., Jensen F.V. and Jensen F. (1989). HUGIN - A shell for building Bayesian belief universes for expert systems. In: Proceedings of IJCAI 89 2, 1080-1985.

Andreassen S., Jensen F.V. and Olesen K.G. (1991). Medical Expert Syst ems based on Causal Probabilistic Networks. In: Int. J. Biomed Comput. 28, 1-30. Elsevier Scientific Publishers Ireland Ltd.

Andreassen S. (1992) Knowledge representation by extended linear models. In: Deep Models for Medical Knowledge Engineering, ed. Keravnou, E. Elsevier.

Hovorka R., Andreassen S., Benn J.J., Olesen K.G. and Carson E. (1992) Causal probabilistic network modelling. An illustration of its role in the management of chronic diseases. IBM Systems Journal 31(4), 635-648.

Lauritzen S.L. and Spiegelhalter D.J. (1988) Local Computations with Probabilities on Graphical Structures and their Application to Expert Systems. J. R. Statist. Soc. B 50(2), 157-224.

Nunn J.F. (1987) Applied Respiratory Physiology, 3rd edition. Buttersworth & Co. Ltd.

Olesen K.G. and Andreassen S. (1993) Specification of models in large expert systems based on causal probabilistic networks. Artificial Intelligence in Medicine. In press.

Pearl J. (1988) Probabilistic Reasoning in Intelligent Systems - Networks of Plausible Inference, 2. edition. Morgan Kaufmann Publishers, Inc.

Siggaard-Andersen O., Gøthgen I.H., Wimberley P.D. and Fogh-Andersen N. (1990) The oxygen status of the arterial blood revised: relevant oxygen parameters for monitoring the arterial oxygen availability. Scand J Clin Lab Invest 50, suppl. 203: 17-28.

Siggaard-Andersen O. and Siggaard-Andersen M. (1990). The oxygen status algorithm: a computer program for calculating and displaying pH and blood gas data. Scand J Clin Lab Invest 50, suppl. 203: 29-45.

Artificial Intelligence in Medecine
S. Andreassen et al. , Eds.
IOS Press, 1993

VIE–VENT: Knowledge–Based Monitoring and Therapy Planning of the Artificial Ventilation of Newborn Infants

Silvia Miksch[1], Werner Horn[1,2], Christian Popow[3], Franz Paky[4]

[1] Austrian Research Institute for Artificial Intelligence (ÖFAI), Schottengasse 3, A–1010 Vienna, Austria
email: silvia@ai.univie.ac.at
[2] Department of Medical Cybernetics and Artificial Intelligence, University of Vienna, Freyung 6/2, A–1010 Vienna, Austria
[3] Department of Pediatrics, NICU, University of Vienna, Währinger Gürtel 18–20, A–1090 Vienna, Austria
[4] Gottfried von Preyer Children's Hospital, Schankenberggasse 31, A–1100 Vienna, Austria

Abstract

We developed a knowledge–based system, VIE–VENT, for monitoring and therapy planning of artificially ventilated newborn infants. One of our aims was to implement clinical and textbook knowledge in VIE–VENT's knowledge base. Therapy planning is based on a combination of transcutaneous and invasively determined blood gas measurements and clinical observations. After the selection and validation of appropriate parameters, these data are transformed into qualitative values. These are used in our model of neonatal respiration for recommending therapeutic actions according to heuristic clinical rules of artificial ventilation. For the weaning process we implemented three possible strategies, which allow adapting different dynamics of weaning (conservative, normal, aggressive).
VIE–VENT is specifically designed for practical use under real–time constraints in the Neonatal Intensive Care Units (NICUs).

1. Introduction

Artificial ventilation has greatly contributed to improve the mortality and morbidity of premature newborn infants [11, 18]. Improved patient monitoring techniques and enhanced knowledge about the pathophysiological mechanisms of barotrauma and oxygen toxicity led to the development of patient–tailored strategies of mechanical ventilation and helped to reduce harmful side effects of respirator therapy. However, the bulk of continuous information arising from complex monitoring systems creates a rising information management problem at Neonatal Intensive Care Units (NICUs).

Knowledge–based system technology may appropriately represent and organize the practical and theoretical knowledge of experienced specialists and help to overcome the suffering from information overload with continuous data selection, data validation and therapy planning [16]. Such a system should therefore be able to support the less experienced physician in the complex decision–making of patient care, and the experienced physician in handling and analysing the complex data arising steadily from the patient monitoring system. During the past decade, several knowledge–based systems were introduced to support clinicians with the monitoring of critical care patients and to assist them with diagnostic decisions and therapy planning. These systems range from simple, intelligent alarming systems to sophisticated systems for knowledge–based monitoring and therapy management (e.g., ventilator management systems).

Starting up with an overview about knowledge–based monitoring and therapy planning for artificial ventilator management, we will describe the essential monitoring and therapy planning tasks which have to be performed. The main part of the paper deals with the architecture of VIE–VENT, a monitoring and therapy planning system for artificial ventilation which we developed at the Austrian Research Institute for Artificial Intelligence (ÖFAI) in cooperation with the Gottfried von Preyer Children's Hospital, the Neonatal Intensive Care Unit (NICU) of the Department of Pediatrics of Vienna's University Medical School, and the Department of Medical Cybernetics and Artificial Intelligence, University of Vienna.

2. Knowledge–based Systems for Artificial Ventilation

During the past decade, several projects were initiated to support clinicians with their information processing needs at ICUs. Uckun's [21] survey of research projects describes 32 projects concerning real–time information management at ICUs in general. Among these, there are nine projects dealing with artificial ventilation management.

A pioneer work in the area of knowledge–based monitoring and therapy planning systems was the Ventilator Manager (VM, [9]), which was designed to manage postsurgical mechanically ventilated patients. VM was developed in the late 1970s as one of a series of experiments studying the effectiveness of the MYCIN formalism.

The recent knowledge–based systems could be classified in two dimensions: the application domain and the system architecture. On the one hand, there are applications which assist patients with adult respiratory distress syndrome (ARDS), like VM [9], VentPlan [14, 15], and COMPAS [17]. On the other hand, projects were developed to support the treatment of neonates, like VMS [3] SIMON [19, 20], and the system of Arroe [1].

The second classification deals with the different system architectures, reasoning tasks and inference methods. For example, VMS [3] used decision trees to formulate therapy recommendations. VentPlan [14, 15] combined qualitative and quantitative techniques (a mathematical model of the physiology of the heart and the lung functions, a belief network to estimate parameter values and a plan evaluator, which ranks the therapy plans). Guardian [2, 12, 13] used a blackboard control architecture to represent the factual and the generic reasoning knowledge about the anatomy and physiology of the lung. It is a 'proof of concept' system, which was not designed for practical use. Finally, SIMON [19, 20] based on YAQ, an ontology derived from Qualitative Process Theory (QPT). YAQ is a combination of qualitative and numerical simulation techniques.

A small number of systems was designed mainly for intelligent alarming and alarm validating (RESPAID [8], PONI [10]). The major goal of these systems is a reduction in the number of false alarms.

From the practical point of view, the usability of all these systems is limited as concerns their monitoring and therapy planning components. Sometimes the therapy component is missing (e.g., in SIMON). Most systems use invasively determined blood gas measurements for therapy planning, which, however, are only discontinuously and infrequently determined. Moreover, therapy planning in a modern ICU is increasingly based on noninvasive continuous measurements of transcutaneous partial pressure of oxygen ($PtcO_2$), arterial oxygen saturation (SaO_2) and transcutaneous partial pressure of carbon dioxide ($PtcCO_2$). Another problem of the systems described is their lack of support of individual artificial ventilation strategies. In addition, data validation modules are simple, and reasoning about the change of parameters over time is missing. Finally, several systems were designed for adults and are therefore not suitable for neonates. Developing VIE–VENT, we tried to overcome these limitations. VIE–VENT is specifically designed for practical use under real–time constraints in the NICU.

3. Tasks of Knowledge–based Monitoring and Therapy Planning

Artificial ventilation of patients at a NICU involves a series of tasks ranging from simple alarming to more complex therapy planning functions. Patient monitoring usually deals with the collection of selected physiological parameters (e.g., blood gases, heart rate) which are registered, displayed and compared to upper and lower limits. The exceeding of these limits usually triggers an alarm.

Knowledge–based monitoring additionally performs analysis tasks [4]. This presupposes an existing system model (e.g., a model of human breathing) and an instantiation of the model using current data values. Data collected by the patient monitor are selected, validated and transformed into qualitative values. The latter are compared with target values derived from the system model. If discrepancies between the system model and the current values are detected, a decision about the proper action(s) has to be made. The precise practical formulation of therapy recommendations is part of the therapy planning module. This component involves the interpretation of the patient's status, the selection of an appropriate therapy and the prediction of its short and long term effects [12, 5, 6].

As shown in Figure 1, the building of a knowledge–based monitoring and therapy planning system can be divided into several steps: feature extraction, data selection, data validation, data abstraction, and therapy planning. Therapy planning consists of interpretation of the patient's status, determination of proper therapy recommendations and the short or long term predictions of the effects of a therapy. All these steps are involved in a single cycle of data interpretation.

4. Architecture of VIE–VENT

Our aim in developing VIE–VENT was to integrate a monitoring and a therapy planning module according to the previously described tasks (Figure 1). According to our philosophy of a practically oriented knowledge–based system, we built the various module components in analogy to the clinical reasoning process.

4.1 Feature Extraction

A feature extraction module handles the task of data storage and retrieval and of low–level signal processing. The monitoring module first selects the data transmitted from various devices (e.g., patient monitor, ventilator) according to its time base of 10 seconds and stores them in a temporary form. Every ten minutes, the arithmetic means of the stored 10–seconds–data are calculated and written in an archiving file.

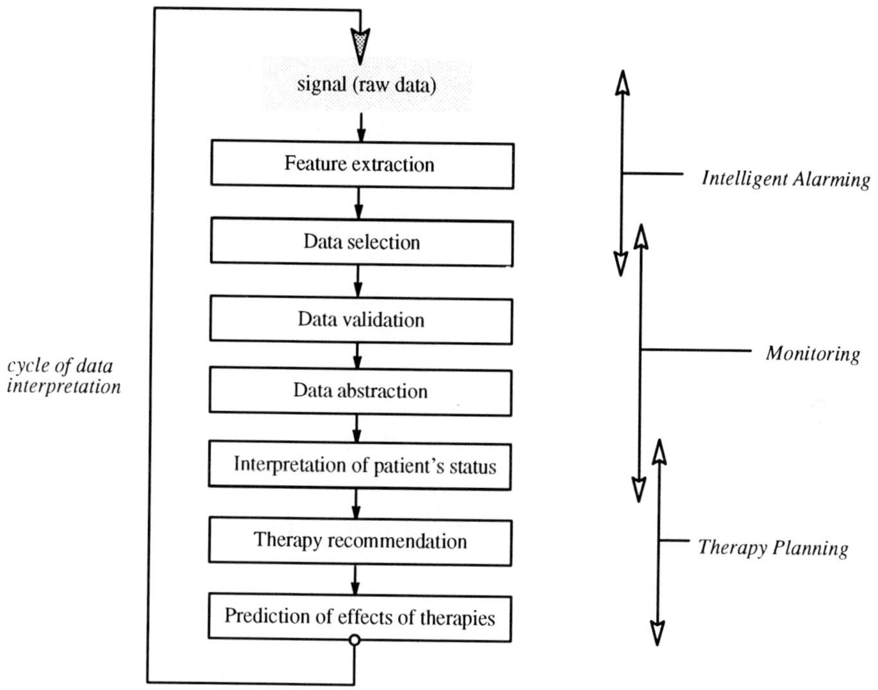

Figure 1: Tasks of knowledge–based monitoring and therapy planning

4.2 Data Selection

The phase of data selection, often the main starting point of the monitoring task, is the process of filtering out context–relevant data for further analysis.

VIE–VENT's whole data set is divided into continuous and discontinuous data. The continuous data are taken from the output of the feature extraction module. The discontinuous data are entered on request to the system, depending on different conditions (e.g., critical ventilatory condition of the neonate, elapsed time intervals). VIE–VENT uses the following parameters:

(a) continuous data:
ventilator settings: F_iO_2, f, PIP, PEEP, t_i, t_e, v_i, v_e, VT
mode of ventilation: IPPV, IMV, CPAP
transcutaneous blood gases: $PtcO_2$, $PtcCO_2$, SaO_2

(b) discontinuous data:
neonate's personal description (e.g., name, sex)
clinical parameters (e.g., weight, age, chest wall expansion, spontaneous breathing effort)
invasive blood gases: pH, PO_2, PCO_2
site of blood gas measurements: arterial, capillary, venous

4.3 Data Validation

The major aim of the data validation process is to arrive at reliable measurements. There are different parts of the data validation process: the checking of plausible measurements, the handling of missing values, the rather complicated process of recognizing artifacts, and the "calibration" of measurements. These four problems are discussed in the following short examples.

– Plausible Measurements

(a) simple checking of ranges: e.g., $15 \leq pCO_2$ (arterial, IPPV) ≤ 130

(b) Reliability of measurements: From the medical and technical sampling point of view, there is a well–defined priority which measurement is more reliable compared to another, depending on different conditions. E.g., for oxygenation: invasive blood gas PO_2 is more reliable than SaO_2 and SaO_2 is more reliable than $PtcO_2$;

– Missing Values

A robust system has to deal with missing values. In VIE–VENT, this problem is solved in two different ways:

(a) using a simplified system model of neonatal respiration during the initial phase when the only reliable measurement is SaO_2 (more details are given in section 4.5.1 System Model of Neonatal Respiration);

(b) context–dependent rules applying defaults for missing values;

– Artifacts

The recognition of artifacts is a rather complicated task. An artifact is a situation where the measured values do not reflect the clinical context. Several monitors have a built–in module for recognizing artifacts, especially those arising from hardware problems. VIE–VENT therefore does not deal with artifacts handled by the monitors. VIE–VENT uses three methods for detecting artifacts:

(a) the measurement is out of range, which is already covered in the item of checking the plausibility of measurements;

(b) rapid oscillations or very fast changing of a single measurement;

(c) cross relations between different measurements

e.g.: the following example shows corresponding values for cross checking of

chest wall expansion		tidal volume (VT)
1 ... small	↔	$VT \leq 5$ ml/kg
2 ... normal	↔	5 ml/kg < $VT \leq 10$ ml/kg
3 ... excessive	↔	$VT > 10$ ml/kg

– "Calibration" of blood gas measurements

One of the benefits of VIE–VENT is the possibility to use continuously assessed transcutaneous blood gas measurements. However, transcutaneous blood gases may deviate from the more reliably but only rarely assessed invasive blood gases. Because therapy planning is essentially based on reliable data, transcutaneous measurements have to be "calibrated" against invasive blood gas measurements. Although there is no strong linear relationship between the two types of measurement, for practical reasons we decided to use a linear calibration factor (e.g., $k = (PCO_2 / PtcCO_2)$; $PtcCO_2$ (new) = k * $PtcCO_2$ (actual)). Calibration is only done in case the qualitative values (see next section) differ by two qualitative categories.

4.4 Data Abstraction

The quantitative data of the observable system are transformed into qualitative values. The qualitative values of the variables are used in our system model of neonatal respiration. The basis of the transformation of the blood gas measurements are schemata, which represent the degree of blood gas abnormalities. These schemata are defined for all kinds of blood gases. They depend on the site of measurement (arterial, capillary, venous, transcutaneous) and the mode of ventilation (IPPV, IMV).

Table 1: Transformation scheme of the degree of blood gas abnormalities

site of measurement: **venous**

KIND OF BLOOD GAS	below target range			Target Range			above target range			mode of ventilation
	s3	s2	s1		TV		g1	g2	g3	
pO_2	10	30	37	40	42	45	50	65	100	
pCO_2	150	65	55	48	45	42	40	30	20	IPPV
pCO_2	150	70	60	55	50	45	40	30	20	IMV
pH	6.6	7.2	7.2	7.23	7.25	7.3	7.35	7.55	7.7	

Explanation of abbreviation:

below target range
s1 ... slightly
s2 ... substantially
s3 ... extremely

TV ... Target Value

above target range
g1 ... slightly
g2 ... substantially
g3 ... extremely

Our classification of the degree of blood gas abnormality (Table 1) is based on a qualitative notation, which abstracts from the quantitative value of the blood gas measurement. In principle, the middle of the table gives the expected normal value range, the target range. "TV" is the target value we are aiming to reach. The term "below target range" means that the amount of artificial ventilation is too low. The term "above target range" means that the amount of artificial ventilation is too high. An example is given in Table 1 for venous pO_2, pCO_2 and pH during intermittent positive pressure ventilation (IPPV) or intermittent mandatory ventilation (IMV). For example the transformation of the venous pCO_2 value of 58 mm Hg, when the mode of ventilation is IMV will result in a qualitative value of "slightly below target range".

One advantage of using qualitative values is their unified usability in the system model, no matter of which origin they are. Adaptation to specific situations can easily be done by using specific transformation tables without changing the model of respiration.

4.5 Therapy Planning

While monitoring deals with the consecutive observation of parameters of a patient, therapy planning deals with the interpretation of the neonate's status and the selection of appropriate therapy recommendations.

Every 10 seconds, VIE–VENT monitors the transcutaneous blood gases and the ventilator settings. In addition, under certain conditions (e.g., critical ventilatory status of the neonate, or elapsed time intervals) the invasive blood gases and qualitative measurements such as chest wall expansion are requested. Therapy recommendations consist of possible and necessary changes of the ventilator settings. These changes depend on the degree of blood gas abnormality and on the three different dynamics of ventilation (e.g., conservative). The therapy recommendations are not formulated every 10 seconds. The frequency of formulation depends on the neonate's ventilatory status, on newly available blood gas analyses, on a very fast change of a measurement, and on different time dependencies.

We will focus on two important parts of VIE–VENT's therapy planning architecture: the system model of neonatal respiration and the dynamics of ventilation during the weaning process.

4.5.1 System Model of Neonatal Respiration

Neonatal respiration in our system model is represented by two processes, ventilation (CO_2 elimination) and oxygenation (oxygen uptake). Ventilation is reflected by the blood tension of CO_2 (PCO_2). Ventilation is increased (and PCO_2 decreased) with an increase of the minute ventilation which is the product of the tidal volume (VT) and the ventilatory rate (frequency, f). The VT is strongly but not linearily related to the peak inspiratory pressure (PIP) and clinically to the extent of chest wall expansion. Independently of the ventilation process, the PCO_2 may be increased due to a poor pulmonary perfusion and to right–to–left shunting. Oxygenation is reflected by the blood tension of O_2 (PO_2). Oxygenation (PO_2) is increased with an increase of the inspiratory oxygen concentration (F_iO_2) and the mean airway pressure (MAP). The MAP increases with PIP, inflation time (t_i) and positive endexpiratory pressure (PEEP). Independently of the oxygenation process, PO_2 is decreased due to right–to–left shunting and an increased pulmonary vascular resistance which itself at least partly depends on the PCO_2.

The target values of pH, PCO_2 and PO_2 for various sampling sites (e.g. arterial, venous) are listed in the transformation schemata for blood gas abnormalities. An example for venous blood gas measurements was given in Table 1.

Description of the different phases of artificial ventilation

Depending on the course of the disease, the monitoring possibilities and the therapeutic goals of ventilation, i.e., the target values of PCO_2 and PO_2, may change. We divided the whole period of artificial ventilation into four phases: an initial phase, a phase of controlled ventilation, a phase of weaning and a phase of returning to spontaneous breathing. Transition from one phase to the next is handled by rules depending on the amount of artificial ventilation (e.g., actual ventilator setting).

During the short *initial phase*, there are only limited monitoring possibilities, when SaO_2 is the single reliable continuously measured variable. At this time, a major goal is to characterize the severity of the disease and to optimize chest wall expansion and SaO_2.

Then follows, depending on the severity of the disease, a more or less prolonged phase of *controlled ventilation* (IPPV), when the main respiratory work is performed by the ventilator. During this phase, the PCO_2 target values are low, aiming to decrease respiratory drive of the patient. Spontaneous breathing efforts should be suppressed by sedation or muscle relaxation if they lead to a poor interaction with artificial ventilation or to an increased oxygen consumption. If during this phase the target values of PCO_2 and PO_2 cannot be reached with reasonable ventilator settings, the target values are adapted accordingly and alternatives to the standard therapies are taken into consideration.

When F_iO_2 can be reduced to a value ≤ 50% and PIP to ≤ 20 mbars, *weaning* (IMV) should be started, where the patient increasingly shares the work of breathing with the ventilator. At this time, higher PCO_2 target values are accepted in order to increase the patient's ventilatory drive.

Finally, at IMV with frequencies of ≤ 10, F_iO2 ≤ 40% and PIP ≤ 15 mbars, the phase of *returning to spontaneous breathing* with positive endexpiratory pressure (continuous positive airway pressure, CPAP) and extubation should be considered.

To illustrate our system model of neonatal respiration, we give a few examples of therapy recommendations during the initial phase and during the phases of controlled ventilation and weaning.

(a) Therapy recommendations during the initial phase

The therapy recommendations during the initial phase represent a very simplified system model, because SaO_2 is the single continuously reliable measurement. There are restricted reactions to decreased oxygenation depending on the degree of abnormality of the SaO_2 and the actual tidal volume (VT). The VT is here estimated by the extent of chest wall expansion.

Qualitative values of "slightly" or "substantially below target range" SaO_2 in combination with a normal or excessive chest wall expansion will cause VIE–VENT to recommend an increase of the F_iO_2. If the chest wall expansion is small, VIE–VENT will recommend an increase of the F_iO_2 and the PIP. Qualitative values of "extremely below target range" SaO_2 in combination with excessive chest wall expansion will cause VIE–VENT to recommend an increase of the F_iO_2 and of the frequency (f). In combination with a normal or small chest wall expansion, it will recommend an increase of the F_iO_2, of the frequency (f), and of the PIP.

(b) Therapy recommendations during the phases of controlled ventilation and weaning

Figure 2 shows the possible reactions to the results of transcutaneous and invasive blood gas measurements ($PtcCO_2$, PCO_2 and pH) in graphical form: no changes of the ventilator settings are recommended if pH or PCO_2 or $PtcCO_2$ are within the target range or if PCO_2 or $PtcCO_2$ is not known. Acidosis and alkalosis, of both respiratory or metabolic origin, will lead to the recommendation of an increase or a decrease of the rate or the MAP. The more severe the problem, the greater the amount of change. This is expressed by proportional changes of the ventilator settings (e.g., for severe problems, as indicated in Figure 2 by status "s3" or "g3", the proportional amount of change is 30%). In addition, this rate is combined with the dynamics of ventilation (see chapter 4.5.2). E.g., if VIE–VENT is used in the conservative mode, only 50% of the maximally allowed amount of change will be recommended. A most common situation of Figure 3 is documented in Rule 1. This notation presents an example of a forward chaining rule as represented in the knowledge base of VIE–VENT.

The oxygenation part deals with possible reactions to SaO_2 and $PtcO_2$ measurements. As pulse oximetry (for noninvasive SaO_2 measurements) is more reliable than $PtcO_2$ measurements, priority is given to SaO_2 measurements. In case of discordant results, a warning to check the sensor sites is released by VIE–VENT. The representation and the interpretation is done in analogy to the ventilation part.

Model: Ventilation, qualitative measurements

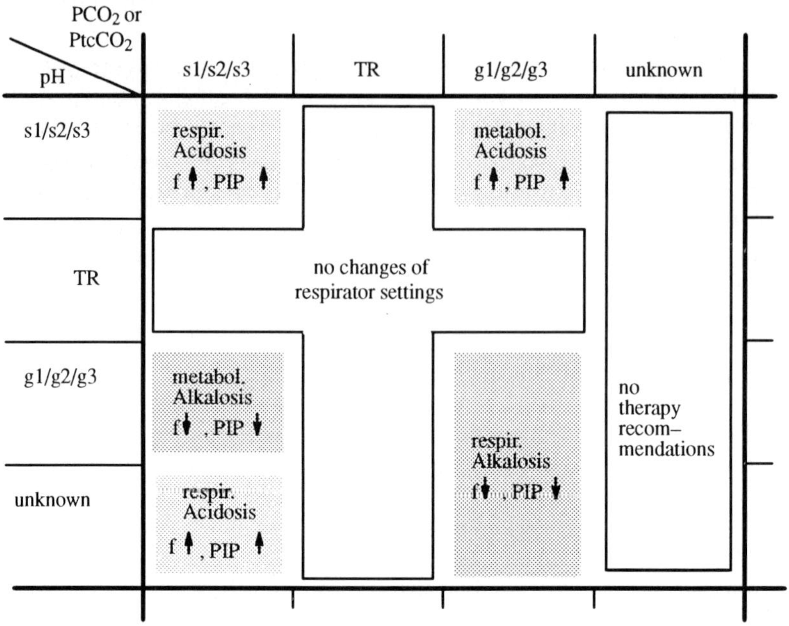

Explanation of abbreviation:

below target range	TR ... Target Range	above target range
s1 ... slightly		g1 ... slightly
s2 ... substantially		g2 ... substantially
s3 ... extremely		g3 ... extremely

f ↑, PIP ↑ increase parameter, depending on degree of abnormalities

f ↓, PIP ↓ decrease parameter, depending on degree of abnormalities

percental change rate:		
	s1 ... 10%	g1 ... 5%
	s2 ... 20%	g2 ... 7.5%
	s3 ... 30%	g3 ... 10%

```
Rule 1: "respiratory alkalosis with extremely_above_target_range of PCO2"
   if (status is therapy_recommendation) and
      (phase_of_ventilation is weaning) and
      (PCO2 is extremely_above_target_range) and
      (pH is (slightly_above_target_range or
             substantially_above_target_range
           or extremely_above_target_range)) and
      (mode_of_ventilation is not aggressive)
   then
      (get mode_of_ventilation aggressive max_amount_of_change) and
      (set mode_of_ventilation is aggressive) and
      (decrease f by (0.3 * max_amount_of_change)) and
      (decrease PIP by (0.3 * max_amount_of_change)).
```

Figure 2: Therapy recommendations during the phases of controlled ventilation weaning.

Table 2: Dynamics of ventilation in the phase of weaning

Recommendations \ Dynamics of Ventilation	conservative	normal	aggressive
react on	blood gases	breathing pattern and blood gases	breathing pattern and blood gases
max. allowed amount of change	50 %	100 %	150 %
changes possible every	30 min.	15 min.	10 min.
change of max. parameters at once	1	1	2
max. number of changes per day	3	8	24
interval recommended between invasive blood gas analyses	24 hours	12 hours	8 hours

4.5.2 Dynamics of Ventilation

The dynamics of ventilation is important in the phase of weaning. There are different restrictions in the case of increasing the respiratory support.

Weaning from respirator therapy is usually performed by gradually reducing the respiratory support (IMV). The rate of reduction depends on the patient's ability to perform more work of breathing and on the physician's judgment on this ability. This judgment is usually based on blood gas analyses, on the observation of the patient's spontaneous breathing effort, and on clinical experience. Moreover, psychological characteristics of the physician, such as more conservative or more vigorous behavior are involved. Therefore various weaning strategies can be chosen and has to be considered in a knowledge–based system. The disregarding of such discrepancies in the weaning strategy has led to poor acceptance of previous therapy planning systems. We have tried to overcome this problem by introducing three different weaning strategies, characterized by psychological categories: conservative, normal and aggressive. These three weaning strategies are implemented in the knowledge base of VIE–VENT, and are represented in Table 2. By default, the normal strategy is used. This may be changed on user's request to a conservative or more aggressive form of weaning.

5. Technical Remarks and Future Enhancements

VIE–VENT was implemented using the knowledge representation language Clips (NASA). We used forward chaining rules for representing the knowledge base. VIE–VENT is running on IBM–compatible personal computers, Apple Macintoshs and UNIX–workstations.

VIE–VENT samples transcutaneous measurements and ventilator settings every 10 seconds. The arithmetic means of these 10–second data are stored every 10 minutes for further analysis.

Enhancements of VIE–VENT cover different levels. VIE–VENT represents an event–driven approach with only limited time representation. Therefore, we are currently expanding our model of artificial ventilation (the neonatal respiration) with a combination of relative and absolute time representation (e.g. "the change of the ventilator's parameter PIP was performed 10 minutes before the neonate's health condition got better", "to improve the ventilation takes longer than to improve the oxygenation").

On the other hand, we are trying to integrate VIE–VENT in the patient data management system used at the NICUs, in order to get on–line data acquisition from the patients' records, the monitor and the ventilator. This will minimize the manual data input. Finally, we would like to enlarge our module for prediction of short and long term effects of the therapeutic strategies and develop a more user–friendly, graphical user interface.

6. Summary of VIE–VENT's Features

VIE–VENT is a knowledge–based monitoring and therapy planning system for artificial ventilation of newborn infants. A context sensitive data validation and therapy planning component were implemented according to practical clinical and textbook knowledge. VIE–VENT uses continuous and discontinuous data input from the patient's monitors, ventilators and the data management systems.

The therapy planning component is based on a combination of transcutaneous and invasive blood gas measurements and qualitative clinical observations (e.g., chest wall expansion). The background knowledge for formulating therapy recommendations is a model of neonatal respiration. This model includes the neonates' delay–time of a physiological reaction to an executed therapy action. Therapy recommendations are released depending on various conditions (e.g., depending on the severity of the neonate's ventilatory status, on newly available blood gas analyses, or on various time dependencies). They consist of a set of possible and necessary changes of ventilator settings. The different strategies of these changes are represented according to the degree of blood gas abnormality. We included three possible dynamics of ventilation (e.g., conservative), according to different strategies of therapy planning, in order to be able to fulfill the requirements of different physicians using the system.

Another very important feature of VIE–VENT is that in case of a poor condition of the neonate, the dynamics of ventilation is automatically set to aggressive. This represents the practical behavior at a NICU, where the physicians have to react to a deterioration of the patient as quickly and much as possible, in order to rapidly improve the situation. At this time, VIE–VENT is clinically tested at two different NICUs.

Acknowledgements

This project is supported by the "Medizinisch–Wissenschaftlicher Fonds" of the Mayor of the City of Vienna, Austria. We also greatly appreciate the support given to the Austrian Research Institute for Artificial Intelligence (ÖFAI) by the Austrian Federal Ministry of Science and Research, Vienna.

References

[1] Arroe M.: A Computerized Aid in Ventilating Neonates, Comp. Biol. Med., 21(1/2), 15–21, 1991.

[2] Ash D., Gold G., Seiver A., Hayes–Roth B.: Guaranteeing Real–time Response with Limited Resources, Artificial Intelligence in Medicine, 5(1), 49–66, 1993.

[3] Boyarsky A.: Computerized Ventilation Management System for Neonates, Journal of Perinatology, 7(1), 1987.

[4] Breuker J.A., Someren M.W.van, Hoog R.de, Schreiber G., Greef P.de, Bredeweg B., Wielemaker J., Billault J.–P., Davoodi M., Hayward S.A.: Model–Driven Knowledge Acquistion: Interpretation Models, University of Amsterdam and STL Ltd., Esprit Project P1098, Memo 87, 1987.

[5] Bykat A.: Intelligent Monitoring and Diagnosis Systems: A Survey, Applied Artificial Intelligence, 5(4), 339–352, 1991.

[6] Coiera E.: Intelligent Monitoring and Control of Physiological Systems, Editorial, Artificial Intelligence in Medicine, 5(1), 1–8, 1993.

[7] Coiera E.: Monitoring Diseases with Empirical and Model–generated Histories, in Keravnou E. (ed.), Deep Models for Medical Knowledge Engineering, Elsevier, Amsterdam, 1992.

[8] Chambrin M.–C., Chopin C., Ravaux P., Mangalaboyi J., Lestavel P., Fourrier F. : RESPAID: Computer–Aided Decision Support for Respiratory Data in ICU, Proc. Eleventh Annual Conf. IEEE Engineering in Medicine and Biology Soc., Seattle, WA., 1989.

[9] Fagan L.M., Shortliffe E.H., Buchanan B.G. : Computer–Based Medical Decision Making: from MYCIN to VM, Automedica, Vol.3., 1980.

[10] Garfinkel D., Matsiras P.V., Lecky J.H., Aukburg S.J., Matschinsky B.B., Mavrides T.G.: PONI: An Intelligent Alarm System for Respiratory and Circulation Management in the Operating Room, Proc. 12th Annual Symp. Comput. Appl. Med. Care, Washington, DC, 1988.

[11] Goldsmith J.P., Karotkin E.H.: Assisted Ventilation of the Neonates, Saunders, Philadelphia, 1988.

[12] Hayes–Roth B., Washington R., Hewett R., Hewett M., Seiver A.: Intelligent Monitoring and Control, in Proceedings of the Eleventh International Joint Conference on Artificial Intelligence (IJCAI–89), Morgan Kaufmann, Los Altos, CA, pp.243–249, 1989.

[13] Hayes–Roth B., Washington R., Ash D., Hewett M., Collinot A., Vina A., Seiver A.: Guardian: A Prototype Intelligent Agent for Intensive–Care Monitoring, Artificial Intelligence in Medicine, 4(2), 165–66, 1992.

[14] Rutledge G., Thomsen G., Beinlich I., Farr B., Sheiner L., Fagan L.M.: Combining Qualitative and Quantitative Computation in a Ventilator Therapy Planner, Proc. 13th Annual Symp. Comput. Appl. Med. Care, Washington, DC, 1989.

[15] Rutledge G.W., Thomsen G.E., Farr B.R.,Tovar M.A., Polaschek J.X., Beinlich I.A., Sheiner L.B., Fagan L.M.: The Design and Implementation of a Ventilator–management Advisor, Artificial Intelligence in Medicine, 5(1), 67–82, 1993.

[16] Shortliffe E.H.: Knowledge–Based System in Medicine, Proc. Medical Informatics Europe 1991, Springer, Berlin, 1991.

[17] Sittig D.F., Pace N.L., Gardner R.M., Morris A.H., Wallace J.: Clinical Evaluation of Computer–based Respiratory Care Algorithms, Int. Journal of Clinical Monitoring and Computing, 7, 177–185, 1990.

[18] Teberg A.J., Hodgman J.E.: Survival of Infants with Birthweight 500–1500g, in Lucey J.F. (ed.), Hot Topics in Neonatology, Proc. Ross Lab. Special Conference, 1992.

[19] Uckun S., Dawant B.M. : Qualitative Modelling as a Paradigm for Diagnosis and Prediction in Critical Care Environments, Artificial Intelligence in Medicine 4(2), 127–44, 1992.

[20] Uckun S., Dawant B.M., Lindstrom D.P.: Model–based Diagnosis in Intensive Care Monitoring: the YAQ Approach, Artificial Intelligence in Medicine, 5(1), 31–48, 1993.

[21] Uckun S.: Intelligent Systems in Patient Monitoring and Therapy Management, Stanford University, Knowledge Systems Laboratory, Report KSL 93–32, 1993.

Artificial Intelligence in Medecine
S. Andreassen et al. , Eds.
IOS Press, 1993

ICONS: Cognitive basic functions in a case-based consultation system for intensive care

L. Gierl[a] R. Schmidt[a] B. Pollwein[b]

[a] Data Processing Centre
[b] Institute of Anaesthesiology

Medical Faculty, University of Munich, Klinikum Grosshadern, Marchioninistr. 15
D - 81366 München, Germany

Abstract

As we have already shown in earlier projects the abstract descriptions of diseases which have been semi-automatically generated from a data base of patients of our Medical Facility produce a better diagnostic accuracy in a case-based consultation system than an equivalent knowledge base compiled from cases in the medical literature. We identified an ordered set of cognitive basic functions which forms a "tool kit" for a consultation process between physician and machine. For the first time, as we can see, there had been defined a mapping from medical basic functions onto the set of case-based and general methods which form the cognitive basis of a cognitive open consultation system. We will use such methods in a consultation system for intensive care.

1. Introduction

It has not yet been possible, even partly to fulfil the hope of making the wide and rapidly-growing medical knowledge available to physicians in form of expert systems. Only a few of these systems have found their way into clinical application. Miller and Masarie [1] summarise over 10 years of experience with the development of the expert system INTERNIST-I, which as a diagnostic consulting system is supposed to cover the whole area of internal medicine, as follows: The attempt has failed to provide physicians with a system yielding a diagnosis with a 65 to 75 percent certainty, as the sole result after a very time-consuming dialogue of between 30 and 90 minutes. The amount of details, the uniqueness of each singular case and the lack of complete and correct data make every result of this kind except for a few classic examples - questionable. Miller summarises his criticism on INTERNIST-1 (and other systems) as follows: 'The style of diagnostic consultation embodied in the INTERNIST-1 program was a "Greek Oracle" model.' As opposed to this, he urges a carefully designed program of building blocks ("tool kit"), which should offer physicians an expert system for supporting their decision-making process: 'Diagnostic decision support systems should provide physicians with a useful set of catalysts for diagnostic reasoning.'

2. Case-based reasoning

Knowledge-acquisition is the bottleneck of building expert-systems. Especially in weak or unstructured domains it is difficult to express the experts knowledge into a set of rules, that can be implemented in a computer language. The method of cased-based reasoning might be an contribution to partly solve this problem. Similarity-based learning, introduced by Winston [4], was developed to case-based reasoning to handle with many cases in memory. Case-based reasoning means to use old experiences to understand and solve new problems. In case-based reasoning, a reasoner remembers a previous situation similar to the current one and uses it to solve the new problem. Case-based reasoning is a methodology for reasoning and learning. A case-based reasoner learns in two ways. First, it can become a more efficient reasoner by remembering old solutions and adapting them. Second, it becomes more and more competent, because of it's increasing experience [5]. The difficulties of this method are to determine the similarity of cases, to efficiently guide the search for similar cases, and to adapt the old solution to the new problem. This results into the three main tasks of case-based reasoning [5]: the similarity-problem, the classification (including the questions of indexing and interpretation) and the adaptation. Solving the similarity problems means to determine the most similar case in memory to the new problem. All the cases in memory have to be compared with the new one by using a measure of similarity. This may be Tversky´s contrast model of features [6] or Rosch´s model of category resemblance [7]. Sometimes the features are weighted. The weight for one feature depends on the importance of the feature to the problem it belongs to. Typically in weak domains no theory exists about these weights. Categories like importance, necessity, typicality of the problem´s features might be used instead of measured weights.

To increase the performance of a case-based system it is necessary to use a memory structure that avoids to determine the similarities for all cases in memory. Therefor it is useful to classify the cases in a hierarchical categorisation tree. The leaves are the cases, at the next higher level are the prototypes and the top levels of the hierarchy are categories, that may be order themselves hierarchically. In the first step the similarities for only the direct successor of the root are calculated. Only the subtree with the greatest similarity must be inspected further. This leads the search through the tree down to a prototype. This prototype possesses all the typical features of his cases. The prototype is a generalisation of his cases.

3. The medical domain of ICONS

ICONS will work in the domain of intensive medicine, first in the part of infectious diseases and fluid balance. The main goals of intensive care for critical ill patients is characterised by (1) monitoring of patients, (2) extensive nursing requirements and (3) constant physician care [8]. Neurologic monitoring, balance of fluids and electrolytes, shock, acute renal failure, hemostasis disorders etc. are sub domains of intensive care. A difficult problem in this domain is the diagnostic of infections, because clear definitions for the various infections are missing. The clinical symptoms are too unspecified. Even very well established definitions of infectious diseases are not used, because the symptoms lead to a wrong interpretation. One of the priority assignments in the domain of infectious diseases is the further development of the definitions of infections. It is necessary to detect the relations of infections, to develop the methods for diagnosis and documentation plans, and to validate the clinical symptoms of infections. The development of infections diagnosis demands the possibility to use intelligent computational programs that are able to process the relevant data quickly.

The balancing of fluid intake and outtake is a domain where causal knowledge is important. Therefore, a combination of case-based methods and deep knowledge is necessary.

4. Cognitive basic functions

The most important factor in evaluating conclusions for the development of expert systems is our *modest knowledge about the cognitive abilities of the human being* especially the efficient use of his "knowledge of the world" (everyday knowledge). But surveys like the ones by Granger and Mc Nulty [9] show elementary cognitive functions. The ability of using every day knowledge was declared by Minsky [10] in respect to specialised agents. All together these agents represent the human spirit. These agents already correspond to the mind operations by Selz [11]. We assume there is no fundamental difference between the problem solving of a doctor and every days problem solving, but the doctor is more specialised and cleverer in his domain.

Following the ideas of Minsky it is useful to reproduce those agents on the computer that are supposed to come up with advantages of accuracy, completeness and cleverness. As the co-ordination with the agents must work well in mind, a co-ordination between artificial and natural agents is absolutely necessary. We defined cognitive basic functions appropriate to the doctors problem solving ability approximately corresponding to Minsky's agents (see Table 1, left row). The basic functions increase in complexity from 1. up to 4. They culminate in the decision of the physician between hypothesis (diagnoses, treatments). In function 4.3 these alternative hypothesis have to be assessed and ordered according to a cognitive preference measure. As a preference measure we applied Tversky´s contrast model and Rosch´s measure of category cohesiveness [6,7].

These cognitive basic functions result from experiences with several expert systems [12, 13]. Gierl [13] describes how this cognitive basic functions are implemented in two expert systems (dysmorphic syndromes and duty roster for physicians). Expert systems with such an architecture are called cognitively open.

5. Mapping of medical cognitive basic functions onto case-based reasoning methods for intensive care

Employing our above defined model of cognitive basic functions we mapped domain-specific instances of such functions onto a set of case-based as well as general methods. The result is presented in Table 1.

Table 1. Mapping of medical cognitive basic functions onto case-based reasoning methods

Medical basic functions	Case-based reasoning
<u>**1.Gathering of facts**</u>	
Input and adoption of facts like findings, medical history etc.	Adoption of data from a clinical communication system (e.g. sodium).
<u>**2. Search**</u>	
2.1 Serial search	
• What diagnosis resp. therapies are present in the system?	List of all prototypes presented to the user.
• What features are present ?	Thesaurus of features (repository).
• What procedures are present ?	Access to ICPM and SNOMED.
2.2 Navigate	
• Methods to provide access to a wide variety of knowledge.	Show all known signs of a case with an infectious disease. Search all former cases with this disease which are not older than two years.
<u>**3. Explanation**</u>	
3.1 Remembering of cases	
• Did a similar case occur ?	Find the former case which is most similar to the current case.
3.2 Identification of associations	
• Essential symptoms.	A set of trigger features assigned to a prototype (e.g. increase of the peripheral leukocyte counts and free air below the diaphragm on x-ray trigger peritonitis).
3.3 Search for explanations of hypothesis	
• Which diseases or therapies are explained by the patients features ?	For instance, increase of peripheral leukocyte counts is explained by peritonitis.
• Refer to multiple diseases of one patient.	Multiple inheritance. It must be possible to assign a case or prototype to several classes or prototypes in a tree of cases and prototypes.For instance, a case has to be assigned to prototypes of renal disorders and infectious diseases because he suffers from both.
3.4 Connect symptoms or hypothesis with known information	

• How should a case be diagnosed or treated that is similar to a known case or prototype?	Adaptation of previous cases or prototypes to the current case. For instance, if CT is used in the most similar case and has established the disease, use it in the current case too.
3.5 Relations for cases, associations or features	
• Provide the features with heuristic attribu-tes like important, safe, less straining et al.	The inference considers heuristic concepts.
• Provide the features with attributes for va-gue knowledge ("very big", "mainly" et al.).	The inference considers vague knowledge (e.g. "high fever").
• Provide the features with attributes for temporal knowledge ("began earlier as", "lasts longer than" et al.).	The inference considers temporal knowledge (e.g. rapid increase of creatinine).
<u>**4.Preference decisions**</u>	
4.1 Comparison	
<u>4.1.1 Compare the features</u>	
• Compare the contents and the semantics of features.	Present the feature thesaurus to the user.
<u>4.1.2 Compare the cases</u>	
• What is the difference between two cases?	Difference tree of those features that are not common between two cases.
<u>4.1.3 Compare hypotheses differences</u>	
• What is the difference between two hypothesis (diagnosis or therapies)?	Difference tree of those features that are not in common between two concepts (e.g. fever oberserved or not observed).
4.2 Assessment	
<u>4.2.1 Split sets (Strategy of discrimination)</u>	
• To which class of diseases does the case belong to ?	Classification process.
• To which class of diseases does the disease belong to ?	Taxonomy of diseases
<u>4.2.2 Discriminate hypotheses (Strategy of elimination)</u>	
• Reasons against a hypothesis (diagnosis or therapy).	Explicit establishment of not existing features by comparing a current case with other cases or prototypes of diseases (e.g. patient has no fever concerning pneumonia).
<u>4.2.3 Strengthen hypotheses (Strategy of confirmation)</u>	

• Reasons for a hypothesis.	Explicit establishment of existing (may be weighted) features by comparing a current case with other cases or prototypes of diseases.
4.3 Serial arrangement using a cognitive measure • Presentation of hypothesis according to a cognitive measure.	Establishment of an ordered set of hypothesis according to Tversky, Rosch and others.
5. Change or examine the preference decisions • Save the conclusions, understandings et al. to lead a renewed consultation dialogue.	Store the findings, diagnoses, therapies (the doctor already decided) on a memory medium.

6. Discussion

Our experience show that case-based systems which combine knowledge acquisition as a machine learning process and the consultation process could give an important contribution to the solution of the knowledge acquisition problem. If the community of AI in medicine goes for capturing and maintaining of the knowledge of the whole medical domain this cannot achieved in a never ending asking of physicians how they are doing their job or delivering double-blind, randomised studies. Furthermore, we are able to show [13] that a knowledge base generated from cases seen and documented in an outpatient clinic can produce a more accurate consultation than a knowledge base compiled from case descriptions in international medical literature of that domain (dysmorphic syndromes). However, the task is still remaining to acquire deep knowledge and meta-knowledge from textbooks and medical experts. The identification of cognitive basic functions provide a framework for the development of a tool kit for generic functions to support the decision process of the physician. It is like a change of a paradigm towards cognitive open systems. Because most work done so far assumes that there is one method in classification or planning a human apply [16, 17]. Often, when a system was developed the designers looked for a domain which fits their methods best. But there is some evidence that humans are rather opportunistic accomplishing problem solving and that they use a wealth of methods based on their abilities to handle general preference problems. It seems to us that the inverse approach in mapping medical cognitive basic functions onto the set of case-based methods available or to develop could cause medical expert systems which will be accepted in routine medical decision making.

7. References

1 Miller R.A., Masarie F.E.: The Demise of the "Greek Oracle" Model for Medical Diagnostic Systems, Meth. Inf. Med 29, (1990) 1-2

2 Puppe F.: Problemlösungsmethoden in Expertensystemen, Berlin (1990)

3 Chandrasekaran B. : Towards a Functional Architecture for Intelligence Based on Generic Information Processing Tasks, IJCAI 87, (1987) 1183-1192

4 Winston P.H.: Learning Structural Descriptions from Examples, in: P.H. Winston, Ed., The Psychology of Computer Vision, McGraw-Hill, New York (1972)

5 Kolodner J.L.: An Introduction to Case-Based Reasoning, in: Artificial Intelligence Review 6, No.1, (1992) 3-34

6 Tversky A.: Features of Similarity, in: Psychological Review 84, (1977) 327-352

7 Rosch E. , Mervis C. B.: Family Resemblance: Studies in the Internal Structures of Categories, Cognitive Psychology 7 (1975) 573-605

8 Gvety J.M., Taylor R.W., Kirby R.R.: Critical Care, Philadelphia, 2nd Edition (1992)

9 Granger H.R., McNulty D.M.: Learning and Memory in Machines and Animals: An AI Model that Accounts for Some Neurobiological Data, in: Kolodner, Riesbeck (Hrsg.): Experience, Memory, and Reasoning, Hillsdale, (1986) 29-45

10 Minsky M.: The Society of Mind, New York (1987)

11 Selz O.: Die Gesetze der produktiven und reproduktiven Geistestätigkeit, Bonn (1924)

12 Gierl L., Stengel-Rutkowski S.: Prototypes as a Core Representation of Medical Knowledge in Diagnosis and Knowledge Acquisition, in: Lun K.C. et al. (Eds.): MEDINFO 92, Amsterdam (1992) 508

13 Gierl L.: Klassifikation mit prototypischen Merkmalsmustern für Expertensysteme in der Medizin, Habilitation Thesis, University Munich (1992)

14 Gierl L.: An architecture for cognitive open medical expert systems using elemental cognitive functions, in: Reichert A. et al. (Eds.): Proceedings of MIE 93, London, (1993) 142-146

15 Clancey W.J.: Heuristic Classification, Artificial Intellignce 27, (1985) 289-350

16 Szolovits P.: Types of Knowledge as Bases of Reasoning, in: De Lotto, Stefanelli: Artificial Intelligence in Medicine, Amsterdam (1985) 209-226

Acknowledgement

This work is part of the MEDWIS-Project (Medical Knowledge Bases) which is funded by the German Ministry for Research and Technology. The project contractor is the GSF MEDIS Institute, Neuherberg.

Artificial Intelligence in Medecine
S. Andreassen et al. , Eds.
IOS Press, 1993

Digital lung mechanics simulator as a validation tool

H. Groß, U. Föhring[2]

Physikalisch-Technische Bundesanstalt
10.33 Lab. für Expertensysteme und Datenbanken
Abbestr. 2-12, D-10587 Berlin, fax: 030-3481-490, elm: hg@lab1033.berlin.ptb.de

[2]Freie Universität Berlin
Klinik für Anästhesiologie und Operative Intensivmedizin
des Klinikum Steglitz, Hindenburgdamm 30, D-12200 Berlin

Abstract

The complex situation of artificial ventilation, especially the consequences of different ventilator settings for the pressure, flow and volume changes of the patients lung with changing mechanical properties, is modeled by a digital lung mechanics simulator. Different lung mechanics properties, designed as RLC circuits, and different ventilator settings can be interactively chosen. Their influences are continuously computed by a transient analysis and then shown as the dynamically updated courses for the pressure, flow and volume parameters. As these calculated curves agree with measured data from patients the system can be used as a component appropriate for the validation of advising systems which give recommendations about better ventilator settings on the basis of measured data from ventilators. The system is a realistic phantom which covers a wide range for the possible different lung mechanics properties in connection with different settings at the ventilator.

Moreover, the implemented models can be used to interpret measured pressure and flow curves from patients in terms of these models, i.e. a quantitative, model based description of the present lung mechanical status is possible by simulation.

1. The Problem

The validation of intelligent monitoring systems in the intensive care unit is a very important task and always has to be solved before any such decision support system will be accepted and used. This is also valid for the development and testing of intelligent respiration programms which should give advice about the ventilator settings on the basis of measured pressure, flow and volume data from the connected ventilator system. Because of the great importance of the artificial ventilation among the therapeutic applications in intensive care, the quality of such advising systems is of great interest. The creation of reproducible test conditions for the many different ventilator settings in combination with different and changing lung mechanic properties is an especially great and usually unsolved problem in the clinical environment.

Therefore, we have developed a digital lung mechanics simulator which is capable of realistically simulating the situations of pressure controlled artificial ventilation. The system acts as data source creating data streams which reflect the time courses of the pressure and flow distribution in the lung for different lung mechanic properties under the influence of different ventilator settings. The simulation system and its object oriented implementation can also be considered as an example for a model based knowledge representation of the situation of artificial ventilation.

2. Methods

The mechanical properties of the lung thorax system in the situation of artificial ventilation can be modeled in a first approach as an electrical circuit analogue: air flow resistance corresponds to an electrical resistance R, the inertance of the air in the bronchial system is represented by an inductance L and the elastic properties of the airways, the alveolar gas and the lung thorax tract by an electrical capacity C. Reasonable values for these R-L-C components are derived from the comparison of the time constants for the pneumatic system and its analogue as a circuit. This comparison leads to a simple one to one conversion between the electrical units (Volt, Ampere, Ohm, Henry, Farad) and the corresponding pneumatic units (mbar, l/s, mbar s/l, mbar s^2/l, l/mbar) [1].

Because of this straightforward relation we use a circuit analysis programm (SPICE2 [2]) to test the performance and quality of RLC models for describing the lung mechanic properties during pressure controlled ventilation. The main benefits are the availability of the complete and approved calculus for analog circuit simulation and the simplicity of the model implementation even for complexer models such as 3 compartment models. With the circuit simulator the pressure controlled artificial ventilation is then realized as a transient analysis, i.e. as the calculation of the response over time to different independent voltage sources. The voltage sources correspond to the different pressure courses created by the ventilator system at the patients mouth.

We have tested two kinds of different RLC models, a one compartment model representing a homogeneous distribution of the resistive, elasitc and inert properties and a three compartment model as a simplified description for an inhomogeneous distribution of the mechanical lung properties. Simular models have been proposed by the studies of Marini et al., Iotti et al. and Heinrich [3-5], but they use only RC components and don't take into account the inertance of the air in the bronchial system. In our models the gas inertance is se-

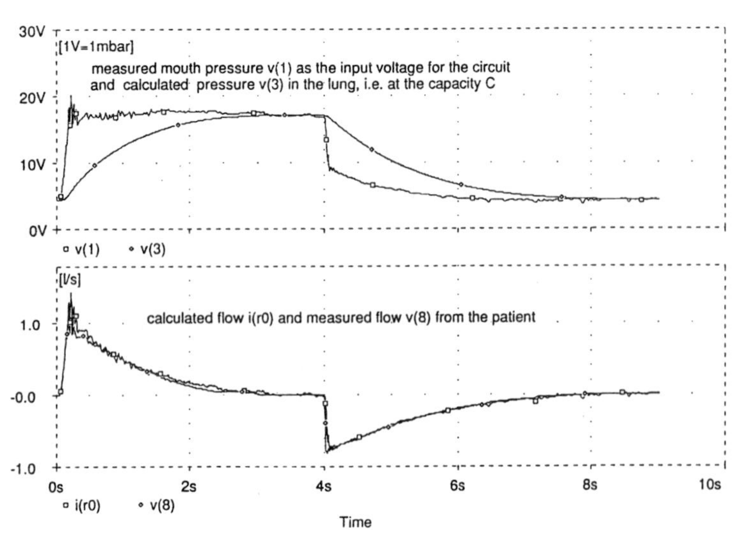

Figure 1: example for a one compartment circuit simulation (R=10Ohm, L=5mH, C=85mF)

parately considered as an inductance component (L). By this completion the shapes of the calculated flow curves become smoother in all time ranges where rapid volume changes occur. The damping influence of the inertance in the higher frequency range is considered.

Figure 1 shows an example for a one compartment circuit simulation compared with a measurement from a ventilated patient with an undisturbed lung function. In the upper part the measured mouth pressure and the calculated course of the pressure in the lung is shown. The measured pressure curve is used as the input voltage source for the RLC circuit. The lower part presents the calculated current which is interpreted as the volume flow and which is compared with the measured flow from the patient (second curve). The RLC parameters were modified until an optimal agreement with this measured flow signal was achieved.

On the basis of these first results we have designed the lung mechanic simulator as a testing tool. It is implemented by an object oriented programming technique. We use the software development environment PROKAPPA on a SPARC station under Solaris and embedded in a MOTIF user interface. The lung mechanic models are programmed as methods of the class 'LungModel', where different lung mechanics models as one or also as more compartment models can be instanciated. Each object of this class has also appropriate descriptive attributes, called value slots, which represent the corresponding physical properties, i.e. presssures, flows and volumes. The values of these slots are continuously computed (t=10ms) by the method slot 'Breath!' and dynamically monitored by images which display the current and proceeding values for a given time window.

Beside the object class 'LungModel' two further object classes, 'Patient' and 'Respirator', exist. The object 'Patient' has, beside others, the descriptive slots r (for resistance), c (for compliance) and l (for inertance) which are used by the method 'Breath!' as input parameters describing the pneumatic properties of the simulated one compartment patient lung. The values of these slots are also continuously monitored but are shown here as vertical slider bars which are able to accept new values by interactively clicking the mouse button.

A further group of input parameters for the method 'Breath!' come from the descriptive slots PEEP (positive endexpiratory pressure), pm (mouth pressure), tcycle (time for one breath) and tinsp (time for inspiration) of the object 'Respirator'. The values of these slots represent the actual settings of the ventilator. They are also monitored by vertical slider bars which accept new input values by a simple mouse click.

3. Results

All curve images and slider bars together are presented in a motif window. A picture of such a window is shown in figure 2. If one or more of the input parameters are interactively changed, the consequences of such variations in the time courses of the pressure, flow, volume and volume versus pressure curves can be immediately defined and determined. These are continuously updated and monitored in their images (see fig. 2). The simulator displays additionally some transient parameters (4 special pressure and 3 special volume values) derived from the inspiratory and expiratory phase of each breath.

In spite of the simple structured lung mechanic models all typical patterns for normal artificial ventilation can be simulated. The pressure, flow and volume courses correspond with our measurements of ventilated patients and with statements from literature, but the model validation has to be completed by a statistical analysis. To simulate also extrem cases of ventilation the models should include special nonlinear effects such as a flow dependency of the resistance and a volume dependency of the lung compliance. This may lead to further improved and thorough models.

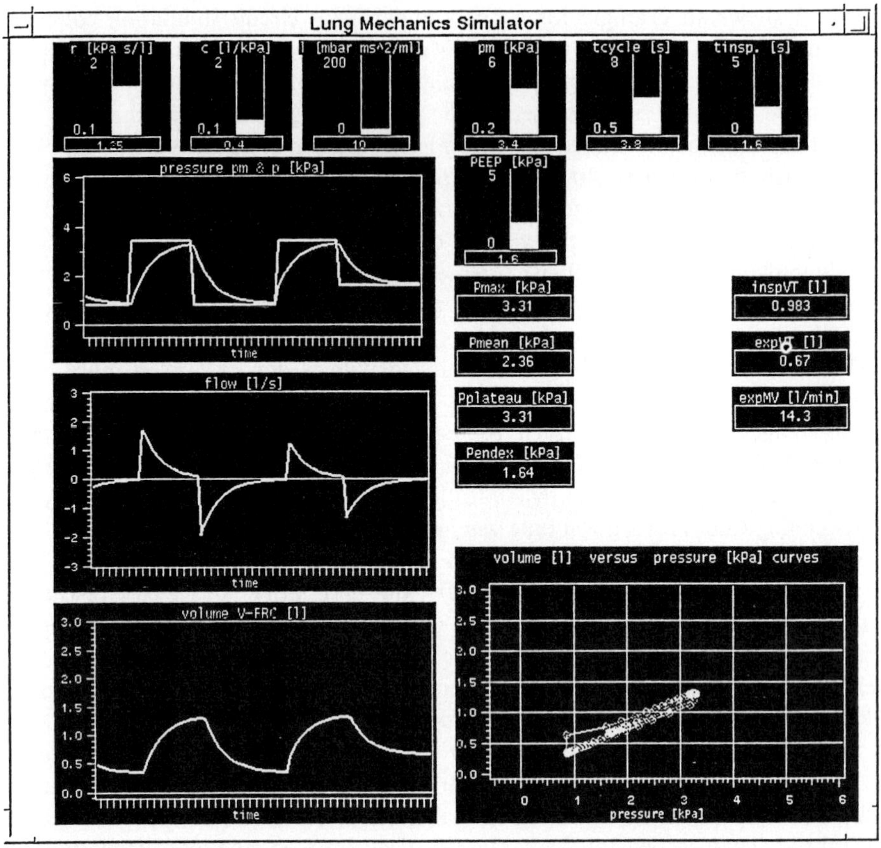

Figure 2: screen copy of the lung mechanics simulator just after an interactive change of the PEEP value from 0.8 kPa to 1.6 kPa;

4. References

1 H Gross, Pressure and flow simulations for artificial ventilation, CCCPM-92, Computers in Critical Care, Pulm. Medicine and Anesthesia, 13. Annual Meeting, 1992, Mainz

2 E Cohen, Program Reference for SPICE2, Memorandum No.M592, June 1976

3 JJ Marini,PS Crooke, JD Truwit, Determinants and limits of pressure-preset ventilation. A mathematical model of pressure control, J Appl Physiol. 67 (1989), 1081-1092

4 G Iotti,A Braschi, JX Brunner,Assessment of Respiratory Mechanics During Total and Partial Ventilatory Support,in Yearbook of Intensive Care and Emergency Medicine (1992), Springer, 331-345

5 W Heinrichs,P Beckmann,D Dany, M Halmagyi, Ein nicht-lineares Zwei-Kompartment-Modell zur Bestimmung von Zeitkonsanten und intrapulmonalen Druckwerten bei Patienten mit ARDS, CCCPM-92, Computers in Critical Care, Pulm. Medicine and Anesthesia, 13. Annual Meeting, 1992, Mainz

Artificial Intelligence in Medecine
S. Andreassen et al. , Eds.
IOS Press, 1993

Interpreting Physiopathological States under Environment Temporal Restrictions

G. Escalada-Imaza[a], J. Jaureguizar-Núñez[a], X. Pastor-Durán[b], G. Fita-Rodríguez[b]

[a]Instituto de Investigación en Inteligencia Artificial. CEAB. CSIC. Blanes 17300, Gerona, Spain

[b]Hospital Clínico y Provincial de Barcelona. Villarroel 170, Barcelona 8036, Spain

Abstract.
We describe a computer model for diagnosing physiopathological states in a dynamic and real time environment, in the domain of a Pediatric Intensive Care Unit (PICU). The approach is based on a graph, using several uncertainty propagation and time restrictions rules.

1. INTRODUCTION

In the PICU, the patient state is continuously monitorized by a set of sensors and devices that measure all the essential biophysical parameters. These monitors activate their own alarms when some conflictive measures are detected. The physician in charge of the patient, must react to the alarm by reading, checking and validating the information. If the measures are validated the physician interprets the patient situation, considering especially the monitorized data, and diagnoses some physiopathological states. After that, the physician makes a decision. This decision can be starting a new round of information acquisition and interpretation, deactivating the alarm, checking the sensors, modifying the alarm boundaries, establishing a treatment, ordering complementary explorations, etc.

Computationally, the described monitoring medical context presents the following features:
1) There exist three types of reasoning processes: capturing-validating the monitor´s signals; quick interpretation the data and diagnosing patient physiopathological states, simple decision making.
2) Great amounts of quick changing information are processed: many data coming from monitors and a few from other sources, must be taken into account at each instant.
3) The character of all the decisions is reactive, (they must be triggered swiftly in response to specific situations): when an alarm is produced, the validating process is activated; when a validated alarm is detected the interpretation process is activated; when a problematic and unexpected physiopathological state is detected a treatment should be quickly executed.
4) A kind of uncertainty reasoning is performed due to the lack of necesary information: a physiopathological state could be asserted with only a certain degree of certainty because for example not all the concerned measures are available, and/or some of them could be erroneous.
5) The process of acquiring information, interpreting the data, diagnosing the state and making decisions is organised in several levels of depth: the information available on a certain level corresponding to that acquired after a certain time, is handled to either take an elaborate decision (e.g. establish a treatment) or to order the acquisition of additional information.

The previous approaches to resolve applications involving some kind of reasoning, based on the classical Expert Systems [1,2] are not well adapted to deal with features involving Real Time processing. On the other side, classical Real Time Softwares developed in Computer Science are not capable of making any kind of reasoning [3].

The work presented in this paper is situated in the line of the recently developed approaches of Real Time Based Knowledge Systems in the Monitoring Medical Context [4,5]. It describes a computer reasoning model for quick interpretation data and diagnosing patient physiopathological states in response to the above mentioned real time and uncertainty features.

2. COMPUTER MODEL

We present the input and output mechanisms, the computing model, and finally, an automatic method for checking two main characteristics of the obtained model, its completeness and consistency.

2.1 Input/output information

The system works in a kind of closed cycle: first it reads the inputs, second a deduction is performed on these inputs and finally the output is obtained. This cycle is repeated infinitely. The inputs come from the validated signal monitoring (≈50 inputs), and from other sources (≈20 inputs) such as laboratories and physical exploration. The outputs consist in the set of deduced physiopathological states together with their corresponding uncertainty factor.

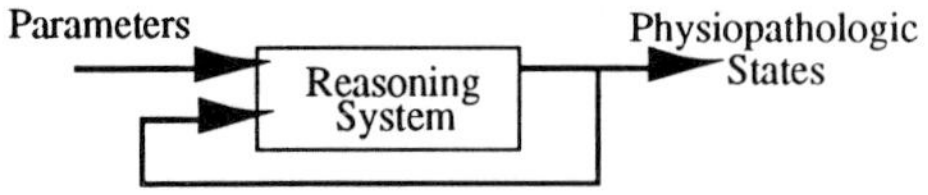

Figure 1. Input/Output Information in the Reasoning System

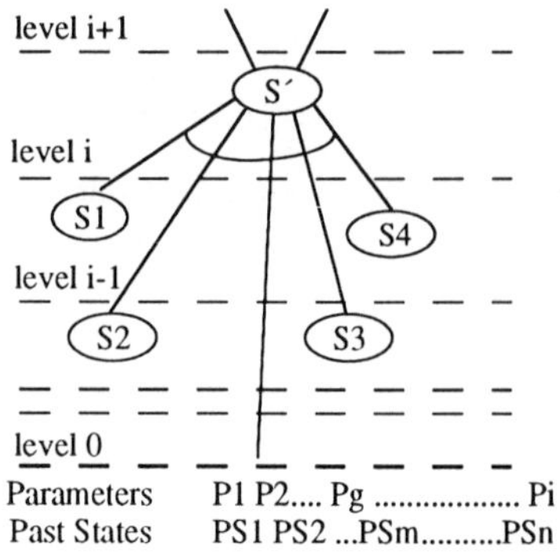

Figure 2. Tree Structuring the Knowledge

2.2 Model of the reasoning process

A kind of feedback exits in the reasoning model: in a first deduction cycle a physiopathologic state can be deduced and this one could be introduced in the next deduction cycle as an input to the system in order to deduce some new states. Figure 1 illustrates this situation.

The physiopathological states can be structured in depth levels. To deduce one particular state at a given instant, the existence of parameter values, and simpler present and/or past physiopathological states has to be verified. Simpler physiopathological states mean that to deduce them a lesser number of parameters have to be considered. This indicates that the sets of states are partially ordered and hence, the relationships between them can be modelled by a *tree* (Figure 2) where:

- Each leaf is associated with a past physiopathologic state PS or a parameter P.
- Each node S is associated with a present physiopathologic state.
- Each arc going from one inferior state S´ (or a parameter P or a past state PS) to a superior one S represents the relation of "S is depending on S´". In a general case, a state S is the father of a connector that has several successor states S1,..,Sk, parameters P1,..,Pi and past states PS1,..,PSn and therefore the set of arcs (S,S1),..,(S,Sk),(S,P1),..,(S,Pi),(S,PS1),..,(S,PSn) indicates that S depends on the set S1,..,Sk,P1,..,Pi,PS1,..,PSn.

Each node is associated with one value. The number of values of the parameters could be at most ten <very high, quite high, high, rather high, normal, rather low, quite low, low, very low>. The number of values (uncertainty degrees) of the states could be at most seven <true, very possible, possible, unknown, little possible, unlikely, false>. This set of values are *ordered* as indicated.

The feedback loop is modelled through a causal relationship where *past states* influence more *recent states*. This causal relationship is of kind: the uncertainty value V of a state depends on the uncertainty value V´ of a past state that occurred a certain time T before the present one and lasted an approximated duration D. The same relation between a past state and an earlier past state could also exist.

For each connector linking a father state to the successor ones, an uncertainty table is handled to calculate the uncertainty degree of the *father node (state)* as a function of the *successor nodes (states or parameters)*. These tables, one for each connector, are given by the physician considering the most relevant and usual combinations of parameter and simpler states to deduce a more complex state.

The tables present the following format: The top X-axis is formed by the different uncertainty degree values of the father node of the connector. The left Y-axis is formed by the parameters and present and past successor states. The item of a cell I(x, y) is as follows. 1) If x is a parameter Px then I(x,y) is a range of parameter values (e.g. Px < High). 2) If x is a present state Sx then I(x,y) is a range of uncertainty degrees (e.g. Sx > possible). 3) If x is a past state PSx then I(x,y) is a range of uncertainty degrees and a triplet (PSj,D,T), where PSj is a past state linked by the causal dependency relationship to Sx, the time T and the duration D, indicating that Sx had to occur a time T before PSj and with a duration D. A standard form of one table is illustrated in Figure 3.

The meaning of the column y-th is:

if the value of each parameter Px is within the range Rx signalled in its respective cell (x,y);
and the uncertainty degree of each state Sx was within a range Rx, happened a time T before a past state PSj and lasted an interval D, where (x,y)=[Rx, (PSj, T , D)];
then the uncertainty value of the father node is the value "y".

The three dimensions of the table is explained by the fact that a *same uncertainty value* of the father node could be found by *several combinations* of parameters´ values and states´ uncertainty degrees.

	Father State	T	VP	P	?	LP	U	F
Parameters	P1	P1<H	.	.	.	.	.	.
	.	.	.	.	.	.	.	.
	Pi	N≥Pi≥L	H≥Pi>N	Pi=VH	Pi=?	— —	Pi=QL	Pi=VL
States	S1	S1=T	.	.	.	.	.	.
	.	.	.	.	.	.	.	.
	Sk	.	.	.	.	.	.	.
	PS1	.	.	PS1=P (0,10,2)	.	.	.	.
	.	PSn=T	.	.	.	.	.	.
	PSn	(Sn,5,5)	.	.	.	.	.	.

Uncertainty State Values : T=True; VP=Very Possible; P=Possible; ?=Unknown; LP=Little Possible; U=Unlikely; F=false.
Parameter values :VH=Very High; QH=Quite high; H=High; RH=Rather High; N=Normal; RL=Rather Low; L=Low; QL=Quite Low; VL=Very Low; ?=Unknow.
— — : the physiscian has not supplied any situation for which the father node is in this uncertainty degree (Low Possible).
(Sn, 5, 5) is a condition meaning that PSn=T should have ocurred about 5 minutes before a Sn state, that should have lasted at least 5 minutes
(0, 10, 2) is a condition meaning that PS1=P should have ocurred about 10 minutes before the present time, and should have lasted at least 2 minutes.

Figure 3. State Table

2.3 Completeness and consistency of the computing model

The complexity to get a right knowledge representation, materialised by a good definition of the tables related to the connectors, makes that the physician could commit two conceptual mistakes:

- *Incompleteness of a table*: there could exist a combination of the successor nodes' values that is not considered in the set of columns of the tables. The input space of the set of successor nodes is defined by the Cartesian product of the sets of possible individual values taken by each successor node. Thus, each column "y" groups a set of points of this space, defined by the specified ranges in the cells (x,y). However, it could be the case that the reunion of the points represented by all the columns do not cover the input values space.
- *Inconsistency of a table*: there could exist a common set of points of the input space, defined by the successor nodes values, which are included in two different columns. That means that a same combination of the successor nodes values is included in the set of points specified by two columns indicating two different values of the father node.

Due to these problems, the system is provided with an elicitation module. Its tasks are to check automatically the completeness and consistency of every table and to indicate to the physician if a combination of input values gives rise to an incompleteness or inconsistency situation. It should be noticed that in a case where the physician has not considered a particular combination, that could be due to two possibilities: the physician has forgotten this values combination or the situation corresponding to this value combination is more unlikely to happen in practice.

Remark: these modules work only on the values of parameter and present states. The completeness of the past states cannot be analysed because the domain of the temporal axis is infinite.

3. THE ALGORITHMS

The system is composed of three mean algorithms: the proper resolution on-line algorithm to determine a set of physiopathological states with their respective uncertainty degree, and the off-line consistency and completeness algorithms. For lack of space, we only give a brief description of the first, the other two are described in [6].

The resolution algorithm employs the tree and the tables associated with each connector. It is based on a bottom-up breath-first strategy. Namely, starting by the present value of the parameters and using the tables corresponding to the connectors linking the parameters with first level states, the algorithm determines in a first step the certainty values of the first level states. The states whose uncertainty degree is below a *fixed threshold* are not considered in the next propagation from the first level to the second one. This propagation from successor nodes, having an uncertainty degree bigger than the fixed threshold, to father nodes of higher order using the associated tables is equally done from any level, now considering present parameters and states and past states.

Let us describe how the tables are used to make the uncertainty propagation throughout a particular connector. The algorithm enters in the table with some concrete values of the parameter and states. Assume that Vx is the value of one of these elements x. Then, for each x the set of columns including Vx in the range Rx defined by the cell (x,y) are retained. This set is intersected with the corresponding similar columns of the others elements x´. The process of intersection is repeated until only one column remains. Then, the value of the father node corresponding to this column is affected to the father state.

The *complexity* of the values propagation throughout the tree is linear in the size of the tree. Also, the propagation throughout a particular connector is linear in the size of the three-dimensional associated table.

4. CONCLUSIONS

We have presented a Real-Time Knowledge-Based System running to simulate the reasoning mechanism of a physician in a PICU. This context imposes the following Real Time features which fulfils the proposed system: a fast reactive diagnosis; a processing of huge quantity of changing input information, an uncertainty diagnosis because imprecise measures have to be considered; and finally, the decomposition by levels of the whole reasoning model.

These features of working are somewhat far of those considered in classical Expert Systems. Also, although the design of the proposed system has been inspired from a medical application, it has carried out in a way that the field of possible extensions should be fairly wide. The tree dividing the model reasoning of physiologic states in layers, and the uncertainty tables between successor and father nodes of connectors in the tree, are general computing elements and so, they open the possibility of applying the system to other areas, as well in medicine as in other different contexts. Indeed, the proposed method presents an adequate trade-off between uncertainty and rapidness of diagnosis, a paradigm that appears as crucial in most Real-Time Knowledge-Based Systems.

5. REFERENCES

[1] Shortliffe EH. Clinical Decision-Support Systems. In:*Medical Informatics, Computer Applications in the Health Care*. Addison Wesley 1990; 466-502.

[2] Miller RA, Pople HE, Myers JD. INTERNIST-I An Experimental Computer-Based Diagnostic Consultant for General Internal Medicine. In: *Computer-Assisted Medical Decision Making*. Springer-Verlag 1985; 139-159.

[3] Korf RE. Depth-Limited Search for Real Time problem Solving. Real Time Systems, May 1990, vol. 2, n1/2; 7-24.

[4] Factor M, Gelernnter DH, Kolb CE, Miller PL, Sitting DF. Real-Time Data Fusion in the Intensive Care Unit. Computer, November 1991; 45-54.

[5] Uckun S, Dawant BM, Lindstrom DP. Model-Based Diagnosis in Intensive Care Monitoring: the YAQ Approach. Artificial Intelligence in Medicine 1993, 5; 31-48.

[6] G. Escalada-Imaz, J. Jaureguizar-Núñez, X. Pastor-Duran, G. Fita-Rodríguez. Medical Reasoning Model for Diagnosing Physiopathological States in a Real Time Environment. The Second World Congress on Expert Systems. Lisbon, Portugal. January 1994.

This study was partially supported by the Spanish Ministry of Education under Grant DGICYT No. PM90/0061 LATIDOα Project , and the CICYT No. TIC 92-0579-C02-01 ARREL Project.

Strategies for Medical Reasoning - Patient Management

Artificial Intelligence in Medecine
S. Andreassen et al. , Eds.
IOS Press, 1993

Medical system design and knowledge acquisition using cooperating intelligent agents
A case study for breast cancer diagnosis

Arturo Ovalle, Emmanuelle Hugonnard and Catherine Garbay

Equipe SIC (Systèmes Cognitifs Intégrés), Laboratoire TIMC - IMAG
Bât. CERMO - BP 53X - 38041 Grenoble Cedex, France

Abstract

Over the past ten years, a significant amount of research has been devoted to the use of Distributed Artificial Intelligence Techniques for Expert Systems Design and Development. The use of Multi-Agent architectures provides several benefits such as modularizing problem-solving knowledge, alleviating the complexity of developing knowledge-based systems by distributing knowledge amongst a group of cooperating agents, or facilitating the integration of heterogeneous knowledge schemes and reasoning mechanisms. However, significant problems yet remain such as how to model the expertise of the medical application domain and incorporate such models within the multi-agent system architecture.

In this paper, we describe our experience in designing cooperating expert systems and distributed knowledge acquisition frameworks specifically to build medical applications. To achieve this, we have developed and proposed a methodology to guide these processes. Concepts dealing with this development methodology become concrete through the design and development of KIDS (Knowledge based Image Diagnosis System), a Multi-Agent Expert System devoted to Breast Cancer Diagnosis.

1. INTRODUCTION

In recent years, there has been an increasing interest in the use of approaches in Knowledge Engineering, Cognitive Science, and Distributed Artificial Intelligence fields. The Multi-Agent paradigm resulting from the synergism of these approaches makes it possible to overcome the drawbacks encountered during the resolution of complex problems. The basis of the Multi-Agent approach is the distribution of tasks and skills among intelligent and autonomous entities that cooperate, pooling their knowledge and their expertise to attain a specific goal [2,3]. In this way, not only the representation of multi-modal knowledge is possible, as well as reasoning schemes handling can but cooperative problem solving as well. In addition, a variety of reasoning schemes emerge which correspond not only to individual behaviour but also to collective behaviour developed within the group of agents.

Early research on multi-agent problem solving concentrated on the blackboard problem-solving approach in which a group of agents (knowledge sources) collaborate by way of a shared database, called the blackboard, in order to reach a solution to the problem [12]. The problem solving protocol is defined here by a central control mechanism that determines which agent has access to the blackboard at a given time. Later research recognised the importance of having autonomous agents capable of engaging in peer-to-peer communication [15]. In this way, diverse cooperation mechanisms between agents can be implemented such as the contract net [20], the partial global planning (PGP) [8], the task sharing or the result sharing [16] protocols.

Few concrete medical applications using multi-agent problem solving approach have been made and specifically applied to the medical diagnosis field. A Blackboard-Based Chromosome Analysis System [19] devoted to chromosome image segmentation was built under the context of SBS, a blackboard system shell. Chromosome and cell models to which images are matched are made explicit by means of a frame-network. A set of SBS experts (knowledge sources) have been conceived, each of which is responsible for a particular domain task in the process of image segmentation and cooperate for solving these tasks. Among the "main" experts (a dozen all in all) we can quote the "cell selection expert", "image enhancement expert" or "statistical chromosome classifier expert".

The distributed knowledge-based system called AMNESIA [15] uses cooperating intelligent agents to diagnose memory related disorder illnesses. AMNESIA was developed using RAPIDO (Rapid, Agent Prototyping DOmain) a rapid agent prototyping environment. Four agents named User (a prototype interface agent), Test Analysis, Drug Effect and Diagnose, correspond to the specialisms identified during knowledge acquisition. After the design analysis step the Diagnose agent was easily separated into two distinct agents since Amnesia-related diseases can be categorised as either 'Slow Onset Amnesias' or 'Rapid Onset Amnesias' depending upon the cause.

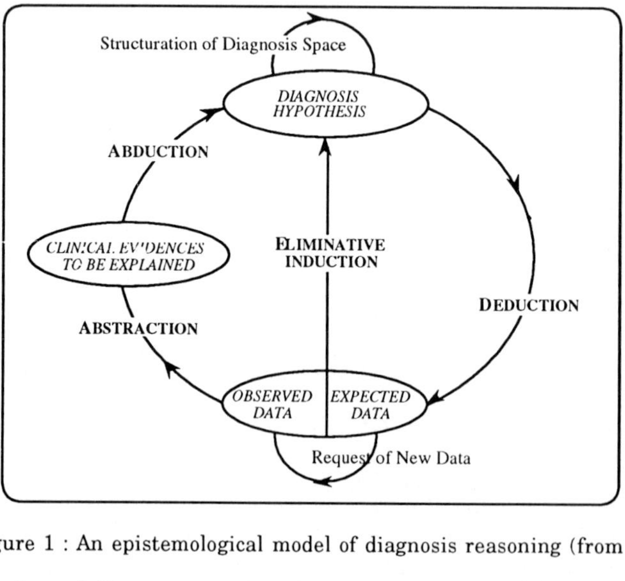

Figure 1 : An epistemological model of diagnosis reasoning (from [14]).

Task-oriented modeling approaches have been proposed which are based on the principle that knowledge may not be separated from its use [4]. The Generic Task [6] approach provides general problem solving methods in conjunction with the knowledge they require. Thus, a generic task is seen as a combination of knowledge structures and inference strategies (know-how) that efficiently solve certain generic types of problems.

An epistemological model of diagnostic reasoning which presents some similarities with the Task-oriented modeling approach is proposed by [14] and defined in terms of abstraction, abduction, deduction and eliminative induction (see Figure 1). The abstraction corresponds to the preliminary identification of the clinical features that diagnosis should be able to explain. The abduction is the inference type that try to identify those initial conditions that deduction-induction will start from. Deduction is the inference type that refers to a logical implication. It allows to derive from each candidate hypothesis what is expected to be true if that hypothesis is true (prediction). At last, eliminative induction is used as a process to reduce uncertainty of infered hypothesis by matching their consequences against observed data.

In addition, a variety of methodologies have been proposed not only for structuring and analyzing knowledge according to rather "formal" knowledge typologies but also for guiding the system design process by studying and following expert cognitive processes. They are totally independent of a technique or system. In KOD methodology [21] two axes are introduced which define models and paradigms to assist the knowledge acquisition process. KADS (Knowledge Acquisition and Design Support) methodology [3,22] permits the user to construct several models, including that of expert knowledge and reasoning, the user / system cooperation, the functional and physical design models.

In this paper, we describe our experience in designing cooperating expert systems and distributed knowledge acquisition frameworks specifically to build medical applications. To achieve this, we have developed and proposed a methodology to guide these processes [18,13]. In the next section, we describe main characteristics of the medical problem domain, before describing the use of our methodology to design and implement the KIDS (Knowledge based Image Diagnosis System) system. Finally, the technical implementation of the KIDS multi-agent system devoted to breast cancer diagnosis is examined. A more detail description of KIDS may be found in [17].

2. MULTI-AGENT SYSTEM DEVELOPMENT METHODOLOGY

It should be noted that there is an outstanding evolution in the Multi-Agent technology. As a result, we have proposed and defined a methodology to design and develop cognitive multi-agent system which consists of three essential steps [18] : the Cognitive Identification Step, the Conceptual Modeling and Formal Specification Step, and the Technological Implementation Step. The aim of Cognitive Identification is to identify the knowledge elements that will be considered within the system design. This identification is based on the use of the two typologies proposed and described in [17].

Once the first step is complete, the second step, called the Conceptual Modeling Step, attempts to define the models which permit the formalization of the domain knowledge and technological components that have been underlined during the previous step. In the third step, the Technological Implementation Step, possible fusions among conceptual models become concrete (see Figure 2). Feedback between steps are indeed possible which permit necessary improvements in the system design.

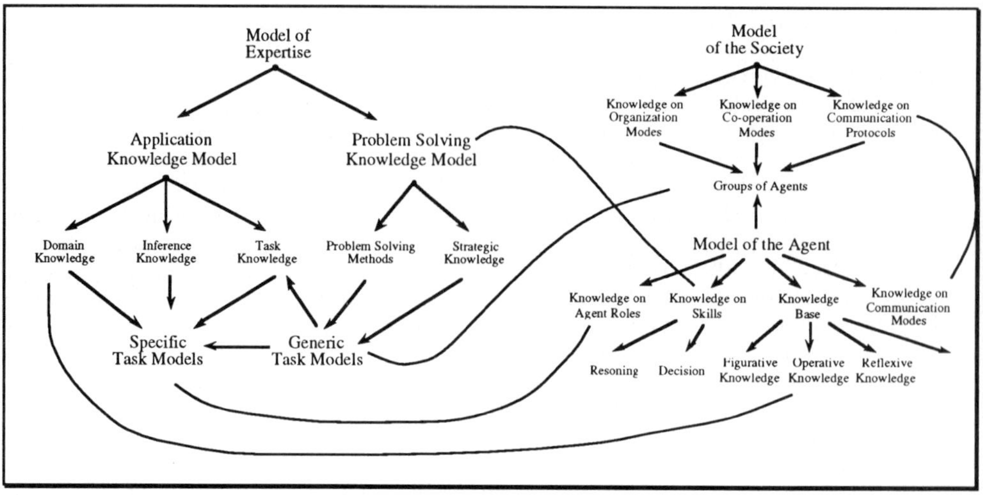

Figure 2 : Fusing Cognitive and Technological models for System Design.

The first and third steps are the best understood in most of the work devoted to cognitive system development. However, much work yet remains to be done on the Conceptual Modeling Step which require multiple models and it becomes necessary to formalize and fuse them. Some of commonest models include the following models : application knowledge, problem solving, generic and specific task, internal structure of the agent, society of agents, communication, ... Each of these models is dependent on several variables or parameters through which models can be completely defined.

However, it is not only necessary to conceive specific models in a formal way but also to carefully analyse the possible links existing among models, especially between cognitive and technological models. In fact, the better the quality in fusing between technological and cognitive models, the better the quality in the system design.

3. COGNITIVE IDENTIFICATION

While using Multi-Agent technology to model the expertise of cytopathological breast cancer diagnosis, technical problems have appeared on the representation of knowledge and reasoning [16]. The need for providing a knowledge/reasoning typology was revealed to be essential to the Cognitive Identification and Conceptual Modeling processes. Our aim at this stage was to propose a cognitive typology for studying expert reasoning schemes according to their intrinsic nature, that is, through the nature of knowledge elements that these reasoning schemes handled.

3.1. The Medical Problem Domain

Clinical cytology concerns the study of cells that have been sampled, stained and fixed upon transparent slides, in order to be observed through a microscope [11]. Various cytological examination styles exist, which apply to a rich variety of organs. It is thus very difficult to exhibit general approach or rules that would apply to any specimen investigation. We have focussed on breast cytology, but hope to be able to exemplify rather general reasoning mechanisms, that would apply to other cytological examinations.

Cytological specimen examination involves two main steps: a preliminary step consisting in material scanning and inspection followed by a decision-making step. The preliminary step, assumed by cytotechnicians, consists in validating the specimen lisibility and significance (Specimen Validation Task) as well as manually marking the significant fields of the slide (Field Selection Task).

The interpretation step, performed by the cytopatologist, must lead to the gathering of morphological evidences, allowing to identify the lesions that might appear on the specimen as benign or malign. This step requires the achievement of three different tasks, namely Morphological Analysis, Cell Type Identification and finally Diagnosis Formulation tasks. The latest task (Validation of Formulated Diagnosis Task) is finally aimed at validating the inferred diagnosis hypothesis : it consists in exploiting additional clinical and administrative data related to the examined patient. Such process leads the pathologist to evaluate the proposed diagnosis hypothesis as fully coherent or not.

- *Cognitive Typology :*

  - Figurative knowledge (i.e. objects) : the specimen image, the observed field, the cellular morphological features, or the diagnosis formulation ;
  - Operative knowledge (i.e. actions) : to describe (e.g. aspect of the specimen, cell morphologies), to select (e.g. field selection), to match and classify (e.g. cell identification, diagnosis formulation) ;
  - Strategic knowledge : random or systematic specimen scanning, prediction / verification strategies ;
  - Tasks : specimen exploration, cell type identification, diagnosis formulation, ... ;

3.2. The Technological Level

Technological Typology introduces a system developer with intrinsic aspects characterizing Multi-Agent environments. Two points of view must be considered : this of the agent and that of the society of agents. Reasoning developed in the society of agents depends on choices made at the individual level (within the internal structure of the agent) and at the social level (tasks and skills distribution modes, communication modes and protocols, and co-operation and organisation modes). By using the technological typology, several categories of heterogeneous elements can be identified.

- *Technological Typology :*

  - Agent roles : to evaluate an information (e.g. field significance, diagnosis likelihood, ...), to acquire or to transmit knowledge (e.g. a specimen image, a cell type identification...), to classify information (e.g. a cell type, pathology, ...) ;
  - Agent groups : different groups of agents can be associated to different analysis phases : exploration, cell type identification, and diagnosis formulation ;
  - Co-operation modes between agents : intermediate results sharing, task and skills distribution, ...

4. CONCEPTUAL MODELING AND FORMAL SPECIFICATION

The aim of the Conceptual Modeling Step is to analyse the models necessary in the system design. Two model classes can be distinguished : the cognitive models, which represent the expertise to be modelled, and the technological models which describe informatic entities to be specified [17].

Three examples of conceptual models are given below along with their associated formal specifications. One cognitive model (the task model for biomedical diagnosis) and two technological models (the internal structure of the agent and the model of the agents society) will be presented.

Table 1. Description of main tasks involved in biomedical cytological diagnosis

Tasks	Input	Output	Objective	Approach	Remarks
T1	Specimen	Specimen Features	Material Inspection & Checking	Random Scanning	*Not Diagnosis Oriented*
T2	Specimen	Selected Fields	Selection of Informative Fields	Systematic Scanning	*Heavily Context Dependent*
T3	Selected Fields	Morphologic Features	Morphologic Description	Low & High Level Examination	*Low Res. may reveal Sufficient*
T4	Morphologic Features	Cell Types	Cell Type Identification	Prediction Verification	*Low Res. may reveal Sufficient*
T5	Cell Types	Diagnosis	Diagnosis Formulation	Evidence Gathering	*Influence further Gathering*
T6	Diagnosis & Patient Data	Diagnosis Confirmation	Diagnosis Validation	Consistency Checking	*May imply Resuming the Analysis*

4.1. Task Model for Biomedical Diagnosis

Cytological Specimen Exploration requires several tasks (Table 1). Il should be pointed out that these tasks as well as reasoning schemes developed inside each task require different kind of knowledge such as : figurative (objects), operative (actions), reflexive (information on the nature of a knowledge element) and heuristic (each knowledge which indicates the conditions for handling a knowledge element and how it is to be done).

4.2. Formal Specification of a Task Model

Based on table 1, we propose the following formal task specification model :

Task Model =
<Name, Objective, Sub-tasks, Approach, Input, Output >

Example of a cytological task :

Name :	Cell Type Identification ;
Objective :	To Identify cell types by using their morphological description ;
Sub-tasks :	- To Describe a morphology ;
	- To Infer a cell type ;
Approach :	Prediction / Verification ;
Inputs :	Morphological Features ;
Outputs :	Cell Types ;

4.3. Model of the Agent Internal Structure

The *internal structure of the agent* comprises four essential parts [9]. The first part describes the agent as a “communicating” and “reactive” entity ; it is responsible for interactions with other agents and the environment. The second part describes the agent as a “rational” entity ; it determines the control mechanisms to be given to the agent : planning possibilities and internal/external task supervision. The third part describes the agent as a "specialist" and is strongly dependent on the application. It thus concerns the expertise of the agent that is its specific skills on the domain. Finally, the fourth part describes the agent as an "intentional" entity in which knowledge is included about itself and others. This aspect requires the ability of the agent to reason with respect to others, and so the ability to model the knowledge of others, their abilities and objectives.

4.4. Formal Specification of the Agent Model

Using the model described above a Formal Specification of the Internal Structure of the Agent can be proposed as follows :

Model of the Agent Internal Structure =
<Communication, Control, Skills, Intentional Knowledge >
Communication = Emission, Reception ; Intentional Knowledge = list of agent links

	Model of the KP Agent	**Model of the KS Agent**
Emission	Messages "Receive, Supply"	Messages "Solve, Process"
Reception	Messages "Solve, Process"	Messages "Receive, Supply"
Control	Solving Strategy (goal driven, data driven), local operative selection, global figurative selection	KB updating, strategy for rule activation, local figurative selection, global operative selection
Skills	(action rules, strategy rules)	(objects, propagation, interrogation & proposition rules)
Int.-Know.	list of acquainted KS agents	list of acquainted KP agents

The two instanciated models given above have been taken from the KP (Knowledge Processor) and KS (Knowledge Server) agent models used within MAPS (Multi-Agent Problem Solver) Shell [1]. They have been used for the technological implementation of the KIDS system.

5. MEDICAL KNOWLEDGE ACQUISITION IN KIDS

In our approach, the duality between KS and KP agents allows any MAPS architecture to be seen alternatively under domain-oriented or task-oriented point of view. This particular feature will be used to guide the elicitation process. In fact, the use of this model provides the basis for a flexible knowledge acquisition environment that should be used to complete various knowledge base of a system such as KIDS : it defines a generic model of problem solving in cytology, and also permits the knowledge acquisition process to be tackled at a certain level of abstraction.

We propose to model knowledge acquisition as a cooperative process based on a multi-agent knowledge model. In fact, a cooperation between elicitation, presentation and resolution modes is provided, in order for knowledge to be kept close to its use, as well as permitting the the flexible alternation between user and system points of view [13]. Moreover, a cooperation between various elicitation and presentation forms is provided, in terms of formal, case-based and task-based approaches (see Figure 3).

The first two approaches are essentially oriented towards the elicitation of domain knowledge, of concepts and properties. Their styles are complementary : they allow to alternate between the elicitation of general and well-structured knowledge, in a rather system-dependent style, with the elicitation of more heterogeneous and sparse knowledge elements, in a more case-dependent style. The third interaction style, so-called task-based approach, on the contrary, offers a more operative point of view in knowledge acquisition, by supporting the elicitation of "causal-like" knowledge. A hypercard metaphor is proposed to drive the interaction.

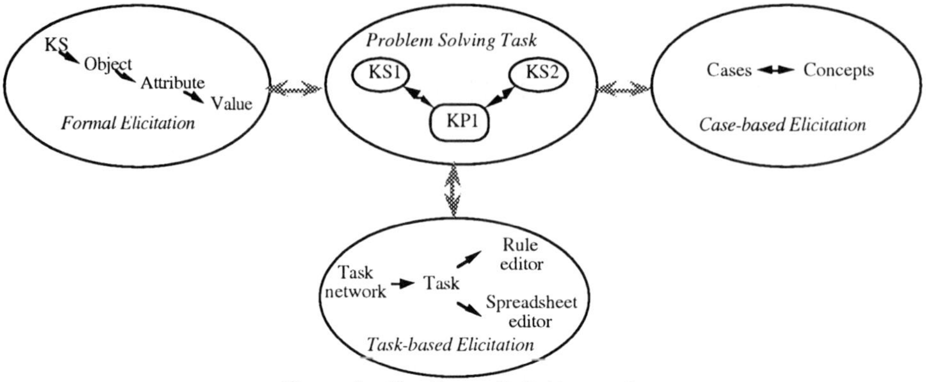

Figure 3 : The three elicitation modes.

5.1. Formal Presentation / Elicitation Mode

The formal mode is devoted to the presentation/elicitation of problem solver resources, according to a rather system-dependent approach. These resources are organized into a hierarchy (agent, objects and rules, attributes and instances), with each element in the hierarchy being accessed through a separate card, and navigation between them being controlled in a flexible way : breadth-first exploration is driven by buttons displayed at the top of each card (a part-of relationship), while depth-first exploration is driven by selecting items in a scrolling list (a kind-of relationship) (see Figure 4). Updating medical knowledge is made by simple list editing : it is clear that such an approach is valid only if a clear, coherent and exhaustive view of domain concepts and properties are available. Rather it might be used to refine an existing knowledge basis, or for the trained programmer as a rapid prototyping tool. Medical knowledge in that case is approached in the form of lists (lists of morphological features, cell types, and diagnoses) : it supports a restricted and figurative view of knowledge.

5.2. Task-based Elicitation Mode

The task-based elicitation approach would draw on MAPS generic task model : it would thus involve interacting with a KP-centered triplet of the form (KS-input, KP, KS-output), the KP agent representing the operative knowledge attached to the task, and the KS agents the input and output domain knowledge handled by the task. Main domain concepts have to be already available for the approach to be usable.

In our approach, it appears that elicitation task may be approached according to two different and complementary points of view, namely a KP-centered and a KS-centered point of view. These points of view respectively allow the direct and indirect elicitation of task-dependent operative knowledge by means of two different interaction tools, namely a rule and a spreadsheet editor. The rule editor is directly linked to the KP agent inference resources, while the spreadsheet editor is provided to facilitate the generation of inference rules ; it allows the cross-association of "input" and "output" domain knowledge. It should be noted that this approach can only be applied when domain concepts have already been elicited.

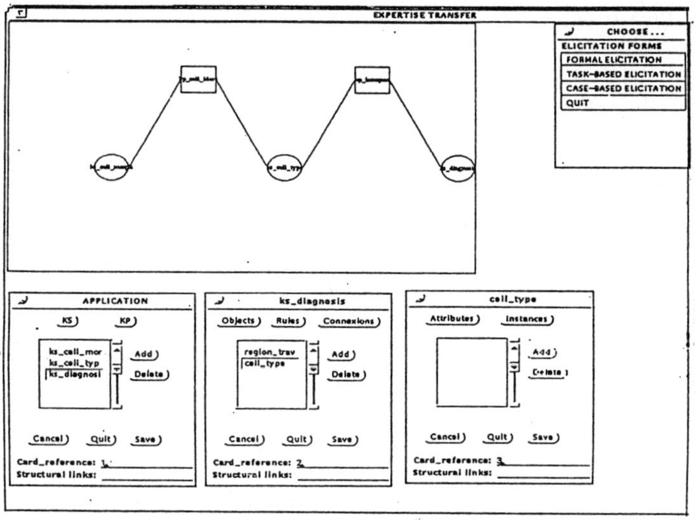

Figure 4 : Formal approach for Medical Knowledge Elicitation

6. THE KIDS SYSTEM IMPLEMENTATION

The technological implementation step attempts to create agents and groups of agents which compose the system architecture. This implementation should specify their resources, which implies defining their skills and interaction modes.

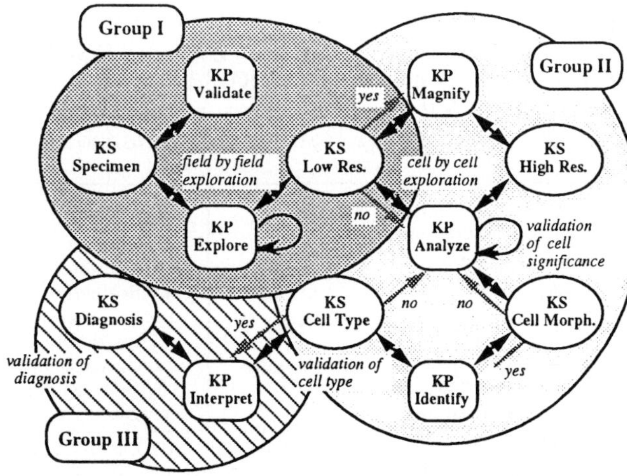

Figure 5 : KIDS architecture comprises three groups of cooperating heterogeneous ES.

The KIDS system has been designed through the KS and KP agent model provided by MAPS. Figure 5 shows the network of cooperating expert systems composing the KIDS system. This network represents a high-level modeling of pathologist expertise. Three different groups of agents can be distinguished which correspond to three generic tasks [5] involved in the Scene Undestanding : Scene Exploration (group I : Specimen Exploration Task), Object Identification (group II : Cell Type Identification Task), and Scene Understanding (group III : Diagnosis Formulation Task) Generic Tasks.

6.1. Specimen Exploration Task

The *task and skill distribution* for Specimen Exploration Task is the following : Specimen Image Acquisition is driven by KS-Specimen agent, Specimen Exploration is managed by KP-Explore agent and Field Selection is handled by KS-Low-Resolution agent. The rule below shows the way in which the selection of relevant fields is made by the KS-Low-Resolution agent based on grey level image analysis.

--> proposition-rule :

IF (1) current-field-image is loaded &
(2) grey level distribution is relevant

THEN propose current-field-image to KP-Analyze
for further investigation

The *Group of* Agents Behaviour for this phase can be described as follows : an image of the specimen is acquired by the KS-Specimen agent and then transmitted to the KP-Explore agent. A particular specimen exploration strategy is implemented in this agent, in the form of a loop which controls the successive sending of fields to the KS-Low-Resolution agent. After reception by the KS-Low-Resolution, user agreement is requested to know whether the analysis of such field is relevant or not, or whether it would need high magnification analysis.

6.2. Cell Type Identification Task

The *task and skill distribution* with respect to the Cell Type Identification Task is the following : Cellular Morphological Analysis is managed by KP-Analyze agent, Feature Computation is handled by the KS-Morphology agent, and Cell Type Identification is driven by the KP-Identify agent. The rule shows below the way in which KP-Analyze agent carries out the field image segmentation sub-task where image features are obtained from the KS-Low-Resolution agent.

--> action-rule : **IF** (1) current-field-image features are obtained from KS-Low-Resolution **THEN** (1) segment current-field-image (*) (2) repeat for each detected cell in current-field-image : - highlight cell contour by a graphical procedure - send detected cell to KS-Cell-Morph for further morphological investigation.	* the image segmentation procedure comprises the following steps : - computation of thresholds by means of histogram analysis (Fisher classification); - image thresholding; - binary closure; - connected component labelling; - geometrical decomposition of cell aggregates.

The *Group of Agents Behaviour* for this phase can be described as follows : after reception by the KP-Analyze agent, the field is segmented and a second loop is implemented, which controls the successive sending of cells to the KS-Morphology agent. The latter is then responsible for collecting relevant morphological information and sending it to the KP-Identify agent for further identification. It should be observed that user agreement is again requested, to determine whether the analysis of the current cell is relevant or not. The various cell features are currently requested of the user : the contour of the current cell is graphically highlighted for this purpose. Cell type identification is afterwards performed by the KP-Identify agent by means of inference rules based on a cross-correlated table in which cell morphologies are assigned to cell types. Such identification may then be validated or not by the user (activation of KS-Cell-Type interrogation rules). In case of acceptance, a scoring procedure is activated as conclusion part of KS-Cell-Type propagation rule. In the opposite case, the next cell is simply proposed for analysis, i.e. control is sent back to loop 2.

6.3. Diagnosis Formulation Task

The *task and skill distribution* for the Diagnosis Formulation Step is as follows : Diagnosis Formulation is driven by the KP-Interpret agent, and Potential Diagnosis Hypothesis Storing is driven by the KS-Diagnosis agent. The following action-rule shows how the KP-Interpret agent concludes a diagnosis hypothesis based on a cross-correlation table tying cell types to pathologies.

```
--> action rule :

IF      (1) fibroblast cell score > N &
        (2) epithelial cell score < M

THEN    send "diagnosis = fibroadenoma" to KS-Diagnosis
```

The *Group of Agents Behaviour* for this phase can be described as follows : the scoring of cell types directly assists the diagnosis formulation that is performed by KP-Interpret. Proposed diagnosis hypothesis is finally received by KS-Diagnosis agent ; activating propagation rules then entails requesting the user to validate the proposed diagnosis or not. Control is sent back to previous steps in case satisfactory diagnosis has not been obtained.

7. CONCLUSION AND FURTHER WORK

We have attempted to outline the advantages of a methodological framework to build medical cooperating expert systems. Our approach makes a distinction between three different steps : cognitive identification, conceptual modeling and technological implementation. The articulation of these steps allows a progressive and controlled design of the system. The main benefits in using Multi-Agent Technology to design and implement medical ES are the following :

- the facility to identify and computer transcribe several classes of reasoning mechanisms comprised in the expertise to be modelled ;
- the potential integration of reasoning mechanisms not only within the generic tasks but also when cooperation between sub-tasks takes place ;
- the possibility of a "constructive" design of intelligent KBS [5] ;
- the alleviating of expert system design tasks by means of better understanding main issues of the Multi-Agent Technology.

In this paper, particular emphasis have been made on the distinction between two classes of agents : the first following a "task-centered" approach as opposed to the second rather "domain-centered" approach. In this way, the elicitation process for knowledge acquisition can be approached under various points of view.

Methodological concepts presented in this paper become concrete through the development of the KIDS system which models the expert approach of cytological specimen investigation. In addition, these concepts attempt to bridge the gap between medical expertise and multi-agent technologies. Even if MAPS shell has been built to offer a set of tools which facilitate the design of cognitive system for complex problem solving additional tools should be developed to further assist the conceptual modeling step.

8. REFERENCES

1 Baujard, O. & Garbay, C.: A programming environment for distributed expert system design. In "ExperSys : Expert System Applications", pp 27-32, (A. Niku-Lari, eds.), Technology Transfer Series, IITT International, (1990).

2 Bond, A.H. and Les Gasser Readings in Distributed Artificial Intelligence. In "Distributed Artificial Intelligence", Morgan Kaufman., Los Altos, (1988).

3 Breuker, A. and Wielinga, B.J. : Knowledge acquisition as modelling expertise : The KADS methodology , Proc. first European workshop on knowledge acquisition for knowledge-based systems (1989).

4 Bylander, T., Chandrasekaran, B, and Josephson, J.R. : The Generic Task Toolset, In "Cognitive Engineering in the Design of Human Computer Interaction and Expert Systems", (G. Salvendy, eds), Elsevier Science Publisher, B.V., Amsterdam, pp. 507-514 (1987).

5 Chandrasekaran, B. : Towards a functional architecture for intelligence based on generic information processing tasks. Proc. 10th IJCAI pp. 1183-1192. IEEE Computer Society Press (1987).

6 Chandrasekaran, B. : Task-structures, knowledge acquisition and learning, Machine Learning (1990).

7 Derder, A, Ovalle, A. and Garbay, C.Towards a Formal Task Model for Biomedical Diagnosis Assistance Proc. 14th. Annual Inter. Conf. IEEE on Engineering in Medicine and Biology Society, pp. 845-846 (1992).

8 Durfee, E.H., Lesser, V.R. et Corkill, D.D. Coherent Coorporation Among Communicating Problem Solving. Proc. of the Distributed Artificial Intelligent Workshop, pp. 231-276 (1985).

9 Erceau J. and Ferber, J : L'Intelligence Artificielle Distribuée, La Recherche, 22, 233, pp. 750-758 (1991).

10 Ferber, J. and Ghallab, M. : Problématique des univers multi-agents intelligents. Actes des Journées nationales du PRC-GRECO "Intelligence Artificielle", pp 295-320.Teknea. (1988).

11 Gompel, C. La cytologie mammaire. Atlas de Cytologie Clinique, pp.125-139. Maloine s.a. éditeur., (1982).

12 Hayes-Roth, B. A blackboard model of control. Artificial Intelligence Vol 26, pp. 251-321 (1985).

13 Hugonnard, E. and Garbay, C.: Elicitation, Presentation and resolution : a multi-agent approach. Numéro spécial "Acquisition de connaissaces", Revue d'I.A., Hermès (eds)., vol 6-n°1-2 : 131-156 (1992).

14 Lanzola, G. and Stefanelli, M. : A specialized Framework for Medical Diagnosis Knowledge-Based Systems. Computer and Biomedical Research, 25, pp 351-365, (1992).

15 O'Hare et al. : AMNESIA - Implementing a Distributed KBS using RAPIDO. In "Research and Development in Expert Systems IX". Proc. 12th. Annual Inter. Conf. of the British Computer Society Specialist Group on ES Bramer & Milne (Eds), pp. 1-29, Cambridge University Press (1992).

16 Ovalle, A. & Garbay, C.: KIDS : A Distributed Expert System for Biomedical Image Interpre-tation.. In "Information Processing in Medical Imaging", pp. 419-433. Lecture Notes in Computer Science, Colchester et Hawkes (Eds), Springer-Verlag (1991a).

17 Ovalle, A.: Contribution to the study of reasoning in Multi-Agent Environments : KIDS, an application for biomedical image interpretation. Ph.D thesis, Computer Science Department, University Joseph Fourier (1991) (in french).

18 Ovalle, A. and Garbay, C.: Towards a Method for Multi-Agent System Design In "Research and Development in Expert Systems IX". Proc. 12th. Annual Inter. Conf. of the British Computer Society Specialist Group on ES Bramer & Milne (Eds), pp. 93-106, Cambridge University Press (1992).

19 Piper, J., Baldock, R., Towers, S. and Rutovitz D. A Knowledge-Based Chromosome Analysis System. In "Automation of Cytology: Advances in Systems and Techniques ", J. Piper and C. Lundsteen (eds), Springer Verlang, Heidel-berg., (1989).

20 Smith, R.G.The contract net protocol : high level communication and control in a distributed problem solver, IEEE Trans Comput, C-29, pp. 1104-1113. (1980).

21 Vogel, C. : Génie cognitif. Paris, Masson, collection science cognitive (1988).

22 Wielinga, B. : KBS Methodologies in Perspective. Tutorial of the 12th. Annual Inter. Conf. of the British Computer Society on Expert Systems, Cambridge (1992).

Artificial Intelligence in Medecine
S. Andreassen et al. , Eds.
IOS Press, 1993

Cooperative Medical Problem Solving*

Wilfried M. Post † ‡, Rudolph W. Koster ‡, Vincent Zocca ‡ and Michael Šrámek ‡

† University of Amsterdam, Social Science Informatics,
Roetersstraat 15, NL-1018 WB Amsterdam, The Netherlands

‡ University of Amsterdam, Academic Medical Center, Cardiology,
Meibergdreef 9 NL-1105 AZ Amsterdam, The Netherlands

Abstract

This paper describes problem solving in a system for the optimization of the prehospital assessment of emergency. This assessment is based on a telephone interview at ambulance dispatch centers and is made by nurses. Since we recognize the knowledge, experience and skills of dispatchers we have build a cooperative system, in which different problem solving steps can freely be distributed among system and user.

1 INTRODUCTION

In this paper we describe how user and system can cooperate in the decision making process of dispatching ambulances in medical emergency situations.

There are clear indications that the assessment of urgency is far from trivial [1,2]. Our own study reveals that more than half of the emergency calls that were judged as urgent and hence resulted in ambulance dispatching did not need an ambulance in retrospect [3]. This apparently low performance has to do with the characteristics of the tasks. These are time pressure, the requirement of high accuracy and the incompleteness and limited reliability of information. The first two points, rapidity and accuracy (especially sensitivity: the identification of urgent cases), are important since human lives are at stake. The third point, the quality of information, is due to the fact that information transfer is hindered by (i) communication problems between medical personnel and laymen, (ii) indirect contact such as with a relative or a bystander and (iii) the intrinsic constraints of communication by telephone.

The need for standard protocols is large, both for dispatchers and for managers of an emergency medical service. However, because of these domain characteristics,

* The research reported here was supported by project 39.006 of the Netherlands Heart Foundation. The production of this paper is partially funded by the AIM program of the Commission of the European Communities as project number A2034.

protocolization of dispatching is hard to accomplish. A protocol should be highly flexible, since the information may be provided by the caller spontaneously and in any order, or has to be asked explicitly otherwise. In addition, lack of protocols means lack of evaluation method. Due to this, the only evaluation criterion is the number of complaints coming from outside the dispatch center. This encourages dispatchers to think "safety first", where safety refers to both the relation with their manager and their client's safety, at the cost of the society's medical budget. This behaviour is one of the explanations of the low performance mentioned above.

Many attempts have been made to tackle triage domains with formal methods and computers (e.g. [2,4]). A more recent system, which is well known because of its outstanding evaluation, is ACORN, which supports the decision to admit a patient to the coronary care unit [5]. Most of these systems are not directly suitable for our domain because of their use of non-verbal information such as the EKG and physical examination. Another problem with these approaches is that they assign to the system a pivotal role and neglect the man-machine interaction aspect. In our view, this man-machine aspect is essential. Our aim is a system that should be used as a *tool* for dispatchers, in contrast to a system as an automated process in which a user is degraded to a service hatchway for questions and answers. Our starting point is that the user has many qualities but that some tasks are less suited to the mental architecture of humans.

In this paper we present a system that can be tailored to the needs of the dispatcher, which requires an effective cooperation and communication between system and user. We start with describing the problem of ambulance dispatching (Sec. 2). Next we describe our model for medical diagnosis (Sec. 3). Subsequently, we describe how cooperation is realized in our system (Sec. 4) followed by a description of an example session (Sec. 5). We end with discussing the current work and our plans for the future (Sec. 6).

2 PROBLEM DESCRIPTION

The task for which our system is meant to provide support is emergency call handling at emergency medical services. It consists of determining the most appropriate medical aid. Two decisions are distinguished:

- Sending an ambulance, and
- Referring the caller to the general practitioner

The scope of application is handling emergency calls placed by citizens (so called "free call"; our system is called after this) dealing with acute thoraco-abdominal complaints and consciousness problems, a domain that covers acute cardio-pulmonary diseases. Emergency calls by professionals such as general practitioner and police are out of the scope as well (these are always awarded). To further narrow down this broad domain we exclude calls for children and external causes such as accidents and intoxication.

The FreeCall system is expected to support emergency call handling in a number of ways: (i) Providing support in the process of interviewing. (ii) Providing a body of biomedical and policy knowledge on which decisions are to be based. Policy knowledge is subjective knowledge: agreements made within an organization (or society) while biomedical knowledge encompasses objective knowledge about diseases, how they develop and how they can be recognized; (iii) Providing support for evaluation by means of standardization and registration of emergency calls.

3 TASK MODEL

The way we provide support to interviewing and decision making is based on existing inference models for diagnosis. These are called 'generate-and-test' in the work of Clancey [6] and Wielinga and Breuker [7], the 'hypothetico deductive method' by Patil [8] and 'Select and Test Model' instantiated for diagnosis by Ramoni et al. [9]. Common in these models are three basic elements, or inference steps: "Generate Hypotheses", "Select Hypothesis" and "Test Hypothesis".

Our inference model is shown in Fig. 1.

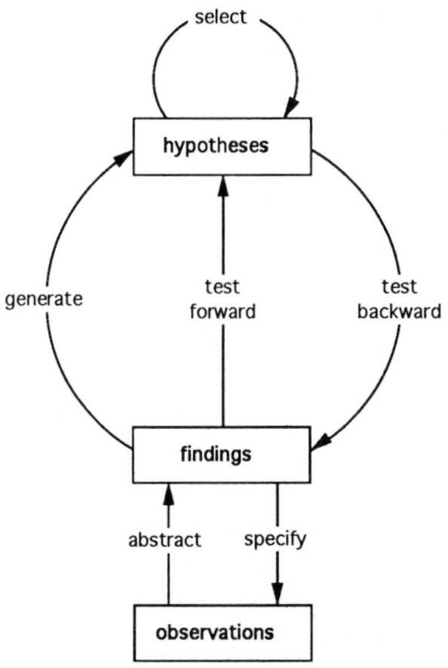

FIGURE 1: The adapted inference model "Generate and Test"

Diagnosing is viewed as a hypothesis driven process. It starts with generating a restricted set of possible solutions, using some available cues. This set of diagnostic hypotheses, called a differential diagnosis, is tested sequentially by selecting a single best hypothesis according to some criteria. During backward testing, expected findings are specified and compared with what is really observed. From this new evidence an other hypothesis may be generated or preferred for backward testing. The "test forward" inference step is directed of from findings to differential diagnosis, which means the forward verification/falsification of a diagnosis starting from the collected findings. The reason for the "test forward" step is twofold: firstly, there are moments when sufficient information is available to infer a certain diagnosis, but if inference is only hypothesis driven, this remains undetected. Due to the "test forward" step in our model, this diagnosis can be inferred immediately. Suppose the leading hypothesis is angina pectoris. Answers reveal that angina pectoris can be rejected since the duration of the pain is already for some hours, although the pain and age are typical for ischemia. This information could infer myocardial infarction immediately, but the selection of this hypothesis may be delayed due to a suboptimal selection heuristic. Secondly, the possibility exists that information is collected by not using this inference model. Especially in our domain much information is provided spontaneously which you would like to enter immediately, without having to wait on a specific question asking for this information. "Forward testing" this information should immediately infer a diagnosis. Cognitive research by Leprohon [10] indeed indicates that nurses in the context of emergency telephone interactions use forward reasoning and pattern recognition strategies in problem solving.

This pattern recognition is related to the two other added inference steps in the model: "specify" and "abstract". We see "specify" as the inverse step of "abstract". In our view, abstraction is information management, fully depending on a viewpoint which is determined by the purpose of this abstraction. Therefore, we see a finding as an abstraction of one or more observations with the purpose to concentrate the information for efficient use. Especially in telephone communication between caller and dispatcher a large amount of information is transferred which should be abstracted for the purpose of better management of all pieces of information. The introduction of both an abstract level and a more concrete level of observations has advantages for man-machine interaction. At the abstract level, the user should have enough medical background to understand the findings and to interpret observations. Interaction is in that case much more efficient. On the other hand, the concrete observation level is suitable for interaction with a less experienced user.

We have taken a model-based approach in describing the domain knowledge. That is, we have developed models for 28 frequently encountered diseases in our domain. The model ontology we used, is partially based on the work of Weiss et al. [11], Console and Torasso [12] and that of Patel et al. [13]. Table 3 and Table 3 give an overview of the types of concepts and relations that are modelled in the system, some instantiations, and their mapping to the inference model.

Table 1
Roles in our inference model, their mapping and some example instantiations

Diagnostic Role	Mapping to Concept Types	Example Instantiations
hypothesis	diagnosis	cardiac asthma; pneumothorax
finding	manifestation	retrosternal pain; orthopnea
	contextual evidence	history of ischemia; risk factors
observation	observable datum	previous infarction; age; gender

Table 2
Inference steps, the relation types used and some example instantiations

Inference Step	Relation Types Used	Example Instantiations
Generate	ASSOCIATES	cyanosis ASSOCIATES status-asthmaticus
Select	heuristic function of priority and probability	
Test	EVIDENCE-FOR	history-of-ischemia EVIDENCE-FOR atherosclerosis
	HAS-AS-MANIFESTATION	ischemia HAS-AS-MANIFESTATION retrosternal-pain
	CLASSIFIES	necrosis CLASSIFIES myocardial-infarction
	CAUSES	atherosclerosis CAUSES ischemia
Abstract/Specify	DEFINES	previous-infarction DEFINES history-of-ischemia

4 TASK DISTRIBUTION

Before we entered the emergency medical service, dispatchers already used a tool: a note-pad on which they often make quick, unordered notes about a call. Apparently, there was a need for an external memory device. A first level of support could be to provide them with a note-pad, but one with relevant entries that would also help in structuring their thought process. In [2] it was found that the mere use of a checklist improved decision making remarkably. An electronic note-pad would have the additional advantage of automatic registration, which is very helpful for evaluation purposes.

The second level of support would be to provide a system that acts as an intelligent note-pad which is able to answer the question "What does this information tell me?". A further extension of this note-pad would be an option to lead the dispatcher through an optimal sequence of entries (depending on the information put in). A final option could be to have the dispatcher find out *why* a certain order is optimal so that he could fill in the checklist in any optimal order himself. The FreeCall system presented here is build according to a continuum with this note-pad concept at one side of a continuum and a fully automated process on the other side. We did not tie up the system to one particular task distribution. In principle, each task can be executed by either the user or the system. Also the order of execution is user controlled.

One aspect of cooperation is the distribution of tasks between agents. Three agents are involved in emergency call handling: the dispatcher, the caller and the manager of the dispatch center.

Dispatchers in The Netherlands are generally highly qualified. They are trained as a nurse and frequently have experience with emergency care, intensive care, ambulatory care and psychiatric care. There are individual differences in knowledge, skills and experience, however, which have to be met. In some centers the dispatchers are no nurses but may be fire brigade employees.

The caller describes the problem and gives answers to questions. Sometimes, the caller should be regarded as a reasoning agent.

She usually presents some complaints (' I have pain in the chest '), but may pose a possible disorder as well (' I think I have a heart attack'), or may exactly understand what information the dispatcher needs. There are different types of callers. One is cooperative and knowledgeable, another obedient but naive. Still another type does not allow discussion but just insists on an ambulance. We distinguish four categories of callers as information sources: (i) the patient (ii) a relative (iii) a witness and (iv) a messenger. These categories determine what questions can possibly be answered. Obviously, the patient is a richer information source than the messenger.

The management evaluates dispatching, eventually adapts its structure or its contents and may initiate additional training. Normally, communication between the manager and the dispatcher does not take place during an emergency call, although in foreign emergency medical services actual calls are sometimes monitored by the management as part of a quality assurance program.

Our system is a fourth agent, both communicating with the dispatcher and caller on the one hand and the management on the other hand. From the point of view of the system, we consider the dispatcher as an extension of the caller. The system will not be equipped with knowledge about the distinction between them. They will be regarded as one and the same agent. In the implementation, the manager will play a passive role in that he only receives the registration of emergency calls but will not provide the system with anything. In reality, the manager is responsible for the refinement and maintenance of the system, which could also be regarded as communication. Fig. 2 shows the communication between the agents as it takes place in reality and as it is implemented.

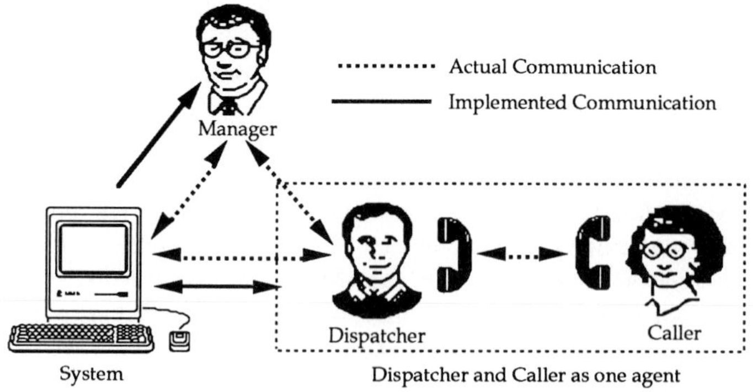

FIGURE 2: Communication between agents

Our aim is a system that acts as a collaborator of the user. Both have strong and weak points in which they can complement each other. A machine is systematic, has a good memory, is specialized in calculation and bookkeeping, while a user has background knowledge and intuitions, and is able to cope with unexpected events. For social and political reasons it is unacceptable that a machine will replace the user. The user will be held responsible for decisions.

In allocating the tasks in emergency call handling to the user and system, we will follow de Greef and Breuker [14]. Tasks that neither can be allocated to one agent, nor can be decomposed further in subtasks, are called "transfer tasks". By using the concepts of "initiative" and the "direction of information flow", they distinguish the following four types of transfer tasks. The flow of information from user to system, which is initiated by the user, is called "Receive". Information flow from user to system, initiated by the system, is called "Obtain". A flow from system to user , initiated by the user, is "Provide" and the same information flow, but initiated by the system is called "Present". The transfer tasks in our system are:

- **Receiving complaints**: the user receives complaints and a problem description from the caller and "provides" these to the system

- **Obtaining answers**: getting the answers from the user. The system needs the answers but the user has to put these in

The tasks that can be freely distributed between the system and the user are:

- **Generate**: the system can generate a set of hypotheses, using some rationale for hypothesis generation, or the system can receive a hypothesis from the user, using his intuition or his ability to recognize)

- **Select**: the system can determine the 'best' hypothesis by using a heuristic or can receive a selection from the user

- **Testing Backward**: the system can generate what findings to look for or the the user can determine the finding of interest

- **Testing Forward**: the system can infer a diagnosis from the entered information, the user can infer a diagnosis also from information that is not or can not be entered

- **Specify**: the system can specify a question to infer a finding, or the user can determine what to ask and how to ask it

- **Abstract**: the system can abstract certain answers, or the user can medically interpret what the caller communicates

Decision making based on the collected evidence is mainly a task for the user (he is responsible) but it can be performed by the system, which will then be referred to as 'Providing Advice'. Different versions of this combination of user/system made decisions are possible. For example, the user could take a decision and ask the system for a critic. If the system derived at an other conclusion, the user can follow or ignore it. If the system could not derive at any conclusion, the user can just acknowledge his decision, can continue interviewing, or can ask the system to take over, until a decision can be taken.

How this cooperation is realized in our FreeCall system is illustrated in the next section

5 EXAMPLE SESSION

In a first window some initial information is collected, such as the the main problem (chest discomfort, abdominal complaints, dyspnea or consciousness problems) and the type of caller. When it has been indicated that vital functions are clearly disturbed or when insufficient information is expected, e.g., because the caller is only a messenger, immediate action should be taken. If not, additional information is obtained by starting a diagnostic interview. Fig. 3 is a screen dump of that part of our system.

The main problem categories in the first window, will each trigger an other set of initial hypotheses. They will be listed on the window 'Differential Diagnosis'. There are five columns associated with each hypothesis. The one indicated with 'a' shows the activated (checked) and deactivated hypotheses. The activated hypotheses are selectable. Hypotheses are deactivated by (i) system inference of the status (e.g., the hypothesis has already been falsified), (ii) deactivation triggers, (iii) deactivation by the user (by clicking on the check box). The column with an 's' indicates the selected hypothesis. The next three columns indicate whether a hypothesis is verified ('+'), falsified ('-'), or inconclusive ('?!'), i.e. definitely unknown to the system (no question remains that could verify or falsify the hypothesis).

After having triggered a set of hypotheses the system selects one using some heuristic and starts to test it. The window 'Controle Paneel' visualizes the process of these inference steps by highlighting the boxes. In line with our cooperative approach, the user can push on the box to initiate an inference step himself, if he wishes. During testing, questions are specified that could determine the status of the selected hypothesis. In the window 'Observatie', the question and answer alternatives are displayed. The system remains to test the current hypothesis until its status has been inferred. After testing, all obtained observations are abstracted to findings, and all findings tested by forward inference: an alternative diagnosis may be inferred now. Then the next round starts with a new 'generate' step, using the newly obtained information.

This 'generate step' can be performed by the user by selecting the hierarchical menu 'Hypothesen'. A disease taxonomy will be presented from which a hypothesis can be selected. The user can also select a group of diseases by selecting an intermediate node. For example, the selection of "ischemic disorder" will put all the subsuming ischemic disorders, such as myocardial infarction and angina pectoris, at

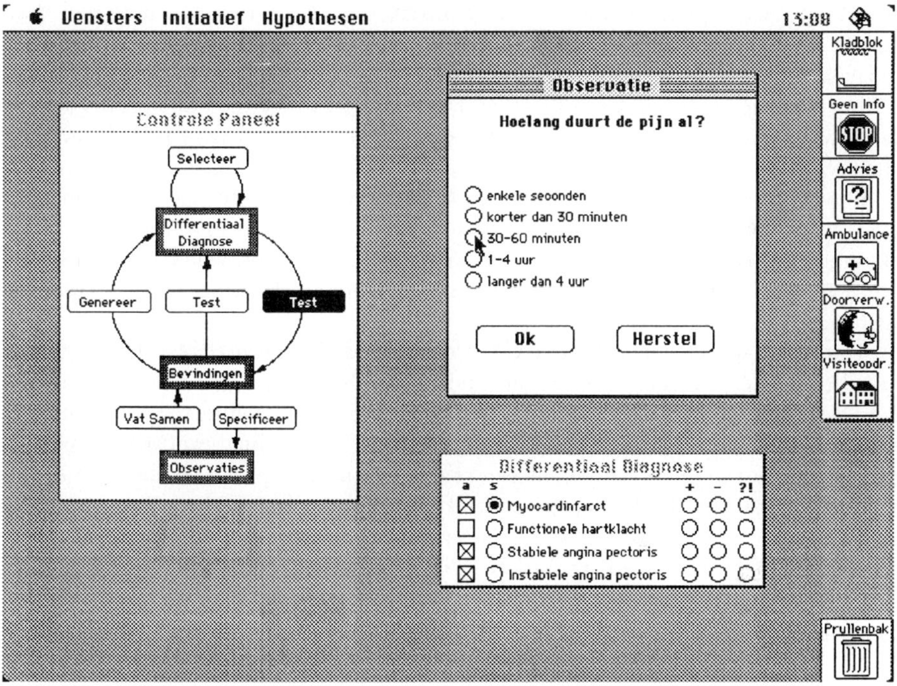

FIGURE 3: Screen dump of a part of the system. The English translation is as follows. Vensters → Windows; Initiatief → Initiative; Hypothesen → Hypotheses; Controle Paneel → Control Panel; Genereer → Generate; Selecteer → Select; Test → Test; Specificeer → Specify; Vat Samen → Abstract; Observaties → Observations; Bevindingen → Findings; Differentiaal Diagnose → Differential Diagnosis; Hoelang duurt de pijn al? → What is the duration of the pain?; enkele seconden → a few seconds; korter dan 30 minuten → less then 30 minutes; 30-60 minuten → 30-60 minutes; 1-4 uur → one to four hours; langer dan 4 uur → more than four hours; Myocardinfarct → Myocardial Infarction; Functionele Hartklachten → Non-organic Chest Pain; Stabiele angina pectoris → Stable Angina; Instabiele angina pectoris → Unstable Angina; Kladblok → Note-pad; Geen Info → No Information available; Advies → Advice; Doorverw. → Referral; Prullenbak → Trash

the differential diagnosis. After having generated one or more hypotheses, the the user can select a hypothesis himself by clicking on a label in the differential diagnosis window. He can test a hypothesis himself by pushing on the note-pad icon in the right-upper corner. This will invoke one of the four note-pad sheets that are associated to each of the main problems. The node pad entries are on the abstract finding level, because the medical relevance of the information should have been recognized before entering, and therefore is already abstracted. Note that the note-pad may well be used without further guidance of the system. The entries are well organized and can be used to structure an interview, either to communicate on an abstract level or by specifying questions to an entry. However, to let the system infer one of more diagnoses from the information entered, a 'Test' button is provided. For the same reason a 'Gererate' button exists. Finally, a 'Take Over' button can be used to hand over the control over diagnosing to the system, that is, to 'generate and test' hypotheses by the system. The note-pad sheets have two additional functions: (i) to enter information that has not been asked for but was provided spontaneously, which frequently occurs, (ii) to visualize all the collected information in a compact (abstract) and structured way.

The user can determine what level of communication he prefers. Questions can be asked on 'observation' level or on 'finding' level. In the second level, questions are abstract and medically oriented, and hence, more goal directed and efficient. However, more expertise is expected from the user. The finding level still provides a way to specify the more concrete observations by pushing on a question icon in the window (or the 'specify' box in the control panel).

The user can set who, he or the system, has initiative in this process of *interviewing*, by using the menu 'Initiatief'. The user can also determine what support he wishes in *decision making*. The row of icons at the right side are used for this. By pushing on the icons 'Ambulance', 'Referral' or 'Visit', the user acknowledges the system of his/her decision. By pushing on 'Advise' the user can ask the system for advice. The system will then tell her own assessment, if she has arrived at a conclusion at that point. The 'Stop' icon is for interrupting the diagnostic process (e.g. no extra information is available, patient's condition has suddenly worsened). Finally, the 'Trash' icon is for quitting a case without saving the information (e.g. in case of training, telephone vandalism). The initiative of decision making can also be dedicated to the system, by using the menu 'Initiatief'. If set to 'system initiative' the system will provide her advice as soon as she can give one. The user can determine to follow it or not.

6 DISCUSSION

Our objective was to optimize the judgement of emergency calls by providing medical knowledge and policy knowledge and by striving for an optimal cooperation between user and system. How well did we reach our goals?

We are currently in the phase of evaluation. In terms of Wyatt and Spiegelhalters' division of evaluation phases [15] we are currently carrying out the laboratory phase. That is, we are collecting with the current system data in the field, both for debugging / refinement and for laboratory testing. Testing will be carried out on a set of cases that has not been used for debugging or refinement. During data collection, the system is only used for supporting the interview, advice is not given. Each emergency call is recorded on tape and the system interactions on disk. This will provide us insight in the man-machine interaction, which is, as explained earlier, a central issue in this study. We trace each emergency call to various hospitals and general practitioners in the service area of the emergency medical service of Amsterdam (which covers 1.2 million inhabitants) in order to determine the "gold standard", in our case one of the 28 diseases we have incorporated in the system, or an additional one. The assessment of urgency will be determined independently by two physicians using the final diagnosis and the information recorded on disk. In the current test phase we do not evaluate our cooperative approach, since many options have been disabled in order to collect cases. The system only supports interviewing on the observation level but does not give advice.

After having adapted the findings of the laboratory test in the system, a new test phase is necessary in which also the cooperative approach is issue of evaluation. Only after that we can start a real field trial.

Informal evaluation about user acceptance has been done by personal interviews. Salient is that the scepticism of the users before implementation has changed to enthusiasm after introduction. Also the management of the emergency medical center has expressed contentment with the result. We are aware that this could be explained by the Hawthorn effect, an effect, due to a change in the environment, that lasts only temporary [15].

Acknowledgements

We gratefully acknowledge the managers and dispatchers of the medical emergency services of Amsterdam and Enschedé for their cooperation during the project. We acknowledge Guus Schreiber for his extensive comments throughout the production of this paper. Gertjan van Heijst, Maarten van Someren and Bob Wielinga gave valuable comments on earlier versions of this work.

References

[1] E. van der Does and J. Lubsen. *Acute coronary events in general practice: the Imminent Myocardial Infarction Rotterdam Study.* PhD thesis, Erasmus University, Rotterdam, 1978.

[2] I.D. Adams, M. Chan, P.C. Clifford, W.M. Cooke, V. Dallos, F.T. deDombal, M.H. Edwards, D.M. Hancock, D.J. Hewett, N. McIntyre, P.G. Somerville, D.J. Spiegelhalter, J. Wellwood, and D.H. Wilson. Computer aided diagnosis of acute abdominal pain: a multicentred study. *Br Med J*, 293:800–804, 1986.

[3] M. Sramek. *FreeCall in Acute Myocardial Ischemia.* PhD thesis, University of Amsterdam, May 1993.

[4] L. Farand, P. Masson, and M. Kalina. The use of artificial intelligence for decision support and teaching telephone triage in the montreal emergency medical services system. *Journal of the World Association for Emergency and Disaster Medicine*, 91, 1987.

[5] J. Wyatt. Lessons learnt from the field trial of ACORN, an expert system to advise on chest pain. In B. Barber, D. Cao, D. Qin, and G. Wagner, editors, *Proceedings MedInfo'89, Singapore*, pages 111–115. North-Holland, Amsterdam, 1989.

[6] W. J. Clancey and R. Letsinger. NEOMYCIN: Reconfiguring a rulebased expert system for application to teaching. In W. J. Clancey and E. H. Shortliffe, editors, *Readings in Medical Artificial Intelligence: the first decade*, pages 361–381. Addison-Wesley, Reading, Massachusetts, 1984.

[7] B. J. Wielinga and J. A. Breuker. Models of expertise. In *Proceedings ECAI-86*, pages 306–318, 1986.

[8] R.S. Patil. Artificial intelligence techniques for diagnostic reasoning in medicine. In H.E. Shobe and AAAI, editors, *Exploring Artificial Intelligence: Survey Talks from the National Conferences on Artificial Intelligence*, pages 347–379. Morgan Kaufmann, San Mateo, California, 1988.

[9] M. Ramoni, M. Stefanelli, L. Magnani, and G. Barosi. An epistemological framework for medical knowledge based systems. *IEEE Transactions on Systems, Man, and Cybernetics*, 22:1–14, 1992.

[10] J. Leprohon. *Nursing Clinical Decision Making in the Context of Emergency Telephone Interactions.* PhD thesis, McGill University Montreal, 1991.

[11] S.M. Weiss, C.A. Kulikowski, S. Amarel, and A. Safir. A model-based method for computer-aided medical decision making. *Artif Intell*, 11:145–172, 1978.

[12] L. Console and P. Torasso. Hypothetical reasoning in causal models. *International Journal of Intelligent Systems*, 5:83–124, 1990.

[13] V. L. Patel, D. A. Evans, and D. R. Kaufman. A cognitive framework for doctor-patient interaction. In D. A. Evans and V. L. Patel, editors, *Cognitive Science in Medicine*, pages 257–312. MIT Press, 1989.

[14] P. de Greef and J. A. Breuker. Analysing system-user cooperation. *Knowledge Acquisition*, 4(1), 1992. Special issue 'The KADS approach to knowledge engineering.

[15] J. Wyatt and D. Spiegelhalter. Field trials of medical decision-aids: potential problems and solutions. In P. Clayton, editor, *Proceedings 15th Symposium on Computer Applications in Medical Care, Washingon.* McGraw Hill Inc., New York, 1991.

Artificial Intelligence in Medecine
S. Andreassen et al. , Eds.
IOS Press, 1993

Demo of FreeCall, a System for Ambulance Dispatching*

Wilfried M. Post † ‡, Michael Šrámek ‡, Rudolph W. Koster ‡ and Vincent Zocca ‡

† University of Amsterdam, Social Science Informatics,
Roetersstraat 15, NL-1018 WB Amsterdam, The Netherlands

‡ University of Amsterdam, Academic Medical Center, Cardiology Department,
Meibergdreef 9 NL-1105 AZ Amsterdam, The Netherlands

This demo presents a system for the optimization of the prehospital assessment of emergency in cases involving thoraco-abdominal complaints and consciousness problems. This assessment is based on a telephone interview at ambulance dispatch centers and is made by nurses. The system has a body of biomedical and political knowledge available to guide the interview and to provide advice. In our approach we emphasize the central role of the knowledgeable dispatcher and strive for an optimal cooperation between dispatcher and system. To this goal we used a variant of the inference models for medical diagnosis that are known as Select-and-Test model [1], 'hypothetico-deductive method' [2] and 'Generate-and-Test' [3,4]. This model can be found in Fig. 1.

We build a system in which each inference step can distributed freely between user and system. The domain knowledge consists of models for 28 diseases, using types of concepts and relations based on the work of [5,6,7]. The knowlegde acquisition has been previously described in [8] and the cooperation aspect can be found in the proceedings of this conference [9]. Fig. 1 is a screen dump of that part of our system.

The demonstration will show a number of aspects of the system. In one setting, the system will generate a series of questions for assessing the emergency of a call. In an other setting, some inference steps are performed by the user and some by the system. In still an other setting the user performs all inference steps but can ask the system for a second opinion.

The system is currently under evaluation.

* The research presented here was supported by project 39.006 of the Netherlands Heart Foundation.

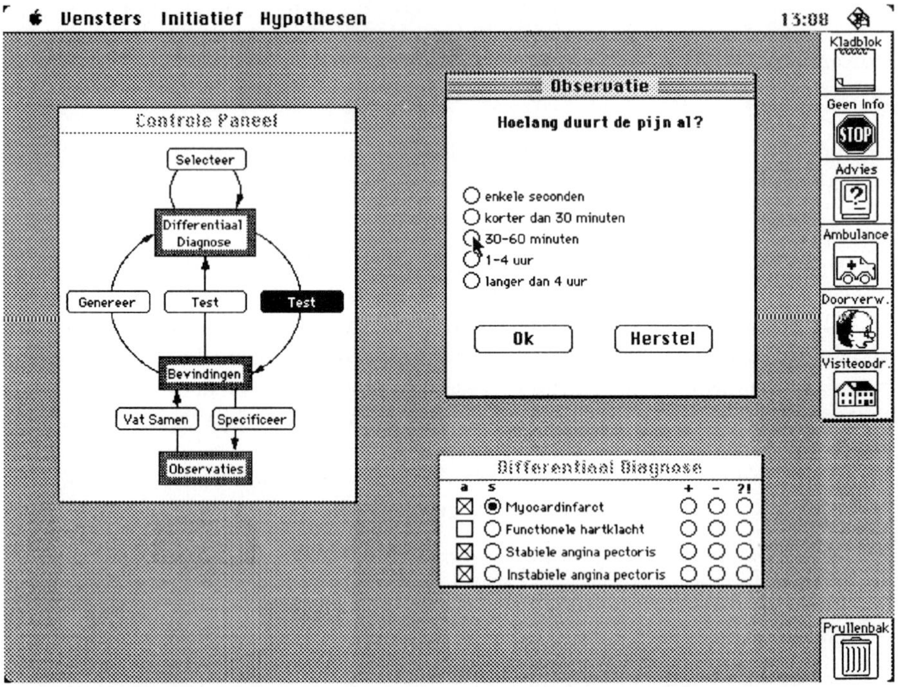

FIGURE 1: Screen Dump of the FreeCall system. The English translation is as follows. Vensters → Windows; Initiatief → Initiative; Hypothesen → Hypotheses; Controle Paneel → Control Panel; Genereer → Generate; Selecteer → Select; Test → Test; Specificeer → Specify; Vat Samen → Abstract; Observaties → Observations; Bevindingen → Findings; Differentiaal Diagnose → Differential Diagnosis; Hoelang duurt de pijn al? → What is the duration of the pain?; enkele seconden → a few seconds; korter dan 30 minuten → less then 30 minutes; 30-60 minuten → 30-60 minutes; 1-4 uur → one to four hours; langer dan 4 uur → more than four hours; Myocardinfarct → Myocardial Infarction; Functionele Hartklachten → Non-organic Chest Pain; Stabiele angina pectoris → Stable Angina; Instabiele angina pectoris → Unstable Angina; Kladblok → Note-pad; Geen Info → No Information available; Advies → Advice; Doorverw. → Referral; Prullenbak → Trash

References

[1] M. Ramoni, M. Stefanelli, L. Magnani, and G. Barosi. An epistemological framework for medical knowledge based systems. *IEEE Transactions on Systems, Man, and Cybernetics*, 22:1–14, 1992.

[2] R.S. Patil. Artificial intelligence techniques for diagnostic reasoning in medicine. In H.E. Shobe and AAAI, editors, *Exploring Artificial Intelligence: Survey Talks from the National Conferences on Artificial Intelligence*, pages 347–379. Morgan Kaufmann, San Mateo, California, 1988.

[3] W. J. Clancey. Heuristic classification. *Artif Intell*, 27:289–350, 1985.

[4] B. J. Wielinga and J. A. Breuker. Models of expertise. In *Proceedings ECAI–86*, pages 306–318, 1986.

[5] L. Console and P. Torasso. Hypothetical reasoning in causal models. *International Journal of Intelligent Systems*, 5:83–124, 1990.

[6] V. L. Patel, D. A. Evans, and D. R. Kaufman. A cognitive framework for doctor-patient interaction. In D. A. Evans and V. L. Patel, editors, *Cognitive Science in Medicine*, pages 257–312. MIT Press, 1989.

[7] S.M. Weiss, C.A. Kulikowski, S. Amarel, and A. Safir. A model-based method for computer-aided medical decision making. *Artif Intell*, 11:145–172, 1978.

[8] W.M. Post and M.W. van Someren. A comparative evaluation of three approaches to the acquisition of medical knowledge. In *AIME-91*, 1991.

[9] W.M. Post, R.W. Koster, V. Zocca, and M. Sramek. Cooperative medical problem solving. In *AIME-93*, 1993.

Artificial Intelligence in Medecine
S. Andreassen et al. , Eds.
IOS Press, 1993

C A R E: A Knowledge-Based System for Assisting the Physician in Patient Management

G. Molino, E. Nicolosi and F. Molino

Dipartimento di Fisiopatologia Clinica, Universita` degli Studi di Torino, Italy.

Abstract

This paper describes CARE, a knowledge-based system prototype for assisting in real-time the medical doctor in the patient management process. CARE (Clinical Advice and Record Entry) is a computer program aimed at providing methodological feed-back and advice at each step of patient management, and making available a recording approach focussed not only on data but also on clinical problems and medical decisions. The actual utility of CARE is threefold: first, used on-line as a decision aid it may improve physician performance in the real clinical context; second, it can be used as an educational tool to train students in clinical methodology; and third, on the base of its recording facilities it can provide well assessed objective decision-mapping databases which might be very useful in evaluating the performance of individual users and in collecting statistical informations about doctor's behaviour.

1. INTRODUCTION

Whenever a patient is admitted to hospital care, attending physicians are expected to provide effective and efficient medical decisions. The fulfilment of such an obvious requirement implies the organization of clinical information and medical actions until the patient is discharged from the hospital, and sometimes even later during patient follow-up.

In particular, the physician is asked to identify existing clinical problems, to rank them according to priority criteria, and to make the proper decisions in a reasonable sequence. General principles of clinical methodology and personal competence make this possible in most cases [1]. However, at least for unexperienced physicians, a decision aid might be useful for optimizing the clinical management of patients and ensuring high quality outcomes. Computer technology can support clinical decision-making by replacing the paper charts with computerised medical records [2,3,4,5] which allow to make more efficient and widely available use of clinical information and retrospective analysis of medical experience. Moreover, the literature on computer-based clinical decision support systems [6,7,8] has shown encouraging effects of these systems on clinical performance and patient outcomes despite the fact that they are very heterogeneous and they have different design.

This is the reason why we designed CARE (Clinical Advice and Record Entry), a computer program aimed at providing methodological feed-back and advice at each step of patient management, and making available a recording approach focussed not only on data but also on clinical problems and medical decisions.

This prototype is concerned with the clinical management of jaundiced patients according to previous papers [9,10,11,12,13,14], and in agreement with the criteria and goals of the AIM Project A2016 "Intelligent Decision-mapping Medical Record (IDMR)". The decision aid is planned in terms of diseases, data and decisions, and constructed from the catalogue of decisions and their data and outcome sets as a knowledge-based system, independent of any particular data collection.

2. METHODOLOGICAL BACKGROUND

Computer-aided feed-back on medical decision-making is based in CARE on a few well assessed principles of clinical methodology, namely on the assumption that: (1) the evaluation of clinical severity is of paramount importance in patient management (e.g., emergency has the highest priority score); (2) diagnosis should be based on well assessed strategies considering first clinical data to activate compatible hypotheses, then finalizing the diagnosis by selected investigations; (3) to attain high quality care, investigations should be accurate, decisional, sufficient, standardized and accessible; (4) therapeutic decisions should be justified, appropriate and carefully weighed; (5) patient care should always include the control of diagnostic and therapeutic efficacy and the prediction and treatment of side effects and complications.

It is worth noting that in CARE the decision aid is featured as a "second opinion" (i.e. provided "after" doctor's decision), aimed at assisting the user in criticizing his own methodological approach to patient care and preventing errors. Accordingly, the program does not provide any facility to support directly the user decision (no automatic conclusion is achieved) or to evaluate his clinical performance (no comment is provided on outcome validity).

3. SYSTEM OUTLINE

CARE is a Knowledge-Based system, written in LPA-386 Prolog running under Microsoft Windows, designed to assist step-by-step the physician in patient management. At each step of the clinical observation the system evaluates the methodological validity of doctor's decisions.

The functions of CARE can be defined as follows: first, the system provides advice about the coherence of the overall process; second, it verifies the consistency of individual decision steps with available patient data and methodological constraints. Aspects considered in CARE are: reliability of the preliminary diagnostic hypothesis and soundness of medical decisions with respect to context, problem and action selection. Evaluations are performed on the base of different approaches, respectively using patient data for hypothesis validation and applying well assessed methodological constraints for evaluating doctor's decisions. In CARE the outcomes of selected actions have no implication for user evaluation, but are simply used to make understandable the reasoning process.

It is worth noting that, according to the above procedure, the critiquing and advisory function of CARE strictly reflects the decisions made by the physician in managing the patient. Thus, the number, type and sequence of decisional steps is determined by the user, and do not depend in any way on the system.

There are very few examples of this kind in the literature, the only one we consider worth mentioning is the paper by Beeler et al [15], which presents a methodology for developing a data architecture for clinical medicine. The resulting model of clinical data architecture shows a lot of commonalities with CARE. For example, the *events* model and the *problem list* model include CARE's concepts of decision blocks and story records which we explain in section 4.

The overall structure of CARE is shown in Figure 1. Three basic ways of interaction are possible in CARE: instantiating a patient management process; consulting existing patient records; and making a cost analysis of existing patient records. While during an instantiation of a patient management process the expert system makes use of both factual knowledge and rules of the domain, during either of the remaining interactions CARE is just using knowledge about specific patients.

4. KNOWLEDGE BASE

The knowledge-base of CARE is composed of factual knowledge and rules of the clinical domain. The factual knowledge includes the patient database and the domain knowledge about concepts and relations between them such as the taxonomy of contexts, problems, and actions and the taxonomy of data concerned with clinical findings, laboratory and instrumental investigations, and the taxonomy of treatment procedures.

The domain knowledge has been represented in CARE by frames, as depicted in Figure 1. Each frame contains a set of slots which represent the features of the frame and it is linked to other frames by either a hierarchical relationship or other type of relationship. The characteristics of a frame are therefore inherited down to the leaves of the hierarchy. Such a structure represents very closely the structure of clinical information.

4.1. Patient Database

There are three types of records associated to each patient: a *patient data* record which includes all the personal information and data; a *leading diagnostic hypothesis* record for each diagnostic hypothesis selected by the user (medical doctor); and a *story record* for each decision block instantiated.

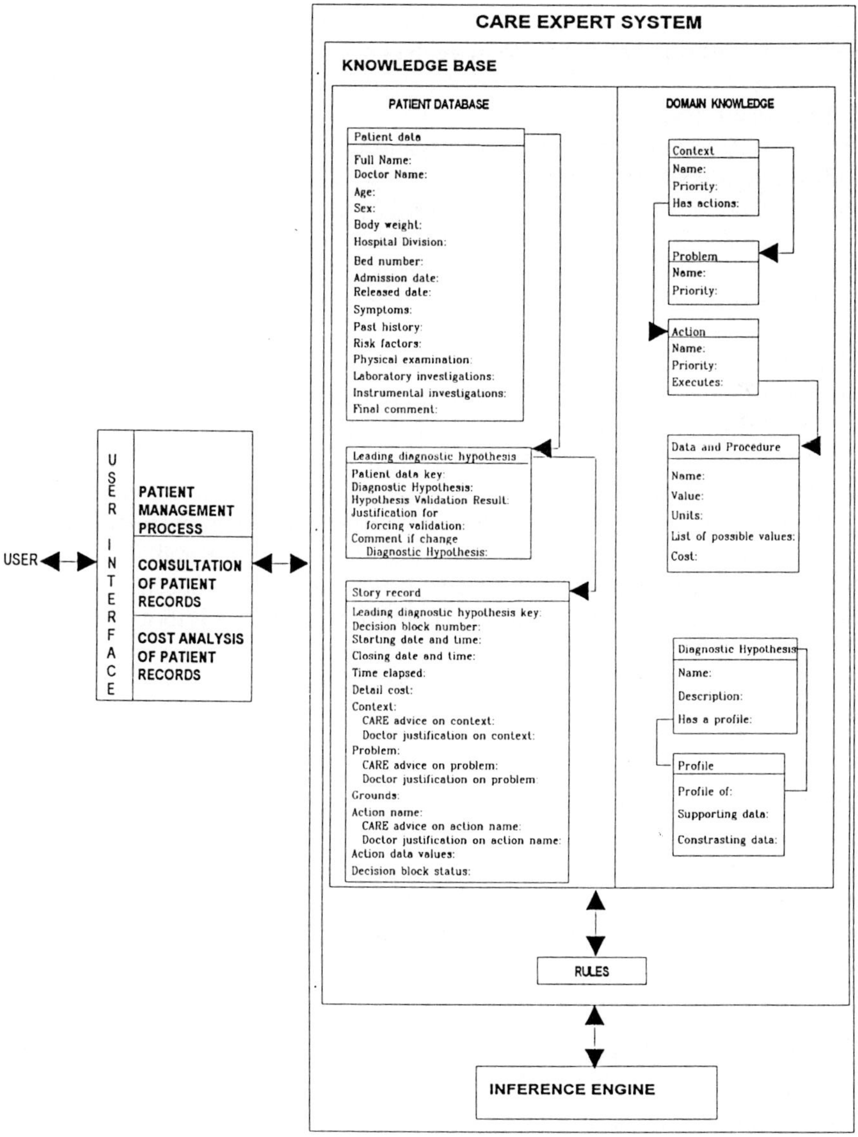

Figure 1. The Architecture of CARE.

Therefore each patient has only one patient data record which is linked to maybe more than one leading diagnostic hypothesis record; and each leading diagnostic hypothesis record is linked to maybe more than one story record.

4.2. Diagnostic Hypotheses

From a structural point of view diagnostic hypotheses are clinical conditions classified into a taxonomy, and described by prototypical profiles (Figure 2) based on clinical findings and a few very simple laboratory investigations.

Data included in the profiles are characterized with respect to each hypothesis by one or more typical values either supporting or contrasting it. Thus profile data are cathegorized in two classes, respectively in favour or against the hypothesis.

4.3. Decisions

The key element in patient management are clinical decisions which are functional blocks defined by a context, a problem and an action (Figure 3).

Contexts can be defined as the environments in which the medical action takes place. They reflect factors associated with the clinical situation, the user and the actual goal. The former are related to technical resources and time available to make the decision; user dependent aspects reflect doctor's competence and skills; goal related factors are concerned with clinical needs which are better specified by problem identification. Each context (Figure 1) is defined by a name, a priority index and has an action associated to it.

The following contexts (decreasing priority order in brackets) are taken into account: emergency (1); diagnosis and treatment of symptoms (2); treatment of disease and control (3).

Problems can be considered as specifications of contexts. Each problem (Figure 1) is defined by a name, and a priority index, which guides the CARE advice in the same way as for context selection.

In addition to contexts and problems, *actions* contribute to the final characterization of decision blocks. Each action (Figure 1) is defined by a name and a priority, it is linked to a specific context and it is characterised by a suitable set of data or procedures.

5. SYSTEM FUNCTIONS

The patient management process of CARE is divided into separate sections corresponding to different aspects featuring the decisional process. They include the management of hypotheses, decisions and outcomes (Figure 3).

5.1. Preliminary Diagnostic Hypotheses

At the beginning of a CARE consultation the user is asked to provide the doctor's full name and the patient's personal details and general data. Then the user has to indicate the diagnostic hypothesis under which the patient management is being performed.

	Datum	Relevance	Supporting Value	Contrasting Value
Symptoms	Jaundice duration	1	< 7	> 30
	Jaundice deepness	1	medium high	
	Jaundice time-course	1	increasing fluctuant	constant
	Pain in abdomen	1	right-upper/epigastric radiates to shoulder or back severe biliary colic single biliary colic multiple	absent
	Feels unwell	1	yes	
	Nausea or vomiting	1	yes	
	Stool pale	1	yes	no
	Urine dark	1	yes	no
	Fever/sweats		yes	
Past history	Pain: similar bouts	1	yes	
	Gallstones known	1	yes	
Physical Examination	Temperature	1	> 38	
	Looks acutely ill	1	yes	
	Gallbladder palpable	1	yes	
	Gallbladder tender	1	yes	
	Liver hard	1	no	yes
	Liver tender	1	yes	
	Liver irregular	1	no	yes
Laboratory Investigations	White blood cells	1	mild increase medium increase	
	Total bilirubin	1	medium increase high increase	normal
	Direct bilirubin	1	medium increase high increase	normal
	ALT	0,8	mild increase medium increase	high increase
	AST	0,8	mild increase medium increase	high increase
	Alkaline phosphatase	1	medium increase high increase	normal
	Gamma glutamil transferase	1	medium increase high increase	normal
	Erythrocyte sedimentation rate	1	mild increase medium increase	

Figure 2. Prototypical Profile of the Diagnostic Hypothesis Gallstone Disease based on clinical findings and routine laboratory investigations.

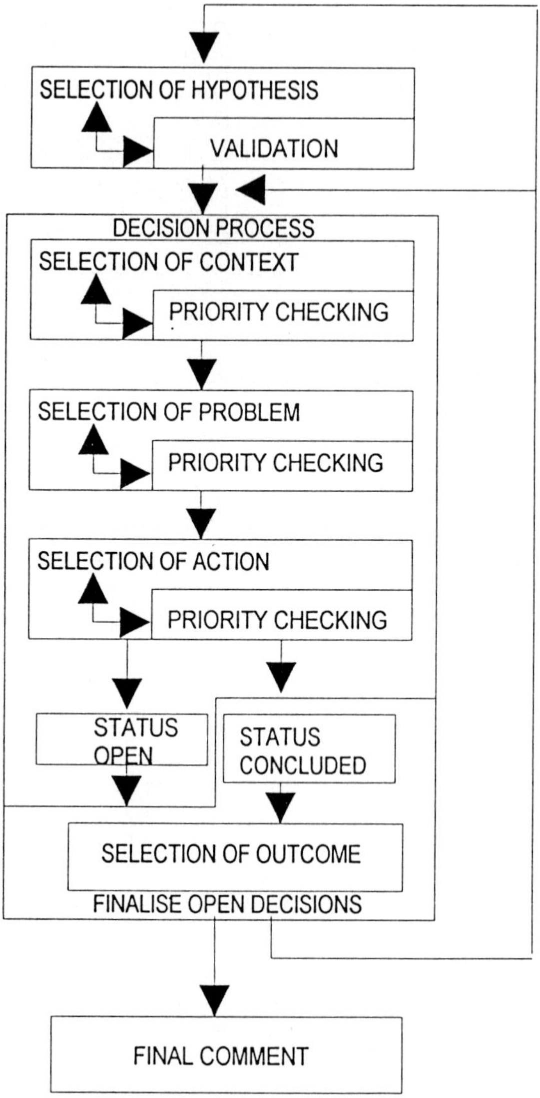

Figure 3. The Patient Management Process in CARE.

This will remain the leading hypothesis, until changed. Once the hypothesis has been selected CARE verifies its acceptability on the base of patient data in a process of validation of the diagnostic hypothesis (Figure 3). The data needed are requested interactively, or retrieved from the database, if already recorded. Since in this phase the goal is essentially to avoid unreasonable investigations or procedures, the validation rules used by the system to confirm or exclude the hypothesis are quite simple and based only on very relevant clinical findings. The rules look for at least 4 existing elements among the supporting and the contrasting data with relevance equal to 1, provided by the profiles (Figure 2), to either confirm or exclude the diagnostic hypothesis respectively. The relevance index indicates the importance of evaluating a particular finding in a specific disease and it is scored (0-1): 0 is irrelevant; 1 is essential.

Whenever the *validity of the selected hypothesis is denied* because of insufficient data then a message is displayed, explanations are provided on request, and the user is allowed to change the leading hypothesis, to provide further data or to force the system advice: this can be done only after providing a short justification which will be recorded in the story record (Figure 4). Patient data with their relevance index are constantly available to the user during this phase of validation of the diagnostic hypothesis. Similarly, if the selected hypothesis is not supported because there are 4 essential data against it, then the user can only change the leading hypothesis or force the system advice.

On the other hand, whenever the *leading hypothesis* is confirmed the user is asked to proceed in the decision process (Figure 3) by opening the first decision block.

In the case the *patient data verify the rules both in favour and against the hypothesis* (which is highly improbable) an advice message is displayed and the user is asked to change the leading hypothesis or to force the system advice. As an example, let us immagine that the hypothesis "acute infectious hepatitis" has been indicated by the user in a jaundiced patient with a recent episode of mononucleosis (not considered in the database), feeling unwell, in which transaminases were found highly increased, with the liver enlarged but hard and irregular and jaundice fluctuant for more than 30 days. CARE will reject the hypothesis because four data are in favour and four against it, respectively. However the user knows that the hypothesis is reasonable: he can force the system conclusion and proceed, simply providing a written justification (possible CMV hepatitis).

5.2. Decision-making

The process of patient management (Figure 3) results in a sequence of decisions the user activates according to priority criteria. Each decision is featured as a functional block characterized by a context, a problem and an action, which can be finalized by a status definition.

As soon as a specific context has been selected by the user, the system verifies if all contexts with higher priority score have already been considered (priority checking in Figure 3). In the case that some of them have been disregarded an advice message is displayed. In this case the user can either change the context or decide to continue within the same context, thus forcing the CARE advice. In the former case the old selection disappears from the screen to be replaced by the new one, but both are recorded in the story record (Figure 4). In the latter the user is asked to provide a short justification which will also be recorded in the story record.

Once the context has been conclusively defined the user must indicate the problem he is going to take into account. Thereafter, CARE evaluates if more important problems have been ignored. Problems disregarded are displayed, submitted to user evaluation, then either accepted or skipped. The same recording procedure used for contexts is here applied to modify the current selection or to force the system advice.

In order to solve the problem selected the user can give the grounds under which the current decision has been taken and must define a proper action, the consistency of which will be evaluated by CARE with respect to the current context and problem, and according to a priority score defined a-priori. Inconsistent actions and actions not achieving the highest priority score level are not directly accepted if preceding ones have not been previously considered. In this case the user is allowed either to change his selection or to by-pass the CARE advice, after providing his written justification. In any case, selected actions (either rejected, changed or accepted) are recorded in the story record.

When context, problem, and action have been defined, a status of the decision block is given by the CARE system. The status is 'concluded' if the action belongs to one of the following classes: intensive care unit, past history, symptoms, risk factors or physical examination. The status is 'open' otherwise (e.g., laboratory investigations, treatments and follow-up procedures).

If the status is 'concluded' a final outcome of the decision block ('problem solved' or 'problem still present') has to be given by the user and the opening and closing times (day and hour) and time elapsed are automatically recorded in the story record (Figure 4). If the status is 'open' the decision block is momentarily suspended until the user resumes it to provide the missing data results, thus finalising the open decisions (Figure 3).

The user can open a new decision block only when either a 'concluded' or 'open' status is given to the previous block. There is no limit to the number of decisions that the user can enter in a single patient management process.

The leading hypothesis can be changed by the user during the consultation after any decision block: in this case the user must provide a written justification, which will be recorded as a comment to the changed hypothesis.

As soon as the patient management process is concluded (i.e. when the last decision block has been finalised and no 'open' decision blocks still exist) the user is asked for a final comment on the process outcome to be used for a posteriori evaluations.

5.3. System outcome

Computerised *medical records* offer important benefits over traditional paper charts [16,17]. They allow a better organization and retrieval of patient data because they capture key information combining coded and free-text formats and they provide fast and simple data entry. They also allow to use patient data easily for

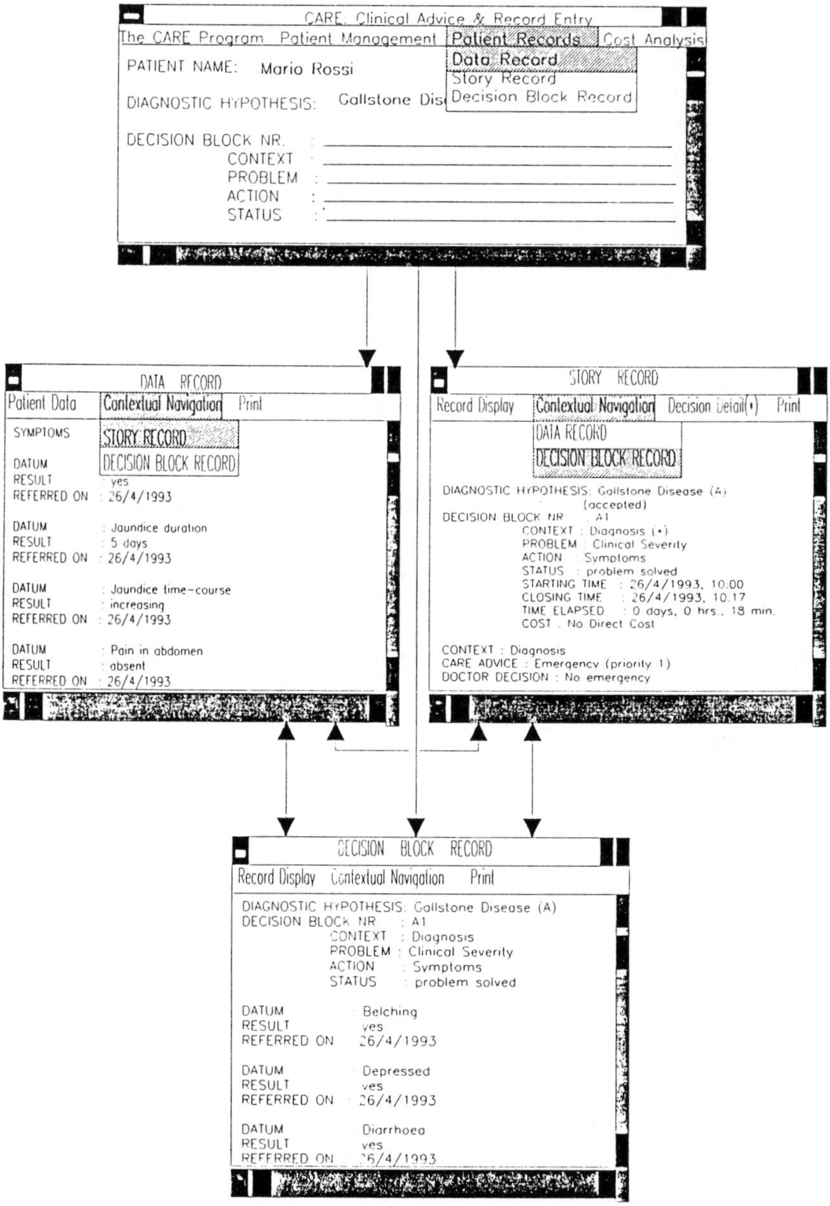

Figure 4. Data, Decision Block, and Story Records produced by CARE.

retrospective analysis and sharing of medical experience in clinical care, administrative and research functions.

In order to provide the physician with a well assessed methodological feed-back on patient management different displays of recorded data are automatically produced by CARE (Figure 4) focussed on data organization (data record), process analysis (story record), and decision analysis (decision block record) respectively. While the *data record* reflects the structure of a conventional clinical record, the *story record* stores the decision blocks chronologically, including the hypothesis validation result, starting and closing time, time elapsed, total investigations cost, CARE advice and doctor's justifications during each decision process. Finally, each *decision block record* shows in detail all referred data or requested procedures with their results or medical reports.

In this way the user, in addition to being adviced during the consultation, is also allowed to return at any time on a structured organization of clinical data and to evaluate a-posteriori his own performance with respect to both soundness of clinical reasoning and efficiency of clinical action. Moreover, the three CARE records can be navigated contextually, which means that from a patient data record the user can select a class of data (e.g., symptoms, laboratory investigations) and look at all the story and/or decision block records in which such a class has been taken as action. Similarly, from a specific story record (decision block record) the user can look at the data record and/or the subset of decision block records (story records) referring to the same action taken in the record from which the contextual navigation has started.

Moreover, the CARE system provides a cost analysis of the whole observation and of each diagnostic hypothesis considered during a patient management process. This cost analysis is a calculation of the time and costs spent in hospital by the patient.

6. FUTURE DEVELOPMENTS

Future developments of CARE include two main activities: the validation of the CARE program; and its development and adaptation to other medical domains.

7. CONCLUSIONS

As outlined above, CARE is essentially concerned with a methodological advice, in that the system does not provide any independent decision, but simply controls and criticises the approach followed by the physician in medical decision-making. Thus, it is a *user-centered system*, since the progression from one step in the program consultation to another is always the consequence of the user decision reflecting his/her responsible choice, while the program runs in the background storing facts and giving advice when necessary. It is therefore not intrusive in the user flow of reasoning but tries to guide the user decisions towards the underlying methodology.

Besides providing a second opinion on medical decision-making, CARE has potential educational properties, since it can improve substantially the user's skill and competence. Another function of CARE is to produce automatically different kinds of records aimed at representing objectively what the physicians actually did in managing the patient. This may be a very useful function since, CARE comments being always provided after user decisions, recorded data can be considered as reflecting the actual user competence.

In summary, the actual utility of CARE is threefold. First, used on-line as a decision aid it may improve physician performance in the real clinical context. Second, it can be used as an educational tool to train student in clinical methodology. Third, on the base of its recording facilities it can provide well assessed objective decision-mapping databases which might be very useful in evaluating the performance of individual users and in collecting statistical informations about doctor's behaviour.

8. REFERENCES

1 L.M. Koran, The reliability of clinical methods, data and judgements, N Engl J Med, 293 (1975) 642-646.
2 M. J. Ball and J.V. Douglas, Hospital information systems: looking into the future, Proceedings of 15th Annual Symposium on Computer Applications in Medical Care (SCAMC), (1991) 224-228.
3 G.O. Barnett, The application of computer-based medical-record systems in ambulatory practice, N Engl J Med, 310 (1984) 1643-1650.
4 M.H. Hodge, History of the TDS Medical Information System, in B.I. Blum and K. Duncan (eds.), A History of Medical Informatics, New York, ACM Press, 1990.
5 M.J. Quaak, R.F. Westerman and J.H. vanBemmel, Comparison between written and computerized patient histories, Brit Med J, 295 (1987) 184-190.
6 K.B. Langton, M.E. Johnston, R.B. Haynes and A. Mathieu, A critical appraisal of the literature on the effects of computer-based clinical decision support systems on clinical performance and patient outcomes, Proceedings of 16th Annual Symposium on Computer Applications in Medical Care (SCAMC), (1992) 626-630.
7 S.M. Speedie, D. McNally, S. Skarupa, R. Michocki, C. Rudo, C. Metge, F. Palumbo and D. Knapp, Evaluating drug prescribing in a large, ambulatory population: application of an embedded expert system, Proceedings of 16th Annual Symposium on Computer Applications in Medical Care (SCAMC), (1992) 621-625.
8 F.J. Zieve and E. Ciesco, Computer-focused modification of physician prescribing behavior, Proceedings of 16th Annual Symposium on Computer Applications in Medical Care (SCAMC), (1992) 617-620.
9 G. Lindberg, A. Björkman and C. Helmers, A description of diagnostic strategies in jaundice, Scand J Gastroenterol, 18 (1983) 257-265.

10 A. Malchow-Möller, C. Thomsen, P. Matzen et al, Computer diagnosis in jaundice. Bayes' rule founded on 1002 consecutive cases, J Hepatol, 3 (1986) 154-163.

11 G. Molino, M. Ballarè, P.E. Aurucci, V. Ripa di Meana, Application of artificial intelligence techniques to a well-defined clinical problem: jaundice diagnosis, Int J Biomed Comput, 12 (1990) 189-202.

12 M.F. Saint-Marc Girardin, M. Le Minor, A. Alperovitch, F. Roudot-Thoraval, J.M. Metreau and D. Dhumeaux, Computer-aided selection of diagnostic tests in jaundiced patients, Gut, 26 (1985) 961-967.

13 R.B. Stern, R.P. Knill-Jones and R. Williams, Use of computer program for diagnosing jaundice in district hospitals and a specialized liver unit, Brit Med J, I (1975) 659-662.

14 J.A. Vennes and J.H. Bond, Approach to the jaundiced patient, Gastroenterology, 84 (1983) 1515-1618.

15 G.W. Beeler, P.S. Gibbons and C.G. Chute, Development of a clinical data architecture, Proceedings of 16th Annual Symposium on Computer Applications in Medical Care (SCAMC), (1992) 244-248.

16 L.L. Weed, Medical records that guida and teach, N Engl J Med, 278 (1968) 593-600.

17 Q.E. Whiting-O'Keefe, D.W. Simborg, W.V. Epstein and A. Warger, A computerised summary medical record can provide more information than the standard medical record, JAMA, 245 (1985) 1185-1192.

ACKNOWLEDGEMENTS

This study has been developed within the AIM Project A2016 "Intelligent Decision-mapping Medical Record (IDMR)".

Knowledge Representation - Protocols

Artificial Intelligence in Medecine
S. Andreassen et al. , Eds.
IOS Press, 1993

CARE PROTOCOLS AND HEALTHCARE INFORMATICS

C Gordon[a], S I Herbert[b], A Jackson-Smale[a] and J-L Renaud-Salis[c]

[a]Advanced Computation Laboratory, Imperial Cancer Research Fund, PO Box 123, Lincoln's Inn Fields, London WC2A 3PX, UK

[b]NHS Information Management Centre, 15 Frederick Road, Birmingham B15 1JD, UK

[c]Fondation Bergonié, Centre Regional de Lutte contre le Cancer, 180 Rue de Saint-Genès, 33076 Bordeaux Cédex, France

Abstract

The paper describes a trans-national generic clinical protocol model designed using a blend of logic engineering and business modelling techniques as part of the CEC AIM programme's DILEMMA project. It will be used to implement protocol use in acute, primary and home care, including the support of shared care.

1 INTRODUCTION

In healthcare consensus guidelines are a topic of growing interest [1,2]. In oncology a detailed care protocol is an essential instrument for ensuring the proper selection and adjustment of therapeutic measures in response to patient characteristics. In primary care in particular, the adoption and dissemination of consensus guidelines promises to provide an efficient way to deliver research-based knowledge to its point of use [3,4]. The definition of protocols is seen as important to the wider use of shared care where specialist expertise is devolved to the primary sector. Guidelines for the collection of standard datasets are also being promoted as aids to clinical audit of process and outcome [5]. Health care service managers see protocols as a way of obtaining value for money, by ensuring the relevant use of specific services. One of the most rigorous applications of protocols is in the drugs trials carried out by pharmaceutical companies. The most widely used protocols are probably the instructions for prescribing and administering drugs published in the various European formularies.

The computerisation of clinical protocols has several potential benefits. Current medical AI technology is capable of recording protocols in knowledge bases which, coupled to an adequate electronic patient record, can be applied to give a care professional precise, reliable advice on the delivery of protocol-based care to individual patients. In healthcare management, a system which identifies care resource needs by applying standard policies on a case-by-case basis would enable more flexible and efficient resource management in "real time" [6].

Knowledge-based systems offer protocol authors and consensus-forming groups a powerful medium for the dissemination and use of their work. But to succeed users' systems should be able to apply knowledge in various domains and from various authors. This in turn entails that computerised protocol information from different sources is expressed in a common logical format. The DILEMMA project funded by the CEC's AIM programme has as a major objective the delivery of guideline-based decision support for shared care in oncology, cardiology and primary care. To date activity has focused on developing a generic model of the clinical protocol. Such a model could be used (via appropriate authoring tools) to construct protocol knowledge bases in such a common logical format.

2 THE TECHNICAL APPROACH USED

Our technical approach to modelling the clinical protocol is informed by two strands of previous work: Logic Engineering [7] and Business Modelling [8].

(a) Logic Engineering draws together the concepts of declarative programming, deductive databases and symbolic decision procedures, with a clean separation between domain knowledge and inference rules. Fox (1993) defines Logic Engineering as "the use of logic programming within a formal life-cycle methodology". In the Oxford System of Medicine project [9], this approach was used to design a decision support system for primary care. In the Bordeaux Oncology Support System (BOSS), the same approach was employed in the design of a first prototype for protocol-based decision support, drawing on the valuable experience gained in the same field by the ONCOCIN project at Stanford University. [10,11]

(b) The Common Basic Specification (CBS) - developed by the UK National Health Service[12] -provides a common framework for defining the informatics needs of clinical activities. The care delivery process is represented as a highly generic business activity hierarchy, the data flows entailed by those activities and a model of the entity types and relations required to support the dataflows. The CBS models all aspects of 'maintaining and improving the health of a population', but

DILEMMA focuses on the delivery of care to a patient. It has made particular use of the clinical view of the CBS provided by the COSMOS project [13]. DILEMMA will also attempt to represent the CBS as a declarative knowledge base.

We have found Logic Engineering a helpful way to address the problem of protocol modelling. That protocols describe clinical *procedures* is, in our view, no reason for not representing their knowledge content in a fully *declarative* format. A protocol definition enumerates a network of operational actions (eg take a blood pressure) and decision actions (eg interpret a finding), their relationships and the criteria determining when, whether and how each one is to be performed. Reasoning services to advise on the application of a protocol to a given case can be implemented in logic programming as a set of declarative, generic inference functions derivable from the protocol model. Business modelling makes a major contribution by providing a proven, flexible vocabulary for the structured representation of activities in organisations. Additionally it helps to determine the patient data required to apply a protocol, and so helps us to design the connections required between protocol-based decision support and a patient record database.

This paper contains an abridged form of the draft DILEMMA generic clinical protocol knowledge model as of July 1993, with emphasis on its use for clinical purposes rather than resource management. The equally essential and concomitant DILEMMA work - see figure 1 - on a protocol authoring tool, a protocol manager, the impact of protocol use on the patient record, and temporal qualification is mentioned only where it is necessary to support the description of the generic protocol model. They are described fully in other DILEMMA material.

Fig 1 The Generic Protocol Model in context

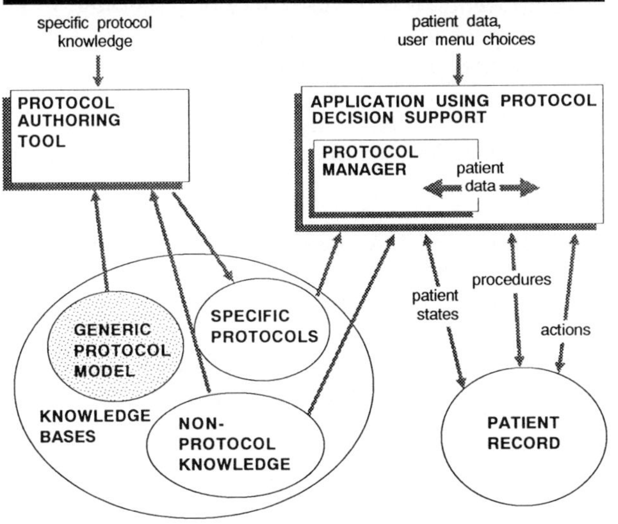

3 THE DILEMMA GENERIC PROTOCOL MODEL

3.1 PROTOCOLS, PROCEDURES AND ACTIVITIES

A *PROTOCOL* is a formal description of a means of achieving an objective or goal that is relevant to a particular class of problem. It is used as a template from which to derive the specific *ACTIVITYs* to be performed for an individual patient with a particular problem and context. It may be a standard, a guideline or a set of options from which the clinician is invited to select one by exercising his clinical judgement. As demonstrated by UK primary care, a single protocols can be a mixture of all three types of element.

Protocols are commonly composite, and at the knowledge level their components are also considered to be protocols, ie descriptions of means of achieving subgoals of the parent composite. A protocol will define the sequence and context in which its components should be executed, and may therefore contain components - eg a randomisation procedure in a treatment trial - to determine which of several succeeding alternative components to do next. A protocol will have an author, be subject to version control and include a definition of the AGENTs who are the intended users. The level of detail in a particular protocol is defined by the expertise the protocol author can assume of its users. A surgeon describing a technique for his peers will usually take as read things that he would explicitly document for his junior colleagues.

The application of a protocol to a specific patient problem at a particular time results in a *PROCEDURE*, its leaf level components relevant to that problem becoming activities to be performed in due course. In the case of protocols that contain conditional components, a procedure may be generated in stages, as the relevance of conditional components may not being known for certain at the outset, or may change during the execution of the procedure.

The *ACTIVITYs* derived from the leaf components of a procedure are executable actions authorised and undertaken by an *AGENT* (or agents), such as a clinician, nurse or patient in order to:

- change or maintain a *SUBJECT*'s - eg a patient's - state, eg by chemotherapy
- find out more about a *SUBJECT*, eg confirm a diagnosis, examine a patient or ask the patient a question

Figure 2 depicts a data model of an activity and the related entity types, and embodies a simple example. It uses entity-relationship modelling (ERM) conventions, which are explained in figure 3.

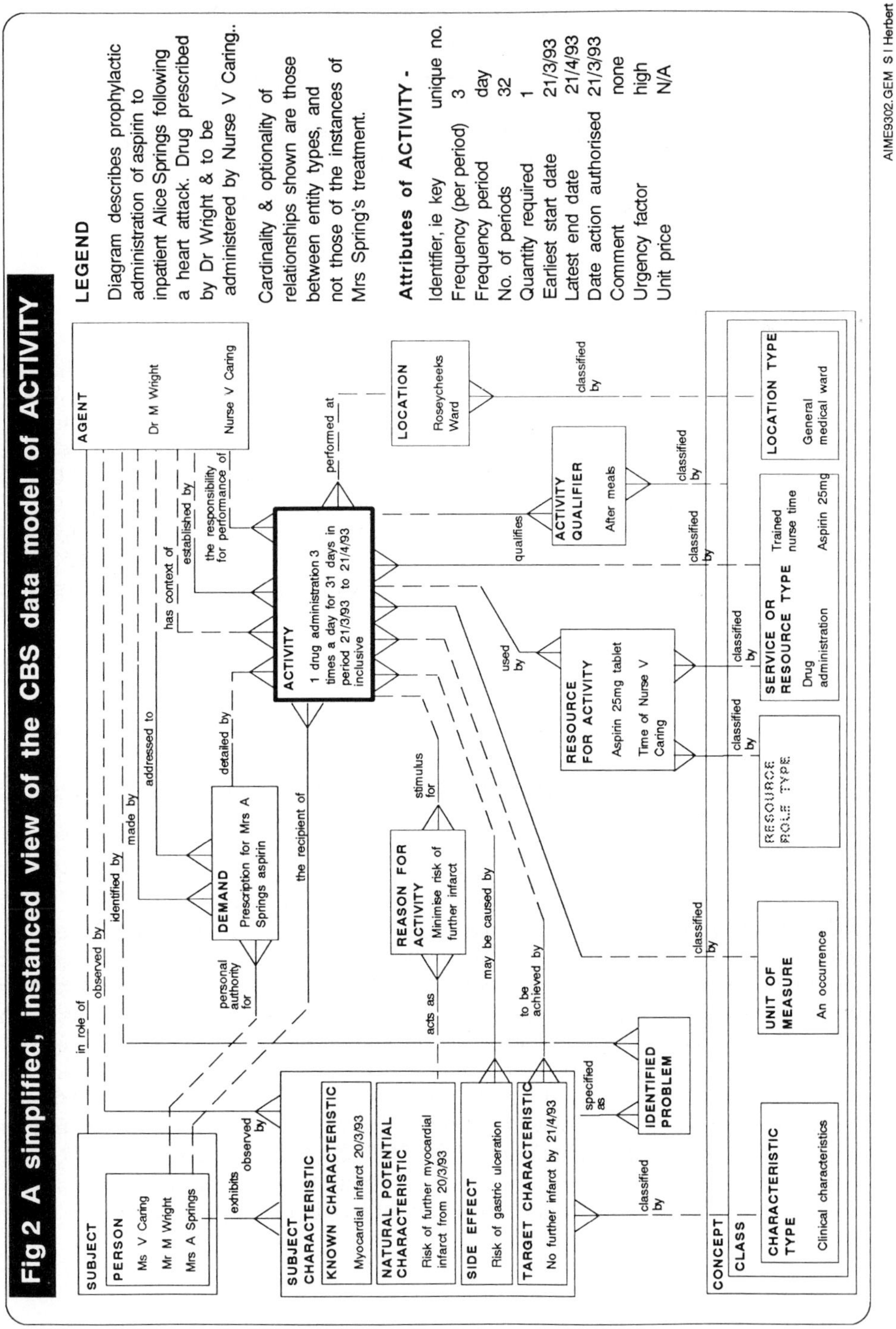
Fig 2 A simplified, instanced view of the CBS data model of ACTIVITY
SUBJECT
PERSON
Ms V Caring
Mr M Wright
Mrs A Springs
AGENT
Dr M Wright
Nurse V Caring
in role of
observed by
identified by
made by
addressed to
has context of
established by
the responsibility for performance of
performed at
LOCATION
Roseycheeks Ward
DEMAND
Prescription for Mrs A Springs aspirin
detailed by
personal authority for
the recipient of
ACTIVITY
1 drug administration 3 times a day for 31 days in period 21/3/93 to 21/4/93 inclusive
REASON FOR ACTIVITY
Minimise risk of further infarct
stimulus for
acts as
may be caused by
to be achieved by
used by
qualifies
ACTIVITY QUALIFIER
After meals
RESOURCE FOR ACTIVITY
Aspirin 25mg tablet
Time of Nurse V Caring
exhibits
observed by
SUBJECT CHARACTERISTIC
KNOWN CHARACTERISTIC
Myocardial infarct 20/3/93
NATURAL POTENTIAL CHARACTERISTIC
Risk of further myocardial infarct from 20/3/93
SIDE EFFECT
Risk of gastric ulceration
TARGET CHARACTERISTIC
No further infarct by 21/4/93
specified as
IDENTIFIED PROBLEM
classified by
CONCEPT
CLASS
CHARACTERISTIC TYPE
Clinical characteristics
UNIT OF MEASURE
An occurrence
RESOURCE ROLE TYPE
SERVICE OR RESOURCE TYPE
Drug administration
Trained nurse time
Aspirin 25mg
LOCATION TYPE
General medical ward
LEGEND
Diagram describes prophylactic administration of aspirin to inpatient Alice Springs following a heart attack. Drug prescribed by Dr Wright & to be administered by Nurse V Caring..
Cardinality & optionality of relationships shown are those between entity types, and not those of the instances of Mrs Spring's treatment.
Attributes of ACTIVITY -
Identifier, ie key unique no.
Frequency (per period) 3
Frequency period day
No. of periods 32
Quantity required 1
Earliest start date 21/3/93
Latest end date 21/4/93
Date action authorised 21/3/93
Comment none
Urgency factor high
Unit price N/A
AIME9302.GEM S I Herbert 6/7/93

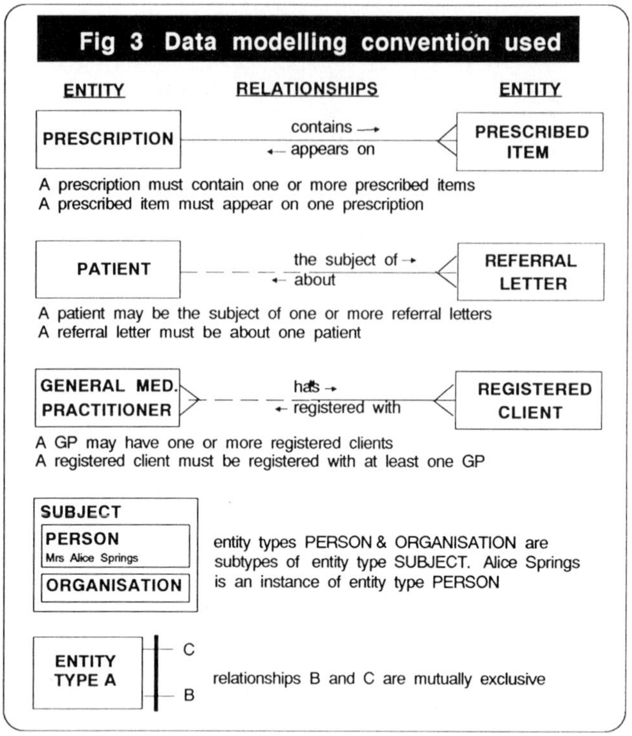

3.2 A GENERIC PROTOCOL ANATOMY

Anatomical components

Figure 4 shows the anatomy of an imaginary protocol, and figure 5 depicts a data model to support this structure.

Discrete components of *COMPOSITE PROTOCOLs* are termed *COMPONENT PROTOCOLs*. Component protocols may be composite, and are either *OBLIGATORY*, ie always performed when the protocol is applied to a patient problem, or *CONDITIONAL*, eg only applied to counter possible side-effects of a related protocol component. A protocol which is not composite is termed an *ATOMIC PROTOCOL*, and becomes a leaf component when used as part of a composite protocol. A protocol which is not a component of another is known as a *SELF-CONTAINED PROTOCOL*. The composite protocol with which a protocol stands in a direct component relationship is termed its *PARENT PROTOCOL*, and the self-contained protocol of which a component protocol is a direct or indirect component is termed the component's *PARENT SELF-CONTAINED PROTOCOL*. A protocol may have a component whose completion is not related in any way to the completion of its direct and indirect parents, viz L and I_2 in figure 4.

The same action, eg 'take a blood pressure', may occur more than once within a composite protocol, but each instance is uniquely identified as a specific component protocol: two such components, I_1 and I_2, appear in figure 4. Appearance of a protocol as a components of itself - recursion - is not allowed.

A protocol may represent the iteration of a task a fixed or variable number of times, and execution of the resultant procedure will produce a number of uniquely identified instances of that procedure. Such a protocol may be represented as two components, one - the parent - representing the whole action, ie the entire set of iterations, and the other - its child - representing the iterated action.

Naming protocols

Every protocol in a knowledge base must have an identifier that is unique within the set of all protocol identifiers in that knowledge base. One way to achieve this is to form the identifier by concatenating the identifiers of all its parents, the main parent first, followed by an identifier for the action it represents eg:

'Myville Hypertension Protocol/Sitting Sphygmomanometer Blood Pressure'.

A repetition of an action on the same path through the parent can then be given a unique identifier by adding a sequence indicator, eg

'Myville Hypertension Protocol/A/Sitting Sphygmomanometer Blood Pressure'.

A protocol, eg for a drug treatment, may of course appear - with different identifiers - as a component in any number of parent self-contained protocols, as well as in its own right as a self contained protocol.

Fig 4 Naming of protocol parts

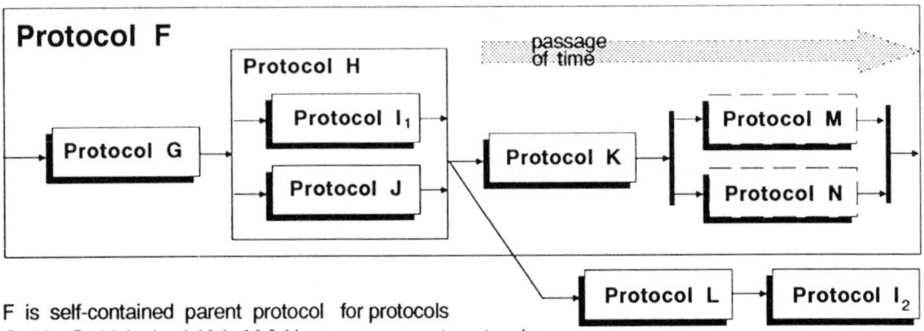

F is self-contained parent protocol for protocols G - N. G, H, I_1, I_2, J, K, L, M & N are component protocols.
M & N are conditional protocols that are exclusive alternatives.
F & H are composite protocols, parents of G - N and I_1 & J respectively.
All protocols except F & H are atomic protocols.

Protocol F components start in the following sequence:
- G, I_1 & J in parallel, K & L in parallel. M or N follows K, and I_2 follows L
When either M or N is completed, F is completed. Completion of L & I_2 are not necessary for completion of F.

Version control
In addition to a unique title, each protocol bears a *VERSION* number and a *STATUS* - 'withdrawn', 'superseded' or 'available'. Revision of a protocol implies the production of a new version of the protocol itself, plus new versions of all other protocols that include it as a component. In figure 4, the revision of protocol J would result in new versions of H and F. The concept 'revision' covers changes to the content of a protocol, or the addition of new entry criteria, but not amendments or deletions of the indications of use (see below). If a protocol for treating stage II breast cancer is now considered to apply only to breast cancer stage IIa, it would become a new protocol, not a new version of a protocol for treating stage II breast cancer. This of course does not preclude the concurrent existence of *different* protocols for dealing with the same problem.

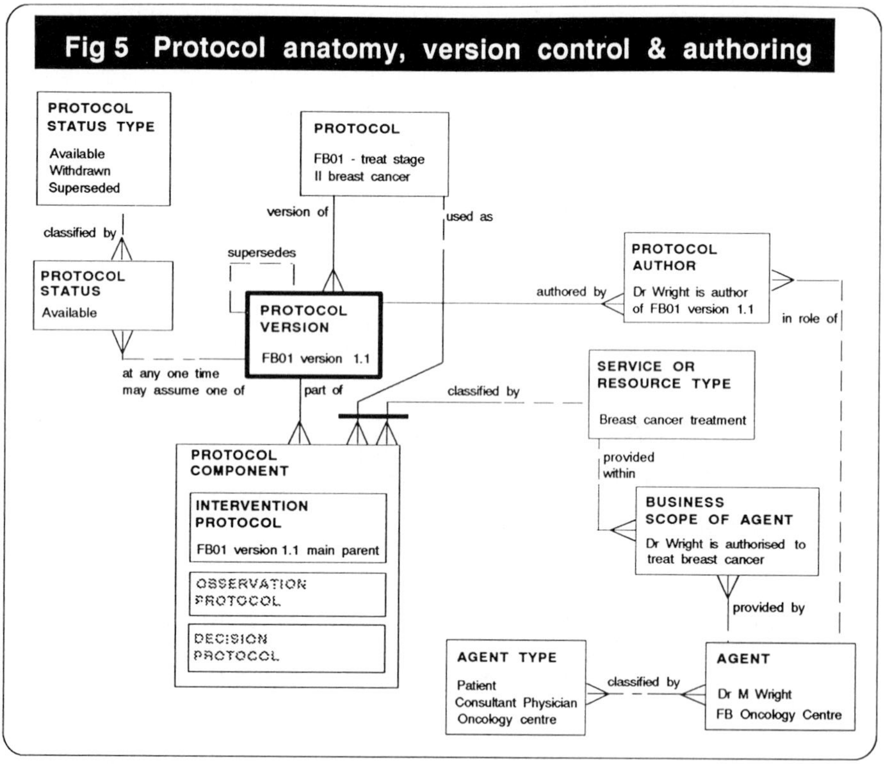

Fig 5 Protocol anatomy, version control & authoring

3.3 SELECTING THE PROTOCOL TO APPLY TO A PATIENT CASE

Selecting a self-contained protocol
Protocol selection is carried out by the DILEMMA protocol manager in two stages. It firstly uses the protocol's *ELIGIBILITY CRITERION* to reason about the

relevance of each protocol to the patient problem under consideration, building a list of the relevant procedures. Secondly it derives possible arguments about the suitability of each relevant procedure from its *SELECTION CRITERION*, checks them against corresponding patient information and uses the results plus data from the *OUTCOME FUNCTION* to inform user choice. It is not envisaged that the protocol manager will make that choice, as in many cases it involves the judgement of the patient and /or clinician about the relative value of the benefits and side effects of treatment, the impact of treatment on other members of the patient's family, and so on.

A model of the data entity types needed to support protocol selection is given in figure 6. It includes examples for each entity type from an intervention protocol to treat breast cancer.

The protocol eligibility criterion
Each self-contained protocol must possess an *ELIGIBILITY CRITERION*, establishing the truth of which for a specific patient problem will lead to the inclusion of that protocol on the 'relevant' list. It must have one or more *INCLUSION PARAMETER*s, and zero or more *EXCLUSION PARAMETER*s.

The *INCLUSION PARAMETER*s must identify at least one *PROBLEM* - 'indication for use' in clinical terms - for which the protocol offers some form of benefit. Each problem will have one *INTENTION* associated with it, eg 'to cure', 'repair', 'replace', 'protection against', 'alleviate', 'observe', 'diagnose', etc. The intention is always a verb, and is constrained by the type of the problem: thus a problem consisting of a patient characteristic classed as 'unknown' would always be associated with an intention 'to observe' it. Taken together, problem and intention define the goal or purpose of the protocol, ie 'to cure stage II breast cancer'.

The eligibility criterion will also identify any *NECESSARY FEATURE*s which the subject - eg patient - must possess to qualify as a suitable candidate for application of the protocol.

The *EXCLUSION PARAMETER*s - contraindications in clinical terms - record features which preclude the use of a protocol in both self-contained and component mode. For example, breast cancer treatment protocols including teratogenic chemotherapy would be contraindicated by concurrent 1st trimester pregnancy, and some would be contraindicated for treatment of (the rare) cases of breast cancer in men. Unless a component protocol is conditional, its contraindications will also apply to the parent self-contained protocol. For any particular patient problem, this will not be true of conditional components found to be unnecessary during the execution of the procedure. DILEMMA is doing further work in this area.

Each *SUBJECT DATA ITEM* referred to in the eligibility criterion will have a corresponding *VALUE*, optionally qualified by a temporal relationship, eg a protocol for treating breast cancer may only be relevant to patients with 'stage II breast cancer confirmed within the last month'.

Fig 6 Protocol relevance and selection

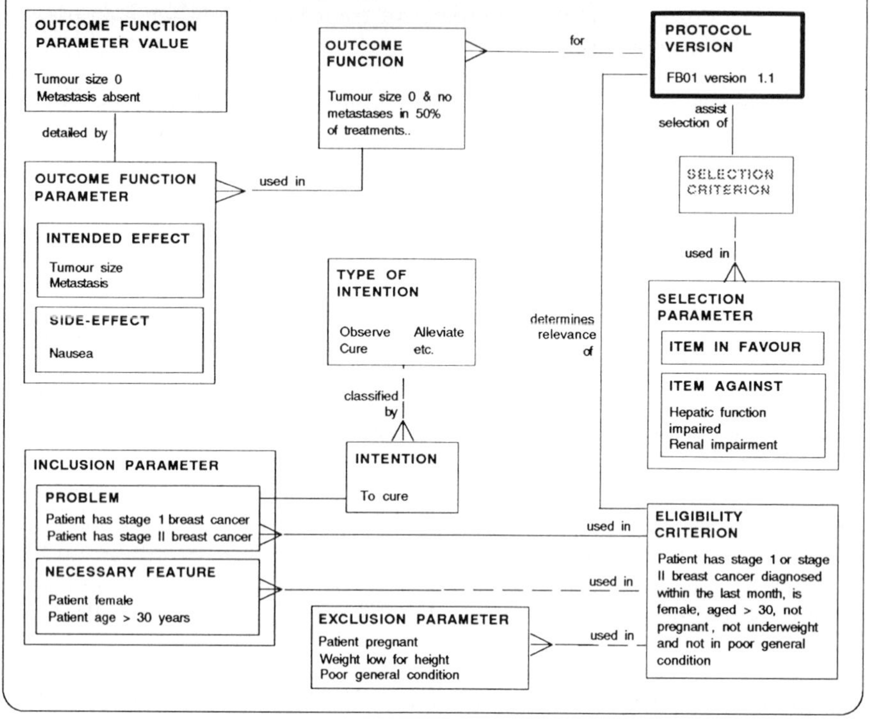

The protocol selection criterion

A protocol may have a *SELECTION CRITERION*, which refers to a value of one or more patient-related feature or the state of an action, with or without a temporal qualification. Each selection criterion has *ITEMs IN FAVOUR* and/or *ITEMs AGAINST* which can form the basis of arguments for and against selecting the protocol that owns it. The 'cautions' given in the prescribing instructions of the British National Formulary are examples of items against. The nomination by formularies of a drug as the 'preferred' treatment without further explanation being given is an example of an item in favour, but they are much less common than items against. As with eligibility parameters, each selection parameter must have a value, and may have a temporal qualifier.

Eligibility and selection parameters must be consistent within themselves and with each other. For example, an indication for use of a protocol may not also be a contraindication or contra-selection parameter of that protocol or its components. DILEMMA is looking at the topic of protocol validation in greater detail, and will provide prototypes that implement the results of this work.

Anticipated protocol outcomes
A protocol will typically have an *OUTCOME FUNCTION* based on subject-related features, by which its potential benefit and practical success can be judged. The type of the outcome function corresponds to its protocol class: diagnoses, for a diagnostic protocol; observed patient characteristics for an observation protocol; resulting subject characteristics, for an intervention protocol. Protocol outcomes are divided into two classes: anticipated intended results - *INTENDED EFFECT*s - and anticipated but undesirable results - *SIDE EFFECT*s. For a breast cancer treatment protocol the intended effects might be tumour size zero, no metastases and a white blood cell count of more than 40,000/mm^3 within 5 weeks of the completion of treatment. At the protocol knowledge level both objectives and side-effects should have a probability of occurrence attached to the value given. Observation protocols may also, like intervention protocols, produce side-effects.

3.4 THE PRIMARY TYPES OF ATOMIC PROTOCOL

An atomic protocol will be of one of two basic types, a *DECISION TASK* - eg 'establish diagnosis' - or an *OPERATIONAL TASK* - eg 'take blood pressure'. The result of a decision task is the choice of one or more from a set of possible options in a given decision.

A *DECISION TASK PROTOCOL* will have a focus (the entity about which a decision is to be taken) and a decision class (eg diagnosis, diagnostic staging, treatment selection, investigation selection). A decision class and the generic decision-making procedure are defined elsewhere[14], and are independent of the specification of particular protocols. These definitions stipulate the form of clinical domain knowledge (eg of the possible stages of a cancer and their definitions) necessary in the protocol (or an associated, general purpose knowledge base) to perform the decision task. This domain knowledge will define case-related criteria for decision options, which are composed of conjunctions and/or disjunctions with or without temporal qualification. Decision task protocols are distinguished from protocol management decisions by their use of domain knowledge applicable both in a protocol and in general clinical decision-making. A draft model of general clinical domain knowledge is given in another DILEMMA publication. The result of a decision task procedure will be recorded in the patient record in the same way as the result of an operational procedure.

An atomic protocol may have attributes and attribute values defining the detail of the action performed: eg a prescribing protocol may have attribute slots for dosage, frequency, and duration. Such attributes may be predetermined, or may be determined or modified in the course of a specific execution. This task will be performed by an associated (preceding) decision protocol.

Another way of determining the characteristics of a protocol is by refinement. A protocol may have other, more specifically characterized versions of itself defined. To execute such a refinable protocol, the eligibility criteria for one of its subclasses must be satisfied in addition to its own. The selected refinement protocol may then be performed, inheriting all the attributes of the refinable protocol.

3.5 PROCEDURE STATES AND INTERSTATE TRANSITIONS

Procedure states

At any time, each procedure - composite or atomic - must be recorded as being in a *PROCEDURE STATE*. Possible states are shown in figure 7. A procedure will progress from the 'relevant' state to 'established' or 'discarded'. Established procedures are then requested - maybe from the establisher him- or herself, accepted, scheduled, started, performed and finally reported. It may exceptionally be cancelled, suspended or abandoned, eg because the patient has died.

Fig 7 Possible procedure states

State	Meaning	Transition to state authorised by
RELEVANT	relevant ro a specific patient problem	requester
ESTABLISHED	a relevant procedure to be applied to a specific patient problem	requester & maybe subject
DISCARDED	a relevant procedure which it has been decided NOT to apply to a particular patient problem	requester & maybe subject
PART-REFINED	a composite procedure that has been partly decomposed into its atomic - ie leaf - components	supplier
REFINED	a composite procedure that has been fully decomposed	supplier
REQUESTED	the supplier agent has been determined & the procedure requested	requester
REJECTED	by the chosen supplier. Action is still regarded as necessary	supplier
ACCEPTED	by the chosen supplier	supplier
SCHEDULED	a procedure with a specific start date & time, performing agent, etc.	supplier
CANCELLED	abnormal finished state for unstarted procedure	requester
STARTED	or restarted after suspension	supplier & maybe subject
ABANDONED	abnormal finished state for a started procedure	supplier
SUSPENDED	started but halted.	supplier
PERFORMED	normal finished state. Its goal may or may not have been reached	supplier
REPORTED	after a normal or abnormal finish	supplier

States in italics are concerned with resource management

Procedure state transitions

Fig 8 shows the legitimate state transitions. The sufficient prerequisites for changing a procedure from one state to another (including its transition to the established state, i.e. its selection) are known as the *STATE TRANSITION CRITERION*. These are held in the definition of the protocol from which the procedure will be derived. There will be one (explicit or default) criterion for each legitimate transition for each procedure. Each criterion may involve a conjunction or disjunction of conditions and subconditions, comprising patient characteristics, states or state transitions of other protocols and temporal expressions. The other protocols whose states form part of such a criterion may (in interests of definitional clarity) be restricted to preceding, component and parent actions.

Fig 8 Legitimate Procedure State Transitions

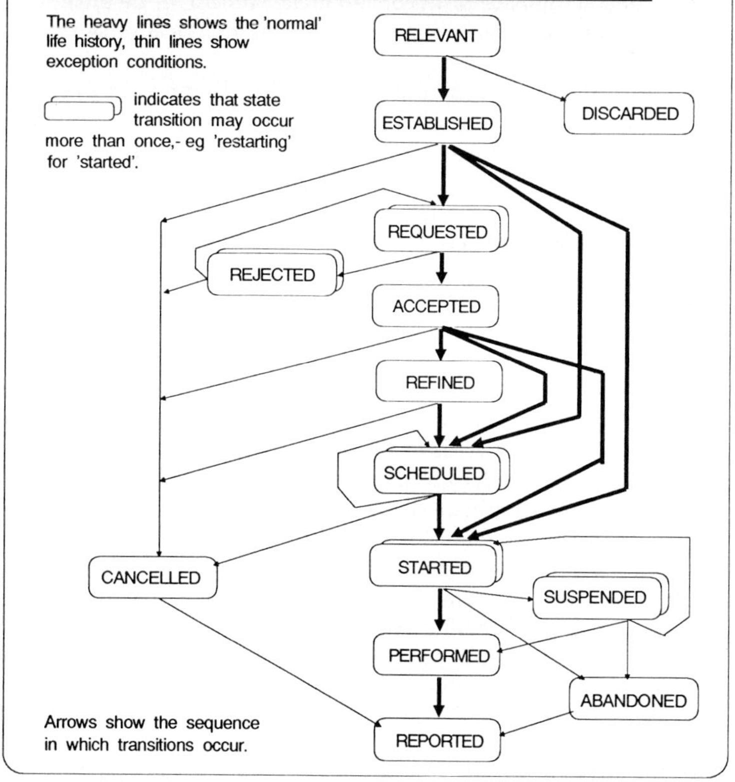

Most state transitions proposed by a protocol decision support system will require explicit authorisation from one or more agents (in some cases including the patient or a proxy) before they may proceed. The user may always change the state of a procedure explicitly via the protocol manager, but only as permitted by the protocol definition.

A state transition criterion for procedure X will have the following attributes:

(One) *CONTEXT*: the identifier of the protocol containing the state transition criterion to be triggered - X.

(One) *STATE TRANSITION* in X which is proposed by the criterion, eg 'scheduled → cancelled'

(One or more) *ASSOCIATED CONDITION*: the condition under which the state transition in X named above will be triggered. The eligibility and selection criterion mentioned in 3.3 are kinds of associated condition, for triggering the (only possible) transitions to the 'relevant' and 'established' states respectively.

A state transition of a composite protocol can either entail, or be entailed by, state transitions of one or more of its components. Some of these entailments can be stated as universal or default rules, while others will be recorded specifically in the state transition criteria of individual protocols. Work is in progress within DILEMMA to determine the general/default rules, and the constraints on other legitimate statements of the interactions between composite and component state transitions.

Decision protocols - and some other categories - may have a more restricted range of possible states and state transitions. A decision procedure normally passes directly from the established state to the reported state, but may be delayed or suspended if insufficient data is found to be available for decision-making. State transition criteria may be defined for a protocol class which will be inherited as default criteria by protocols belonging to that class. A specific state transition criterion for a given transition overrides any criterion for that transition inherited from a superclass, so that individual protocols may only be able to assume a subset of the possible states and state transitions. Thus a protocol which contains actions to be invoked and performed by a general practitioner within a single consultation by him- or herself would not involve resource management decisions, and so its components would pass straight from the 'established' to 'started' state, without making the transition to the 'requested', 'accepted', 'rejected' or 'scheduled' states. Figure 9 contains a model of the protocol data needed to support state transition criteria. It includes the previous instances shown for transition to the 'relevant' and 'established' state shown in fig 6.

3.6 SUCCESSION RELATIONSHIPS BETWEEN COMPONENTS

We have now defined sufficient knowledge to control the flow of execution of the components of a procedure, as well as the selection of parent main protocols described in 3.3. Succession relationships between component procedures - eg B and C, both components of A - are expressed by means of criteria for a state

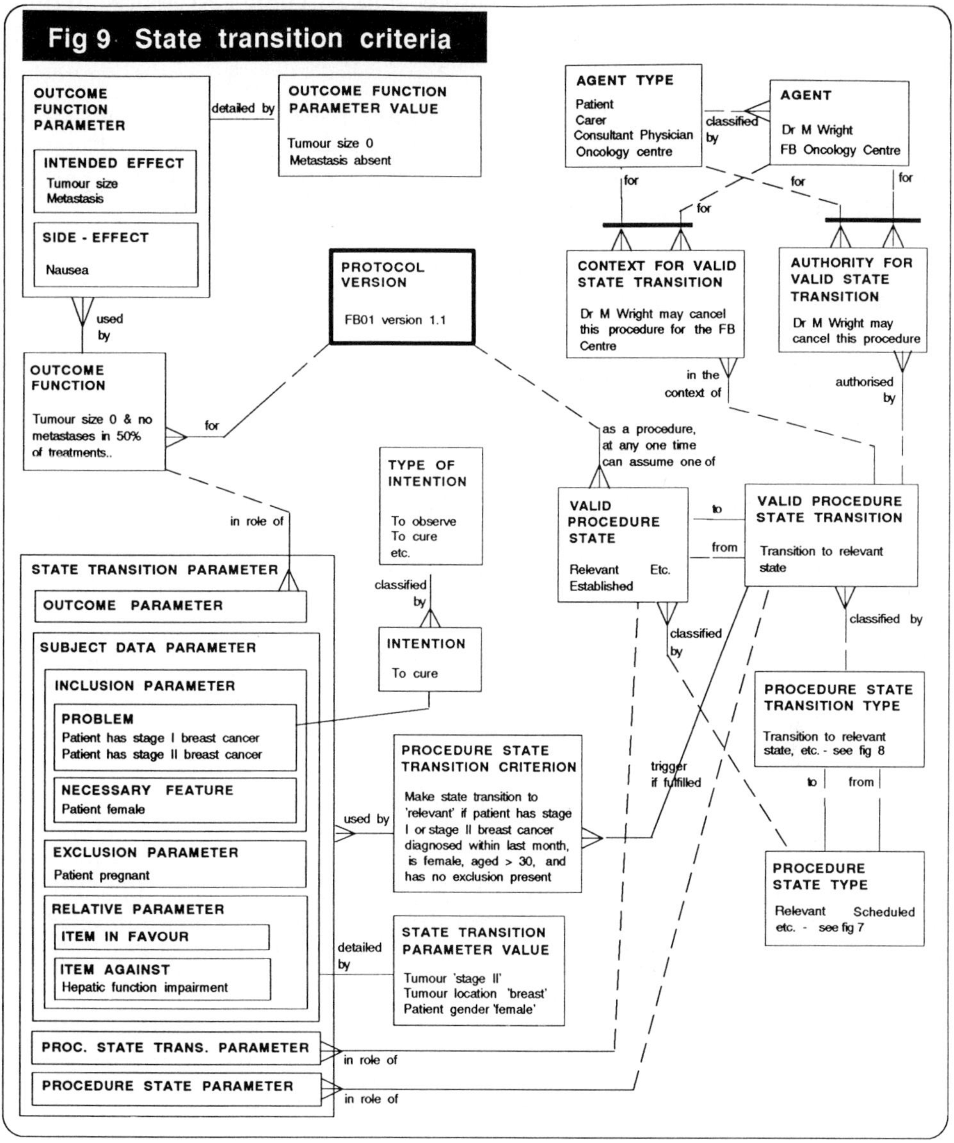

transition in C which lists the relevant state transition in B as one of its preconditions. In the simplest - and commonest - case, completion of B would allow C to start. Detection of a triggering event (ie a 'preceding' state transition in another protocol or a patient data item mentioned in the criterion) will cause the protocol manager to evaluate the condition of its potential successor(s) in full. The condition may be found to be satisfied immediately, or it may become satisfied at a subsequent time as a result of a subsequent event.

One (or more) component of a composite protocol will have an initial state transition criteria - typically for transition to the 'established' or 'accepted' state - which is triggered - wholly or in part - by the establishment of the parent protocol. These are the initial components of the composite protocol.

Multiple successor and predecessor protocols
Mention of a specific predecessor in several subsequent components' state transition criteria allows the predecessor to have more than one successor component, and - unless they are all mutually exclusive - allows two or more of these to be performed in parallel. Conversely, execution of a component protocol may be triggered by state transitions of more than one possible predecessor, either as exclusive alternatives or in combination. This will be indicated by including each necessary component state as a part of the state transition criteria for the triggering of a state transition in the successor protocol. Thus a component protocol for discharging an inpatient will only be able to start when all the parallel strands of activity involved in the treatment have attained the 'reported' state.

Conditional protocols
A component may be optional or one of a number of exclusive alternatives. The conditions involved will form state transition criteria for the change to the initial state of the successor action. It is also possible for any other state transition to be conditional if required.

The transition to the 'cancelled' or 'abandoned' state
Where a component protocol can be used on its own, its exclusion parameters - ie contraindications - are automatically used as state transition criteria for transition to the 'cancelled' or 'abandoned' states. Thus if the component was a protocol for drug prescription and administration, the drug's contraindications are used to determine whether the treatment should proceed or not, along with any criteria specific to the particular state transition and component protocol.

4 VALIDATION OF THE PROTOCOL MODEL

Examples from France, Holland and the UK have been used in the development of the model. The French examples are concerned with the treatment of breast cancer, and have been developed - and are used - by a regional tertiary cancer treatment centre in Bordeaux, the Fondation Bergonié. The Dutch material is the work of the national programme for primary care protocols developed by the NHG, Utrecht, and monitored by the Centre for Quality Assurance Research (CQAR) at the University of Nijmegen. The protocols are for problems commonly presented to primary care where treatment is known to vary widely and a national consensus about the elements of care is attainable. The protocols include examples to deal with ankle distortion, diabetes mellitus type II, oral female contraception, urinary tract infection, etc.. From England we have used primary care protocols for detecting colo-rectal cancer and treating hyperlipidaemia (courtesy of the ICRF General Practice Research Group and the Oxford Lipids Centre respectively), and an angina protocol written at a tertiary cardiology hospital, the Royal Brompton National Heart & Lung Hospitals, London. A prototype repository for a subset of the generic model has been implemented using a logic engineering toolset and a knowledge authoring tool- EDITH - developed by DILEMMA. A comprehensive implementation will be available by late 1993.

Ongoing work within DILEMMA involves the representation of more test material from all these organisations, including the prescribing and administration rules for about ninety of the commonest generic drugs used in two practices of the ICRF GPRG. Protocols for asthma and hypertension developed by the GPRG will be entered when they are finalised. The ICRF and the CQAR will exchange primary care protocols, and enter them into their respective knowledge bases. Implementation of a prototype protocol manager using the model, based on logic engineering principles and linked to a hospital information system, should be complete by the time this paper is presented. A general practice version of protocol decision support will be implemented in the UK and France by mid-1994.

5 MODEL-BASED IMPLEMENTATION OF PROTOCOL DECISION SUPPORT SYSTEMS

The objectives

Our aim is that the generic model outlined above should be capable of representing many different protocols and provide the basis for a knowledge representation format shareable by many medical KBS implementors. In this section, we outline our own approach to the use of such a model in designing a family of clinical decision support applications.

5.1 DETERMINISM AND CLOSURE

Applying KBS technology to help healthcare professionals choose and execute protocols promises to be a practical and useful exercise. Compared to some of the deeper AI problems encountered in medical informatics, it is relatively tractable. The point of a protocol is that the operational implications of the knowledge it contains are deterministic. A protocol rarely caters for all the events that could affect it and so may not be infallible, and the execution of a given protocol may not always be the optimal clinical choice in a given case. On the other hand, the raison d'etre of a protocol is that it gives precise recommendations for any individual case. Consequently a protocol decision support system (DSS) has no requirement to implement any form of reasoning under uncertainty. Furthermore, given that each protocol has precise indications of use and entry criteria identifying the cases to which it may safely be applied, the brittle behaviour encountered in classic medical expert systems functioning near the borders of their speciality is unlikely to be a problem. *However a clinician applying a protocol remains responsible for ensuring that actions carried out according to its recommendations are clinically safe in the individual case.*

A more advanced type of DSS than that being developed in DILEMMA might be able to offer high-quality advice on situations where it may be advisable to override or customise a protocol, on whether a given protocol is the best course of action for a patient, or on how to concurrently apply more than one protocol to a single patient. We are interested in using Logic Engineering to address these more challenging tasks. In the meantime, a DSS which can help to apply a protocol accurately and correctly appears to have a legitimate and useful place in clinical practice.

5.2 INFERENCE SERVICES

A protocol comprises a collection of inferences and decision criteria governing the execution of a set of actions. Criteria are designed so that their truth may be inferred from the available data. The design of a protocol DSS is therefore centrally concerned with the specification of inference functions for this purpose. These functions can appropriately be implemented as an event- and data-driven monitoring service which repeatedly determines - for any newly known state of the world - whether any criterion for a currently possible action state transition has become true. A prerequisite for system design is the definition of a protocol-oriented model of patient data, such that any finding concept (patient characteristic) contained in the definition of a protocol criterion can be proved or disproved by inferences from that data. Particular attention is needed here to the modelling of temporal knowledge and data representation, and of the associated inference capabilities (such as to be capable of inferring the truth of criterion expressions such as "at least 3 episodes of leucopenia in the last 21 days"). In the broader context protocol decision support will place new functional requirements on the electronic patient record, which will have to hold a complete record of the stages of execution of protocol-derived procedures and their components (probably including a record of the reasons why given actions were performed/not performed).

5.3 PROTOCOLS AND DECISIONS

The kernel of a protocol-based DSS will thus consist of advice about what actions are at any time determined as being required by the application of a clinical protocol. Such a system will include aids for collecting data and results that are currently relevant, aids for viewing the protocol-oriented record in terms of performed, outstanding and potential future care actions, and ways to browse the protocol being applied.

Does the deterministic nature of protocols make the use of a symbolic decision procedure unnecessary? We have not found it to be so. It is true not all of the reasoning about protocol actions is most naturally represented in terms of a decision procedure: this comment arguably applies to much or all of the inference involved in answering the questions "what should be done now?" and "what should be done next?". On the other hand, where part of a protocol represents the performance of a specific clinical decision act (such as diagnosis or choosing a treatment strategy), knowledge representation and the consequent delivery of clinically intelligible decision support are enhanced if such decisions, their rationale and the knowledge they use can be expressed in an explicit, declarative form. The DILEMMA generic protocol model proposes formats for embedding these decisions within the action structure of the protocol. This approach should also provide a favourable basis for adding in the future more advanced decision support services for protocol users, based on non-deterministic reasoning.

ACKNOWLEDGEMENT

This paper is published by kind permission of the DILEMMA consortium. The organisations involved are:

Advanced Computation Laboratory, Imperial Cancer Research Fund, London, UK
General Practice Research Group, Imperial cancer Research Fund, Oxford, UK
Hewlett-Packard Research Laboratories, Bristol, UK
Royal Brompton National Heart & Lung Hospitals, London, UK
Fondation Bergonié, Bordeaux, France
The NHS Information Management Centre, Birmingham, UK
Deutsches Krebsforschungszentrum, Heidelberg, Germany
MDA Group, Linköping University, Sweden
UNINOVA, Lisbon, Portugal
WOK (CQAR), Nijmegen University, Netherlands

REFERENCES

1 David M Eddy, A Manual for Assessing Health Practices and Designing Practice Policies. The Explicit Approach. American College of Physicians. Philadelphia, 1992

2 David M Eddy, Designing a practice policy: standards, guidelines and options. JAMA. 1990:263, 3077-3084

3 Jackson-Smale, A The Dilemma Project and Computerised Primary Care Guidelines in the UK and Holland, British Journal of Healthcare Computing, 1993 (forthcoming).

4 Beckers W P A, Vries Robbe P F de, Haring E J van der, Zwaard A M, Mokkink H G A, Grol R P T M, Automation of medical Audit in General Practice. Proceedings of the Third Conference on Artificial Intelligence in Medicine, ed. Stefanelli et al. Berlin: Springer, Lecture Notes in Medical Informatics, No 44, 129-139.

5 Ginzler M and Pritchard P The Oxford System of Medicine in trans-national markets. AIM project LEMMA, Biomedical Computing Unit, Imperial Cancer research Fund, November 1990

6 Mackenzie Tribbeck Associates Ltd Real-time Resource Management. Report published for the NHS Management Executive, 1990

7 Fox, John On the soundness and safety of expert systems. Artificial Intelligence in Medicine 5 (1993) 159-179.

8 The CBS in 1992. NHS Information Management Centre. Birmingham, UK, 1992.

9 J Fox, C Gordon, A J Glowinski and M O'Neil, Logic engineering for knowledge engineering: The Oxford System of Medicine, Artificial Intelligence in Medicine 2 (1990), 323-339.

10 Tu S W, Kahn M G, Musen M A, Ferguson J C, Shortliffe E H, Fagan L M. Episodic Skeletal-Plan Refinement Based on Temporal Data, Communications of the ACM 32(12) (1989), 1439-1455.

11 Shortliffe E H, Scott A C, Bischoff M B, Campbell A B, Van Melle W, Jacobs C D, Oncocin: An expert system for oncology protocol management. Proceedings of IJJCAI,81, Vol 1, 876-881 (1981).

12 The Common Basic Specification Generic Model, 3 vols. NHS Information Management Centre. Birmingham, UK, 1992.

13 The clinical view of the Common Basic Specification: the COSMOS project clinical process model version 2.0. NHS Information Management Centre. Birmingham, UK, 1993.

14 J Huang, J Fox, C Gordon, A Jackson-Smale. Symbolic Decision Support in Medical Care. To appear in an issue of Artificial Intelligence in Medicine devoted to logic programming in October 1993.

Artificial Intelligence in Medecine
S. Andreassen et al. , Eds.
IOS Press, 1993

Generic GP-guidelines and reasoning

W.P.A. Beckers[a], P.F. de Vries Robbé[a], P.E. Zanstra[a], A.M. Zwaard[b]

[a]Medical Informatics and Epidemiology, University of Nijmegen, POBox 9101, NL 6500 HB Nijmegen, The Netherlands

[b]Centre for Quality Assurance Research, Department of Family Practice, University of Nijmegen, POBox 9101, NL 6500 HB Nijmegen, The Netherlands

Abstract

In The Netherlands guidelines for General Practitioners (GPs) have been developed to meet the needs of quality assurance and expertise improvement. The development of the decision support program RAP to promote dissemination and implementation of these guidelines in general practice was facilitated by the uniform concept behind these guidelines. Definition of different reasoning methods using that uniform concept was simplified and the reasoning methods became highly transparent for system developers and -users.

In previous papers the emphasis was on the evaluation of the program. This paper focuses on the reasoning strategies.

1. DUTCH COLLEGE OF GP'S GUIDELINES POLICY

In Primary Health Care in The Netherlands the need for quality assurance and expertise improvement led in 1988 to the development of national guidelines for Primary Health Care (PHC). [1] The policy of the Dutch College of General Practitioners (NHG) is to standardize GPs medical action-taking using guidelines for so-called prototypical situations (=patient problems). These guidelines are developed through consensus meetings by expert GPs and are based on the scientific literature for the specific topics. The guidelines are to be seen as practical tools for use in daily general practice. The NHG has identified 50 prototypical situations and diseases for which to develop guidelines. So far 30 standards have been published.

The NHG-guidelines prescribe the medical procedure which has to be carried out in the standard patientcase and they do not allow for individual deviations. They are strictly meant to describe the best common procedure for the relevant prototype situation. [2] In that sense these guidelines should, because of their intended (in)flexibility, be characterized as standards. [3]

Dissemination and local implementation of these standards can be improved if they are embedded in a broader program that addresses the need for interpretation and implementation. [4] Quality assurance and expertise will benefit from immediate feedback in practice, especially where this feedback supports the individual practice procedures of GPs. [5]

2. DISSEMINATION AND IMPLEMENTATION OF GP-STANDARDS

To facilitate dissemination and implementation of these standards a project - the Guidelines Automation Project - was started to develop a computer program named RAP. RAP was intended to support quality assurance of medical action-taking in PHC on the basis of the NHG-standards. [6]

RAP provides two functions:

- evaluation and assessment:
  - GPs submit their patient-related actions, and then receive feedback on the correctness of those actions;
  - assessment of GPs in continuing medical education: the program makes comparison between trainees in general practice possible;
- continuing medical education:
  - transfer of standards on the basis of relevant casuistry.

Evaluation of the RAP program has shown that:

- its structure, unambiguity and user-friendliness have provided very satisfactory;
- although the format of the feedback was at first sight complicated, users rapidly got used to it;
- individual well-reasoned deviation from the standards cannot be supported by the program (this of course does not mean that such deviations are not allowed in practice!);
- computerized assessment is a convenient method to become acquaint with the NHG-standards and to encourage their use. [7]

3. GENERIC FORMAT OF NHG-STANDARDS

The procedure for taking medical action in all NHG-standards is based on the consultation-process in General Practice. Analysis of the current NHG-standards showed that they all comprised five parts: history-taking, examination, evaluation, course of action and providing patientinformation. This mirrors the normal structure of a consultation. All five parts can contain sub-parts, i.e. part-hierarchies. History-taking- and examination-hierarchies have as end-points the possible results or values of specific history/examination-items. Evaluation-, course of action- and patient-education-hierarchies end with specific sub-parts.

History-taking, examination and patient-education tasks were either obligatory or conditional. Evaluation and course of action components always appeared to be conditional. The following model appears to represent the textual NHG-standards:

```
NHG-standard
      ├─history
      │  └─specific question
      │     └─result
      ├─examination
      │  └─specific examination
      │     └─result
      ├─evaluation
      │  └─specific evaluation
      ├─course of action
      │  └─specific course of action
      └─patient education
         └─specific patient education
```

Fig. 1: Abstraction of a typical NHG-standard format

which can be condensed to the following generic format:

```
NHG-standard
          ▲
          └─part of standard (phase)◄──┐
              ▲                         │  (condition)
              └─possible result─────────┘
```

Fig. 2: Generic format of a typical NHG-standard

This generic format formed the basis for representing NHG-standards in a knowledge based system using a developmentkit for knowledge based decision support systems.

4. DEVELOPMENT OF THE RAP-PROGRAM

The RAP-program was implemented in the Relation Oriented Inference System (ROIS). The ROIS tool consists of three layers: a basic network engine, a subshell and a domain. [8] The basic building blocks for the knowledge representation and the primitive inference functions are defined at the system level. The knowledge representation resembles a semantic network. Basic building blocks for this representation are nodes, links, and attributes. Primitive inference functions are used at the level of the subshell to specify the reasoning method. In these methods it is then determined which parts of the semantic network are to be instantiated.

The semantic net represents concepts as nodes, and links between those concepts as labelled directed arcs. [9] The network can be seen as a directed knowledge graph, in the sense that links can have different meanings depending on the directions in which they are traversed. The role of each link in the reasoning process must be explicitly defined. This is done at the level of the subshell where the types of links and nodes that are being used also have to be specified.

For representation of the NHG-standards in a semantic network, a template was constructed on the basis of the former generic format.

```
NHG-standard
          ▲
   KO     │
          │
specific NHG-standard
              ▲
       PO     │
              └─part of standard (phase)◄──┐                 KO = Kind Of
                  ▲                         │                 PO = Part Of
          RO      │                         │  IT             RO = Result Of
                  └─result──────────────────┘                 IT = If . . Then
```

Fig. 3: Template for knowledge representation in domain

5. FACILITIES OF THE RAP-PROGRAM

The RAP-program [6] offers GPs facilities for:

- case creation and case modification
- self-assessment for a single case, accompanied by an explanation

- self-assessment for all cases:
  - for single NHG-standard
  - for multiple NHG-standards
- advice on the best next step in accordance with the relevant NHG-standard.

6. REASONING IN THE RAP-PROGRAM

The generic format formed the basis for the specification of reasoning methods using the primitive inference functions. Determination of the parts of the semantic net that will have to be instantiated were defined using the generic format. This format facilitates definition of the role each link has to play in the reasoning process. [10]

The RAP-program supports the GP with the following reasoning methods (tasks):

- case workup:
  - input of case data (not guided by the NHG-standard)
- self-assessment (single case)
- self-assessment (multiple cases)
  - for one NHG-standard
  - for multiple NHG-standards
- advice
  - advice only
  - input of case data (guided by the NHG-standard).

6.1 Case workup

Case workup involves the following steps:

- choice of standard (if not already in case)
- choice of a consultation phase (eg. history, examination, evaluation, course of action, patient education)
- choice of all possible items (obligatory and conditional).

Case workup stops if all NHG-standard items are completed or if the user stops the input.

This task shows the GP the NHG-standard items plus other actions commonly but mistakenly carried out for the type of patient problem dealt with by that standard. This mode of use is made possible by including both NHG-standard and non-standard actions in the domain knowledge base. Patient data already known are taken into account.

6.2 Self-assessment single case module

For case assessment the particular patient case must be selected. Execution of the Assessment task generates feedback for the selected case by matching the case items with the relevant NHG-standard. Depending on the recommendations stated in the standard, the program determines whether the case items match the prescribed actions and their sequence. Reasoning takes place in two steps:

- collection of all case items
- justification of actions considering the prescribed NHG-standard procedure.

6.2.1 Collection of NHG-standard items from domain and case

- NHG-standard in patient case

a collect all case-items

b obligatory actions

1 determine all obligatory actions from domain

2 determine performed obligatory actions from the case

c conditional actions
 1 determine all conditional actions from domain
 2 determine cond. actions from the domain triggered by all case items
 3 determine performed conditional actions from the case
 4 determine conditions of conditional actions from domain
d determine mistakenly performed actions, from the domain.

6.2.2 Justification of actions considering the prescribed NHG-standard procedure
(Feedback is shown between quotes.)

- standard in question
"I in accordance with the NHG-standard you did"
  - b.2
  - intersection c.2, c.3
"II according to the NHG-standard you should have done"
  - difference b.1, b.2
  - difference c.2, c.3
    - "of which the following are obligatory"
      - difference b.1, b.2
    - "and the following dictated by the conditions present in the case"
      - c.4 belonging to difference c.2, c.3
"III according to the NHG-standard you did superfluously"
  - difference c.3, c.2
  - intersection a, d
    - "because the following conditions are missing in the case"
      - c.4 belonging to difference c.3, c.2
    - "and the following actions do not belong to the standard"
      - intersection a, d

6.2.3 Feedback as shown to the user
An example of the actual feedback as generated by the above described procedure is shown in the next three figures. The user may scroll forwards and backwards through the feedback, which in the example shown occupies three screens.
Assessment of a single case starts with selection of the case. The assessment process then matches the case items - and the sequence in which they occur - with the contents of the NHG-standard. A sample of the feedback output by RAP is shown in figures 4-6.

```
File Case Advice Options Help  Consultant 2.11

Assessment
THE STANDARD IN QUESTION
   NHG-standard diabetes mellitus type II

A. IN ACCORDANCE WITH THE STANDARD YOU DID
         history
          ├well being ?
          ├physical complaints ?
          ├weight ?
          ├diet problems ?
          ├medication problems ?
          └enough exercise ?
         examination
          ├Quetelet's rule
          └blood glucose

B. ACCORDING TO THE STANDARD YOU SHOULD
   HAVE DONE
         examination
          └Quetelet's rule > 6 months
         course of action
          ├referral to dietician
                                            Advice
```

Figure 4: Feedback as result of the task 'Assessment' (first screen)

```
File Case Advice Options Help  Consultant 2.11

         ├continue current diet therapy
         └follow-up appointment 3 months
        patient information
         ├inform about DM type II, ther,ass
         ├advise for foot hygiene
         └possibility of self control

 B.1 OF WHICH THE FOLLOWING ARE OBLIGATORY
        Quetelet's rule > 6 months
        follow-up appointment 3 months
        inform about DM type II, ther, ass.
        advise for foot hygiene
        possibility of self control

 B.2 AND THE FOLLOWING DICTATED BY CONDI-
     TIONS IN THE PRESENT CASE
        referral to dietician
         └diet problems: yes
        continue current diet therapy
         ├Quetelet's rule: < 25
         └blood glucose (fasting): < 6,7
                                        Advice
```

Figure 5: Feedback as a result of the task 'Assessment' (second screen).

```
File Case Advice Options Help  Consultant 2.11

C. ACCORDING TO THE NHG-STANDARD YOU DID
   SUPERFLUOUSLY
      history
       ├micturation frequency
       └polydipsia ?
      examination
       └glucosuria screening
      course of action
       └advise for exercise and sport

    C.1 BECAUSE THE FOLLOWING CONDITIONS ARE
        MISSING IN THE CASE
             advise for exercise and sport
              ├enough exercise: no
              └Quetelet's rule: > 27

    C.2 AND THE FOLLOWING ACTIONS DID NOT
        BELONG TO THE STANDARD
             micturation frequency ?
             polydipsia ?
             glucosuria screening
                                        Advice
```

Figure 6: Feedback as result of the task 'Assessment' (third screen).

6.3 Self-assessment all cases one standard module

Self-assessment of all patient cases concerning one NHG-standard needs aggregation of the assessment results of all those cases. This task searches the case database for all cases that match the chosen NHG-standard and aggregates all feedback items. Feedback here informs the GP about his action-taking for all concerning cases, which means an overall view as opposed to the 'individual assessment' concerning one single case. As the feedback is aggregated, RAP cannot give any explanation of the assessment results.

Reasoning here takes place in two steps:

- collection of all case items for all patient cases belonging to the chosen NHG-standard
- justification of actions considering the prescribed NHG-standard procedure.

6.3.1 Collection of NHG-standard items from domain and cases

- select an NHG-standard
- compare NHG-standard with first patient case
  if they match continue, otherwise go to next case, etc.

a collect all case items
b obligatory actions
  1 determine all obligatory actions from the domain
  2 determine performed obligatory actions in each case
c conditional actions
  1 determine all conditional actions from the domain
  2 determine cond. actions from the domain triggered by all case items
  3 determine performed conditional actions from the case
d determine mistakenly performed actions from the domain.

6.3.2 Justification of medical actions

(Feedback is shown between quotes.)

- standard in question {nr. of cases}

"I actions according to the standard"
  - b.2 {nr. per specific action}
  - intersection c.2, c.3 {nr. per specific action}

"II actions that should have been done"
- difference b.1, b.2 {nr. per specific action}
- difference c.2, c.3 {nr. per specific action}

"III superfluous actions that have been done"
- difference c.3, c.2 {nr. per specific action}

"IV actions that don't belong to the standard"
- intersection a, d {nr. per specific action}

Repeat until case-file doesn't contain cases of the concerning standard. If action already in I, II, III and IV: add one up, if not: add action.

This feedback is shown when the whole database has been searched for matching patient cases.

6.4 Self-assessment multiple cases, multiple standards module

Self-assessment of patient cases involving multiple NHG-standards needs aggregation of the assessment results of all those cases. This task searches the case database for all matching patient cases and aggregates all feedback items. As specific actions differ from standard to standard, feedback only concerns the respective consultation phases, for example 'history', in which these actions were performed.

Reasoning here takes place in two steps:
- collection of all case items for those patient cases belonging to the chosen NHG-standards
- justification of actions considering the prescribed NHG-standard procedures.

6.4.1 Collection items from domain and cases
- select NHG-standards
- compare NHG-standard to first patient case
  if latter matches former continue, otherwise go to next case, etc.

a collect all case items

b obligatory actions
  1 determine all obligatory actions from the domain
  2 determine performed obligatory actions from the case

c conditional actions
  1 determine all conditional actions from the domain
  2 determine cond. actions from the domain triggered by all case items
  3 determine performed conditional actions from case

d determine mistakenly performed actions, from the domain.

6.4.2 Justification of medical actions
(Feedback is shown between quotes.)

- standard in question {nr. of cases}

"I in accordance with standard"
- consultation phase of b.2 {nr. actions per phase}
- consultation phase of intersection c.2, c.3 {nr. actions per phase}

"II should have done according the standard"
- consultation phase of difference b.1, b.2 {nr. actions per phase}
- consultation phase of difference c.2, c.3 {nr. actions per phase}

"III done superfluously"
- consultation phase of difference c.3, c.2 {nr. actions per phase}

"IV not belonging to the standard"
- intersection a, d {nr. per specific action}.

Repeat until case-file doesn't contain cases relevant to the standard concerned. If action already in I, II, III and IV add one up; if not add action.

This feedback is shown when the whole database has been searched for matching patient cases.

6.5 Advice module

For advice concerning a case the particular patient case must be selected. Execution of this task generates advice about which actions must be undertaken at the present stage of the consultation. Depending on the recommendations stated in the standard, the program determines which prescribed actions are appropriate now. Reasoning again takes place in two steps:
- collection of all case items
- determination of actions according to the prescribed NHG-standard procedure.

6.5.1 Collection items from domain and case

- NHG-standard in patient case
  if not in case select a NHG-standard

a collect all case-items

b obligatory actions
  1 determine all obligatory actions from the domain
  2 determine performed obligatory actions from case

c conditional actions
  1 determine cond. actions from the domain triggered by all case items
  2 determine performed conditional actions from the case
  3 determine conditions of conditional actions from the domain.

6.5.2 Determination of medical actions

(Feedback is shown between quotes.)

- "the following actions must be done"
  - difference b.1, b.2
  - difference c.1, c.2
    - "from which the following are obligatory"
      - difference b.1, b.2
    - "and the remainder should have been done according to the known data in this particular case"
      - c.3 belonging to difference c.1, c.2).

7. CONCLUSION

As demonstrated in section 6 the reasoning process can be declared in terms of 'spreading activation' followed by 'set operations' on the network. Although we still do not have a formalism to construct and reason about protocols, this work represents an important step towards establishing a common model for protocols, at least in general practice.

All the published NHG-standards embody the same abstract description of the consultation process. This description could be conceptualized in a generic format, representing the concept underlying all these standards. The generic format resembles a template: it was used to guide domain building (not described further in this paper), and also provided a basis for defining reasoning methods that are valid for all NHG-standards. As the RAP-program was initially developed as an assessment tool, the generic format and the convenient procedural inference functions of ROIS both facilitated the additional development of reasoning methods, such as Advice.

Both domain building and defining of reasoning methods, benefit from this generic format. Although definition of reasoning methods in the current version of ROIS still is more complicated than we would like it to be, the concept of each reasoning method is highly transparent to developers and users of DSS-programs that use semantic networks as formalism.

8. REFERENCES

1 Grol, R.P.T.M. (1990). National standard setting for quality of care in general practice: attitudes of general practitioners and response to a set of standards. British Journal of General Practice, No. 40, pp. 361-364.

2 Zwaard, A.M., Mokkink, H.G.A., Hofstra, M., Grol, R.P.T.M., Tielens, V. (1991). Interim-rapportage: Ondersteuning van kwaliteitsbewaking voor het medisch handelen (in Dutch) (interim-report: Support in quality assurance for medical action-taking). Nijmegen: Nijmeegs Universitair Huisartsen Instituut.

3 Eddy, D.M. (1990). Designing a practice policy: Standards, Guidelines, and Options. JAMA, Vol. 263, No. 232, pp. 3077-3084.

4 Lomas, J., Anderson, G.M., Domnick-Pierre, K., Vayda, E., Enkin, M.W., Hannah, W.J. (1989). Do practice guidelines guide practice? The effect of consensus statement on thc practice of physicians. The New England Journal of Medicine, Vol. 321, No. 19, pp. 1306-1311.

5 Sheldon, M. (1983). Micr9ocomputers in medical audit and continuing education. Update, No. 26, pp. 463-469.

6 Beckers, W.P.A., Vries Robbé, P.F. de, Haring, E.J. van der, Zwaard, A.M., Mokkink, H.G.A., Grol, R.P.T.M. (1991). Automation of medical audit in general practice. In: Stefanelli, M., Hasman, A., Fieschi, M., Talmon, J.L. (Eds.), Proceedings of the Third Conference on Artificial Intelligence in Medicine 91. Berlin: Springer Verlag. Lecture Notes in Medical Informatics, No. 44, pp. 129-139.

7 Beckers, W.P.A., Vries Robbé, P.F. de, Zanstra, P.E., Zwaard, A.M. (1992) Self-assessment in general practice. In: Lun., K.C., Degoulet, P., Piemme, T.E., Rienhoff, E. (Eds.), Proceedings Medinfo 92. Amsterdam: North-Holland.

8 Vries Robbé, P.F. de, Zanstra, P.E., Beckers, W.P.A. (1989). The MEDES subshell: towards an open architecture for decision support systems. Talmon, J.L., Fox, J. (Eds.), Proceedings of the workshop "systyem engineering in medicine" 89. Berlin: Springer Verlag. Lecture Notes in Medical Informatics, No. 47, pp. 106-114.

9 Charniak, E., McDermott, D. (1985). Introduction to artificial intelligence. Reading: Addison-Wesley.

10 Vrics Robbé, P.F. de, Zanstra, P.E., Hartkamp, S.F., Beckers, W.P.A. (1989). MEDES as a tool for different reasoning strategies. Hunter, J., Cookson, J., Wyatt, J. (Eds.), Proceedings of the Second European Conference on Artificial Intelligence in Medicine 89. Berlin: Springer Verlag. Lecture Notes in Medical Informatics, No. 38, pp. 308-314.

Artificial Intelligence in Medecine
S. Andreassen et al. , Eds.
IOS Press, 1993

Sharing and reusing therapeutic knowledge for managing leukemic children

Silvana Quaglini[a], Riccardo Bellazzi[a], Mario Stefanelli[a], Franco Locatelli[b],
[a]*Dpt. Informatica e Sistemistica - Università di Pavia, 27100 Pavia, Italy*
[b]*Clinica Pediatrica - IRCCS Policlinico S. Matteo, Pavia, Italy*

Abstract

Managing complex medical problems requires the ability to execute different medical tasks: diagnosis, therapy planning and monitoring. Moreover, therapeutic plans have to be modified several times along the patient's progress according to his/her conditions. In this paper we propose a method useful both for representing the management knowledge and for individuating pieces of knowledge that can be shared and reused in a knowledge based system. The methodology is illustrated by using a challenging clinical example: the management of leukemic children.

1 Introduction

Therapeutic planning may be required at different times along the patient's progress. Therapeutic actions are sometimes well-codified according to patient's conditions, but, more often, they involve trade-offs. In the latter case, taking a decision, often imply evaluating, more or less precisely, possible outcomes of subsequent decisions. The amount of a patient's data is increasing during his/her clinical course and, for this reason, early decisions have to be taken with *limited* information, as compared to the information needed to solve the whole problem. Nevertheless, differently from data, the *structure* of decisional problems can be defined and assessed from the beginning. The consequence is that the same pieces of therapeutic knowledge may be *shared and/or reused* at different levels of specialization. The concepts of *sharing and reusing* are well defined by a recent paper of Mark Musen [1]. We propose slightly different definitions:

As *knowledge sharing* we intend the use of the same inference model and medical entities, with different knowledge roles, if required, across different tasks; for example a certain disease may be a hypothesis to be tested within the diagnostic task, or it may be an already inferred abstract problem feature within the therapeutic task.

As *knowledge reuse* we intend the utilization of the same piece of knowledge in different contexts or tasks; for example a set of production rules may be used to generate abstractions useful for both therapy planning and diagnosis, or a certain therapeutic decision may be faced several times, in dependence of the patient's clinical course, so that the same Influence Diagram may be exploited repetitively, with different variable instatiations.

The goals of the present work are the following:

1. to propose a method for representing management knowledge, that is to define in an explicit way when a task, diagnosis or therapy planning, has to be executed;

2. to illustrate how a piece of knowledge can be shared and reused within the same system.

These concepts are illustrated through a real-world example, namely the treatment of patients with Acute Myeloid Leukemia (AML).

2 The clinical problem

AML in childhood represents a heterogeneous group of diseases, classified according to French-American-British criteria (FAB) into 7 groups (M1 to M7) [2], and accounting for approximately 20% of acute leukemias in childhood. At present, treatment strategy could be allogeneic Bone Marrow Transplantation (BMT) and chemotherapy. BMT can undoubtely be a curative procedure, but can be followed by severe long term effects, especially in children, where the growing organism is particularly vulnerable to the consequences of chemo-radiotherapy, used as BMT conditioning regimen, and graft-versus-host-disease (GVHD), which represents a peculiar life threatening event of marrow transplant. The acute form (A-GVHD) affects outcome and event-free survival at least as frequently as any other complication [3]. Nevertheless, the reaction of donor cells against recipient may also affect leukemia cells. In fact, an immune-mediated anti-leukemia effect of GVHD, named Graft versus Leukemia (GVL), is reported. This indicates that GVHD may be determinant for the success of BMT [4]. However, in patients where a benefit could derive from GVL, namely poor prognosis leukemic patients, it is important to avoid severity of the complication, that could be fatal. According to severity, GVHD is classified into four degrees. Only I and II grade GVHD are associated with a significant advantage in terms of event-free survival in the above described situation. Patients given BMT generally need some kind of A-GVHD prophylaxis. The chronic form of GVHD (occurring about 100 days after BMT) is also well known, and it can follow A-GVHD, with or without a disease-free interval, or in a third of cases it can present *de novo.*

GVHD physiopathology has not yet been completely understood and both occurrence and severity cannot be surely predicted.

In addition to GVHD and long term side effects, affecting the quality of life of survivors, the BMT option must take into account the low risk of graft failure (1-2% of cases). Therefore, it is a fundamental axiom in pediatric oncology to apply allogeneic BMT only when conventional, more riskless procedures based on chemotherapy have been proven to be inferior.

3 Management Knowledge Representation Issues

Managing *AML* patients requires the execution of different fundamental medical tasks, such as diagnosis, therapy planning and monitoring. Each of them can be executed by knowledge-based-systems (KBS) where an inference model exploit domain knowledge, organized according to a well-defined ontology [5].

The *ontology* represents the conceptual model of entities and relationships structuring the knowledge in the application domain. The most specialized and domain oriented part of the ontology describes the features typical of the problem at hand. The ontology is *shared* among the different tasks.

The *inference model* is the conceptual description of the operations to be made over the ontology to solve a problem. The inference model we adopt is domain and task independent.

Moreover, this inference model may be broken down into two different phases: first, initial information is employed to *select* plausible hypotheses, and then these hypotheses are used as starting conditions to forecast expected consequences that should be matched with the state of affairs in the patient in order to confirm or falsify those hypotheses from which they come. This model of medical reasoning has been called *Select and Test Model* (ST-Model) [5].

From a computational point of view, each task can be implemented through a *Blackboard Control Architecture* [6], that uses different *knowledge sources* to execute the successive inference steps as defined in the ST-Model. These knowledge sources may be represented using different formalisms, such as frames, production rules, and Influence Diagrams. The knowledge sources may be *reused* by the different tasks.

4 The Task Planning Diagram

The problems encountered by a physician in the management of patients with AML are represented in Fig. 1: it illustrates which tasks have to be executed along all the possible clinical courses of a given patient, following the two possible therapies and the main BMT side effect, namely GVHD. Thus, this diagram does not cover all possible therapeutic problems of a AML patient, but only a portion of them. On the other hand, it can be outlined that this diagram holds for any type of leukemia, only the knowledge sources being disease-tailored.

Circles represent possible *patient's clinical states*, while diamonds represent *therapeutic actions*; arcs denote *transitions among states*. Two types of transitions can be defined, precisely *free transitions*, denoted by arcs connecting directly two states, and *action-driven transitions*, denoted by arcs passing through a diamond node. For example, when a patient is in the clinical state defined as AML, three transitions may occur: one of them is *free* and leads to death (in other words, if no action is undertaken, the patient will die); the other ones are action-driven, where possible actions are chemotherapy or BMT, possibly leading to different remission states. If therapy fails, no transition occurs, and patient sojourns in the AML state. As a matter of fact, the result of an action is not certain, so many arcs are in general leaving a diamond node.

If we interpret this diagram as a pictorial representation of a KBS for patient management, involving different diagnostic and/or therapeutic tasks to be performed, it can be called *task planning diagram*.

Patient management problem solving can be in one of the indicated states, according

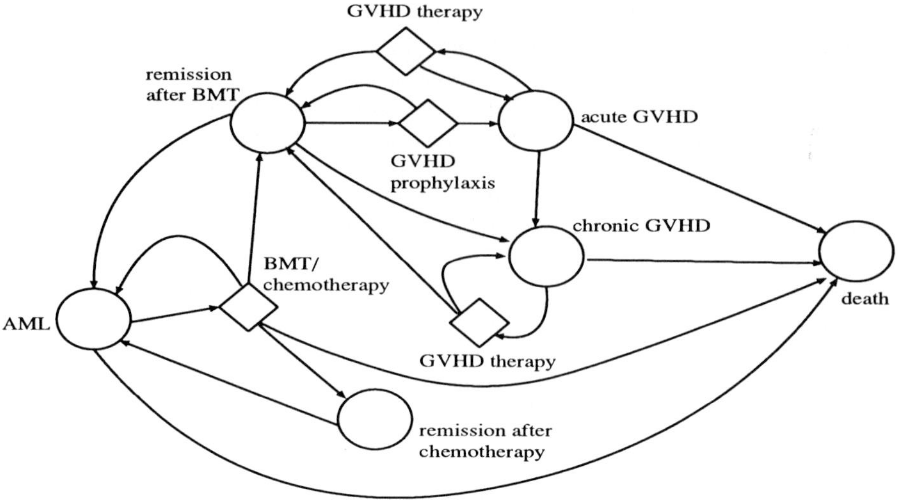

Figure 1: The task planning diagram.

to the patient's clinical time course. For each current state, and according to patient's past history and actual context, one or more *goal states* do exist, and the aim of the therapeutic tasks is to reach them (for example, when the current state is *acute GVHD* the goal state is *remission/BMT*). A therapeutic task may require to *choose among competitive therapies*, or to establish a *drug dosage*: the decision may result in different subsequent clinical states, or simply modify the probability of reaching the same clinical state.

For example, when AML has been diagnosed, BMT and chemotherapy are competitive choices: once a decision has been taken, the future of the patient is described by different portions of the graph. On the contrary, just after BMT the only possible action is the GVHD prophylaxis, that is basically a matter of drug dosage assessment and that modify the probability of GVHD development. Particularly, such a task requires to establish dosages of two drugs, Cyclosporine (Cs-A) and metothrexate (MTX), to avoid GVHD or to induce GVL.

When an action leads to different subsequent paths, it must take into account the complete future progression of the patient. Thus a single choice may need to take into account multiple decision problems, and a large number of different paths.

The diagram above introduced is both an instrument for the physician to clarify the possible epochs of the patient's disease and the basis for a system able to present automatically the successive decision problems that an 'intelligent manager' has to cope with.

The task planning diagram may share medical entities and provides a comprehensive view of the whole management problem. From the implementation point of view, it can be thought as a set of metarules which activate, in turn, diagnostic or therapeutic tasks:

each of these is represented by a suitable instantiation of the ST-Model. For example, an S-T model will perform the diagnostic task of individuating a relapse condition, another will choose the therapy for the A-GVHD.

In other words, the task planning diagram is used to select the succession of the tasks to be performed in the patient management. Moreover, it explicitly clarifies that, when solving a task, a system must take into account also the tasks that could have to be analyzed in the future. The 'long-term' perspective allowed by the task planning diagram, enables the system manager to easily understand which tasks could share and/or reuse a set of knowledge sources.

For example, from the task planning diagram of Fig. 1, it is clear that the therapy choice between BMT and chemotherapy must take into account the outcomes of the possible future A-GVHD prophylaxis. This imply that the knowledge sources related to A-GVHD prophylaxis will be use a first time when deciding the primary therapy and will be re-used if a patient will be transplanted, in order to decide the A-GVHD prophylaxis on the basis of the patient's data after BMT. It is clear that the results from the same knowledge source will be in general different, depending on the time of its use, because the amount of patient's data is changing in time.

In the following we will show how to share and to reuse therapeutic knowledge sources during AML patients management.

4.1 Managing AML patients

Referring to Fig. 1, let us suppose that the first diagnostic task inferred the diagnosis of *AML*. The diagram shows that a therapeutic choice has to be done between the two actions BMT and chemotherapy. This activates an S-T model for therapy planning. As widely described in [6], the first inference step of a therapy planner consists in defining data abstractions called *therapeutic problems*. In the AML case, three different therapeutic problems can be defined, as the basis for subsequent therapy choice: low, medium, and high risk of relapse. Simple rules perform such abstractions, as in the following examples:

rule 1

```
IF AML-type = M4 AND (White Blood Cells < 200.000 OR hypereosinophylia)
THEN risk of relapse = medium
```

rule2

```
IF AML-type = M1
THEN IF presence of auer rods OR trisomy 8
        THEN risk of relapse = medium
        ELSE IF White Blood Cells > 200.000
              THEN risk of relapse = high
```

In the cases of low and high risk of relapse, the decision is straightforward: *chemotherapy* for the former, and *BMT* for the latter. On the contrary, for medium risk patients, there is no clear indication in favour of one of the two choices. The decision requires a

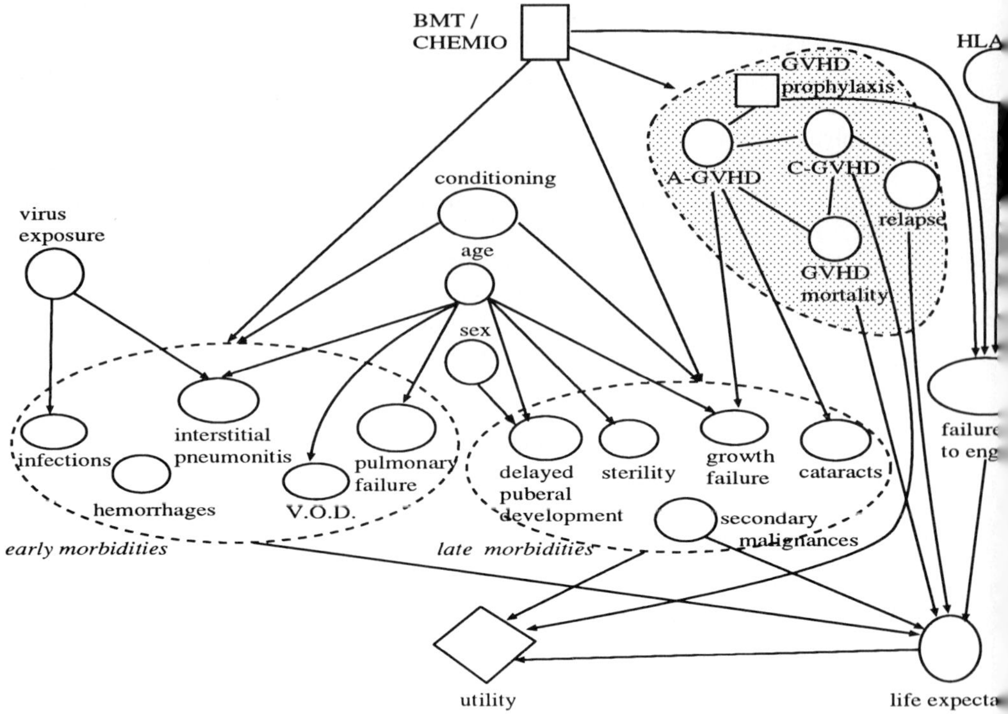

Figure 2: The ID for choosing between BMT and chemotherapy. The shaded area represents a *special node* (see text). An arc pointing to a dotted circle is intended to point to all included nodes.

more complex analysis, involving uncertain outcomes and trade-offs. The suitable formalism to cope with this problem is that of *influence diagram (ID)* [7, 8]. The proposed ID is reported in Fig. 2, and it will be referred to as *BMT/CHEMO ID*.

The BMT/CHEMO ID

Choosing between BMT and chemotherapy is difficult because of the following uncertain outcomes:

1. as previously mentioned, the major complication of BMT is A-GVHD, whose probability of occurrence and severity is modulated by the prophylaxis. In addition A-GVHD is a risk factor for the development of chronic GVHD;

2. BMT may fail to engraft, depending also on GVHD prophylaxis;

3. the probability of relapse depends in general from the disease status and donor/patient match, and it is reduced by the beneficial GVL effect in case of BMT;

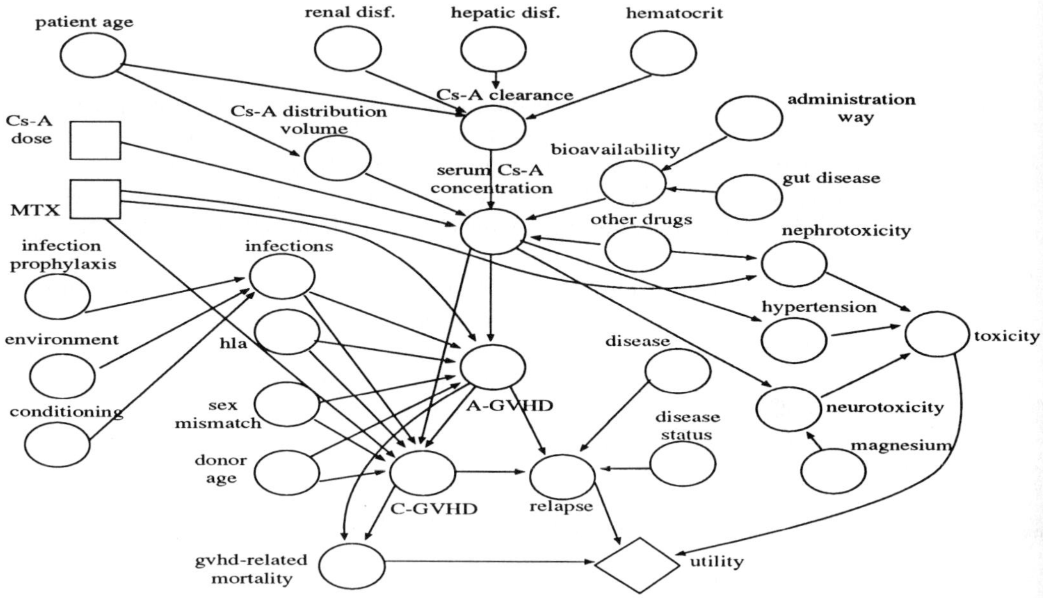

Figure 3: The ID for choosing A-GVHD prophylaxis.

4. both therapies may involve early and late morbidities. All of them, with the exception of chronic GVHD, are common to BMT and chemotherapy, although with different conditional probabilities. Each morbidity may have specific risk factors (for example *sex* and *age* for *delayed puberal development*);

5. the life expectancy is mainly affected by the probability of relapse (for both therapies) and failure to engraft (in the case of BMT), but also by morbidity occurrence;

6. finally, the utility is expressed in terms of both quantity and quality of life, considering this latter affected by late morbidities.

As it is clearly shown in Fig. 1, and also explicitly reported in the *BMT/CHEMO ID*, solving the decisional problem between BMT and Chemotherapy, involves a guess about A-GVHD prophylaxis and an estimate of the probability of A-GVHD occurrence and leukemia relapse. But, deciding this prophylaxis is itself a complex task. This is the meaning of the shaded area grouping these three nodes in Fig. 2. We choose the *ID* formalism also to represent this second decisional problem, as shown in Fig. 3. In the following we will refer to it as *A-GVHD ID.*

The A-GVHD ID

Three main subproblems are involved in A-GVHD prophylaxis [3]. The first one deals with the determination of the appropriate dosage of Cs-A, in order to reach a therapeutic range of drug serum concentration. As regards Cs-A, a number of factors influence its clearance and distribution volume, particularly age, renal and/or hepatic disfunctions and hematocrit. In addition, bioavailability and interaction with other drugs affect serum concentration. A second problem concerns avoiding too severe side effects, mainly nephrotoxicity, neurotoxicity and hypertension. The third problem consists in forecasting GVHD development and severity, starting from prophylaxis, compatibility between patient and donor, and a number of context variables, such as patient's conditioning regimen and isolation procedure (evironment). Finally, on the basis of the prognosis, physician has to judge the opportunity of avoiding or inducing A-GVHD, and this involves the setting up of a utility model. In fact, there is low utility of developing A-GVHD in standard risk leukemic patients and high utility in patients with more advanced neoplastic disease, due to the GVL effect mentioned above.

The methods used for quantification and evaluation of the *A-GVHD ID* are extensively described in [9], where the ID performance is also presented. In summary, the predictive accuracy is about 80% on a data base of 50 patients (see Table 1), and the ID has been shown to be a useful tool for reasoning about real cases, by means of sensitivity analysis and result explanation facilities.

Table 1 - The performance of the A-GVHD ID

	GVHD development (50 cases)		
system prediction	No (25)	grade I-II (16)	grade III-IV (9)
No	23	4	1
grade I-II	1	11	2
grade III-IV	1	1	6

Reusing the GVHD-ID

As mentioned before, the problem related to A-GVHD may have to be faced in two different moments: when AML is diagnosed, to decide among BMT and Chemotherapy (because the A-GVHD prpphylaxis problem belongs to the path following BMT decision), and when the patient is in remission after BMT, in order to actually prevent or to induce mild A-GVHD.

More precisely, when the decisional process starts (just after the diagnosis of leukemia), specific data, such as those related to donor, or patient's condition at the transplant moment, are not available yet. Nevertheless, the physician, more ol less explicitely, takes into account the possibility of a future GVHD prophylaxis and its outcomes. Normally, he/she derives an estimate about the type of prophylaxis and the probability of GVHD development by considering *mean values* from both personal experience and reported data. However, given that a knowledge source exists, the *A-GVHD ID*, able to predict GVHD development and, consequently, to choose prophylaxis, a convenient procedure would consist in evaluating that ID, even with limited amount of data. Results obtained will anyway represent the best possible decision, on the basis of decision theory: in the worst hypothesis, when no data at all are available, given that nodes representing patient's data are given prior probabilities that reflect population characteristics, the

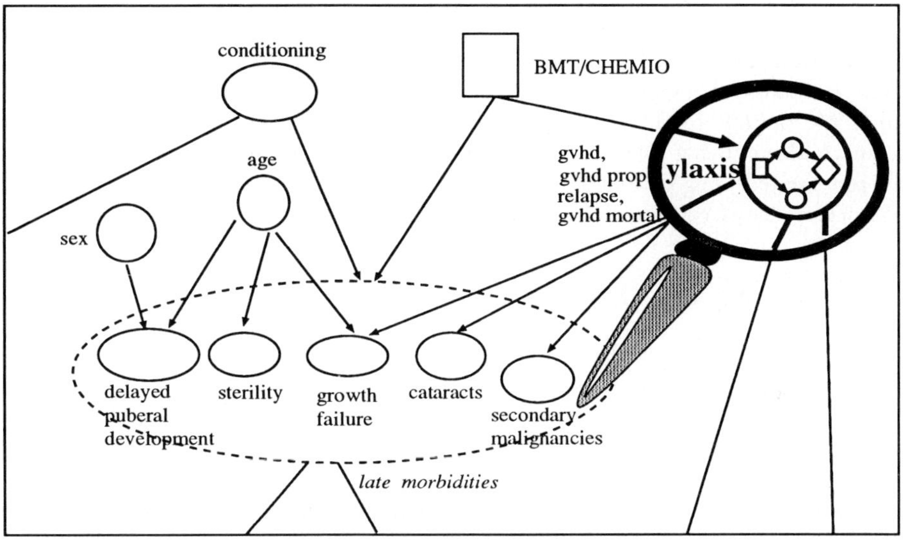

Figure 4: Showing nested decision problems. A special node is quantified by solving another knowledge source.

decision will be the best one for the *generic patient*. More and more data about the specific patient will allow the decision to be more and more patient tailored.

When the *A-GVHD ID* is used for deciding the GVHD prophylaxis, after BMT, all the patient's and donor's characteristics are known, so the suggested decision will be more reliable.

From these observations, the nodes *A-GVHD prophylaxis*, *A-GVHD*, and *Relapse* in the *BMT/ CHEMO ID* can be viewed as a part of a *special node*, hidding a further *decisional problem*, somewhere already described. The undirected link between these nodes mean that their true conditional dependences are shown only within the representation of the hidden decisional problem.

Fig. 4 is a pictorial representation of this concept. How IDs containing special nodes can be quantified? Normally, each ID's node is given a prior or conditional probability; moreover, when the ID is to be evaluated, available patient's data are used to instantiate nodes representing patient's characteristics. Moreover, each node is given a prior or conditional probability. Obviously, if an ID embeds special nodes, performing these quantifications will be more complicated. In fact, a special node must call the associated knowledge source, that will provide either a value or a conditional probability for the nodes composing it. After these computations, these nodes become conditionally independent.

For example, when solving the *BMT/CHEMIO ID*, the evaluation of the special node (and hence the *A-GVHD ID*) gives the probability distribution of *A-GVHD* and *relapse* and the value of *GVHD prophylaxis*.

This is an example of knowledge reuse. As a matter of fact, the same knowledge source is reused by different tasks that are progressively executed during the analysis of the patient's life paths. This implies that the same knowledge source will give different conclusions when evaluated in different patient's states.

The remaining therapeutic problems outlined in the task planning diagram are related to the therapy of GVHD (acute and chronic). They do not involve complex decisional problems, being solvable through standard therapeutic protocols. They can be easily represented using production rules where therapeutic actions are chosen according to the occurrence of certain clinical conditions.

5 Running the System

This section illustrates how the system could work on a real case. Particularly we are going to examine a limited life portion of a patient whose state is diagnosed as AML. Thus the patient 'enters' the task planning diagram of Fig. 1. Let the patient be affected by AML of type M4 with hypereosinophylia. The therapeutic task *leukemia therapy*, i.e. *choice between BMT and chemotherapy* is called. The first inference step is the abstraction performed by the rules as described in section 4.1. These rules check the patient's data, and, in this case, *rule 1* asserts the condition of *medium risk*, that requires a decision analysis. The *BMT/CHEMO ID* is invoked during the deduction-induction step of the ST-model, by a rule of the type:

rule 3

```
IF BMT is a possible therapy AND
    CHEMOTHERAPY is a possible therapy AND
    an ID is associated to BMT AND
    the same ID is associated to BMT
THEN perform ID evaluation
```

This ID, as previously described, embeds a special node, composed by *A-GVHD prophylaxis*, *A-GVHD*, *C-GVHD*, *GVHD-related mortality* and *relapse*: the best possible prophylaxis and the consequent probability of GVHD occurrence and mortality and relapse will be obtained by solving the *A-GVHD ID.*

At this time, in our example, the patient's and donor's characteristics considered by the *A-GVHD ID* are only partially known. For example, we cannot infer data about hepatic or renal disfunction, hematocrit, gut disease and magnesium level, because these features may rapidly change and have to be assessed just at the BMT time.

With the available data *conditioning, infection prophylaxis, patient and donor age*, the *A-GVHD ID* gives the following results:

- the best prophylaxis is found to be *Low dose Cs-A* without *MTX*, as shown in Table 2 (data not between parentheses). This result represents the best compromise in order to avoid a too severe GVHD and to induce the GVL effect;

- under the optimal prophylaxis, we found: *p(no occurence of A-GVHD)=0.47, p(grade I-II A-GVHD)=0.31, p(grade III-IV A-GVHD)=0.23, p(C-GVHD)=0.14, p(GVHD-related mortality)=0.035, p(relapse)=0.19.*

Table 2 - Expected utility values of the different prophylaxes, obtained by evaluating the GVHD-ID within the first therapeutic decision and within A-GVHD prophylaxis assessment (data between parentheses)

		Cyclosporine-A dose			
		low	medium	high	very high
Metothrexate	no	0.43 (0.48)	0.37 (0.42)	0.36 (0.41)	0.34 (0.37)
	yes	0.4 (0.47)	0.33 (0.40)	0.32 (0.39)	0.31 (0.35)

The solution of the *A-GVHD ID* allows to quantify the special node: *GVHD prophylaxis* is given the value *Low Cs-A without MTX* while nodes *A-GVHD*, *C-GVHD*, *GVHD-related mortality* and *relapse* are given the probability values reported above. Now the *BMT/CHEMIO ID* can be solved, thus suggesting an option on the basis of the expected quality adjusted life years. The result shows a preference towards BMT, the solution effectively adopted by the physician.

As shown in Fig. 1, after BMT has been performed, the patient can follow one out of three transitions: to death (therapy related mortality is reported from 15 to 40%), to AML because of graft failure, and to remission. The patient we are analysing reached the clinical state *remission after BMT*. In addition to sojourn in this state, she can relapse or develop acute or chronic GVHD. The transition toward A-GVHD is action-driven, through a possible prophylaxis.

A second therapeutic task, associated to the problem of A-GVHD prophylaxis, is called. Its deduction step utilizes, once again, the *A-GVHD ID*. During this second evaluation, the best choice may change with respect to the one previously obtained, because all patient's and donor's findings are now known. In this particular case the choice suggested is the same, although with slightly different probabilities and utilities (shown in Table 2 between parentheses).

6 Discussion

This work represents the first step towards a new method for the design of KBSs, that explicitly takes into account the problem of the whole patient's management. The task planning diagram above proposed is a design tool allowing a change of perspectives in a KBS building, describing both the patient evolution and the task plan to be executed during the patient's follow up. As a matter of fact, this diagram describes the management knowledge necessary to allow the correct succession of the tasks, and suggests what piece of knowledge may be reused during the clinical course of the patient at hand.

In this paper we have focused our attention on sharing and reusing therapeutic knowledge sources during therapeutic tasks solutions, but the method proposed here may be useful for any type of medical task.

Future work on this topic will concentrate on giving to the task planning diagram a well-defined semantics, in order to have an instrument for automatic acquisition of management knowledge.

Last, but not least, the methodology proposed here is applied to a challenging clinical problem, the management of leukemic children. This project, developed in collaboration with the I.R.C.C.S. Policlinico San Matteo of Pavia, is actually involving physicians and computer scientists in order to assess the utility of a decision support in a very complex domain.

Acknowledgments

This work is partially supported by the European Community, through the AIM project 2034 GAMES II - A General Architecture for Medical Expert Systems.

References

[1] Musen MA. Dimensions of Knowledge Sharing and Reuse. Computers and Biomedical Research, 1992, 25:435-467.

[2] Bennet JM, Catovsky D, Daniel MT. Proposed revised criteria for the classification of Acute Myeloid Leukemia. A report of the French-American-British cooperative group. American Internal Medicine 1985, 103:620-625.

[3] Ferrara JLM, Deeg HJ. Graft-versus-host disease. New England Journal of Medicine 1991; 310:667-674.

[4] Atkinson K, Farrely H, Cooley M et al. Human marrow T-cell dose correlates with severity of subsequent acute graft-versus-host disease. Bone Marrow Transplant 1987; 2:51-79.

[5] Ramoni M, Stefanelli M, Magnani L, Barosi G. An epistemological framework for medical knowldge based systems. IEEE Transactions on Systems, Man, and Cybernetics, 1992, 22 (6):1361-1375.

[6] Quaglini S., Bellazzi R., Berzuini C., Stefanelli M., Barosi G. Hybrid knowledge-based systems for therapy planning. Artificial Intelligence in Medicine 4 (1992) 207-226.

[7] Pearl J. Probabilistic Reasoning in Intelligent Systems. Palo Alto (CA):Morgan Kaufmann, 1988.

[8] Oliver RM, Smith JQ, ed. Influence Diagrams, Belief Nets and Decision Analysis. Chicester:John Wiley and Sons, 1990.

[9] Quaglini S, Bellazzi R, Locatelli F, Stefanelli M, Salvaneschi C. An Influence Diagram for Assessing GVHD prophylaxis after Bone Marrow Transplantation in Children. submitted for publication to Medical Decision Making, 1993.

Artificial Intelligence in Medecine
S. Andreassen et al. , Eds.
IOS Press, 1993

A decision support system for test request screening

E.J.L. de Wilde,[a] P. Pop,[b] A. Hasman,[a]

Dept. of Medical Informatics, University of Limburg, P.O.Box 616, 6200 MD Maastricht, The Netherlands[a]
Diagnostic Coordinating Centre, AZM, P. Debyeplein 25, Maastricht, The Netherlands.[b]

In this contribution a computerized feedback system is described that provides GP's feedback about the adequateness of their test requesting behaviour. This system is developed in the framework of the AIM-programme OPENLABS. The requests are stored in a database that is part of the laboratory decision support system. The other part of the decision support system, an expert system, retrieves the request data (including patient data) from the database, screens the requests for adequateness and provides feedback when necessary.

1. INTRODUCTION.

The purpose of this contribution is to present a computerized feedback system as it is developed in Maastricht, the Netherlands. This feedback system provides GP's with information about the adequacy of their test requesting behaviour. At the moment the system is manual. Because the manual feedback system appears to be effective but work intensive a project was started in the framework of the AIM-programme OPENLABS to automate the screening procedure.
First the experience with the manual personal feedback system in Maastricht will be described. Then a prototype of the decision support system that will be used for the delivery of automatic feedback will be presented. The last section contains the conclusions.

2. THE MAASTRICHT APPROACH

The Diagnostic Coordinating Centre (DCC) Maastricht provides personal feedback to about 80 GP's concerning their requesting behaviour as a health care activity since 1985.
The feedback is based on data recorded on the DCC test request form by the GP when he orders tests to be performed in the Academic Hospital Maastricht (AZM). The GP's can order clinical chemistry tests (blood or urine), faeces tests, tests in the area of haematology, serology, virology, bacteriology, etc.
Apart from the test requests the GP adds clinical information about the patient:

o Problems/complaints of the patient
o Results of physical examination
o Possible diagnosis
o Medication
o Reason for request
 * Confirmation of a disease
 * Ruling out of a disease
 * Screening for unclear pathology
 * Monitoring of known disease
 * Check-up
 * For reassurance
 * On patient's request

Twice a year personal feedback concerning their requesting behaviour is provided by the specialist-coordinator of the DCC to the GP's. This feedback concerns a selected month in the preceding half year.
The structured feedback reports contain the following items:

o the number of requests of the GP during one month; a comparison with earlier analyses and with the average of the colleagues in the same periods
o a judgement on the adequateness of the information provided about the patients
o the number of specific tests and the reasons for request
o a discussion both of the requested tests in general and concerning individual patients more specifically
o a number of questions concerning the policy of the GP after receiving results of laboratory investigations, X-ray investigations, etc.
o the question to answer the posed questions and to comment on the feedback.

About 70% of the GP's reacts in writing, via telephone or by visiting the DCC. The GP's usually are positive about the provided feedback.

Since 1985 (start of providing feedback) a decline in the number of requests has been observed. A comparison was made with a similar laboratory elsewhere in the Netherlands [1,2]. Differences in the use of 47 tests were investigated. It could be shown that the number of tests requested per 1000 patients was increasing in the other area. Another study has shown that feedback not only results in a decline of the number of test requests, also their quality increases. The usefulness of a personal feedback system was therefore proven.

3. DECISION SUPPORT SYSTEM.

In the framework of OPENLABS a decision support system is being developed that will automatically screen the test requests coming from GP's. The decision support system consists of a database system and an expert system. The database system was designed for storing incoming request data, related patient data and test results. The data are either entered manually from the request forms or automatically making use of EDI.
The data in the database are accessed by the expert system. This expert system is built

using the in-house developed shell SYMPLEXIS [3]. This is a rule based system using a three-valued logic (the rule's conclusion can be either true, false or unknown). The system allows the use of different types of rules. Although in expert system's jargon a rule is commonly considered to be an 'if-then' directive that is as a whole always a true proposition in our case when we speak of a rule we refer to the rule's conclusion. So the rule COMPLAINTS tells us whether the patient has any complaints. The value of the rule (or of the consequent of the rule in the expert system's jargon) can be true, false or unknown. One type of rule that is most equivalent to 'if-then' rules is the evaluation rule:

```
COMPLAINTS: 'Does the patient have any complaints?'
WEIGHTINCREASE OR WEIGHTLOSS OR...
```

The above rule says: if the patient has increased in weight (WEIGHTINCREASE is true) or the patient has lost weight (WEIGHTLOSS is true) or ... then the patient has complaints (COMPLAINTS is true). We refer to the above rule as rule COMPLAINTS but COMPLAINTS is actually the consequent of the rule. WEIGHTLOSS and WEIGHTINCREASE can be the consequent of other rules.

ASK rules ask questions from the user, who can either answer with 'y', 'n' or '?' (these answers are internally translated into true, false or unknown). In our application the data are directly obtained from the database and not from a user. An example of an ASK rule is the following:

```
WEIGHTINCREASE: 'weight increase'
ASK
THEN FA: WEIGHTLOSS
```

In ASK rules the consequent is determined by the answer of the user. In this example also another feature of SYMPLEXIS is presented. If according to the answer WEIGHTINCREASE is assigned the value true then at the same time WEIGHTLOSS, the value of which in principle can also be determined by another ASK rule, is given the value false. This means that in this case the latter ASK rule does not have to be executed.

Another type of rules are the TEST rules. These rules perform tests on available data:

```
HYPERSCORE: 'score hyperthyroidism'
TEST
  score := 0;
  if t(_PALPITATIONS)      then score := score + 2;
  if ....
  ...
  if score > 15 then                 TEST := TR else
  if (score >= 7) and (score <= 15) then TEST := PO else
  if score < 7 then                  TEST := FA
ENDTEST
```

In this case the TEST rule HYPERSCORE tests through the use of a scoring system whether hyperthyroidism is present, possibly present or absent. In this example PALPITATIONS is another ASK rule that inquires about the presence of palpations. In this example if palpitations are present (the function t is then assigned the value true) the

score will be raised by 2 points. The rule HYPERSCORE is given the value true when the variable TEST is assigned the value true, etc.
The database is implemented using the BTRIEVE record management system. When screening the requests the expert system accesses all new request records sequentially. Since all the data are stored in the request database no ASK rules are used by the expert system. Instead TEST rules are used.
In the case of the above mentioned rule COMPLAINTS for example the rules WEIGHTINCREASE and WEIGHTLOSS are now implemented as TEST rules. In the body of these TEST rules PASCAL or C code is used to check whether the rules WEIGHTINCREASE respectively WEIGHTLOSS are true by inspecting data from the retrieved request record.
At the moment the work agreements and guidelines concerning thyroid disease and allergies that are now used in the manual feedback system are translated into rules.
The results indicate that a representation consisting of rules can be used for screening the test requests. Although the work agreements and guidelines cannot always be directly translated into rules our first experience is that with some additional information it is possible to implement the work agreements in the form of rules.
At the moment a large number of test requests combined with the relevant patient data have been entered into the system in order to be able to evaluate the quality of the screening and the feedback.

4. DISCUSSION.

A more rational requesting behaviour of physicians is important both to enhance the quality of health care and to reduce its costs.
A number of studies evaluated the effects of feedback, educational programs and audits. The results of these studies are equivocal. It can be concluded however that continuous individual feedback can foster a rational requesting behaviour. In the Netherlands a continuous feedback program has been shown to be effective. The feedback was provided twice a year and concerned the requesting behaviour of a selected month from the previous half year. It was deemed essential to provide the feedback on a more regular basis. This can only be achieved when the screening process can be automated. The decision support system described here will serve that purpose.

REFERENCES.

1. P. Pop and R.A.G. Winkens, J. Coll. Gen. Pract. 39 (1989) 507.
2. R.A.G. Winkens, P. Pop, R.P.T.M. Grol, A.D.M. Kester and J.A.Knottnerus, B.M.J. 304 (1992) 1093.
3. J.A. Blom, The SIMPLEXYS experiment; Real time expert systems in patient monitoring, PhD thesis, Technical University Eindhoven, 1990, ISBN 90-9003296-7.

Knowledge Representation - Terminology

Artificial Intelligence in Medecine
S. Andreassen et al. , Eds.
IOS Press, 1993

Interfacing Conceptual Graphs (CG) and the Galen Master Notation (MN) for medical knowledge representation and modelling

Alpay L, Baud R, Rassinoux A-M, Wagner J, Lovis C, Scherrer J-R

Centre d'Informatique Hospitalière, Hôpital Cantonal Universitaire de Genève, 24 Rue Micheli du Crest, 1211 Genève 14, Switzerland

Abstract

At the Hospital of Geneva, conceptual graphs (CG) have been applied successfully to extract and represent semantic information from medical texts. In the context of the European AIM project Galen, the Galen Master Notation (MN) based on a semantic network representation is being developed, and the need to interface the two knowledge representations - the Galen MN and CG - has emerged. This paper reports on a first experiment which shows that the mapping between these two representations is feasible, and on the development of an interface conversion module which enables an automatic translation from one representation to the other. The process of relating these two representation methods brings relevant issues for modelling and representing medical terminology which are also discussed in this paper.

1. THE CONTEXT

The work reported in this paper has been carried out in the context of the AIM (Advanced Informatics in Medicine) project entitled Galen (Generalised Architecture for Languages Encyclopedias and Nomenclatures in Medicine). Its purpose is to establish the foundations for the next generation of coding systems to support integrated clinical information systems. The heart of Galen is a Semantical Encyclopaedia of Terminology (SET). The SET consists of a generative Galen Master Notation (MN), and a Coding Reference (Core) Model for medical terminology formulated in that notation. The SET also contains information modules providing multilingual lexicons, and conversions to and from existing coding systems. The SET is to be encapsulated by an application programming interface to form a general Terminology Server for use by other applications in a client-server environment.

In the Galen project, the work of the Geneva group is focused on the Natural Language Processing (NLP) side [1]. More specifically, one of the modules of the Galen architecture which is being developed at the Hospital of Geneva is the Multilingual Information Module. This module contains a text generator whose purpose is to generate natural language from expressions in the Core Model. The generator is based on the NLP analyser developed at the Hospital of Geneva, and uses information produced by the NLP analyser [2]. The Multilingual Information Module does not work directly on the Galen Master Notation, since it uses the knowledge representation which has been adopted for the NLP work based on conceptual graphs (CG). Hence, in order to comply with the Galen notation, we have investigated its link with the NLP representation based on conceptual graphs and the feasibility to develop automatic tools to interface the two representations.

Figure 1. illustrates the links between the Galen MN, CG and free text which are discussed in this paper, with a special focus on the relationship between the Galen MN and CG (see Figure 6. and Figure 7. as summary examples).

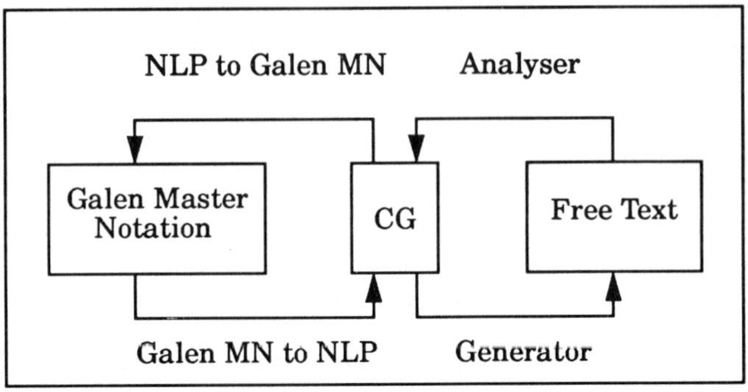

Figure 1. Links between the Galen Master Notation, CG and free text

This paper is organised as follows. The second and third sections briefly introduce CG and the Galen MN respectively. The fourth section presents the initial experiment which was carried out with the Galen Master Notation and discusses the differences and similarities of mapping the two knowledge representations. The next section reports on the development of a prototype to interface CG and the Galen MN. Finally, some interesting implications of this translation process are discussed.

2. CONCEPTUAL GRAPHS

During the past three years, a broad experience with NLP and CG in the field of medicine has been acquired at the Hospital of Geneva [1]. A NLP system [2] which is able to analyse sentences from medical texts written in French and in English has been further developed in the context of the AIM project HELIOS-2 (Hospital Object Software Tools) [3,4]. This original system uses a set of syntactical and semantical procedures which gradually build the semantical representation of the natural language input. Hence, the system uses a two phase process 1) an integrated, syntactical and semantical analysis based on proximity processing rules, and 2) a knowledge representation based on conceptual graphs. This proposed approach is robust in that it allows for irregular structures and medical jargon which are frequently used by physicians. In addition, this method is less dependent on a specific European language because it is principally driven by semantics.

Conceptual graphs as defined by J. Sowa [5], are a means to represent the contents of a text. They constitute, nowadays, a complete model for knowledge representation insofar as they are a generalisation of various previous approaches to the representation of the semantic relationships beween words, such as semantic networks, semantic case grammar, conceptual dependency, frames, scripts and object oriented formalisms. A conceptual graph is a directed graph with two kinds of nodes: a) concept nodes, representing entities, and b) conceptual relationship nodes representing semantic relationships among concepts. A simple graph would be:

[Concept1]-> (Relation) -> [Concept2].

An example of a CG for the phrase 'abdominal pain' is:

[Pain] -> (LOC) -> [Body_Part: abdomen].

A concept is defined by the type and the reference: [<type> : <reference>]. The type specifies the conceptual class of the concept, and the reference an instantiation of that class. When the concept is generic (such as pain), the instantiation is omitted. At present, the NLP system contains about 160 concepts in the hierarchy of concepts, and about 60 relationships.

Knowledge representation in the form of conceptual graphs presents some strong points. CG are grounded on First Order Logic, and they allow a uniform representation insofar as sentences, which convey the same semantics, have a unique representation. Furthermore, this representation is independent of text words, as it is based on the corresponding concepts.

3. THE GALEN MASTER NOTATION

In the framework of the Galen project, the building of a Terminology Server, which is able to conciliate a number of classifications and nomenclatures, requires a powerful knowledge representation schema and accordingly a representation language. The Galen Master Notation is such a language, primarily intended to model terminology. It is used in the development of medical domains, and one of the final goals is to design a large medical model in the form of a semantic network. The Galen Master Notation formalism is described in full in [6].

The following is a summary of the main features of the Galen Master Notation. It should be noted that the vocabulary of the Galen Master Notation has evolved over the past few months. In the present paper, we have kept the vocabulary that was used at the time that the work reported here was carried out. However, we point out the vocabulary which has been referred differently.

The Galen Master Notation can be used to create new compound entities (e.g. Carcinoma, Disease) called *prototypes*. The creation of these new compounds is controlled by *triples* (also referred to as *statements*). A triple represents a relationship between specified entities. Moreover, triples are controlled through layers of qualifiers such as *grammatical, possible* (also referred to as *sensible*) and *necessary.* This sanctioning mechanism allows the specification of what is sensible to say at different levels, depending on the qualifier. The *grammatical* qualifier allows an expression to be said (e.g. a disease is located in a body part); a *possible* qualifier expresses what is medically possible to say (e.g. a temperature can be high); and a *necessary* allows necessary expressions (e.g. a fracture is located in a bone). Using triples and qualifiers, we can say for example, *BenignNeoplasm triple hasCellTissueType GlandularCell possible.* From these triples, a complex entity can be generated using a *which* clause to form a prototype. In other words, a which operation defines an entity according to an expression. This complex entity may be given an explicit name if required. For example, we can say *(BenignNeoplasm which hasCellTissueType GlandularCell) name Adenoma.*

Additional control is represented through inheritance and cardinality of attributes. Inheritance affects whether or not triples based on the attribute, for a particular entity, are seen by the subsumptions (i.e. the children) of that entity. The cardinality of an attribute determines whether triples using that attribute and its inverse can have one or many values. In the Galen Master Notation, inheritance occurs along subsumption pathways, and subsumption occurs either explicitly i.e. it is stated as a fact, or formally i.e. due to an entity's structure.

The tools which have been developed to implement and use the Galen Master Notation are described in [7]. At present, the set of tools that the user can work with include: 1) a Knowledge Engineer (KE) browser which displays information about an entity's criteria sets, the triples which the entity inherits and those that have been asserted about it directly; 2) a statement editor which is an interactive editor allowing triples about an entity to be asserted or retracted. 3) There is also a graphical browser which displays the subsumption hierarchy in a graphical form and allows triples to be asserted about entities.

4. EXPERIMENTING WITH THE GALEN MASTER NOTATION

An initial experiment was carried out with the Galen Master Notation at the Hospital of Geneva. The objectives were to model the NLP knowledge with the Galen Master Notation formalism and to investigate the similarities and differences between the Galen Master Notation and the NLP semantical representation based on conceptual graphs. Specifically, the aim was to establish the level and types of correspondence between the two formalisms. The knowledge of the NLP system which was the starting point to experiment and model with the Galen Master Notation includes: the hierarchy of conceptual classes and their instances, the relationships, and semantical knowledge of the NLP system. The following describes this modelling process. It should be noted that the examples of the CG side given here are in the form of Prolog clauses since the NLP system has been implemented in this programming language.

Modelling NLP conceptual classes and instances: The concepts of the NLP hierarchy were modelled as entities of the Galen Master Notation. They were entered manually into the semantic network using the Galen Master Notation tools. Figure 2. shows the similarity between the CG and the Galen MN representations for defining subsumption. The Galen Master Notation network contains basic entities from which other entities are built. Hence, the parent nodes of the NLP hierarchy are viewed as subsumptions of these basic entities of Galen Master Notation. For example, the NLP concept *Actor*s was entered under the Galen Master Notation entity *TopIndividual,* and *Events* under the Galen Master Notation entity *World*. This gave in the Galen Master Notation: *TopIndividual newSub Actors,* and *World newSub Events* (*newsub* is also referred to as *subsume*).

Instances of an NLP conceptual graph were also modelled as subsumptions. For example, *Ablation* which is an instance of the class *SurgicalTreatment* was modelled as *SurgicalTreatment newSub Ablation* in the Galen Master Notation.

CG	Galen Master Notation
Class1 *is* Class2.	Class2 *newSub* Class1.
SurgicalTreatment *is* Treatment.	Treatment *newSub* SurgicalTreatment.

Figure 2. Modelling NLP concepts into entities of the Galen MN

Modelling NLP relationships: Figure 3 shows the modelling of an NLP relationship into an attribute of the Galen Master Notation. The possible value for the inheritance of an attribute was systematically set to *allAll* since inheritance is not implemented in the first version of the Galen Master Notation. However, the possible values for cardinality were chosen by the builder of the network, depending on the NLP relationship.

CG	Galen Master Notation
thematic_rel([Relation]).	attribute *newAttribute* identifier1 identifier2 inheritance cardinality.
thematic_rel([EXPER]).	Attribute *newAttribute* HasExper IsExperOf allAll oneOne.

Figure 3. Modelling NLP relationships into attributes of the Galen MN

A relationship in the NLP system is defined as a single identifier and its category e.g. EXPER (for the experiencer), and the bidirection of the relationship is implicit in the representation of the graph. In the Galen Master Notation, one needs to define explicitly the bidirection of an attribute e.g. HasExper IsExperOf. A remark should be made regarding the unary relationships of the NLP system (e.g. PAST, NEGATION). By definition a unary relationship has only one direction, whereas an attribute in the Galen Master Notation needs to be entered as a bidirectional relationship. At present, NLP unary relationships have been entered as pseudo binary relationships in the Galen Master Notation.

Modelling NLP semantical knowledge: There are three types of semantical knowledge in the NLP system: semantics of the words found in the dictionnaries, semantical compatiblities and CG schemas.

Each entry in the dictionary has three arguments: the word itself, the syntactical argument and the semantical argument. For example, the word appendectomy in the dictionary is given by the clause: *mot_lex(appendectomy, noun(no,sing),['SurgicalTreatment':ablation,['THEME'('Organ':appendix)]]).* Modelling of the CG present in the semantical argument of words in the dictionaries was carried out as follows: The first two steps were 1) to enter the conceptual classes and their instances of the given graph as entities, and 2) to enter the relationships of the graph as attributes (as shown in Figure 2. and Figure 3.). Triples and prototypes in the Galen Master Notation were then built.

Semantical compatibilities, which are used to group words of a sentence by proximity, have also been modelled in the Galen Master Notation, in a similar way to CG in the dictionnaries. These compatibilities are semantical associations between the concepts which in some cases are linked to the syntax of a natural language. The semantical compatibility rules of the NLP system have a correspondence with the triples in the Galen Master Notation since they also play a sanctioning role.

CG

A semantical compatibility rule to handle "feverish patient":

compasem(Num,[syntactical structure], class1, class2,
[link between class1 and class2]).

compasem(97, [adjective, inverse complement], Patient, Symptom,
n2 modifies_by rel('EXPER', n1)).

Galen Master Notation

Triples: Symptom *triple* HasExper Patient *grammatical.*
(Symptom *which* HasExper Patient)
triple HasSyntax adjective *grammatical.*

Prototype: (Symptom *which*
< HasExper Patient HasSyntax adjective >)
name CompaSemRule97.

Figure 4. Modelling an NLP semantical compatibility rule

Modelling semantical compatibilities showed that some syntactical information which is in the NLP rule needs to be made explicit in the Galen Master Notation formalism. Figure 4. shows an example of a semantical compatibility rule. It should be pointed out that *triple* and *which* clauses can be combined. For instance, we can see in Figure 4. that from a *triple* clause, a *which* clause can then be generated, which in turn is combined with another *triple* clause. In the Galen Master Notation, the attribute HasSyntax/IsSyntaxOf was created to model the syntactical structure of the adjective. Even though we have introduced a syntactical information for this example, by creating the attribute HasSyntax, we need to investigate further whether or not syntactical information should be included in the Galen Master Notation, and the desirable way to do it. If this is not the case, this syntactical information should be generated by hand.

CG schemas of the NLP system are used to describe semantical knowledge. Modelling of the general as well as specific CG schemas in the Galen Master Notation was carried out in a similar manner to the CG in the dictionnaries and the semantical compatibilities. Figure 5. illustrates an example of modelling a general CG schema into triples and prototypes of the Galen Master Notation.

CG

CG schemas:
cg_schema(PhysicalExamTest, [AGENT (Doctor), EXPER (Patient)]).

Galen Master Notation

entity1 *triple* attribute entity2 qualifier.
PhysicalExamTest *triple* HasAgent Doctor *grammatical.*
(PhysicalExamTest *which* HasAgent Doctor) *triple* HasExper Patient *gramm.*

entity *which* criterion qualifier *name* Name.
(PhysicalExamTest *which* < HasAgent Doctor HasExper Patient>)
name graphSchemaPhysicalExamTest.

Figure 5. Modelling NLP CG schemas into prototypes of the Galen MN

Conclusions of this first experiment: This first experiment in modelling NLP knowledge into the Galen Master Notation has determined some similarities and convergence as well as differences between the CG and the Galen MN representations. It has also highlighted a few restrictions which require further investigations. Nevertheless, the results obtained in the modelling process are encouraging. The examples presented in this section illustrate the high level of equivalence betwen CG and the Galen MN. Moreover, this experience successfully demonstrates how one can model CG into the Galen MN. The main conclusion of this first experiment is that the testing made with the Galen MN tool has been positive, and that the mapping between the Galen MN and CG representations is feasible.

5. INTERFACING AUTOMATICALLY CG AND THE GALEN MN

Following the first experiment with the Galen Master Notation (reported in section 4), the aim has been to build some automatic tools that would transform a conceptual graph into the Galen Master Notation and vice versa. This section presents the conversion processes which have been implemented, and describes some problems that have been encountered. At the moment, the interfacing of CG and the Galen MN is as follows. The Galen Master Notation is implemented with SmallTalk and the interface module in Prolog. For the conversion from CG to the Galen MN, the system produces a file which contains clauses in the Galen Master Notation. This resulting file can then be input and used with the Galen Master Notation tools. In the reverse process, the Galen Master Notation file that contains the clauses is used as input to the prolog module.

Converting from CG to the Galen Master Notation: The system uses CGs (produced by the NLP analyser from free text) as input, and generates a Galen Master Notation syntax, which consists of a complex entity in the form of a prototype as output (see Figure 6.).

Initial free text phrase accepted by the NLP analyser: a vesicle lithiasis

From a CG

graph(Cgnumber,Type1:Reference1,[Type1:Reference1,
Relation(Type2:Reference2)]]).
graph('13 | 1',disease:lithiasis,[disease:lithiasis,['LOC'(organ:vesicle)]]).

To a prototype in the Galen MN

(Reference1 *which* Relation Reference2 Qualifier) *name* Name.
(lithiasis *which* hasLOC vesicle) *name* grph13_1.

Figure 6. Conversion from a CG to the Galen MN

There are a number of testing procedures which check whether the concepts and relationships in a given CG already exist in the Galen Master Notation model. In other words, the system checks for *newSub* and *triple* clauses. Regarding the subsumptions, the current issue (mentioned in section 4) is that in a CG, an instance of the class such hospitalisation is treated as a subsumption (i.e. a newSub) in the Galen Master Notation. Thus, for instance in the Galen Master Notation we have *GeneralTreatment newSub Hospitalisation*. Changes are made from the CG side to resolve that aspect so that NLP instances are considered as NLP classes. That is, each instance in the NLP system becomes a class confined to one element.

Regarding the attributes, the inheritance type of a relationship is automatically set to *allAll* (as explained in section 4). For the cardinality, a table that matches an NLP relationship to an attribute of the Galen Master Notation has been used. In the Galen Master Notation, if an attribute has a cardinality of *one*, then one can only apply a triple based on that attribute once to an entity. For example, hasColour should have a cardinality of *one*, since nothing can be two different colours simultaneously. On the other hand, the attribute hasPart should have a cardinality of *many*, since some entities can have many different parts. Since there is not that kind of restriction on the NLP relationships, to a certain extent the Galen Master Notation cardinality for the NLP corresponds to *manyMany*. Concerning the triples, they are checked against the Galen Master Notation model, with the different levels of qualifiers. From these, the system can generate *which* expressions to form prototypes of the Galen Master Notation.

From expressions in the Galen MN

NewSub: Disease *newSub* Inflammation.

Triple: Inflammation *triple* HasTheme Gallbadder *grammatical*.

Prototype: (Inflammation *which* HasTheme Gallbladder)
name Cholecystitis.

To a CG representation

For a newsub: graph(_,disease:inflammation,[disease:inflammation]).

For a triple: graph(_,inflammation,[inflammation,[THEME(gallbladder)]]).

For a prototype: graph(_cholecystitis,disease:inflammation,
[disease:inflammation,[THEME(gallbladder)]]).

Free text produced by the NLP generator: a cholecystitis

Figure 7. Conversion from clauses of the Galen MN to CG

Converting from the Galen Master Notation to CG: The system uses expressions in the Galen Master Notation as input, and generates CG as output (see Figure 7.). The system can take any kind of expression in the Galen Master Notation (e.g. newSub, triples, combinations of both, prototypes) and transform it into a CG representation.

There are also a number of procedures for checking that the entities of the Galen Master Notation exist in NLP. For this transformation process, the main issue centres around the extra information that is brought from the Galen Master Notation, and how it needs to be represented within the CG representation. This additional information includes the qualifiers of the Galen Master Notation (i.e. grammatical, possible and necessary), as well as the cardinality and inheritance of attributes. Intuitively, it seems that each level of qualifiers corresponds to a type of semantical knowledge of the NLP system. The semantical compatibilities can be viewed at the grammatical level, while the CG schemas can have an equivalence with the possible and necessary levels. Finally, CG in the dictionnaries can also be seen at the necessary level. Nevertheless, this issue needs to be clarified and investigated further.

Link with the NLP system: The link between the NLP analyser and the interface conversion module has been establised. The NLP analyser takes a sentence or a file with natural language sentences, and produces one (or more) CG. These graphs are in turn treated by the conversion module which generates a file containing the CG in the Galen Master Notation representation. This link has an interesting implication as it is a means of testing the conversion process to generate correctly one or more clauses of the Galen Master Notation from a CG. For example, given the phrase *acute pain,* the NLP system generates the graph, *graph(graph1, 'Pain', ['Pain',[INTENSITY('Acute')]]).* Then, the conversion module produces from that graph the clause in the Galen Master Notation *('Pain' which hasINTENSITY 'Acute') name graph1.* This link with the NLP analyser offers the possibility to feed the model using natural language medical expressions. However, the technical feasibility of such a process does not allow immediate contribution to a carefully developed model, without testing procedures and other precautions.

6. IMPLICATIONS AND CONCLUSIONS

The prototype for interfacing CG and the Galen MN which has been developed shows promising results with respect to the transformations it can perform from one representation to the other. Even though, some problems remain to be solved and further work needs to be done to consolidate the current prototype, the translation module is able to capture common and important aspects expressed by the two representations.

It is clear that when comparing an expression in the Galen MN to a CG, it appears that both representations are vehicles for knowledge with a converging expressiveness. In fact, the Galen Master Notation belongs to the large class of structured knowledge representation systems which also include semantic networks. Hence, all the systems like the Galen Master Notation and CG are closely related. The differences are partly of substance and partly of notation. The results obtained from comparing and interfacing the Galen Master Notation and CG representations have not only demonstrated, but also emphasised their closeness and strong connections. Moreover, the interfacing between the two notations does not disadvantage one representation or the other. In fact, in the conversion process from CG to the Galen MN, there is no significant loss of information from the representation of the graphs. In comparison, in the conversion process from the Galen Master Notation to CG, there is a contribution of information from the Galen Master Notation formalism to the graph representation.

The converting process from the Galen MN to CG is of direct interest to the Multilingual Information Module of the GALEN architecture (see section 1). The generator that it contains uses expressions of the Galen Master Notation model via the Terminology Server as its input. The expressions in the Galen Master Notation are then transformed into CG, from which natural language expressions are generated.

More importantly, the translation module CG/Galen MN has stronger implications. Indeed, the process of interfacing CG and the Galen MN constitutes the first step towards a bridge between natural language understanding (NLU) and knowledge base modelling. This is an important issue which is described in [8]. The benefit of this automatic translation is of twofold. The first benefit is a potentialisation of the Galen Master Notation model, which has access to natural language input and output. In the converting process from CG to the Galen MN, a validation of the Galen Master Notation model is made. In other words, the NLP knowledge is checked against the Galen Master Notation expressions, and declared whether or not it is sensible in comparison to the Galen Master Notation model. The second benefit is a potentialisation of the NLP system, being grounded by a solid source of knowledge before generating its dictionaries. The model knowledge is viewed as a source of data to populate new entries in the NLP dictionaries. This potentialisation of the NLU can be helped by the converting process from the Galen MN to CG.

7. REFERENCES

1 Baud RH, Rassinoux A-M, Scherrer J-R. Natural Language Processing and Semantical Representation of Medical Texts. Methods of Information in Medicine, Vol.31, 2/1992.

2 Rassinoux A-M, Baud RH, Scherrer J-R. Conceptual graph model extension for knowledge representation of medical texts. MEDINFO92, K.C. Lun et al (eds), Elsevier Science Publishers B.V.

3 Rassinoux A-M, Alpay L, Baud R. HELIOS-2 Deliverable 1: Goals of the NLP part within the HELIOS-2 project. 1992.

4 Rassinoux A-M, Alpay L, Baud R. HELIOS-2 Deliverable 2 : Goals and functionalitites of the Natural Language Processing part within the HELIOS-2 project . 1992.

5 Sowa JF. Conceptual structures: information processing in mind and machine. Addison-Wesley, Reading, MA, 1984.

6 Rector A, Nowlan A, Glowinski A, Matthews G, Rush T, Pakarinen V. GALEN Deliverable 6: The Master Notation, version 1. 1993.

7 Rector A, Piumarta I, Matthews G, Zantra P. GALEN Deliverable 7: Consolidated Terminology Engine and SET Tools, version 1. 1993.

8 Baud R, Lovis C, Alpay L, Rassinoux A-M, Scherrer J-R, Nowlan A, Rector A. Modelling for Natural Language Understanding. Submitted to SCAMC 93.

Artificial Intelligence in Medecine
S. Andreassen et al. , Eds.
IOS Press, 1993

Compositional Classification Based on Conceptual Graphs

J. Bernauer and H.Goldberg

Institute for Medical Informatics, University of Hildesheim, Samelsonplatz 1
31141 Hildesheim, Germany, e-mail: bernauer@rz.uni-hildesheim.de

Abstract

For the structured representation of medical record data a formalism is in demand that both is expressive and supports classification. Common classification and coding systems in medicine make a compromise on these aspects. This paper proposes a model for compositional classification that is based on restricted conceptual graphs. Basic elements are primitive concepts that can be composed to composite concepts via roles. In contrast to the full expressiveness of the conceptual graph formalism the model restricts composite concepts to connected tree-like graphs without quantification, or specification of referents. The model emphasizes a clear distinction between subsumption and part-of relations. Definitions are given that solely base on the structure of composite concepts, and explicit subsumption and part-of relations between primitive concepts. The composition of concepts is constrained by the domain and the range of a role, and by global and local role restrictions. A global restriction limits the range of a role for a primitive concept, a local restriction limits the range of a role for a primitive concept in the context of a composite concept. The model is applied to the AO classification of fractures of long bones. This outlines how a conventional combinatorial coding system can be represented in terms of a compositional classification system.

1. Introduction

Conventional tools for the representation of patient specific information, i.e. mono-hierarchical classification systems (i.e. ICD), combinatorial coding systems (i.e. [1]) and multi-axial nomenclatures (i.e. [2]), are shortcoming in several respects: In general, concept formation in mono-hierarchical systems suffers from combinatory explosion if new types of characteristic are to be considered. Combinatorial coding systems and multi-axial nomenclatures are a means for coping with that problem, but in general, they do not support the formation of meaningful concepts, and are mostly limited to simply structured concepts by a strict composition formalism. Additional limitations arise if concepts in multi-axial systems are not throughout atomized or if the structure of the concept system is constrained by decimal coding. For each tool classification under aspects that are different to the a prior implemented is not supported and can be difficult.

These structural weaknesses may be overcome by taking knowledge representation techniques for the modelling of medical concepts and by incorporating both terminological knowledge and domain knowledge into medical classification systems. Knowledge representation formalisms in the KL-ONE tradition [3,4] propagate the strict separation between terminological knowledge (T-Box) which contains the definitions of concepts on the basis of primitives, and assertional knowledge (A-Box) which contains empirical knowledge in an axiomatic form by using the concepts defined in the T-Box. Classification is restricted to purely terminological information. In [5] Doyle and Patil argue against the restricted classification thesis, that representation systems should restrict taxonomic classification to terminological definitions alone. They show that restrictions on the concept-definition language limit the expressive power of the representation system in such a significant way that important classes of medical concepts become inexpressible. Instead, they call for general-purpose knowledge representation systems with fully expressive languages, tolerance of incomplete classification, terminological classification over relevant contigent as well as definitional information, allowing also "approximate" classification, and give preference to rational management of inference tools.

The SMK formalism [6] argues on both formal and pragmatical grounds for the separation of different types of medical knowledge within representation systems. The one is called conceptual knowledge which is knowledge about terminology, but extended over the T-Box knowledge: It contains in addition conventional knowledge which is indefeasible and cannot be overridden, and descriptive knowledge which is knowledge of concrete relations among concepts. The second knowledge type has been called general inferential knowledge which is usually expressed in first order logic or a rule-based formalism. SMK is a generative formalism for defining complex composite concepts in terms of elementary concepts. Its application aims to the representation of basic knowledge on anatomy, pathophysiology and therapeutics to form a common core model of medical conceptual knowledge, that can reside in medical information systems around which to integrate clinical systems.

This paper proposes an approach for compositional classification which combines terminological and empirical knowledge within one formalism. This proceeding is motivated by the hypothesis that for conceptualizing clinical observations, manifestations etc. the formal definitions of the related concepts are of minor interest: people are commonly using concepts effectively even if those are not exactly defined. But, more important for terminological representation systems is the way how people refine and modify concepts by other concepts in generating meaningful composite concepts.

2. Representation of Medical Concepts by Conceptual Graphs

The formalism proposed for compositional classification is based on conceptual graphs, a notation introduced in [7]. The conceptual graphs notation is equivalent to the predicate calculus, but is more readable. It stands in the tradition of semantic networks. Conceptual graphs have been applied to medical knowledge representation from several perspectives [8-13]. The principle idea is to form complex propositions by connecting primitive concepts via semantic relations. Here, for the purpose of compositional classification the expressiveness and compositionality of the notation in [7] has been restricted.

2.1 Primitive concept

The primitive concept is the conceptual unit of a compositional classification system (*CCS*). In a *CCS* primitive concepts are not further decomposable into semantical components. In this connection the linguistic designation of a concept is irrelevant. Thus, even complex or compound terms also with attributive phrases are permissible designations of primitive concepts. In this paper the designation of primitive concepts is written in `Courier` as one-word string. The concepts `long_bone`, `more_than_three_intermediate_fragments` can be seen as primitive concepts. The set of primitive concepts of a *CCS* is finite and called *PRIMC*.

2.2 Role

A role characterizes the semantical relationship between two or more concepts. Roles are representable as monadig, dyadig or n-adig relations and correspond to types of characteristic in concept systems. Designations for roles are written in `Courier` with a leading colon. The role `:loc` has the meaning of 'has location'. The role `:morph` has the meaning of 'has morphology'.

In general the set of roles of a *CCS* depends on the concept field and must be chosen with respect to the relevant types of characteristic. However, there are two roles that have fixed semantics: The one is `:neg` which is for denying an instance of a concept and which is the only monadig role. The other is `:part` which has the meaning of 'which is part of'. The set of roles of a *CCS* is finite, disjoint to *PRIMC* and called *R*.

2.3 Composite concept

A composite concept is formed by connecting primitive concepts via roles. Composite concepts can be represented by conceptual graphs. Conceptual graphs are finite, directed, bipartite graphs consisting of concept nodes that correspond to primitive concept elements and conceptual relation nodes that correspond to roles. In contrast to the expressiveness of the original notation composite concepts of a *CCS* have restricted structure: A conceptual graph representing a composite concept is (1) connected, (2) has a tree-like structure, i.e. every concept element has at most one in-going role, and (3) all the out-going roles of a concept element have different types. The set of composite concepts of a *CCS* is called *COMPC*. The set of primitive concepts *PRIMC* is a subset of *COMPC*.
Figure 1 gives an example of a conceptual graph representing a composite concept.

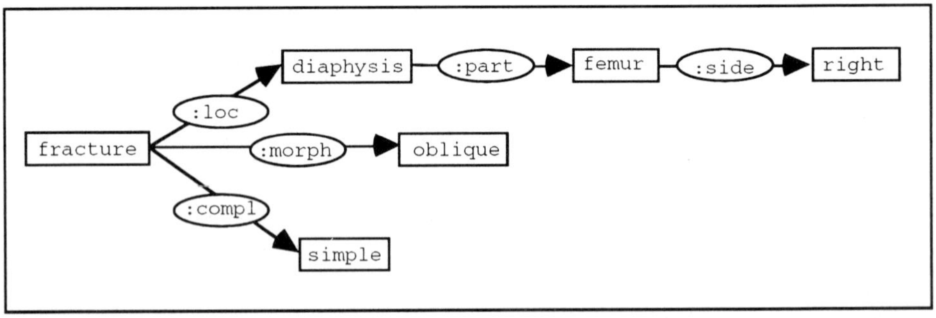

Figure 1: Conceptual graph representing the concept 'simple oblique diaphyseal fracture of the right femur'.

For better writing the equivalent linear notation for conceptual graphs is used which represents a concept as a nested list. The linear notation of the concept of Figure 1 is:

```
(fracture
      (:loc (diaphysis (:part (femur     (:side (right))))))
      (:morph (oblique))
      (:compl (simple)))
```

It follows from the structural restrictions that every composite concept is composed by a root, which corresponds to a primitive concept, and a tail which is a set of 2-tuples each corresponding to a role and a composite concept:

$\forall c \in COMPC\colon\ c = (root(c),\ tail(c))$
where:
$root\colon\ COMPC \rightarrow PRIMC,\quad tail\colon\ COMPC \rightarrow 2^{R \times COMPC}$

The out-going roles of the root of a concept are partitioned into at most one `:part` role, that links to a whole concept, and several non-`:part` roles, that link to refining concepts. The *whole* of a composite concept is the concept, that is linked by the root via a `:part` role. The *rtail* (refining tail) of a composite concept is the subset of *tail* which corresponds to the non-`:part` role linkages:

$$whole\colon COMPC \rightarrow COMPC, \quad whole(c) = \bar{c} \;\Leftrightarrow\; \exists(\texttt{:part},\bar{c}) \in tail(c)$$

$$rtail\colon COMPC \rightarrow 2^{R \times COMPC}, \quad rtail(c) := \{(r,c') \mid (r,c') \in tail(c) \wedge r \neq \texttt{:part}\}$$

Both the *whole* and the *rtail* of a concept may be empty.
For the concept 'lateral condyle of the right femur':

```
(condyle
      (:part       (femur       (:side (right))))
      (:orient     (lateral)))
```

the *whole* concept is: `(femur (:side (right)))`,
and the *rtail* is: {(`:orient, lateral`)}

3. Classification of concepts

Concept systems are based on hierarchical relations between concepts. There are two kinds of hierarchical relations. Both are essential for medical classification systems: generic and partitive relations. The generic ordering mostly applies to concepts that relate to diseases, findings, tissue types, procedures etc. where subordinate concepts can be organized under superordinate concepts. The partitive ordering is appropriate to concepts that relate to objects having a spatial, temporal or conceptual extension. Here, partitive concepts can be organized under comprehensive concepts. In medicine partitive ordering applies to anatomical structures, body regions, functional systems, processes etc.

Typically, medical classification and coding systems implicitely mingle both hierarchical ordering principles. For instance, in disease classifications there are commonly subsets of concepts organized according to partitive relationships. Anatomical topographies often show some generic subdivisions. This mixing of hierarchical principles may be intuitive, adequate for navigating through concept systems, and efficient for manual classing and coding. But, in general it disguises the interrelationship between concepts and the inheritance of properties. This becomes apparent if a selection of concepts across to the hierarchy is asked for.

Compositional classification systems are a means to deal explicitely with the relationships of concepts, both by representing subsumptive (generic) and part-of (partitive) relationships between primitive concepts a prior, and by representing these relations also in the structure of composite concepts in form of roles.

3.1 Subsumption between primitive concepts

The primitive concepts of a *CCS* are explicitely organized in a subsumption hierarchy. This hierarchy realizes is-a or kind-of relationships. Subsumption is designated by <.
For $c_1, c_2 \in PRIMC$ $c_1 < c_2$ has the meaning: c_1 is subsumed by c_2, i.e. c_2 is superordinate concept of c_1 (c_1 is subordinate concept of c_2). The subsumption relation is reflexive, antisymmetrical and transitive, and imposes a partial ordering on *PRIMC* with $\top$ as top element. Examples for subsumption relationships between primitive concepts are:
`femur < long_bone, fracture < trauma.`

3.2 Subsumption between composite concepts

In contrast to subsumption between primitive concepts, which is explicit, subsumption between composite concepts is defined solely by the structure of composite concepts and primitive subsumption between their elements. Subsumption between composite concepts is designated by $\lessdot$ and is defined in the following way:

$$\forall c_1, c_2 \in COMPC: \; c_1 \lessdot c_2 :\Leftrightarrow$$

$$root(c_1) < root(c_2) \wedge \forall (r'', c'') \in tail(c_2) \; \exists (r', c') \in tail(c_1): \; r' = r'' \wedge c' \lessdot c''$$

Figure 2 gives an example of subsumption between composite concepts.

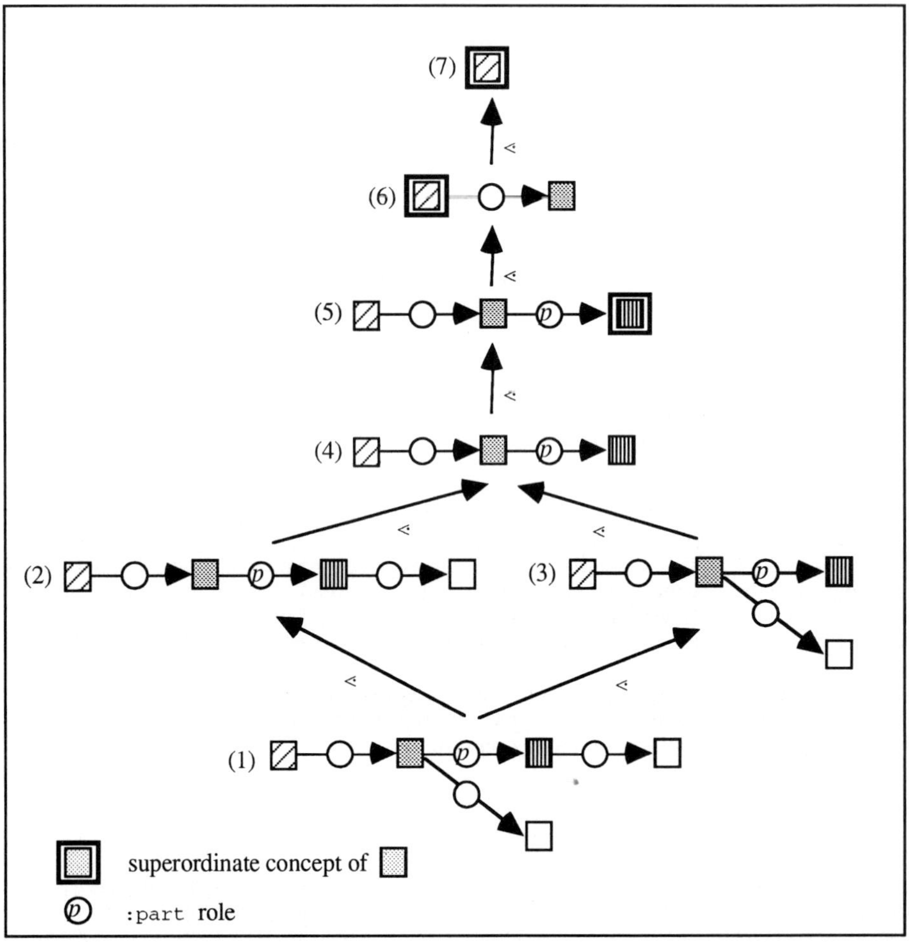

Figure 2: Subsumption between composite concepts. (1) fracture of the lateral condyle of the right femur, (2) fracture of a condyle of the right femur, (3) fracture of the lateral condyle of a femur, (4) fracture of a condyle of a femur, (5) fracture of a condyle of a long bone, (6) trauma of a condyle, (7) trauma

3.3 Part-of relation between primitive concepts

Primitive concepts may have explicit partitive relationships. The partitive relation between primitive concepts is designated by $<_p$.

$c_1 <_p c_2$ has the meaning: the object related to c_1 is part of the object related to c_2 , or c_2 is a whole of c_1 . Like primitive subsumption primitive part-of is reflexive, antisymmetrical and transitive. Examples for part-of relationships between primitive concepts are:
`major_trochanter` $<_p$ `femur`, `femur` $<_p$ `lower_extremity`,
`bone_marrow` $<_p$ `hemopoetic_system`.

3.4 Part-of relation between composite concepts

Like subsumption the part-of relation between composite concepts is defined solely by the structure of composite concepts and primitive part-of relation between their elements. The part-of relation between composite concepts is designated by $\lessdot^*_p$ and is defined in the following way (see also Fig.3):

$\forall c_1, c_2 \in COMPC\text{:} \quad c_1 \lessdot^*_p c_2 \; :\Leftrightarrow$

$whole(c_1) = c_2 \; \vee \; (\; root(c_1) <_p root(c_2) \; \wedge \; tail(c_1) = tail(c_2) \;)$

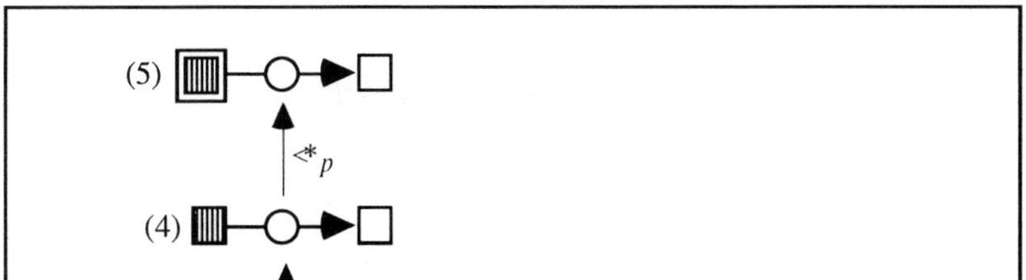

Figure 3: Part-of relationships between composite concepts. (1) joint surface of the lateral condyle of the right femur, (2) joint of lateral condyle of the right femur, (3) lateral condyle of the right femur, (4) right femur, (5) right lower extremity.

3.5 Part-of-sensitive subsumption between composite concepts

In general, subsumption is independent from partitive relations. Sometimes this may be too strict: For instance, 'fracture of the neck of the femur' may be seen as subordinate to 'fracture of the femur'. For that reason, part-of sensitive subsumption is introduced which takes also part-of relations into account. Part-of sensitive subsumption between composite concepts is designated by $\lessdot_p$. $c_1 \lessdot_p c_2$ ($c_1, c_2 \in COMPC$) has the meaning: c_2 subsumes c_1, but elements of the tail of c_2 are permitted to be wholes of the corresponding elements of the tail of c_1. $\lessdot_p$ is defined in the following way (see also Fig.4):

$$\forall c_1, c_2 \in COMPC: \; c_1 \lessdot_p c_2 \; :\Leftrightarrow$$

$$root(c_1) < root(c_2) \; \wedge$$

$$\forall (r'', c'') \in tail(c_2) \; \exists (r', c') \in tail(c_1): \; r' = r'' \; \wedge \; (c' \lessdot_p \; c'' \; \vee \; c' \lessdot^*_p \; c'')$$

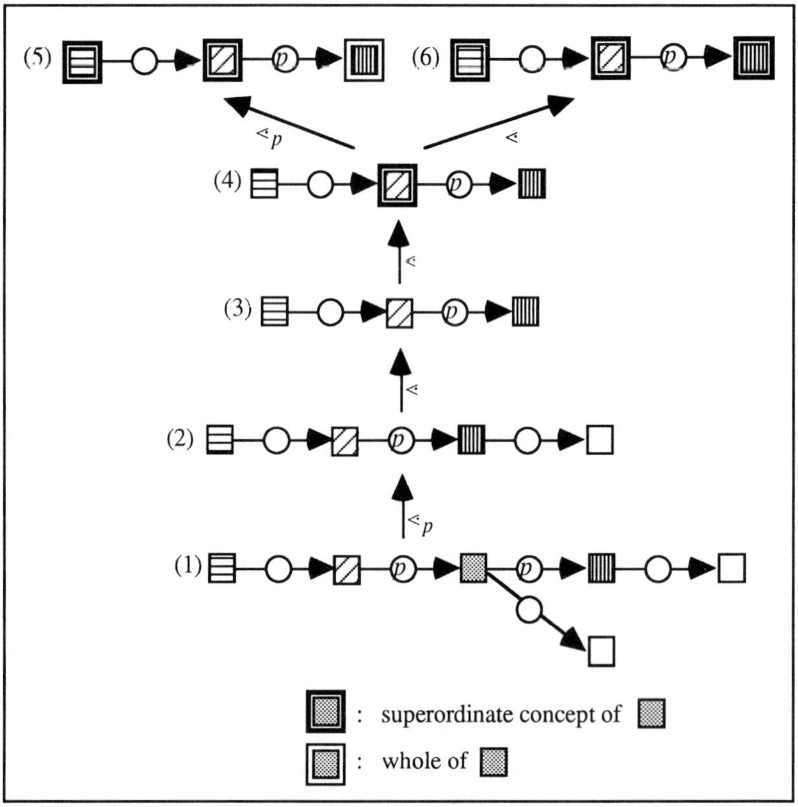

Figure 4: Part-of sensitive subsumption between composite concepts. (1) lesion of a joint surface of a lateral condyle of a right femur, (2) lesion of a joint surface of a right femur, (3) lesion of a joint surface of a femur, (4) lesion of cartilage of a femur, (5) trauma of cartilage of a lower extremity, (6) trauma of cartilage of a long bone

4. Role Restrictions

Not every combination of concepts that meets the restricted graph structure is per se a meaningful concept. In order to ensure the sensible combination of concepts the application of roles is restricted by the domain and range of a role, and potentially by global or local role restrictions.

4.1 Domain / range of a role

In principal, the application of a role is restricted by its domain concept (*domc*) and range concept (*rangec*): It is only permitted to link a concept of the extension of the domain concept (i.e. the domain concept or subordinate) to a concept of the extension of the range concept.

$domc\colon R \rightarrow PRIMC, \quad rangec\colon R \rightarrow PRIMC$

For example, the domain and range concept of the `:loc` role ('has_location') are:

domc`(:loc)= path._entity,` *rangec*`(:loc)= anatomical_structure`

4.2 Global role restriction

A global role restriction restricts the range of a role for a primitive concept to a subset of the extension of the role range. Global role restrictions are defined by *grestr*.

$grestr\colon R \times PRIMC \rightarrow 2^{PRIMC}$

For example, the global role restriction: *grestr*`(:loc, fracture) := bone` restricts the application of the `:loc` role for the pathological entity 'fracture' to the anatomical structure 'bone'.

Global role restrictions must be restrictive along the primitive subsumption hierarchy: a global role restriction for a particular concept must be a subset of global role restrictions for the same role on superordinate concepts.

4.3 Local role restriction

A local role restriction restricts the range of a role for a primitive concept in the context of a composite concept to a subset of the extension of the role range. Local role restrictions are defined by *lrestr*.

$lrestr\colon R \times PRIMC \times COMPC \rightarrow 2^{PRIMC}$

For example, the application of the `:morph` role for `fracture` in the context of the concept

```
c:= (fracture      (:loc       (diaphyse    (:segment    (long_bone)))
                   (:compl     (simple)))
```

is restricted by the local role restriction:

lrestr`(:morph, fracture, c) := {spiral, oblique, transverse}`

to the concepts `spiral, oblique,` or `transverse.`

For local role restrictions the following conditions must hold: (1) A local role restriction for a primitive concept must be a subset of global role restrictions for it, or superordinate concepts of it. (2) A local role restriction for a primitive concept in the context of a composite concept must be a subset of local role restrictions for superordinate concepts of the primitive concept in the context of superordinate concepts of the composite concept.

5. Compositional classification of fractures of long bones

For illustration, the model is applied to the classification of fractures of long bones given in [1], in form of a combinatorial coding system. Figure 5 presents a fragment of this classification.

- fracture of long bone
  - diaphyseal fracture
    - diaphyseal fracture of humerus, femur, tibia
      - simple diaphyseal fracture
        - spiral, oblique, transverse
          - femur, humerus
            - proximal
            - middle
            - distal
          - tibia
            - fibula intact
            - fibula fractured at an other level
            - fibula fractured at the same level
      - wedge fracture
        - spiral wedge
        - bending wedge
        - fragmented wedge
      - complex fracture
            - pure diaphyseal
            - proximal diasphysio-metaphyseal
            - distal diaphysio-metaphyseal
        - spiral
          - two intermediate fragments
          - three intermediate fragments
          - more than three intermediate fragments
        - segmental
          - an intermediate fragment
          - an intermediate fragment and additional wedge fragment(s)
          - two intermediate segmental fragments
        - irregular
          - two intermediate fragments
          - three intermediate fragments
          - limited shattering
          - extensive shattering

Figure 5: Fragment of the classification of fractures of long bones according to [1].

The following section represent the fragment in terms of a compositional classification system as outlined above. Definitions are provided for subsumption of primitive concepts, part-of relations, roles, global role restrictions, concept definitions, and local role restrictions:

<u>subsumption of primitive concepts:</u>

```
{humerus, femur, tibia} < long_bone < bone < anatomical_structure

fracture < trauma < path._entity

{simple, wedge, complex, extra-articular, partial_articular,
complete_articular} < fracture_complexity

{fracture_morphology, wedge_morphology, fragment_morphology} < morphology

{spiral, oblique, transverse, segmental, irregular} < fracture_morphology
```

```
{spiral, bending, fragmented, non-fragmented} < wedge_morphology

{one_intermediate_fragment,
one_intermediate_fragment_and_additional_wedge_fragment(s),
two_intermediate_fragments, three_intermediate_fragments,
more_than_three_intermediate_fragments, limited_shattering,
extensive_shattering} < fragment_morphology

{fibula_intact, fibula_fractured_at_an_other_level,
fibula_fractured_at_the_same_level} < fibula_condition < condition

{pure_diaphyseal, proximal_diaphysio-metaphyseal, distal_diaphysio-
metaphyseal} < diaphyseal_extension < extension
```

part-of relations:

{proximal_diaphysis, middle_diaphysis, distal_diaphysis} $<_p$ diaphysis

roles:

domc(:loc)= path._entity	*rangec*(:loc)= anatomical_structure
domc(:morph)= path._entity	*rangec*(:morph)= morphology
domc(:compl)= path._entity	*rangec*(:compl)= complexity
domc(:part)= anatomical_structure	*rangec*(:part)= anatomical_structure
domc(:qual)= path._entity	*rangec*(:qual)= condition
domc(:fragm)= fracture	*rangec*(:fragm)= fragment_morphology
domc(:extens)= path._entity	*rangec*(:extens)= extension

global role restrictions:

grestr(:loc, fracture) := bone
grestr(:morph, fracture) := fracture_morphology
grestr(:compl, fracture) := fracture_complexity
grestr(:morph, wedge) := wedge_morphology

concept definitions:

```
diaphyseal_fracture           :=
(fracture   (:loc (diaphysis (:part (long_bone)))))

simple_diaphyseal_fracture    :=
(fracture   (:loc (diaphysis (:part (long_bone))))
            (:compl (simple)))

simple_diaphyseal_tibia_fracture    :=
(fracture   (:loc (diaphysis (:part (tibia))))
            (:compl (simple)))

diaphyseal_wedge_fracture           =
(fracture   (:loc (diaphysis (:part (long_bone))))
            (:compl (wedge)))
```

```
complex_diaphyseal_fracture  :=
(fracture   (:loc (diaphysis (:part (long_bone))))
            (:compl (complex)))

spiral_complex_diaphyseal_fracture :=
(fracture   (:loc (diaphysis (:part (long_bone))))
            (:compl (complex))
            (:morph (spiral)))

irregular_complex_diaphyseal_fracture    :=
(fracture   (:loc (diaphysis (:part (long_bone))))
            (:compl (complex))
            (:morph (irregular)))
```

local role restrictions:

lrestr`(:compl, fracture, diaphyseal_fracture) :=`
`{simple, wedge, complex}`

lrestr`(:morph, fracture, simple_diaphyseal_fracture) :=`
`{spiral, oblique, transverse}`

lrestr`(:qual, fracture, simple_diaphyseal_tibia_fracture) :=`
`fibula_condition`

lrestr`(:morph, wedge, diaphyseal_wedge_fracture) :=`
`{spiral, bending, fragmented}`

lrestr`(:morph, fracture, complex_diaphyseal_fracture) :=`
`{spiral, segmental, irregular}`

lrestr`(:extens, fracture, complex_diaphyseal_fracture) :=`
`{pure_diaphyseal, proximal_diaphysio-metaphyseal,`
`distal_diaphysio-metaphyseal}`

lrestr`(:fragm, fracture, spiral_complex_diaphyseal_fracture) :=`
`{two_intermediate_fragments, three_intermediate_fragments,`
`more_than_three_intermediate_fragments}`

lrestr`(:fragm, fracture, irregular_complex_diaphyseal_fracture) :=`
`{two_intermediate_fragments, three_intermediate_fragments,`
`limited_shattering, extensive_shattering}`

6. Conclusion

A model for the compositional classification of concepts has been proposed based on restricted conceptual graphs. Subsumption and part-of relations can be defined for composite concepts from their structure, and subsumption and part-of relations between primitive concept elements. The composition of meaningful concepts is supported by global and local role restrictions. It can be shown that a conventional hierarchical classification system can be represented in terms of compositional classification.

7. References

[1] Müller M.E., Nazarian S., Koch P., Schatzker J., The Comprehensive Classification of Fractures of Long Bones. Springer-Verlag, 1990

[2] Côté R.A., (ed.), Systematized Nomenclature of Medicine. College of American Pathologists, Illinois, 1977

[3] Brachman R.J., Schmolze J.G., An Overview of the KL-ONE Knowledge Representation System, Cognitive Science 9 (1985) pp. 171-216

[4] Von Luck K., Nebel B., Peltason C. et al., The anatomy of the BACK system. Tech. Rept., Technische Universität Berlin, Berlin 1987

[5] Doyle J., Patil R.S., Two theses of knowledge representation: language restrictions, taxonomic classification, and the utility of representation services. Artificial Intelligence 48 (1991) pp. 261-297

[6] Rector A.L., Nowlan W.A., Kay S., Conceptual knowledge: The core of medical information systems, in: Lun K.C., Degoulet P., Piemme T.E., Rienhoff O., (eds.), MEDINFO 92, North-Holland, 1992, pp 1420-1426

[7] Sowa J.F., Conceptual Structures: Information Processing in Mind and Maschine, Addison-Wesley, 1984

[8] Campbell K.E., Musen M.A., Representation of Clinical Data Using SNOMED III and Conceptual Graphs. In: Frisse M. (ed.), Proc. 16th SCAMC,1992, McGraw-Hill, 1993, pp 354-358

[9] Schröder M., Knowledge Based Analysis of Radiology Reports Using Conceptual Graphs. In: Pfeiffer H.D. (ed.), Proceedings of the Seventh Annual Workshop on Conceptual Graphs, New Mexico State University, Las Cruces, New Mexico, 1992, pp. 213-222

[10] Baud R.H., Rassinoux A.M., Scherrer J.R., Natural Language Processing and Semantical Representation of Medical Text, Meth Inform Med, 2, 1992

[11] Bernauer J., Conceptual graphs as an operational model for descriptive findings, in Clayton PD (ed.), Proc. 15th SCAMC, Washington DC,1991, McGraw-Hill, 1991, pp 214-218

[12] Bernauer J., Gumrich K., Kutz S., Lindner P., Pretschner D.P., An interactive report generator for bone scintigraphy, in Proc. 15th SCAMC, Washington DC,1991,McGraw-Hill, 1991, pp 858-860

[13] Bernauer J., Taphorn F.J., Pretschner D.P., A model for composing medical descriptions from fragments, in: Lun K.C., Degoulet P., Piemme T.E., Rienhoff O., (eds.), MEDINFO 92, North-Holland, 1992, pp. 1395-1401

Artificial Intelligence in Medecine
S. Andreassen et al. , Eds.
IOS Press, 1993

Needs and constraints in modelling medical knowledge using semantic networks: A medical point of view

Lovis C, Baud R, Alpay L, Rassinoux A-M, Wagner J and Scherrer J-R

Centre d'lnformatique Hospitalière, Hôpital Cantonal Universitaire de Genève, 24 rue Micheli-du-Crest, 1211 Genève 14, Switzerland

Abstract

The point of view discussed here is that of a clinician in the Medicine Department of the Geneva University Hospital. This is a non computer scientist approach of a generalised representation of medical knowledge. Two important issues are discussed in this paper. The first issue is concerned with defining the necessary contents of what should be modelled. An attempt is made to define domains that should be included in the model. The extent of the model may be defined in two ways. Horizontally, by meaning the various domains to be included such as anatomy, therapy, and vertically to define the granularity or the precision with which each domain will be defined. The knowledge included in such a model may cover natural language processing, expert and alert systems, coding schemes and bibliographic retrieval.

The second issue discussed in this paper is how to model medical knowledge. One of the features of the medical knowledge is its relative evolution, which needs good maintenance tools. The validation and coherence of such a model will be difficult to maintain, depending on the experts in charge. Furthermore, such a model will probably need to be built by medical people rather than by computer scientists. This requires a user-friendly interface for entering new data and for control tools. The system must include a knowledge browser, a coherency and redundancy checker and tools to put together different models built on the same platform. In order to stand any chance of imposing itself on the various actual coding schemes, such a system must be language and hardware independent. As a concrete example, the Geneva experience with a modelling system called the Galen Master Notation, developed in the context of the European project Galen, is described.

1. CONTENTS OF MEDICAL KNOWLEDGE

1.1. Overview of the application domain: A philosophical approach

What does medical knowledge mean ? Although at first this would appear to be a well defined discipline, i.e. “a large amount of textbooks", it soon becomes a real challenge to have a well-defined survey of what "Medical Knowledge" implies.

In contrast to a clear, exact science, such as physics or biology, medical knowledge covers a great amount of "natural" human knowledge, known as common sense knowledge [1]. Hence, the medical domain can be separated into five parts:

i) Basic medical science, containing fundamental medical knowledge (such as anatomy, physiology, biology).

ii) Complex medical science, including pathology, surgery, therapies, psychiatry, etc.

iii) Paramedical knowledge, including knowledge directly linked to medical knowledge (such as devices, various actors or geographic locations).

iv) Temporal reasoning, which plays a major role in medical applications and remains difficult to solve [2].

v) Finally, common sense knowledge, which is basic knowledge that everyone has, before learning anything about medicine. This knowledge will be used everyday to understand or describe a particular medical situation. This domain of knowledge is much more difficult to describe. It includes "semantic" information, e.g. pregnancy is not a disease or old people are sick more often than young people, etc. Furthermore, there is some trivial but important knowledge, like for example that a knife wound causes a haemorrhage or that a girl very probably takes the pill.

1.2. Which support to medical knowledge ?

Due to the huge amount of knowledge in medecine, and the highly interconnected medical subdomains, a good representation is found in semantic networks. Such a model allows a lattice of high density of concepts and relationships, with inference and combinatorial effects. It provides the use of a formal language with validation on instances and conversion capabilities by explicit rules.

1.3. An attempt to define what should be modelled

To such a question, one could reply: everything ! This answer would further lead to two questions: what is everything ? how is it possible to model everything ?

The problem of defining what a general model of medical knowledge should contain is an ongoing problem and depends on the applications to be supported. This problem is not an academic question. The medical community needs information exchange, KB systems, decision support aids, and administrative and financial tools. All these needs imply the use of a common language. The various applications that could benefit from medical knowledge representation are:

a) Medical records

The huge quantity of data contained in hospital and practitioners' archives probably represent the largest amount of sensible medical information known. However, this information remains almost useless, as it is mainly represented by paper archives. These archives are very difficult to consult. The need for *electronic-readable* and *computer-understandable* medical record is urgent. It will allow the exchange of information between hospitals for travelling patients, for teaching purpose and for scientific studies. To achieve this goal, a common representation of the sensible information contained in a medical record is needed. This is far from easy to resolve, as long as medical records represent heterogeneous data. Moreover, sensible data are not always strictly medical data, often involving general knowledge or patient history.

With relation to the medical knowledge representation as semantic networks, it should be borne in mind that the diversity of the domains represents the horizontal developments and the depth of knowledge in each domain, the vertical development. Given these definitions, we can therefore consider that a complete representation of medical records needs both vast horizontal knowledge and deep vertical knowledge.

b) Natural language processing

The discussion about medical records largely justifies the need for natural language processing (NLP) tools. They should provide valuable facilities for recording and translating free text medical records into a conceptual representation of their content. The work carried out in NLP at the Geneva Hospital, based on the conceptual graphs paradigm [3], has demonstrated the necessity for a good represention of the semantic knowledge contained in free texts [4]. Such a model must include a good horizontal knowledge, whereas the vertical detailed information seems to be less important. Hence, for example, in most cases, it is enough for a NLP model to know that kidneys are organs in order to resolve local, syntactical ambiguities.

c) Knowledge based systems

Knowledge based systems require not only conceptual or descriptive knowledge, but also formal knowledge. In this case, one of the difficulties is to determine, at least, where pragmatic knowledge begins. Therefore, it is necessary to decide what belongs exactly to the knowledge model and what belongs to the inference mechanism of the expert system. For example, the fact that diabetes is a kind of disease belongs to conventional knowledge. The fact that diabetes may by caused by Coxsackies B4 virus is part of the descriptive knowledge. Formal knowledge could be that non-insulin dependent diabetes is a kind of diabetes. Finally, one could add in one of the above groups that diabetes is a risk factor for cardiovascular or infectious diseases, or that pregnant diabetic women will have overweight children, etc.

d) Bibliographic retrieval

Bibliographic retrieval knowledge is a mixture of medical records and natural language processing knowledge. Three main problems are eminent in electronic processing of medical literature. The first involves the introduction of articles, that could benefit from natural language processing. The second involves the indexing problems that are currently done "by hand". Last but not least, the development of an efficient query language that is keyword oriented has proved to be very difficult. This leads to "noise", inducing the system to give information that is irrelevant. More dangerously, this leads to "silences", i.e. sensible information is not taken into consideration by the query. The following two examples illustrate this: a) if one is interested in all problems involving the hand, one probably wants to receive anything involving fingers, and b) if one makes a clear distribution between "allergy to drugs" and "drugs for allergy", a search with two indexes, like [drug, allergy] will fail to solve this problem.

These problems could probably be avoided with a good semantic representation of the bibliographic data. In this case, a knowledge representation must be both horizontal large and vertical deep.

e) Coding schemes

The reproduction of the contents of current coding schemes is a pitfall that should be avoided. This would only cause more confusion in the "market" of coding schemes. The new model must be better, faster and more exhaustive, even if this represents a kind of "chimera" as explained by Alan Rector [5].

A current problem in medicine is the difficulty to compare various groups of patients collected in different places, whose medical problems are coded using different coding schemes. Whereas it is not possible to represent Lung Carcinoma in the ICD-9 coding scheme [6], with SNOMED it is possible through linking concepts (lung T - 28000 + carcinoma H - 80103). In contrast, there is a redundancy in EMTree [7], where two different codes could represent "blood wessel" (A 7.30 et A 7.10.30) [8, 9].

It is therefore necessary to use each coding scheme for the specific purpose, for which it has been designed. So, ICD-9 is a classification of disease for statistical purpose, whereas MeSH is a thesaurus for concept retrieval and SNOMED is a standardisation of medical expressions.

A medical knowledge model should at least be able to represent the current coding schemes and to resolve the coherency and redundancy problems between them. It could either have its own coding scheme by representing exactly the semantic content of a diagnosis for example, or give the equivalent or near equivalent canonical form for each different coding scheme. This requires a large horizontal representation of the knowledge (to support SNOMED or MeSH [10] for example) and a deep vertical representation (to support DSM-3 in psychiatry for example).

This preliminary remark leads to the first conclusion. This model would be a main improvement on the existing coding schemes and thesauri. Moreover, such a model would be an ambitious project, using powerfull tools, and should be able to represent the vast domains described above. In this case only, it would really benefit the medical community and, furthermore, the scientific community, the economic and administrative people, and, at last but not least, the patients !

2. MODELLING MEDICAL KNOWLEDGE: The Galen Master Notation

Geneva's experience with medical knowledge modelling was gained with the tools developed in the GALEN Consortium. GALEN is an AIM project (Advanced Informatics in Medicine A2012 of the CEC). It is an acronym for "Generalised Architecture for Languages Encyclopaedias and Nomenclatures in Medicine".

Among other things, the main work was to develop a semantic network and to implement a formalism and tools to allow medical knowledge representation. The language developed is called the Galen Master Notation [11].

2.1. The portability: a successful goal

Hospital Information Systems, general practices and economic structures use a variety of computer platforms. Therefore, the system that supports the model should run on different kinds of hardware. The Galen Master Notation is based on Smalltalk which has been used successfully in Geneva on various UNIX workstations and on two PC-based systems (Windows and Macintosh). This leads to a first, fundamental comment: the portability of the Galen Master Notation is remarkable. It works, and it works well. However, one question remains: is it possible to have such a semantic network in paper form, for those who are currently coding medical reports from coding schemes using books?

2.2. The Galen Master Notation formalism: a convivial language !

One of the problems faced by medical experts concerning informatics is that they do not have computer training. Therefore, the formalism used to introduce knowledge into the model must be easily understandable. It should be as near as possible to the natural way of expressing knowledge. This is one of the main goals of the GALEN project, as long as it is necessary to have medical experts in charge of populating the model.

The GALEN formalism is a step forwards achieving this goal. The basic components are divided into two groups: entities, like *Arm* or *Device* and relations like *isPartOf* or *isContainedln.* It is possible to create generic subsumptions, such as *Device* subsumes *Catheters.* Rules and qualifiers can then be used to link Entities. Qualifiers are *[grammatical],* which just allow something to be said. For example, it is grammatically true to say that a disease is located in a part of the body, whereas it is untrue to say that a disease is located in a colour. A more constraining qualifier is *[possible].* This qualifier expresses what is medically sensible to say. For example, it is *[possible]* for a temperature to be high. Finally, the more constraining qualifier is *[necessary].* This one could be considered as a kind of defining qualifier, since it puts definite attributes to the entity. Thus, for example, it is *[necessary]* for a fracture to be located in a bone. The Galen Master Notation allows the definition of simple and compound objects to be made. For example, to express that tachypnea is related to the respiratory system, and consists of accelerated breathing, one can say:

(Finding which < isSignOf RespiratorySys isFunctionOf (Ventilation which hasState Increased)>) name Tachypnea.

Although it is difficult to write, it is easy to read. It is obvious that such a definition is clear and very close to natural language, allowing any medical person to understand this formalism.

2.3. The Galen Master Notation philosophy: an unusual way of thinking for medical people

The first model built in Geneva using the Galen Master Notation was based on the idea that classifying knowledge is like "Russian dolls". Hence one could say that the respiratory system contains lungs, which contain lobes, which contain alveolus, etc. This structure could be compared to object oriented structures, the main semantic contents of which lie in the structure itself and the succession of entities with the inheritance concept. This kind of structure has been widely used in current mono or multiaxial coding schemes like ICD-9 or SNOMED. This method has rapidly shown certain limits. Hence, for example, once it has been said that the Pancreas belongs to the digestive apparatus, it is difficult to add that it also belongs to the endocrine apparatus.

The Galen Master Notation resolves all these problems, as it allows a lattice to be built, rather than a tree. Therefore, multiple inheritance of properties is possible. A very important and decisive step was taken when we realised that giving properties or definitions to entities is much easier using relations between the entities than using the structure itself. For example, we first made a list of infectious agents and, only after, gave them properties using relations. This way, one could easily resolve the problem brought by the multiple inheritance of pancreas. This can be done by building pancreas as an organ, *that* belongs to the digestive, exocrine and endocrine systems. Hence, one can say "I create a new Organ, that belongs to digestive system and to endocrine and exocrine system". In the syntax of the Galen Master Notation, it is written as follows:

(Organ newSub Pancreas)
triple belongsTo DigestiveSys [necessary];
triple belongsTo EndocrineSys [necessary];
triple belongsTo ExocrineSys [necessary]; ...

Once the concept Pancreas has been created (although incompletely in this example), one could now be interested in defining two subgroups of this concept, namely the part that involves endocrine or exocrine functions of pancreas. In this way, it is then possible to attribute to each subpart the equivalent SNOMED code:
(Pancreas which belongsTo EndocrineSys) triple hasSNOMED2
"T-99000" default
(Pancreas which belongsTo ExocrineSys) triple hasSNOMED2
"T-59000" default.

Hence, a good, but unusual way to model medical knowledge, was to create a flat list of Organs using subsumption. Their respective definitions and properties were then given by using attributes, relations and qualifiers.

2.4. Method and experience

The requirements for defining the model developed at the Geneva Hospital is based on a model of infectious diseases of the urinary system. What appears to be a little model at first glance, rapidly gives a list of problems when building a semantic network. Detailed examples will be used as much as possible to illustrate the problems and advantages encountered when modelling with the Galen Master Notation,

- Defining the knowledge to be first modelled

Describing knowledge needs knowledge! A common pitfall in modelling is to "put something in the machine and see what happens ...". This pragmatic way of working is hopeless ! To illustrate this, some anatomical considerations about the genito-urinary system in the model: There are normally two kidneys, symmetrically disposed on the right and left hand sides at the back of the abdomen. In this example, there are very different elements. The kidney is an organ, the abdomen is a topographical part of the body, right and left are general topographic concepts. Hence, these three general groups of concepts will need to be modelled before the kidney itself. The result might be:

(Organs newSub Kidney)
triple hasLaterality Bilateral[necessary];
triple IsStructuralComponentOf Abdomen [necessary];

This would express the fact that "A new organ exists, whose name is kidney, which is necessarily located bilaterally in the abdomen".
The same remark applies for the entire knowledge domain. For example, the model has to "know" about blood cells before you can model the alteration of blood elements, etc.

- Horizontal or vertical expansion ?

An important problem encountered in modeling a specific domain is the constant necessity to refer to knowledge other than that contained in the model. This leads to the conclusion that, to build a deep vertical model, good horizontal knowledge is required. This is particularly true if the model has to remain consistent for further domains. To illustrate this, in the case of infectious urinary diseases, it is evident that infectious agents must be present in the model. It requires a model of bacteria's, fungi and viruses, and some of their respective properties. It implies some physiological, functional concepts, like an infection generally leads to increased white blood cells. The latter example shows that a model of blood is needed, and therefore of bone-marrow where blood cells are produced, and so on. Often, a vertical expansion in a particular domain leads both to horizontal expansion as well as further vertical expansion in all the other domains. This is, in fact, only the result of the high level of interconnection in medical knowledge. To illustrate the problem of verticality and the depth of knowledge in our model, let us take an example where we had to enter information about urinary diseases involving immunological, biomolecular and genetic knowledge. This example is about Lowe's disease (also known as oculo-cerebro-renal syndrome), which is an X-linked recessive form of the Fanconi syndrome. This syndrome is characterized by a constellation of transport defects in the kidneys and, therefore, has a complex clinical presentation. The example shown below models some properties of the Lowe's syndrome, and then "adds" this syndrome to the model as "kindOf" Fanconi disease:

a) definition of Lowe's syndrome and some characteristics
Disease newSub [OculoCerebroRenalSyndrome]
triple hasEponym "LoweSyndrome" default
triple isDiseaseOf UrinarySystem [necessary];
triple isDiseaseOf NervousSystem [necessary];
triple hasGeneticComponent
(XLinkDisease which <
hasTransmission Recessive
hasChromosomeLocus Xq25>) necessary];
triple hasPhysicalSign Cataract[necessary];
triple hasPhysicalSign Glaucoma [necessary];
triple hasPhysicalSign Nanism [necessary];
triple hasPhysicalSign Rachitism [necessary];
triple hasPsychicalSign WeaklQ [necessary];
triple hasBiologicalSign
(Urine which<
abnormalContains Glucose
abnormalContains AminoAcids >) [necessary]...

b) Telling the model that Lowe's Syndrome is "a kind of" Fanconi Syndrome:
FanconiDisease addSub OculoCerebroRenalSyndrome.

- The "atomisation " state, or degree of detail

The term atomisation means the degree of fragmentation of each piece of knowledge. For example, a catheter could simply be defined as a kind of device with some properties. One could also fragment catheters into different kinds of catheters, with various lengths, diameters and compositions. Each kind of catheter could then respectively be linked with its properties and usage. In fact, the degree of atomisation is, in our model or in any model, imposed both by the kind of knowledge needed and the discriminative properties of each concept. Let us take bladder catheters as example. There are two main kinds of urinary bladder catheters. The first one enters the urinary bladder using the natural routes, through the urethra. In contrast, the second one goes through the skin and the abdominal wall directly into the urinary bladder. These two kinds of catheter are obviously different. In our model, it is unnecessary to describe the physical properties of these catheters, like length or diameter. It is of great importance, however, to define that the first one goes via the natural routes whereas the second breaks the skin and therefore the natural barriers against infectious diseases.

Moreover, the microbiological analyses that can be carried out with these two catheters are different. The catheter that goes via the natural routes will provide urine that has been in contact with air, whereas the suspubian catheter will not. Hence, it is futile to search for bacteria that are killed by air in the urine coming from the first catheter, and it is sensible to perform these analyses with urine coming from the second one. This example illustrates both the horizontal and the vertical knowledge necessary to model these two kinds of urinary catheter. In English, this could be expressed as follows :

1) "A urine collecting catheter exists, that goes via the natural routes and collects urine that has been in contact with air", and 2) "A urine collecting catheter exists, that goes through the skin and abdominal wall, collecting urine that has not been in contact with air". In the Galen Master Notation, this can be expressed as follows :

```
1) (Device newSub UreteralCatheter
        triple isDeviceFor UrinarySys [necessary];
        triple passBy Uretera [necessary];
        triple hasBodyProduct
            (Urine which hasAnalyze AerobeGerms) [necessary].


2) Device newSub SusPubianCatheter)
        triple isDeviceFor UrinarySys [necessary];
        triple passBy Skin [necessary];
        triple hasBodyProduct
            (Urine which <
                hasAnalyze AerobeGerms
                hasAnalyze AnaerobeGerms>) [necessary].
```

2.5. Coherence and validation

Coherence and validation are two different problems. The coherence control of a knowledge model can be subdivided into two subproblems. The first subproblem may be called "self-coherence". This means the coherence of the model itself, i.e. the coherence of the concept structures of the model between them. The second coherence type relates to the coherence between the model and the world. Whereas it is possible to have some machine rules to help the maintenance of self-coherence, only the review of the knowledge model by knowledge experts can assure the coherence between the model and the outside world.

As an example, let us take the problem of fractures. If it is modelled that any part of the body may suffer from a fracture, it is then self-coherent to say that an eye may have a fracture. However, it is obvious that such a concept is incoherent in reality.

An interesting fact about self-coherence is that it can be partly automatized by a few rules. These mechanisms help the knowledge modeller to build a coherent model. In fact, it appears that coherency tools are essentially constraining rules. The Galen Master Notation currently supports two main mechanisms that help to maintain self-coherence:

i) The constraint qualifier of an attribute. For example, it can be expressed that the location of a fracture is definitely a bone: *Fracture triple asLocation Bone [necessary].*

When such a rule is given, the application of the concept *Fracture is* constrained to the concept *Bone,* and it is therefore no longer possible to say *Fracture which hasLocation Eye.* Therefore, the qualifiers of attributes are a good way of limiting the use of these attributes to the appropriate concepts.

ii) The cardinality constraint of an attribute. The cardinality represents the numbers of similar concepts that could be linked to the right and left sides of an attribute. Let us give some examples to clarify the use of cardinality. The most constraining use of cardinality is the situation where an attribute can link one concept to another. This could be illustrated with the attribute *hasAtomicNumber.* Hence, any chemical element has only ONE atomic number and each atomic number corresponds to only ONE chemical element. Therefore, the cardinality of *hasAtomicNumber* would be *oneOne.* In contrast, the concept *Severity* can be applied to any disease, whereas a specific disease can only have one *Severity* at the same time. Therefore, the attribute concept *hasSeverity* would have a *ManyOne* cardinality. It means, MANY diseases can have the same severity, but only ONE severity can apply to a specific disease at one time. The self-coherence of a model remains a problem. The need for new tools to help maintain this coherence is urgent and they still have to be developed. The problems involving the development of such tools are yet to be resolved.

The coherence between the model and the external world has to be maintained by the knowledge builder and independent validation instances.

2.6. Validation

The problem of validation is of much greater importance than the self-coherence of a model, since it implies the coherence between the model and the reality of medical knowledge. Therefore, it will not be possible to automatize such a process, other than by using comparison tools between various models. This would only transfer the problem to another model. The necessity for external validation, in our case, medical experts, is therefore clear. Such independent validation will probably be easy for fundamental knowledge, since it will be possible to use current coding schemes to estimate the extent of knowledge contained in the model. Hence, the evolutive part of medical knowledge needs constant adaptation. The debate about this problem is far from being resolved, and is beyond the subject of the present paper. What can be said is that a model based on a clear, understandable formalism, such as the Galen Master Notation, will greatly help the capacity to rapidly adapt the model to new knowledge. This remains particularly true when the knowledge builder is not a computer specialist.

3. CONCLUSIONS

The conclusion is divided in two parts. First, the modelling problem of medical knowledge. Second, the results obtained with the Galen Master Notation formalism.

The modelling of medical knowledge implies a huge amount of knowledge, either of medicine or common sense. In order to have any chance of really being used, the knowledge model should cover the various applications that need medical knowledge, i.e. medical records, bibliographic retrieval, expert systems, coding schemes and natural language.

It should provide common exchange bases for physicians, scientists and economists. This implies a large horizontal and vertical extent of the model. Due to the evolutive characteristics of medical knowledge, the tools used must allow fast and easy modification or extension of the model, with redundancy and coherency checking tools. Entering knowledge must be simple and as close as possible to natural knowledge understanding, because this information will usually be introduced by non-computer scientists. Finally, the hardware and software support must be usable on multiple hardware platforms.

The Galen Master Notation formalism developed in the GALEN project provides a possible answer to all the constraints summarized above. This formalism supports multiple platforms either in the UNIX world as well in the personal computer world. The way to introduce data is close to natural language and a physician may be enrolled for this task. The use of rules, qualifiers and definition concepts allows a very fine definition of medical knowledge. However, some problems that have to be resolved in this formalism remain, such as the use of negation in inheritance structures, the development of coherence checkers, especially between similar concepts, and finally, tools to automatize the merge of two models into one developed in the same formalism.

4. REFERENCES

1 Lenat D B, Guha R V, Building Large Knowledge-Based Systems: Representation and Inference in the Cyc Project, Addison-Wesley Publishing Company, 1989.

2 Kahn M, Modelling Time in Medical Decision-support Programs, Med Decis Making, 1991, 11:249-264.

3 Sowa J, Conceptual Structures: Information Processing in Mind and Machine, Addison-Wesley Publishing Company, 1984.

4 Baud RH, Rassinoux A-M, Scherrer J-R. Natural Language Processing and Semantical Representation of Medical Texts. Methods of Information in Medicine, Vol.31, 2/1992.

5 Rector AL et al., Conceptual Knowledge: The core of medical information systems, Medinfo 92.

6 ICD - 9, World Health Organisation, Geneva, 1977.

7 EMTree, Elsevier Publishing Company.

8 Lorino F, the GALEN Consortium, WP1.2.3, the Code Conversion Module: Functional Specifications, January 1993.

9 The Galen Consortium, Deliverable 5: Setting up the Decomposition Database for the Population of the Core Model, Jan 1993.

10 National Library of Medicine, MeSH Medical Subject Headings, NLM Bethesda, Maryland (yearly).

11 Rector A, Nowlan A, Glowinski A, Matthews G, Rush T, Pakarinen V. the GALEN Consortium, Deliverable 6: The Master Notation, version 1, 1993.

Artificial Intelligence in Medecine
S. Andreassen et al. , Eds.
IOS Press, 1993

A Model of Patient Related Data and a Structure of Medical Terms for Knowledge–Based Systems in Medicine

J. Stausberg, T. Diedrich, A. Wormek and P. Hucklenbroich

GSF - Forschungszentrum für Umwelt und Gesundheit GmbH, Institut für Medizinische Informatik und Systemforschung, Neuherberg, Ingolstädter Landstr. 1, 85764 Oberschleißheim, Germany

Abstract

Modelling medical knowledge is still a significant problem in Artificial Intelligence in Medicine. The topic of our project is to develop a general reference model for medical knowledge and decision making. This development requires a thorough analysis of the structure of patient related data. To support modelling patient related data, we also developed a repository for all relevant medical terms. For both we defined a model, derived a frame–like representation and coded a prototype implementation.

In the repository, terms are described by specialisation, components, attributes, and possible values. The implementation of the repository also consists of an acquisition tool and a definition browser. The model of patient related data is represented in a frame–like form, the Case–Data–Sheet. Case–based–data can be formalized in the Case–Data–Sheet by simple object–attribute–value–triples as well as by more complex structures with iterated attributes and multiple attributes. The above complex structures can be augmented by context–dependent information about patient–object and/or object–object relationships.

We developed our prototype implementation to evaluate whether our model of patient related data is adequate and complete. This implementation consists of a comfortable user interface, that lets the user enter information about a patient with familiar terms and generally accepted descriptions. Our system then creates Case–Data–Sheets as necessary and automatically transforms the user's input into the corresponding data structures. The models for both, the patient–related data and the repository of terms, are implemented fairly straightforward in Smalltalk/V on PC. Future research should investigate, whether these models and the derived structures can be an adequate base for the formalization of patient related data in medical knowledge–based systems.

1. Introduction

The work presented in this article is part of an ongoing project at the GSF–MEDIS–Institute carried out by the research group on *Methods of AI*. Background of this project and related work is the KliniC approach which briefly will be described in the following. The KliniC approach is a methodological model of medical decision making incorporating all phases of the medical decision making process on the basis of the diverse information structures and kinds of knowledge that are used in medical practice (KliniC model). KliniC is based on work of Hucklenbroich on the methodological and theoretical foundations of medicine [1,2]. It is intended to become a reference model for the development of medical knowledge bases and knowledge-based systems. But so far, KliniC is just a rather informal, verbally formulated, model. It has to be transformed into a formal model to be useful as a reference model. To reach this goal, we are implementing parts of the model as computer programs. Developing and evaluating this programs can support the further specification and correction of the model. Alternating phases of experiment and theory should lead to a formal, experimental validated, model. The work presented in this paper is part of this approach.

The KliniC model distinguishes four case related information structures in medical decision making: *facts, diagnostic hypotheses,* the *indicated* and *contraindicated measures (diagnostic, therapeutic* or *preventive),* and the *resulting decisions.* These four information structures are used and modified within an argumentation strategy which is common in clinical medicine but also specific for the domain of medicine. This strategy controls every part of diagnostic and therapeutic decision making. The static medical knowledge is differentiated into various kinds of knowledge which are organized in a such a way, that they support the control process. For details of the KliniC model we refer to [3].

As described above, the overall project goal is the development of a formal knowledge model. In this respect it can be compared with other approaches, like the KADS methodology [4], the GAMES/GAMES II project [5], and the MACCORD model [6]. There are major differences between each of these approaches and the KliniC model which are briefly described below:

- In the KADS approach it is presupposed that problem solving competence can be formulated and formalized independent of the underlying application domain. This assumption is not shared in KliniC. Rather the KliniC model formulates and describes problem solving strategies and kinds of knowledge that are specific for the domain of medicine.

- The Select and Test model (ST-model) [7] of Stefanelli et.al. starts from the paradigm of abstract logic. It distinguishes (according to Peirce) *abduction, deduction,* and *induction* as the three main inference types. Cyclic applications of these concepts lead to models for medical tasks, namely *diagnosis, therapy,* and *monitoring.* In contrast to this approach, KliniC integrates diagnosis, therapy, monitoring, and in addition prevention and rehabilitation, within one single argumentation model. The interactions between these tasks thus can be modelled explicitly within KliniC.

- The MACCORD model is not a model of medical argumentation in the same sense that KliniC is. It neither contains information structures that are specific for medicine nor a procedural model for argumentation and decision making. It rather can be viewed as a heuristic classification system for the various kinds of medical knowledge and medical subtasks.

2. Problem

As mentioned above, we are implementing example computer prototypes of parts of the KliniC model in order to evaluate and formally specify the model. The first step within this complex task was the implementation of the model of patient (case) related information (patient data and other relevant facts). Using this implementation, we can enter real case histories to prove the completeness and correctness of this subsystem and of other subsystems. The part of our work dealing with the subsystem for patient related information is subject of this paper.

Patient related facts and data include all medically relevant information a physician or a clinic is collecting with regard to an individual patient. This information is usually documented in the medical report of the patient. It contains statements on the patients symptoms, signs, findings, diagnoses, diagnostic and therapeutic procedures etc. Moreover it may include information about the patients social relationships and behaviour and all kinds of conclusions the physician is drawing concerning the patient (cf. section 4). In modelling patient related information (facts and data), two components have to be distinguished:

1) modelling the overall structure (syntax) of fact descriptions, and

2) defining and structurally characterizing all medical terms that can be used within patient related fact descriptions.

The former component contains the definition of an information structure whereas the latter constitutes the first stage of a medical knowledge base. Although by now our main concern has been the implementation of the information structure, the term definitions turned out to be a necessary prerequisite for the intended subsystem. The structural characteristics of a term (e.g. the value range of a certain quality) were intended to automatically drive the generation of input menus for the case entry. To be able to prove the completeness and correctness of the information structure and the user interface design, we therefore had to define a reasonable number of medical terms. Besides a prototypical user interface, two data structures form the basis of the implementation: the *Case–Data–Sheet* (the information structure, cf. section 4) and the *Repository* (a dictionary of medical terms and their definitions, cf. section 5).

We implemented our system on a PC using the object-oriented programming environment Smalltalk/V for Windows. Case–Data–Sheet and Repository have been designed using object-oriented methods [8]. The user interface consists of two main components: one module for the input of case related data and one module for the input of medical term definitions. Besides, there is an ascii-interface to link the system to external data bases and knowledge bases. However, the user interface and the Repository are not intended to become useful and really used in real medical practice. They are just an aid for the development and evaluation of the information structure rsp. the underlying model.

3. Methods

The Case–Data–Sheet is a frame-like structure which implements a model of patient related information. The elements of the knowledge base are intended to be represented as frames, too. The resulting structural equivalences are supposed to simplify the management of the interrelations between data and knowledge. Before starting with the implementation, we tested the structure of the Case–Data–Sheet manually using real case histories. These preliminary tests had positive results.

We did not try to develop a model of patient related information which incorporates processing of natural language structures. Natural language processing is still a significant and not completely solved research problem. Steps towards that direction with respect to patient related data were done by Baud et.al. [9] and Bernauer [10] using conceptual graphs. Besides, we also did not try to develop a general architecture for medical terminology as it is currently done in the AIM-GALEN project (AIM Project 2012). However, the structures of the Repository and the Case–Data–Sheet are so flexible, that they could integrate the existing medical terminologies and nomenclatures.

4. A Model of Patient Related Data

A model of patient related information that comes into question as a reference model for medical knowledge bases must be so complete and flexible that every medically sensible piece of patient related information can be formulated in the model. It must take into consideration various kinds of information:

- Every piece of information is related to a certain individual patient. This relation has to be expressed by the model.
- A major part of patient related information can be viewed as a state, aspect or parameter of a patient ("object") which has some qualitative or quantitative, possibly nested, properties ("attributes") with specific values. Therefore, the model must incorporate simple object-attribute-value tripels as well as multiple and iterated attributes and values.
- An important subinformation is the "status" of a piece of information. That includes information on whether a certain question has already been investigated or not, or whether a piece of information is known, doubtful, unknown or wrong, or whether a procedure is possible, impossible, carried out or not carried out.
- Other kinds of information are the source of the data (intellectual or according to the supply), the causal relations of a fact to other facts, and the uncertainty of a piece of data.
- Finally, there are kinds of information dealing with specific relations between data, like *x can explain y* or *x is result of y*.

The Case–Data–Sheet is a frame-like structure which contains all these kinds of information in its slots and subslots. Moreover, every Case–Data–Sheet contains system information in order to manage various instances of Case–Data–Sheets within a patient data base.

5. Repository

To be able to enter patient related data menu driven, we developed the Repository. The Repository consists of medical terms and definitions. It can be viewed as the first part of a clinical knowledge base. A term in the Repository is defined by:

1. The term's denotation together with an id-number which is unique throughout the system.
2. Optional is a verbal description and the declaration of synonyms of the term, and

3. a conceptual characterization which can include:

    (a) specializations of the subject to be characterized (which constitutes an *is–a* lattice),

    (b) parts of the subject (which constitutes a *part–of* lattice)

    (c) identification of the qualities (attributes) of the subject,

    (d) identification of possible values of the subject, like *numeric, boolean, date* or *term.*

Terms can denote diseases, symptoms, signs , findings, and qualities like *location* or *intensity.* The specializations, parts and qualities of a term are expressed by lists of terms. *Pain* is a specialization of *symptom*, the *finger* is a part of the *hand* and *pain* can have the qualities *location, duration, radiation* etc. Qualities like *intensity* are themselves defined as terms for which possible values like *high, low, increasing* or *decreasing* can be declared. The characteristics described above automatically constitute a semantic network of terms. Five terms have been defined to be the root nodes of the *is–a* lattice (that means, they do not have generalizations): *anamnesis* (including common information like *age* and *sex*), *physical examination, diagnostics, diagnosis* and *therapy.* The implementation of the Repository consists of a knowledge aquisition tool and a definition browser (cf. fig. 1). With the definition browser it is possible to inspect the network of terms as well as every single term definition. An ascii-interface has been implemented to be able to interchange data with external data bases and knowledge-based systems.

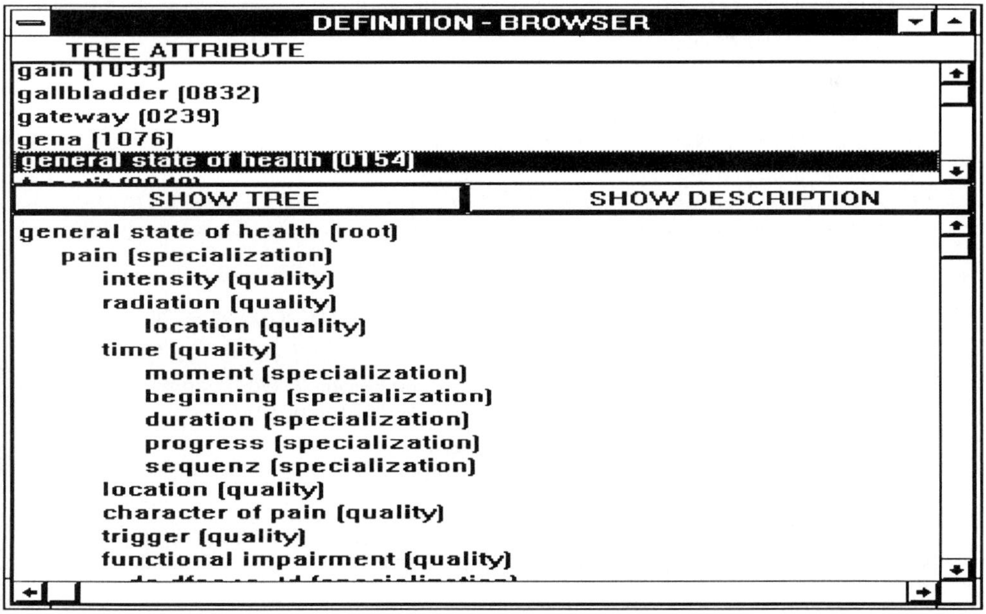

Figure 1: screen of the definition browser

6. Conclusions and Future Work

Preliminary results of our research have revealed that our models and corresponding representation structures for patient related data and the term repository can serve their purposes adequately. Further evaluation steps will focus on correctness and completeness of mapping of input information to internal structures. To perform the proper tests, we are now collecting and analysing appropriate case histories and clinical records. Certain important aspects of the model for patient related data need to be worked out and refined in more detail. The most significant of these aspects are context-dependend information, basic relationships, and the representation of time and uncertainty. The principal goal of our project is the development of a general reference model for medical knowledge and reasoning. The results achieved so far (the model of patient related data, the term repository, and the prototype implementation) will serve as modules for data entry and knowledge management of a future exemplary knowledge-based system based on such a general reference model.

7. References

1 Hucklenbroich, P.: *Künstliche Intelligenz und medizinisches Wissen*
Habilitationsschrift Münster 1989

2 Hucklenbroich, P., Toellner, R. (Hrsg.): *Künstliche Intelligenz in der Medizin*
Klinisch-methodologische Aspekte medizinischer Expertensysteme
Gustav Fischer Verlag Jena, New York 1993

3 Hucklenbroich, P.: *Modellierung unterschiedlicher klinisch-medizinischer Wissensarten*
Biometrie und Informatik in Medizin und Biologie 23 (1992), 43

4 Wielinga, B. J., Schreiber, A. Th., Breuker, J. A.:
KADS: A Modelling Approach to Knowledge Engeneering
Knowledge Acquisition 4 (1992) 5-53

5 Stefanelli, M., Bellazzi, R., Berzuini, C., Ironi, L., Quaglini, S.:
Towards a General Architecture for Medical Expert Systems
Working Notes of the AAAI Spring Symposium Series, Stanford University, 1992, 105-11

6 Mannebach, H., Kraus, D., Petkoff, B.:
Methodologie der Klinischen Medizin:
Voraussetzung für die Konstruktion eines medizinischen Expertensystems
in Hucklenbroich, P., Toellner, R. (Hrsg.): *Künstliche Intelligenz in der Medizin*

7 Stefanelli, M., Ramoni, M.: *Modeling Medical Knowledge Based Systems*
Biometrie und Informatik in Medizin und Biologie 23 (1992), 215

8 Coad, P., Yourdon, E.: *Object-Oriented Design*
Prentice Hall, Englewood Cliffs, New Jersey 1991

9 Baud, R. H., Rassinoux, A. - M., Scherrer, J. R.:
Natural Language Processing and Semantical Representation of Medical Texts
Methods of Information in Medicine 31 (1992), 117

10 Bernauer, J.:
Konzeptuelle Graphen als Semantisches Modell für den Medizinischen Befund
Biometrie und Informatik in Medizin und Biologie 23 (1992), 228

Artificial Intelligence in Medecine
S. Andreassen et al. , Eds.
IOS Press, 1993

The knowledge-based management of medical acts in NUCLEUS

M. Joubert [a,b], H. Kanoui [a]

[a] IIRIAM. Technopôle de Château-Gombert. Europarc, bat. C. 13453 Marseille Cedex 13. France
[b] CERTIM. Faculté de Médecine. Boulevard P. Dramard. 13326 Marseille Cedex 15. France

Hospital information systems are currently required to provide an intelligent support to the daily professional activity. A semantic model is presented which is intended to represent the knowledge about the acts that are practised, the resources they involve and the consumable objects they need We show how this knowledge is used to structure the patients records.

1. INTRODUCTION

The hospital information systems (HISs) designers are now required to allow an intelligent support to the daily professional activities of health care in the hospitals [1]. The health care professionals (HCPs) - the actual end-users of the information system - require a high-level of customisation with respect to: (1) the procedures and the rules that govern activities such as patients management, medical and nursing care, and (2) the knowledge related to the medical practice achieved by the HCPs which may be specific to a hospital service, a health care unit or a medical speciality.

The knowledge-based management of the medical acts in a HIS was introduced in the framework of the RICHE project (ESPRIT II n° 2221). It is enhanced and refined in the frame of the NUCLEUS project (AIM n° 2025). In the frame of RICHE, the fundamental notion was the concept of act and relies on the requester-performer schema [2]. The management of acts supports the HCPs activity in a hospital. The knowledge about the acts deals mainly with the management of the acts and the resources necessary for their performance [3]. The description of the classes of acts and their environment is a part of the domain knowledge as opposed to the information relying to patients data and actual acts content.

NUCLEUS adds the notion of the patient reference dossier (PRD) which is the structured set of all the recorded acts for a given patient. The PRD data constitute the way to structure the acts of a given patient according to the knowledge that apply on the classes from which they are instanciated. Specially, links connect acts between themselves or with resources necessary to do them. These links are instances of the semantic relationships that apply on the classes of related objects. The user has not only the capability to structure sets of acts, as PRDs, but also to query and navigate in PRDs while being guided and controlled by the domain knowledge [4].

2. THE SEMANTIC MODEL OF NUCLEUS

The knowledge model of NUCLEUS is designed to provide functionalities at different levels according to the architecture presented in the figure 1: (1) a general high-level layer of knowledge which describes all the system basic class models and constitutes a meta-model for the NUCLEUS classes of objects, (2) a layer of knowledge which constitutes the structured model of NUCLEUS objects whose classes are instanciated from the above layer, and (3) the data layer: the actual data stored at this level are instances of the classes of the latter layer.

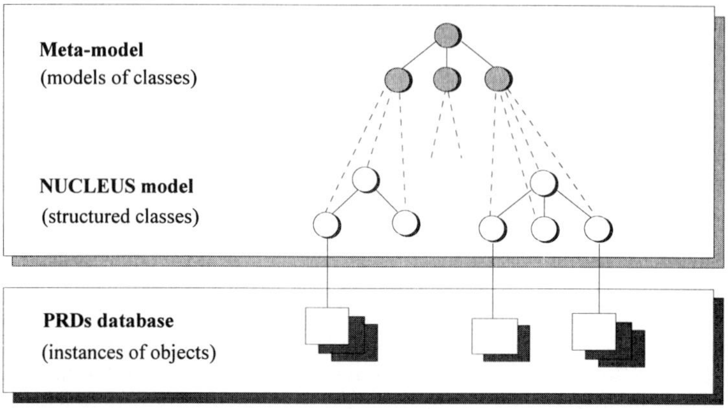

Figure 1. An overall view on knowledge and data in NUCLEUS

2.1. The meta-model

The models of classes defined at the upper level are generic and constitute a meta-model for the classes of NUCLEUS. They are: (1) *Node*: the class of nodes in a semantic network, (2) *Relationship*: the class of both structural and binary semantic relationships in this network. The nodes and the semantic relationships that apply on them are the very basic elements of a semantic network [5]. Then, with the definition of structural, relationships between nodes it is possible to define tree-structures, called taxonomies, that organise nodes and provide them with typed properties [6].

The structural relationships are: (1) *Gen/Spec* which applies on nodes only and organises them in more generic and more specific ones in taxonomies, (2) *Composition* that applies on nodes only and serve to group sets of nodes into new classes of compound objects. Attributes and methods of this class will be further refined to express constraints on instances of this class such as temporal and physical applicability.

These classes of structural relationships serve to define new sub-classes of Node: the class of taxonomies and the class of compound objects. Thus, the sub-classes of Node are: (1) *Elementary Object*: the class model of all the basic nodes of information in the HIS, (2) *Compound Object*: this class model defines the objects that are grouped by the mean of Composition links to create new classes of objects, and (3) *Taxonomy*: the class model which defines what is a taxonomy, that is a hierarchical organisation of objects of a same class structured by Gen/Spec links.

2.2. The NUCLEUS model

It is then possible to define the classes of objects and relationships of NUCLEUS. This will be achieved in two steps: (1) the first step consists in the definition of the class models of objects that are necessary to express the knowledge involved in the management of acts in the information system, (2) the second step will concern the adaptation of the system to a given hospital. That is the customisation by the performers of the acts they are able to provide in the hospital and the constraints they imply. The engineering aspects of this latter process are detailed in [4].

Among the general classes of objects involved in the implementation of NUCLEUS is the class model *Act*: the class model of all acts that can be practised in a hospital. It is a sub-class of Node. Sub-classes of the Act class are Medical Act, Nursing, and so on. The body of an act refers to the actual data its instances will contain. Consumable Object, Resource, and other class models are defined at this level. Each one of the above classes can be specialised into specific sub-classes according to the wished level of detail. This process leads to a hierarchical conceptual model of classes.

It is then possible to define semantic relationships, as instances of the previously described Relationship class model, between some of the above classes of objects. Among these relationships we can notice: (1) *Needs* whose origin is a sub-class of Medical Act and whose destination is a Resource, (2) *Precedes*: the semantic relationships that apply on two classes of medical acts, (3) *Consumes* that applies on a Medical Act, as the origin, and on a Consumable Object, as the destination, (4) *Diagnoses* which links a class of Diagnostic Procedure and a class of Diseases. Other semantic relationships are defined in a same way. These semantic relationships serve both to express the relations which exist between objects, such as: «a surgical act treats a disease», and to precise the respective roles and constraints in compound objects, such as «an anesthesia precedes a surgical act».

2.3. The structured PRDs database

This knowledge is exploited to structure the PRDs database. The figure 2 presents a part of a PRD for a given patient. This latter consists in a collection of actual acts featured by squares. Each actual act is an instance of a class of acts.

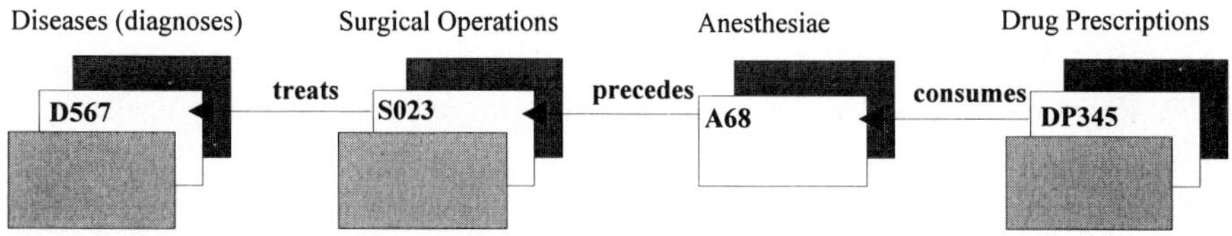

Figure 2. An example of a PRD organisation

The setting of a link labelled «treats» between the act #S023 and the act #D567 is authorised because there exists the semantic relationship «treats» between the classes Surgical Act and Diseases. Similarly, a link labelled «precedes» is set from the actual act #A68 to the act #S023, because it is said that a general anesthesia precedes a coronary artery bypass, at the knowledge level. This example shows how the patient dossier is structured and organised with the help and under the control of the domain knowledge.

3. DISCUSSION

The semantic model that we presented and discussed here operates in two complementary ways in the system NUCLEUS. First, it is the support for the knowledge related to the objects that the hospital information system manipulates, mainly the acts practised on patients and the resources needed by their performance. Secondly, it provides the mean to structure the actual acts stored in the PRDs database according to the semantic network defined at the knowledge level. The actual data of a given patient are then organised in a network of acts linked by instances of the semantic relationships.

A language has been designed to query both the knowledge bases and the PRDs database. By reference to the so-called SQL, it has been named XQL (X for eXtended). In this way, the above semantic model and XQL appear as an extension of the relational databases model. This kind of extensions are currently under investigation [7]. Two directions are emerging today. The first one tries to provide integrated models of both object-oriented models and databases. A second way of investigation, which seems attractive in the medical domain, consists in the definition of a semantic conceptual model of a relational database. The system PENGUIN illustrates well this kind of research [8]. This work goes clearly in this latter direction.

REFERENCES

1. Olsen PS. Flexibility of hospital insformation systems. In: Bakker AR, and al. (eds), Towards new hospital information systems. North-Holland 1988; 25-31.
2. van der Werff A, and al. Towards a European framework reference model and architecture for the development of open hospital information systems. In: Lun KC, and al. (eds), MEDINFO 92. North-Holland 1992; 188-193.
3. Riouall D, and al. The customisation of the RICHE HIS: the role of knowledge servers. In: Lun KC, and al. (eds), MEDINFO 92. North-Holland 1992; 194-198.
4. Kanoui H, and al. Customisation environment for an act-based hospital information system. In: Reichert A, and al. (eds), MIE 93. Freund Publish. 1993; 241-245.
5. Woods WA. What's in a link: foundations for semantic networks. In: Bobrow D, Collins A (eds), Representation and understanding: studies in cognitive science. Academic Press 1975; 35-82.
6. Woods WA. Understanding subsumption and taxonomy. In: Sowa JF (ed), Principles of semantic networks: exploration in the representation of knowledge. Morgan Kaufmann Publish. 1991; 45-94.
7. Cattell R. Object data management: object-oriented and extended relational database systems. Addison-Wesley, 1991.
8. Barsalou T, and al. Management of complex immunogenetics information using an enhanced relational model. Computers and Biomedical Research, vol. 24, n° 5, 1991.

Knowledge Acquisition, Representation & Learning

Artificial Intelligence in Medecine
S. Andreassen et al. , Eds.
IOS Press, 1993

Knowledge Representation and Modelling in HYBRIKON

Oliver Brendel[1], Rolf Widdig[1], Frank Piron[1], Diedrich Graf von Keyserlingk[2]

[1] Institute for Computer Science and Society, University Freiburg, Friedrichstraße 50, 79098 Freiburg

[2] Institute for Anatomy I, RWTH Aachen, Pauwelstraße, 52074 Aachen

Abstract

HYBRIKON is projected as a knowledge based system for Neuroscience with clinical relevance. In this paper we describe a three level knowledge acquisition method for heterogeneous neuroanatomical knowledge. The acquisition method integrates logical representation and ER-Models. We apply our techniques to the representation of important parts of the brain topography. As first results we present a logical theory for the brain topography and an ER-Model for neuroanatomical facts. In a parallel task a formal approach to literature knowledge is given. Finally we discuss the problem of different nomenclatures and show how to cope with it.

1. Introduction

One of the most prominent problems in Neuroscience is the localization in the CNS respectively the topographical mapping from functions to anatomical structures in brain and spinal cord. In Neurology the local diagnosis precedes the diagnosis of disease. Questions like "where is the problem" or "where is the lesion" are posed before naming the disease [19]. Laboratory medicine has grown impressively in the last decades but nevertheless neurological topical diagnosis keeps its central position [9].
The structural complexity of the CNS exceeds the functional one. There seems to be no unique mapping function for any part of neurology. The relation between structure and function is many to many and moreover we have to cope with fuzzy and partially inconsistent data in the literature. The several, differently structured anatomical nomenclatures (functional, histochemical, systematical etc.) give an additional problem.

In our project HYBRIKON (Hybrider Konsiliar für die Neurowissenschaften[1]) the aim is to conceptualize and to implement a knowledge based system for neurology and neurosurgery. For the above reasons our main difficulty is to represent spatial topographical knowledge and to relate it to higher brain functions respectively dysfunctions.

Our knowledge base is modular structured. There is a central module containing the topography which gives our main structuring principle surrounded by modules for several higher brain functions. In the actual state of the project we include modules for language, memory and motorial functions due to the speciality of our clinical partners. All modules are able to maintain incomplete, overlapping and inconsistent knowledge and to associate it with various nomenclatures. In the development and representation of these modules we use a logical approach in which we separate factual knowledge from background knowledge in a very early state of modelling and formalize it according to its internal structure.

The neuroanatomical knowledge module is the center of our system and has as the other modules a logical representation. So it was not possible to adapt one of the former representation methods on this subject (see e.g. [12], [18], [23]).

The methodical distinction between factual and background knowledge is maintained until the implementation. The main advantages are in a systematical consistency check of the background knowledge and a dynamical management of the factual knowledge.

Our first completely developed module is the topography model described in what follows. It contains knowledge about brain area hierarchies, neuronal connections, classifications according to nomenclatures, all based on neuroanatomical facts.

2. Methods

To represent relevant parts of neuroanatomical knowledge in a structured, accessible form on a computer we think it is not sufficient to restrict oneself on one single representation formalism. For that very reason we choose a heterogeneous representation formalism which can be derived from a uniform one. Picture 1 gives a general view on our representation process from "Rational Reconstruction" of the domain (see [24]) to the implementation on a digital computer.

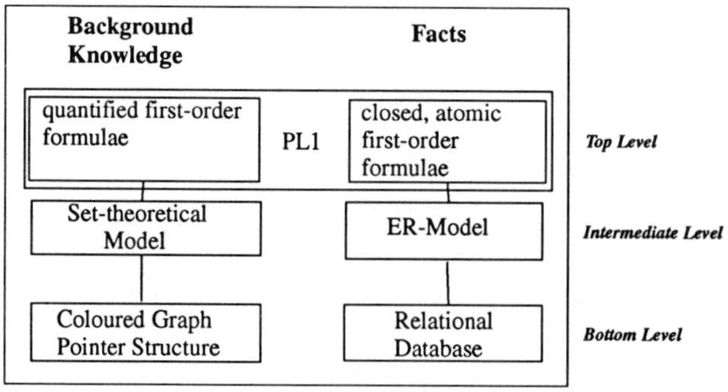

Picture 1

1 Hybrid counsellor for the neurosciences

Picture 1 shows a structure which is divided into two parts in horizontal direction and into three parts in vertical direction. The horizontal division reflects the heterogeneous nature of our knowledge domain. We draw a distinction between background knowledge and factual knowledge. Both kinds of knowledge are transformed along the vertical lines from the top to the bottom. The bottom level consists of the implemented data structures and algorithms. The three levels of picture 1 correspond to different levels of knowledge representation from abstract high level descriptions down to machine oriented structures. The division in three distinct, successive representation tasks is similar to the KADS-Methodology (see [5]) but has to be more concrete to develop a real software-application.

2.1 Top Level

Lets start with an explanation of the top level of picture 1 and define the concepts of Background Knowledge and Factual Knowledge. We use some concepts from logic and model theory which are all explained in [7] .

The Background Knowledge is the set of all logical and geometrical-topological facts concerning the objects of the domain and their relations. We give a simple example :

"If brain area 1 is a part of brain area 2 and if brain area 2 is a part of brain area 3, then brain area 1 is a part of brain area 3"

formally:

$$\forall \mathbf{a_1,a_2,a_3([Sub\_Struc(a_1,a_2) \wedge Sub\_Struc(a_2,a_3)] \rightarrow Sub\_Struc(a_1,a_3))}$$

For more complex examples see chapter 3 Results. The example shows that we represent background knowledge on the top level by quantified first-order formulae and until now all our background knowledge is axiomatized by universal quantified Horn-formulae which are equivalent to PROLOG-Rules.

The Factual Knowledge is the set of all individual neuroanatomical facts known about brain areas, tracks and all other objects and relations in the knowledge domain. Again we give a simple example:

"Brain area 1 is connected to brain area 2 by track 1"

formally:

$$\mathbf{Connection(A_1,T_1,A_2)}$$

Note that representation of factual knowledge on the top level is done by closed, atomic formulae.

In our opinion there are two main advantages of a logical representation:

- Logical formulae are universal in that one can derive other formalisms like frames ore semantic nets from them, depending on the structure of the formulae.

- In a logical representation it is possible to build clusters of formulae, characterized by their syntactical structure. In a second step one can map these clusters on suitable machine oriented representation forms as we do later.
In our case the two most important clusters are the quantified formulae and the closed, atomic formulae.

The result given by our top level representation is a logical first-order theory $\mathbf{T} = \mathbf{B} \cup \mathbf{F}$ consisting of a background theory B and a set of facts F.

2.2 Intermediate Level

On the intermediate level of picture 1 we have no more uniform representation like on the top (first-order logic). From the background theory B we construct a set-theoretical model in the sense of model-theory (see [7]), the facts F are described by an Entity-Relationship(ER)-model (see [8]). The set-theoretic model gives us a consistency proof for the background theory B and we can use it as an "Implementation Guide" for the final data structure. This model contains general knowledge about the substructure - or Part_Of relation- on brain areas and about the connection of brain areas.
The ER-model which consists of Entities and certain Relations between them (in analogy to the individual objects and relations of a set-theoretical model) represents elementary restrictions on an atomical, logical level. So for example: "In a fact of the form Connection(x,y,z) at least two argument positions have to be instantiated". Furthermore the ER-model reflects functional dependencies on the argument positions of the relations.

Now what are the advantages of the bidivision of modelling on the intermediate representation-level? What are the advantages of set-theoretical respectively ER-models?

- The division into two classes of models enables us to modify and extend different kinds of knowledge according to their structural properties. The background theory for example which contains general knowledge about the topography of the brain is represented by one closed model. The structure of the factual knowledge, represented in an ER-model can be translated in a relational database scheme.

- If we use suitable models for the background theory B (in fact we use saturated structures) it is possible to embed the facts (precisely: the individual constants which are contained in the facts) in these set-theoretical models. So we get a consistency check of the factual knowledge relatively to the background theory.

For more details concerning model construction and consistency proofs see [4], [3] and [15].

2.3 Bottom Level

Finally on the bottom level of picture 1 we implement the data structures and algorithms. The set-theoretical model of the brain-topography is to be translated into a coloured graph which pictures the general topology of brain areas. We have to say here that we do not represent spatial relations and information concerning metrics.
The coloured graph is the "Implementation Guide" for a pointer structure in the programming language C++. For such data structures and their algorithms see [22].

Also on the bottom level we translate the ER-model of facts into a relational database scheme. For this task we make use of ORACLE-CASE-TOOLS (see [1]). But it is worth to note that this is an interactive - rather than an autonomous process.

The connection between the pointer structure and the relational database scheme is realized by the embedding described above. Individual names for brain areas and tracks are mapped on the corresponding nodes and edges of the coloured graph.

3. Results

Now we show how our representation methods apply on the construction of a module for neuroanatomical, topographical knowledge. When several structured interviews with experts in neuroanatomy and some clinical partners specialized on neurology and neurosurgery were done and the relevant literature (e.g. [6], [2], [16], [17], [21]) was studied, the following demandmends on the topography model emerged.

- The representation of anatomical items with PNA-name, synonyms, abbreviation and other names like physiological names.

- The embedding of anatomical items in different nomenclatures, respectively to give a complex structure-nomenclature relation.

- To represent hierarchies of brain areas with the possibility to show partial views on hierarchy trees connected with given nomenclatures.

- A structured list for every brain area containing its subareas and superareas.

- A representation of connections together with initial area, name of the connecting track and destination area. Furthermore for every area a list of its afferences and efferences.

- mechanical derivation of complex, multistaged connections.

- A pointer on the literature respectively on one or more references in a separate literature database for every entry in the knowledge base. A single author or expert name as a reference for isolated entries.

3.1 The background theory of the topography

Now we show the most important parts of our background theory. We skipped the relations for literature and nomenclature and the corresponding axioms.

System of Axioms

alphabet:

a) junctures, quantors, bracketsymbols,

b) variables : $a, a_0, a_1, a_2, \ldots$ (variables for areasymbols)
$t, t_0, t_1, t_2, \ldots$ (variables for tracksymbols)

c) funtionsymbols

- 0-dim (constants) : $\varepsilon_a, \varepsilon_t$

d) relationssymbols

- 2-dim : Neuro_Path, Norm_Path, Sub_Path
Part_Of, Sub_Struc,
- 3-dim : Connection

$$\forall a \left(\neg \text{Sub\_Struc}(a, a) \right) \tag{1}$$

$$\forall a_1 a_2 \left(\text{Part\_Of}(a_1, a_2) \rightarrow \text{Sub\_Struc}(a_1, a_2) \right) \tag{2}$$

$$\forall a_1\, a_2\, a_3 \left([\text{Sub\_Struc}(a_1, a_2) \wedge \text{Sub\_Struc}(a_2, a_3)] \rightarrow \text{Sub\_Struc}(a_1, a_3) \right) \tag{3}$$

$$\forall a_1\, a_2\, t \left(\text{Connection}(a_1, t, a_2) \rightarrow \text{Norm\_Path}(a_1, a_2) \right) \tag{4}$$

$$\forall a_1\, a_2\, a_3\, t \left([\text{Connection}(a_1, t, a_2) \wedge \text{Norm\_Path}(a_2, a_3)] \rightarrow \text{Norm\_Path}(a_1, a_3) \right) \tag{5}$$

$$\forall a_1\, a_2\, a_3 \left([\text{Sub\_Struc}(a_2, a_1) \wedge \text{Norm\_Path}(a_2, a_3)] \rightarrow \text{Sub\_Path}(a_1, a_3) \right) \tag{6}$$

$$\forall a_1\, a_2\, a_3 \left([\text{Norm\_Path}(a_1, a_2) \wedge \text{Sub\_Struc}(a_2, a_3)] \rightarrow \text{Sub\_Path}(a_1, a_3) \right) \tag{7}$$

$$\forall a_1\, a_2\, a_3\, a_4 \left([\text{Sub\_Struc}(a_2, a_1) \wedge \text{Norm\_Path}(a_2, a_3) \wedge \text{Sub\_Struc}(a_3, a_4)] \rightarrow \text{Sub\_Path}(a_1, a_4) \right) \tag{8}$$

$$\forall a_1\, a_2 \left([\text{Norm\_Path}(a_1, a_2) \vee \text{Sub\_Path}(a_1, a_2)] \leftrightarrow \text{Neuro\_Path}(a_1, a_2) \right) \tag{9}$$

We use the relation symbols Part_Of and Sub_Struc to define area hierarchies respectively heterarchies. The interpretation of Part_Of is an input relation with arguments superarea and subarea, the derived relation Sub_Struc may reflect multistaged paths in the hierarchy. The axioms (1) - (3) say that Sub_Struc is an irreflexive partial ordering containingPart_Of. Part_Of is axiomatized as an irreflexive antisymmetric relation.

Norm_Path contains the transitive closure of the input relation Connection (axioms (4) and (5)). For a proof you may verify by induction on n:

$$\left[\bigwedge_{i=1}^{n-1} \text{Connection}(a_i, t_i, a_{i+1})\right] \Rightarrow \text{Norm\_Path}(a_1, a_n)$$

For that reason Norm_Path represents more complex connections. It is not defined explicitly irreflexive, because it shall describe nervous feedback too.

To motivate the axioms (6) - (8) we take a look at picture 2:

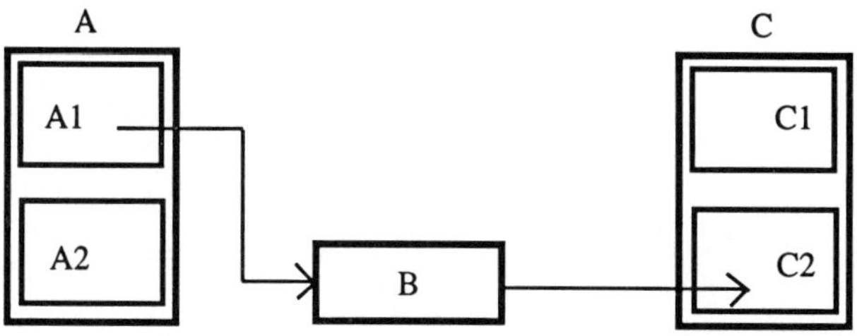

picture 2

There is a Norm_Path from A_1 to B finally reaching C_2. Of course this implies that there is also a path from A to C_2, from A_1 to C and from A to C. For semantic reasons we separate these paths (called Sub_Path), which contain at least one real step in the hierarchy from the Norm_Paths.
Axiom (9) says that we cannot compose connections and hierarchy steps arbitrarily. Superareas inherit the connections of their subareas and therefore all other properties like e.g. functional topographical facts.
Axiom (9) restricts the set of path, which can be inferred by the system. Note that Neural_Path is not a transitive relation (see picture 3):

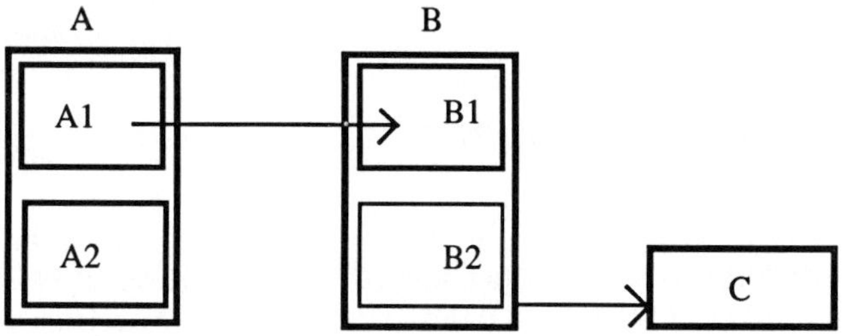

picture 3

There are Neural_Paths from A to B and from B to C . But there is no evidence for a Neural_Path from A to C because we do not know the roots of the neural path from B to C. They may completely lie in B_2 separated from B_1.

3.2 The ER-Model of the topographical facts

As earlier mentioned in the method part we represent the factual knowledge using ER-models separated from the background theory. Due to our modular system architecture the graphical ER-models remain transparent and so may give a foundation for the discussion with the medical experts in the phase of conceptualization.

For the graphical standards used in the ER-diagram (picture 4) see [1].
The subentities are given by an inheritance method. General features are modelled as attributes and associated with the main entity. More special features are associated with the subentities.

Picture 4 shows a model of the topographical factual knowledge. Relations with more than two arguments are represented as a combination of an entity and an association. This is necessary if we want to respect the convention only to use binary associations.
Additionally we resolve in a later step many-to-many relations for consistency reasons.

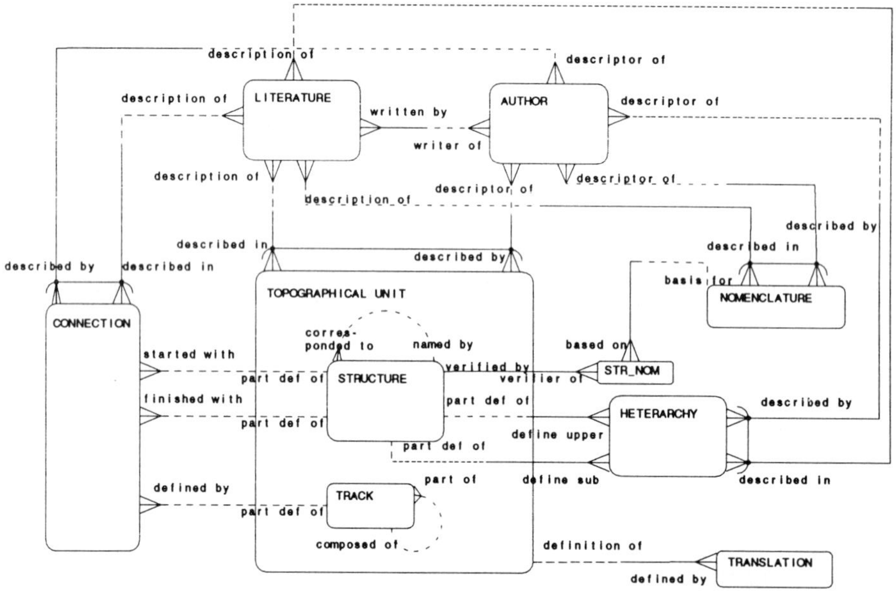

picture 4

The technical entity STR_NOM connects STRUCTURE with NOMENCLATURE. CONNECTIONS, STRUCTURES or TRACKS (TOPOGRAPHICAL UNIT), area hierarchies respectively HETERARCHIES and NOMENCLATURES are associated to one or more references (LITERATURE) or alternatively to a single author name (AUTHOR). This improves the citability of the system entries.

3.3 Data acquisition

Currently we acquire a database of about some hundred facts concerning the human Thalamus. There are several nomenclatures concerning the Thalamus. For the human Thalamus see [10], [13], [25], for the monkey see [20]. Hirai and Jones [11] make a detailed comparison of the nomenclature of Hassler, Jones and Olszewsky. With Hassler as a reference the naming of the several thalamus nuclei in the different nomenclatures is compared and synonyms and abbreviations are given. Furthermore they show that the different nomenclatures induce hierarchies with different granularity of partition into subnuclei. It is also shown that there are gaps in some of the nomenclatures.
For the parallel or even overlapping use of nomenclatures in our system we have collected all practical relevant cases which emerge if we embed one nomenclature in another. The formalizations of these cases are embodied in our model. For example we have 1:1-correspondences, different refinements of structures in the several nomenclatures and overlappings of structures. [26] contains a detailed description of all cases.

4. Discussion

Our results show, that relevant parts of neuroanatomical knowledge can be formalized. To perform this task, our three level representation method was a good tool because it kept the process of formalization transparent and manageable. The partition in analogical modelling techniques like coloured graphs on the one hand and normalized ER-models on the other hand makes it possible to manipulate heterogeneous knowledge in a flexible manner. We have shown that multistaged projections even in the hierarchy of brain areas can be derived. A concrete theory was given as a set of logical axioms. Furthermore we have maintained neuroanatomical facts in a relational database scheme.
In future work we will formalize functional modules with our representation method and we will connect our symbolic knowledge base with a digital brain atlas (see e.g. [14])

5. Acknowledgement

The project HYBRIKON is part of the MEDWIS programme (Wissensbasen in der Medizin[2]), which is financed by the federal ministry of research and development.
We specially like to thank Prof. Dr. Britta Schinzel for her continuous support of our project and for her ideas, which she has contributed.

---

[2] knowledge based systems in medicine

6. References

1 Barker, Richard: CASE*METHOD: Entity Relationship Modelling. Addison-Wesley, Reading, Mass. 1990.

2 Benninghoff, Alfred: Makroskopische und mikroskopische Anatomie des Menschen. Urban & Schwarzenberg, München, Wien, Baltimore 1985.

3 Brendel, Oliver: Funktioneller Hirnatlas - Axiomatisierung und Repräsentation der Topographie. Technical Report 7/1992, Institute of Computer Science and Society, University Freiburg.

4 Brendel, Oliver; Widdig, Rolf; Piron, Frank; Schinzel, Britta: HYBRIKON - Bericht Oktober 1992. Technical Report, Institute of Computer Science and Society, University Freiburg, 1992.

5 Breuker, J.; Wielinga, W.: KADS: Structured Knowledge Acquisition for Expert Systems. Proc Expert Systems and their Applications, Vol. 2, 1985, pp. 887-90.

6 Bucher, Otto; Wartenberg, Hubert: Cytologie, Histologie und mikroskopische Anatomie des Menschen. Verlag Hans Huber, Bern Stuttgart Toronto1989.

7 Chang, C.C.; Keisler, H.J.: Model Theory, North-Holland, Amsterdam 1973.

8 Chen, P. S.; Knöll, Heinz-Dieter: Der Entity-Relationship-Ansatz zum logischen Systementwurf: Datenbank- und Programmentwurf. BI-Wiss.- Verlag; Mannheim, Wien, Zürich,1991.

9 Duus: Neurologisch-topische Diagnostik. Thieme Verlag, Stuttgart, New York 1988.

10 Hassler, R.: Anatomy of the thalamus. In G. Schaltenbrand and P. Bailey (eds.) Introduction to Stereotaxis with an Atlas of the Human Brain. Thieme, Stuttgart 1959, pp. 230-290.

11 Hirai, T.; Jones, E.G.: A new parcellation of the human thalamus on the basis of histochemical staining. Brain Research Reviews 14, 1989, pp. 1-34.

12 Horn, Werner: Utilizing detailed anatomical knowledge for hypothesis formation and hypothesis testing in rheumatological decision support. Artificial Intelligence in Medicine 3, 1991, Elsevier, pp. 21-39.

13 Jones, E.G.: The Thalamus. Plenum, New York 1985.

14 Keyserlingk, Diedrich Graf von; Niemann, Klaus; Wasel, Josef; Maurer, K.: Digital Brain Atlas for Structure Localization in CT Combined with EEG Mapping. Psychiatry Res. 29, 1989, pp. 461-462.

15 Klomp, Frank: Funktioneller Hirnatlas - Die Datenbankkomponente. Technical Report 1/1992 of the Institute of Computer Science and Society, University Freiburg.

16 Nieuwenhuys, R. : Chemoarchitecture of the brain. Springer, Berlin, Heidelberg, New York 1985.

17 Nieuwenhuys, R.; Voogd, J.; van Huijzen, Chr.: Das Zentralnervensystem des Menschen. Springer Verlag, Heidelberg 1991.

18 Niggemann, Jörg: Analyse und Repräsentation neuroanatomischen Wissens. Technical Report 8/1989, Fraunhofer Institute für zerstörungsfreie Prüfverfahren, Hauptabteilung Medizintechnik.

19 Nyce, James M.; Graves III, William: The construction of knowledge in neurology: implications for hypermedia system development. Artificial Intelligence in Medicine 2, 1990, Elsevier, pp. 315-322.

20 Olszewsky, J.: The Thalamus of the Macaca mulatta. An atlas for use with the Stereotaxic Instrument. Karger, New York 1952.

21 Poeck, Klaus: Neurologie. Springer, Berlin, Heidelberg, New York 1990.

22 Sedgewick, R.: Algorithms. 2. ed., Addison Wesley, Reading, Mass. 1988.

23 Spitzer, Klaus; Stein, Volker; Thie, Andreas; Kunze, Klaus: NERVTRACK- A neuroanatomical Data Bank. Computers and Biomedical Research, 22, 1989, pp. 181-189.

24 Stegmüller, Wolfgang : Rationale Rekonstruktion von Wissenschaft und ihrem Wandel. Reclam, 1986.

25 Waldeyer, Anton; Mayet, Anton: Anatomie des Menschen, Band 2, 16. neubearbeitete Auflage, bearbeitet von Diedrich Graf v. Keyserlingk. Walter de Gruyter, Berlin, New York, 1993.

26 Widdig, Rolf; Brendel, Oliver; Piron, Frank; Schinzel, Britta : HYBRIKON - Jahresbericht 1992. Technical Report, Institute of Computer Science and Society, University Freiburg, 1993.

Artificial Intelligence in Medecine
S. Andreassen et al. , Eds.
IOS Press, 1993

Knowledge Organisation in Medical KBS Construction*

A. Th. Schreiber †, G. van Heijst †, G. Lanzola ‡ and M. Stefanelli ‡

† University of Amsterdam, Social Science Informatics
Roetersstraat 15, NL-1018 WB Amsterdam, The Netherlands

‡ University of Pavia, Medical Informatics
Via Abbiategrasso 209, I-27100, Pavia, Italy

Abstract In this paper we present an analysis of the structure of medical knowledge for the purpose of the construction of knowledge based systems. We discern three different views on knowledge that each have a different but complementary function with regard to reusability. We show that each of these views suggests distinct activities in the knowledge engineering process. The reported knowledge organisation is a key element of the GAMES methodology for the construction of medical knowledge based systems.

1 Introduction

In this paper, we discuss structuring principles of medical domain knowledge in knowledge-based applications. We take a knowledge-level [1] viewpoint, abstracting from potential symbolic representations of the knowledge. We distinguish three views on medical knowledge, namely (i) the *vocabulary* of basic medical terms, (ii) the knowledge *types* distinguished in an application, comprising the *ontology* of the application, and (iii) the knowledge *roles*, pointing to the way in which knowledge is used during problem solving.

Multiple views on medical knowledge are useful for a number of purposes. In this paper we focus on two aspects:

- The identification of generic, reusable knowledge elements.
- The rationale for specifying activities in knowledge-based system (KBS) construction.

The organisation of medical knowledge as discussed in this paper in one of the corner stones of the AIM project GAMES-II. The goal of this project is to develop a methodology,

* The research reported here was carried out in the course of the GAMES-II project. This project is partially funded by the AIM Programme of the Commission of the European Communities as project number A2034. The partners in this project are SAGO (Florence, Italy), Foundation of Research and Technology (Crete, Greece), Geneva University Hospital (Switzerland), the University of Amsterdam (The Netherlands), University College of London (UK), the University of Pavia (Italy) and the University of Ulm (Germany).
This paper reflects the opinions of the authors and not necessarily those of the consortium.

including theory and practical tools, for structured medical KBS construction (see [2] for an overview of the GAMES methodology). This paper reports on ongoing work and results within GAMES in the area of knowledge organisation and ontologies. We do not claim that all this is novel. In fact, our aim is to integrate results from knowledge engineering research and specialise these for use in medical applications. In the area of knowledge reuse our ideas are very much in line with [3].

In Sec. 2 we discuss in more detail the notion of knowledge-level modelling and the multiple views of medical knowledge used in GAMES. Subsequent sections describe how this view can be exploited for defining generic libraries of knowledge elements (Sec. 3) and for describing knowledge engineering activities (Sec. 4). Sec. 5 discusses related work and sketches a research agenda that follows from this work.

2 Knowledge Organisation

2.1 Background: knowledge-level modelling The first generation knowledge-based systems employed one relatively simple *inference engine* working on a knowledge base in a particular representational format, usually production rules. Clancey showed in his analysis of the prototypical system of this generation, MYCIN that such a knowledge base hides various important properties of the reasoning process, and of the structure of the knowledge in the application domain [4]. Certain rules, or parts of rules, fulfill particular roles in the reasoning process which remain implicit in such a KBS organization. This implicitness of underlying structures impairs the acquisition and refinement of knowledge for the KBS as well as the reuse of the system, its explanatory power and the assessment of its relation with other systems.

It is fair to say that this problem was not specific for the field of knowledge engineering. Similar problems were being identified in the broader area of knowledge representation. Clear evidence of this was brought forward by Brachman and Smith through the results of their SIGART questionnaire [5].The aim of this questionnaire was to get data on various knowledge representation approaches in order to perform a comparative study. About the results of their analysis of the huge amount of data received, they remark:

> "Perhaps more than anything else, it has emerged as a testament to an astounding range and variety of opinions held by many different people in many different places." [5, p. 1]

Everyone seemed to be speaking a different language: a true Babel.

In response to this confusion, Newell coined, in his presidential address to AAAI-80, the "knowledge-level hypothesis". The key point underlying his argument was that the confusion arose because AI research was too much focused on detailed representational issues. What was missing was a description of the rationale behind the use of AI techniques. He pleaded for a shift of emphasis in AI research from the "how" questions to the "why" questions. The knowledge-level was his proposal for realizing a description of an AI system in terms of its rational behaviour: why does the system (the "agent") perform this "action", independent of its symbolic representation in rules, frames or logic (the "symbol level").

2.2 Multiple views on medical domain knowledge During the last decade, a number of proposals have been put forward in knowledge engineering research for describing knowledge-level models [6,7,8,9,10,11,12,13,14,15]. A common distinction that is being made is between (i) domain knowledge, defining a declarative theory of the application domain, and (ii) control knowledge which specifies how to use domain knowledge to solve a problem.

In this paper we focus on the description of domain knowledge and its relation with control knowledge. Although terminology varies, there appear to be at least three descriptive levels of domain knowledge that can be found in most approaches:

Application ontology

The application ontology, in short "ontology" [1], specifies the structure of the domain knowledge in terms of a number of (domain) knowledge *types*. It characterises the types of objects and expressions that one finds in the domain knowledge.

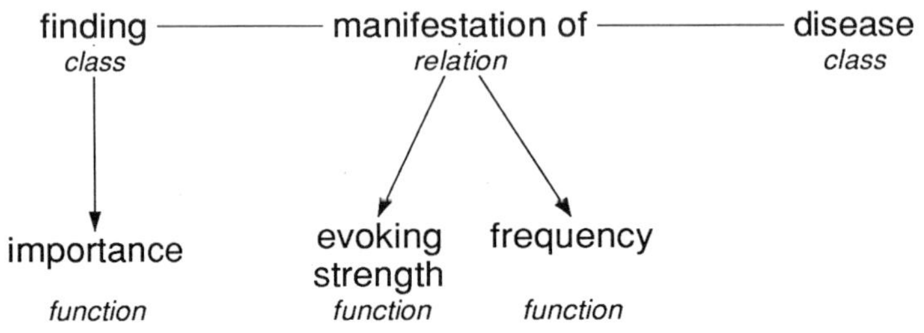

FIGURE 1: Example domain knowledge types, derived from the ontology underlying INTERNIST-1 [17]

Fig. 1 shows a partial example ontology, derived from the way in which domain knowledge is described in INTERNIST-1 [17]. As [18] point out, there is an additional underlying ontological commitment in such an ontology, namely the representational primitives that are used for describing the ontology. In GAMES we have chosen the primitives used by Gruber in Ontolingua [19]: classes, relations and functions.

Application knowledge

The application knowledge constitutes the "actual" domain knowledge. Roughly, it consists of two parts:

1. *Domain vocabulary* The set of terms that the application employs to describe the application domain. Example medical terms are "liver size", "enlarged" and "veno occlusive disease".
2. *Domain models* Domain models are sets of expressions about how domain terms are related. An example expression is the statement that the finding that the "liver size" is "enlarged" is a manifestation of "veno occlusive disease". Domain models contain relation tuples and function expressions of which the underlying structure is defined in the ontology.

From a logicist stance the domain vocabulary and the domain models can respectively be termed the universe of discourse and sets of axioms about elements of this universe.

[1] In a previous publication [16] the first author favoured the term "schema" above "ontology" to stress that it is product of engineering, and does not necessarily imply a faithful description of the real world. The use of the second term has, however, become predominant in the literature.

Loosely speaking, one could view the application knowledge as an instantiation of the ontology. However, one should realise that medical terms are objects in their own right. The fact that some term, say "headache" is viewed as being of type "observable" is dependent on the application domain. In some other application, it might well be a disease! Thus, it is probably more correct to view the relation between the application knowledge and ontology as a mapping relation.

Knowledge roles

Knowledge roles are names for domain knowledge elements that characterise their role during problem solving. Example role names are "hypothesis" and "expected datum". Knowledge roles are linked to the ontology to specify which elements can play this role. For example, in a diagnostic application the role "hypothesis" will usually be linked to an ontological type "disease", which in turn can be mapped on a set of medical terms representing the diseases in the domain.

Knowledge roles specify how domain knowledge is manipulated by the control knowledge. In GAMES this control knowledge consists of an *inference model* that specifies the basic inference steps, and a set of task descriptions specifying how inferences can be ordered to reach a problem solving goal (see for more detailed descriptions [15]). Knowledge roles are part of the inference model. Fig. 2 shows the generic version of the inference model used in GAMES.

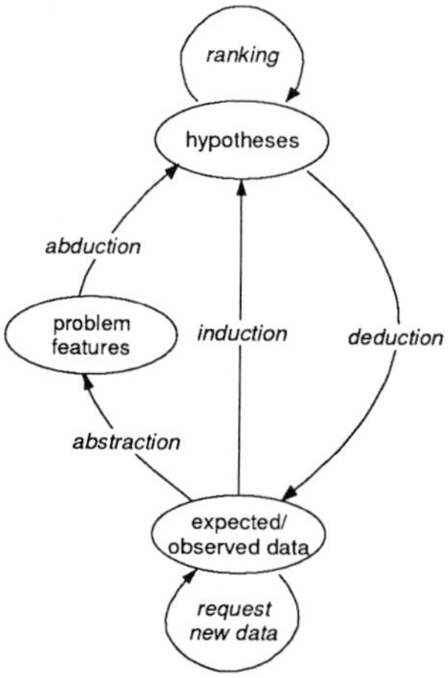

FIGURE 2: General "Select and Test" (ST) model of problem solving used in GAMES. The names within the ellipses represent knowledge roles. Italic names denote inference steps. See for a detailed description [15]

Fig. 3 summarises the three views by organising them in three levels and indicating typical mappings between these levels. The levels can be seen as *attributing various types of semantics* to domain knowledge elements. This is in contrast with the the traditional logicists view of model-theoretic semantics, which implies a description of semantics at one level.

1. The *vocabulary* of the application knowledge defines medical terms that are used in the application. Although the particular set of terms in a vocabulary is geared

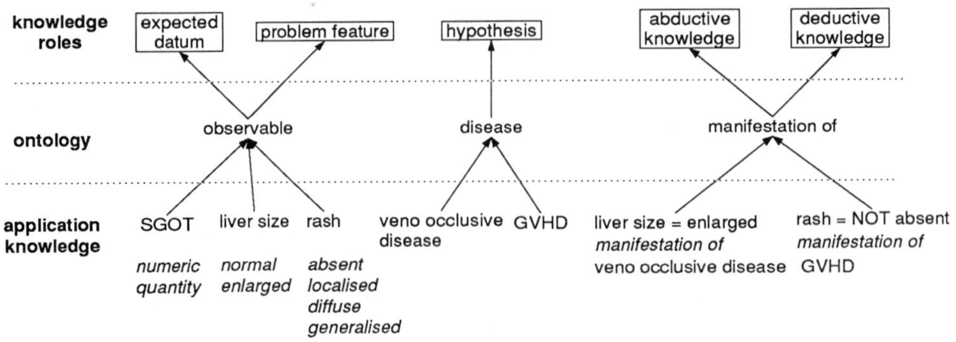

FIGURE 3: Example knowledge elements illustrating the three-level organisation of medical domain knowledge

towards the application, the terms *themselves* are expected to belong to the field of medicine in general. The semantics of terms like "lateral side of the femur" is determined by general medical knowledge, in this case anatomical knowledge. We will argue in the next section that this effects the way in which we should view reusability of medical terms.

2. The *ontology* defines additional semantics of application knowledge. We say that some term like "liver size" is interpreted as an "observable" in our application domain. Unlike the vocabulary, the conceptualisations that we chose for an application ontology are dependent both on the medical sub-domain, e.g. liver diseases, and on the problem solving task, e.g. diagnosis.
3. The *knowledge roles* specify the semantic interpretations that we attach to knowledge elements during problem solving. For example, the finding "liver size = enlarged" can play the role of expected datum for the hypothesis "veno occlusive disease", and be used to disconfirm or strengthen the belief in this hypothesis.

In the following sections we elaborate on how these different levels of knowledge description can be employed to aid the process of knowledge engineering.

3 Reusability

KBS construction is a time-consuming activity. Even building simple systems requires a considerable effort. Reusing parts of previously built KBSs is potentially a powerful approach to overcome these problems. Reuse changes the nature of knowledge engineering from a pure construction activity to a selection and refinement process of existing components. It helps turning knowledge engineering from an art into a real engineering discipline. In fact, it is probably fair to say that reuse is a necessary condition for building the complex systems we are ultimately aiming at.

It has been recognised that the knowledge-level stance is particularly useful for reusability purposes [19,3,16]. For reusability of knowledge, it is necessary to abstract from the symbol-level pecularities of knowledge representation. Knowledge-level descriptions are intended to provide precisely this abstraction. In this section we consider how the knowledge organisation as sketched in the previous section can be employed to support reusability.

Library of problem solving methods Knowledge roles are part of an abstract model of how problem solving should be performed. In the literature such a model is called a *problem solving method* (PSM) [20,21,12]. The Select and Test model in Fig. 2 is the general PSM supported by GAMES. In addition, three specialised versions of this PSM were developed that are specific for prototypical medical tasks: diagnosis, therapy planning, and monitoring. These PSMs are used in GAMES as a *library* of PSMs from which the knowledge engineer can choose a PSM to realise a medical task in the application domain. Each PSM contains a set of specific knowledge roles for this task.

Library of ontologies In GAMES we have taken the position that it is not possible to fix in advance the ontology for applications. As pointed out in the previous section, the ontology is usually application specific and is dependent on the application task and the medical sub-domain. Fixing the ontology would constrain the task of building an adequate knowledge base containing adequate epistemological distinctions too much. However, each application ontology contains definitions which reappear in other applications. The approach we have taken in GAMES is to supply the knowledge engineer with a library of predefined partial ontologies. Through a process of selection and refinement, this library can be used to support the construction of the application ontology. We distinguish four kinds of reusable ontologies:

Ontologies for general medical entities With this we mean the terminology that is related to the medical practice. Here objects such as disease, observable, finding and therapy, and relations between these objects are defined. The ontology in Fig. 1 is ax example of such an ontology.

Generic medical and physiological ontologies These are ontologies which are domain dependent in the sense that they are related to medical domains, but which are generic in the sense that the same ontology is required in many different application areas of medicine.

Generic basic ontologies With these we mean ontologies which are reusable across a large number of domains. Examples of these are number-theory, scales and scale conversions, and time ontologies.

Meta-ontologies These ontologies are general systems for organising the world. An example of such an ontologies is the "frame ontology" underlying Ontolingua [19] which defines primitive notions such as classes, objects, functions and relations. For practical purposes meta ontologies are usually fixed, but making them explicit facilitates extension and modification when required.

Fig. 5 in the next section shows a snapshot of part of a tool that was built in GAMES to support the selection and refinement process of partial ontologies.

Library of standard medical terms Currently, most knowledge-acquisition front ends for building medical KBSs simply ask a domain expert to type in a name when eliciting, for example, possible diseases in the domain. They do not check the correctness of the name (other than syntax or internal name clashes). They rely on the expertise of the user to enter correct medical terms. This situation seriously hampers the reuse and sharing of knowledge bases. Medical terminology contains many slight variations, such as the language used (Latin, native language), the position of words in composite terms such as "lateral side of the femur", etcetera.

There is a large amount of research in the field of standardising medical vocabulary, e.g. [22,23]. It is outside the scope of GAMES to do any work in this area. Instead, our aim is to provide the necessary anchor points that enable the construction of bridges with terminological knowledge bases to ensure that terms in the application knowledge are consistent and potentially sharable. This is also one of the reasons why a clear distinction between application vocabulary and ontology is important.

4 Knowledge Acquisition Activities and Tools

It will be clear that in the GAMES view "knowledge acquisition" comprises more that just entering medical domain-specific knowledge such as the set of diseases and findings. A major part of knowledge acquisition concerns the knowledge-level description of the structure and the use of this domain knowledge during problem-solving. In GAMES the full knowledge-level model (comprising the three types of descriptions of domain knowledge plus the instantiated problem solving methods) is called the *epistemological model* [15].

The multi-level knowledge organisation and their associated generic libraries provide also a rationale for identifying knowledge acquisition activities that need to be performed when building an application. Fig. 4 gives a schematic overview of these activities. We discuss each of these briefly, indicating also support tools for activities.

Task model construction The phrase "task model" is used in GAMES to refer to the control-knowledge description of some application. This activity uses the library of PSM specifications in order to build an inference model and a set of task definitions for the application. At the University of Pavia, a prototype system has been built that supports the construction of a task model using a metarule language with an associated metarule editor [24,25]. The syetem provides standard sets of metarules, representing the different library tasks. These metarules can be edited to meet specific demands of applications.

It should be noted that the task model of an application often contains a combination of PSMs. Many real-life medical tasks are combinations of the generic medical tasks represented in the library. For example, the task of managing graft-versus-host disease (GVHD) after bone marrow transplantation involves both a diagnostic task (establishing the presence of GVHD; grading of GVHD) as well as therapy planning activities. Typically, this involves multiple mappings between the ontology and the knowledge roles. For example, GVHD takes the role of "hypothesis" during diagnosis, but is considered a "problem feature" during therapy planning. Such multiple mappings constitute an additional rationale for the explicit distinction we make between ontological elements and knowledge roles.

Ontology specification The goal of this activity is to define a schematic description of the medical knowledge in some domain: the application ontology. This needs to be done by the knowledge engineer or an informed expert that takes the role of knowledge engineer. It is supported by a predefined library of ontology descriptions. The idea is that the knowledge engineer does not build the ontology from scratch, but can use existing ontologies from the library, and, if necessary, tune these to meet the demands of the

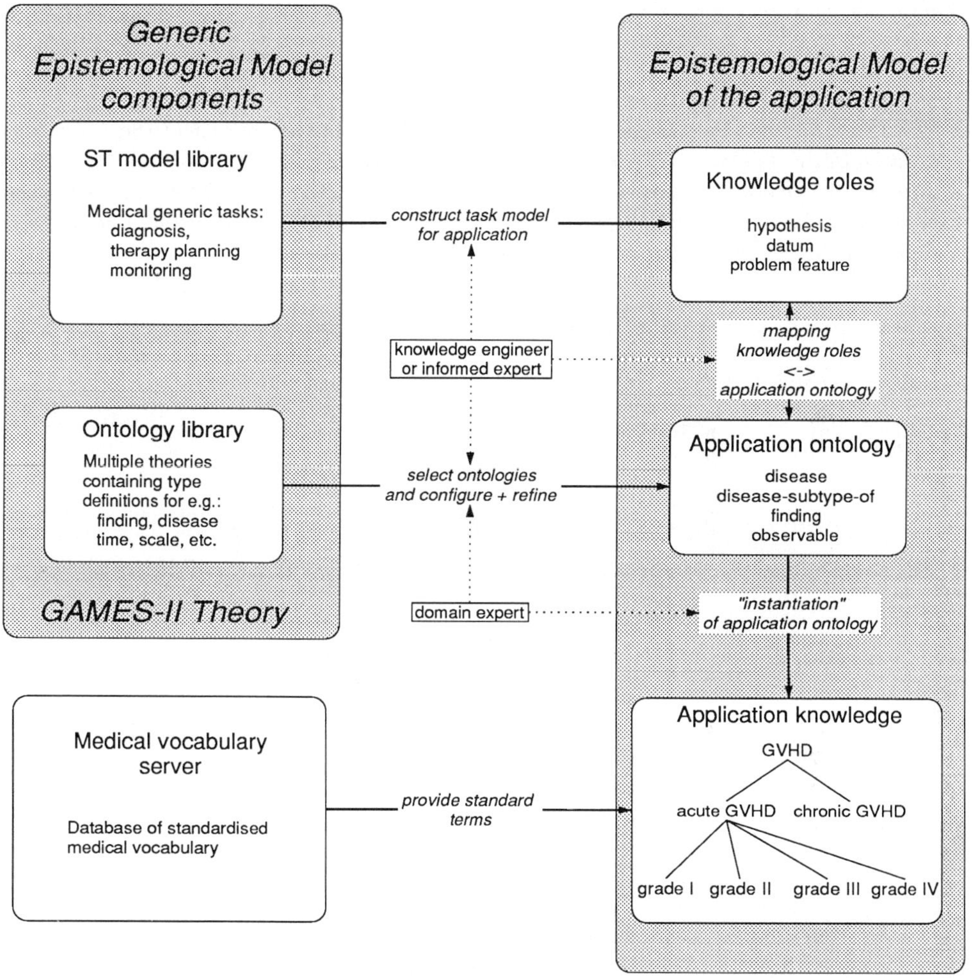

FIGURE 4: Schematic overview of the domain knowledge organisation in the GAMES epistemological model. The right-hand side represents the model of an application; the left-hand side denotes corresponding generic knowledge. GAMES supports the upper two types of generic knowledge (libraries of PSMs and ontologies). The solid arrows represent knowledge acquisition activities that need to be performed when building an application. The dotted arrows indicate the type of agent that is expected to carry out some activity

application. For example, several ontologies of time exist, each with varying degrees of complexity. Monitoring applications usually require a much more explicit representation of time than diagnostic ones. Typically, the knowledge engineer will select the simplest time ontology required by the application.

In GAMES we use the Ontolingua language developed in the context of the knowledge sharing initiative in the US [26,19] to represent ontologies. We have built a tool that acts as a front-end to Ontolingua representations and allows both the construction of ontological theories as well as the selection and fine-tuning for a particular application. Fig. 5 shows the part of the tool that supports viewing and refining a theory (partial ontology) in the library.

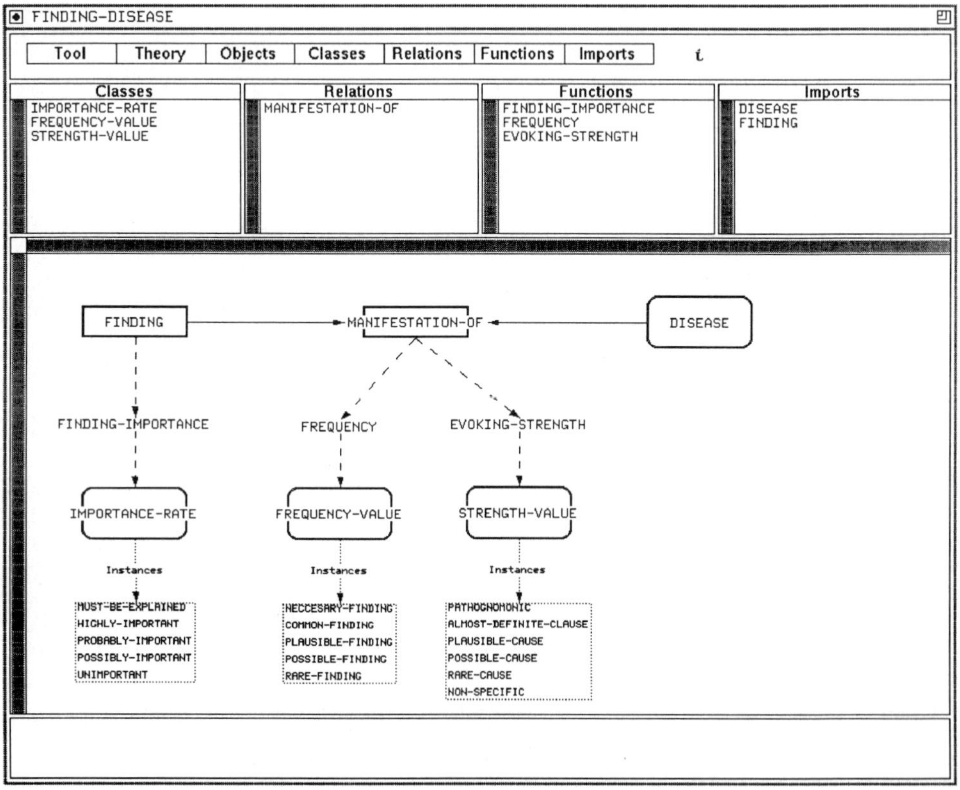

FIGURE 5: Screen dump of the part of the GAMES ontology editing tool that supports viewing and refining a theory (partial ontology) in the library. The ontology shown is derived from INTERNIST-1 (see also Fig. 1)

Role mapping This activity defines how the elements of the medical ontology map onto roles in the inference model. This is largely predefined by the GAMES theory [15], but can be modified by the knowledge engineer, This activity requires detailed knowledge of the GAMES theory and should thus be carried out by the knowledge engineer. The mapping is represented in the task model (see above) and is achieved in the prototype system through metarules.

Entering application knowledge The ontology defines the *format* for the application knowledge. The actual specification of the application knowledge in this format is a separate knowledge acquisition activity. This activity can and probably should be carried out by the domain expert. This activity has often been viewed as the only real "knowledge acquisition" activity. This was mainly due to the fact that the formats that were used by medical KBSs were fixed by the symbol-level representation of knowledge and their associated inference regimes.

The aim of the GAMES approach is to allow experts to interact with a knowledge acquisition tool in a vocabulary that is meaningful to them. Similarly to OPAL [20], we aim for a dialogue with the expert in terms of the ontology ("What are diseases in this domain?"), rather that in terms of knowledge roles ("What are hypotheses in this domain?") as in systems like MOLE and SALT [10].

One point that arises from the discussion on standardised medical vocabulary in the previous section, is that one would like to support the entering by the expert of medical terms with tools that browse and/or search through terminological databases. This would ensure the presence of correct and potentially sharable terms in the knowledge base of the application. One of the longer term research goals of GAMES is to make such additional facilities available to the GAMES user.

5 Discussion

We have described the framework employed by the GAMES project for organisation of medical knowledge. This framework is intended to support maximisation of reusability and to provide a rationale for identification of KBS-construction activities.

In this paper we concentrated on knowledge-level modeling, focusing on the contents of the knowledge instead of the form (the symbol level). However, some words are in place on the computational aspects. In order to build a running KBS the selection of representation formalisms and reasoning techniques needs to be addressed as well. In GAMES we account for these decisions through the *computational model*: the symbol level counterpart of the epistemological model. The structure of the computational model is loosely based on the notion of a control blackboard architecture [27], where the knowledge sources implement the inferences in the ST model. In principle, the knowledge sources can be realised with different problem solvers, thus allowing the use of multiple representations and multiple reasoning techniques in one KBS. We are currently experimenting with qualitative simulation techniques, causal-probabilistic networks and rule and frame based reasoners. Construction of the computational model involves two steps, namely (i) selecting appropriate problem solver for the inferences, and (ii) translating the ontology and the domain knowledge into the particular representation formalism of that problem solver. Note that we select the problem solvers after we have constructed a knowledge level model. This allows us to select problem solvers that are both epistemologically and computationally adequate for the knowledge and the task at hand. This form of integration, which we call *knowledge-level integration*, should be contrasted with the approach in hybrid systems because integration is realised on the basis of the contents of the knowledge instead of the form. The use of Ontolingua allows us to use the associated translation architecture for automatic translation of the application ontology and the application knowledge into the specific formalisms.

As pointed out in Sec. 1, the framework for knowledge organisation as described in this paper is derived from recent work in knowledge engineering. A relevant development in this field is the Sisyphus initiative [28] of which the aim is to come up with a common framework for describing problem solving methods and the ontologies these methods employ, which allows sharing and reusing PSMs across research groups. Our aim is to extend and specialise this research in a medical context. We view the following items as major research topics for further work in this area:

- Construction, validation and refinement of a library of PSMs that are specific for the medical domain.
- Construction, validation and refinement of a library of partial ontologies that are relevant in the medical domain. Example elements of such a library include partial ontologies of medical data, causal networks, disease taxonomies, time, etc.
- Experiment with links between knowledge acquisition tools and terminological databases.
- Establish the relationship between medical knowledge bases and medical information systems.

  In practice, KBSs are not used in isolation but have to be integrated with more conventional information technology such as hospital information systems. The framework outlined in this paper provides clear anchor points for establishing bridges between medical knowledge bases and databases, e.g. through shared ontologies.

Ultimately, this should pave the way the way for building a new generation of KBSs that meets the demands of medical practice.

Acknowledgements We are grateful to the other members of the GAMES-II consortium for fruitful discussions on the ideas presented in this paper.

References

[1] A. Newell. The knowledge level. *Artificial Intelligence*, 18:87–127, 1982.

[2] G. van Heijst, G. Lanzola, A. Th. Schreiber, and M. Stefanelli. Methodological foundations of medical KBS construction. Technical Report GAMES-II/T1.1/UvA/PP/009/1.0, University of Amsterdam and University of Pavia, 1993. Available from: University of Amsterdam, Social Science Informatics, Roetersstraat 15, NL-1018 WB, Amsterdam, The Netherlands.

[3] M. Musen. Dimensions of knowledge sharing and reuse. Report KSL-91-65, Knowledge Systems Laboratory, Stanford University, California, 1991. To appear in *Computers and Biomedical Research.*

[4] W. J. Clancey. The epistemology of a rule based system -a framework for explanation. *Artificial Intelligence*, 20:215–251, 1983.

[5] R. J. Brachman and B. C. Smith. Special issue on knowledge representation. *SIGART Newsletter*, 70:1–138, 1980.

[6] W. J. Clancey. Heuristic classification. *Artificial Intelligence*, 27:289–350, 1985.

[7] R. Neches, W. R. Swartout, and J. D. Moore. Enhanced maintenance and explanation of expert systems through explicit models of their development. *IEEE Transactions on Software Engineering*, 11:1337–1351, 1985.

[8] B. J. Wielinga and J. A. Breuker. Models of expertise. In *Proceedings ECAI-86*, pages 306–318, 1986.

[9] B. Chandrasekaran. Generic tasks as building blocks for knowledge-based systems: The diagnosis and routine design examples. *The Knowledge Engineering Review*, 3(3):183–210, 1988.

[10] S. Marcus, editor. *Automatic knowledge acquisition for expert systems.* Kluwer, Boston, 1988.

[11] M. A. Musen. *Automated Generation of Model-Based Knowledge-Acquisition Tools.* Pitman, London, 1989. Research Notes in Artificial Intelligence.

[12] L. Steels. Components of expertise. *AI Magazine*, Summer 1990.

[13] A. Th. Schreiber, B. J. Wielinga, and J. A. Breuker, editors. *KADS: A Principled Approach to Knowledge-Based System Development.* Knowledge-Based Systems Book Series. Academic Press, London, 1993. ISBN 0-12-629040-7.

[14] B. J. Wielinga, W. Van de Velde, A. Th. Schreiber, and J. M. Akkermans. Towards a unification of knowledge modelling approaches. In Jean-Marc David, Jean-Paul Krivine, and Reid Simmons, editors, *Second Generation Expert Systems.* Springer-Verlag, 1993.

[15] M. Ramoni, M. Stefanelli, G. Barosi, and L. Magnani. An epistemological framework for medical knowledge based systems. *IEEE Transactions on Systems, Man and Cybernetics*, 22:1361–1375, 1992.

[16] B. J. Wielinga, A. Th. Schreiber, and J. A. Breuker. KADS: A modelling approach to knowledge engineering. *Knowledge Acquisition*, 4(1):5–53, 1992. Special issue 'The KADS approach to knowledge engineering'. Reprinted in: Buchanan, B. and Wilkins, D. editors (1992), *Readings in Knowledge Acquisition and Learning*, San Mateo, California, Morgan Kaufmann, pp. 92-116.

[17] R. A. Miller, H. E. Pople, and J. D. Myers. INTERNIST-I: A general computer-based diagnostic consultant for general internal medicine. *New England Journal of Medicine*, 307:468–476, 1982. Also in: *Readings in Medical Artificial Intelligence: The First Decade*, W. J. Clancey and E. H. Shortliffe (eds.), Addison Wesley, Reading, MA, 1984.

[18] R. Davis, H. Shrobe, and P. Szolovits. What is a knowledge representation? *AI Magazine*, Spring:17–33, 1993.

[19] T. Gruber. Ontolingua: A mechanism to support portable ontologies. version 3.0. Technical report, Knowledge Systems Laboratory, Stanford University, California, 1992.

[20] Mark A. Musen, L. M. Fagan, D. M. Combs, and E. H. Shortliffe. Use of a domain-model to drive an interactive knowledge-editing tool. *Int. J. of Man-Machine Studies*, 26:105–121, 1987.

[21] J. McDermott. Preliminary steps towards a taxonomy of problem-solving methods. In S. Marcus, editor, *Automating Knowledge Acquisition for Expert Systems*, pages 225–255. Kluwer, Boston, 1988.

[22] R. A. Coté, editor. *Systematized Nomenclature of Medicine.* College of American Pathologists, Skokie, Illinois, 1982.

[23] M. Tuttle, D. Sherertz, N. Olson, M. Erlbaum, D. Sperzel, L. Fuller, and D. Nelson. Using Meta-1 – the first version of the ULMS metathesaurus. In R. A. Miller, editor, *Proc. of the 14th Annual Symposium on Computer Applications in Medical Care*, pages 131–135, Washington DC, 1990. IEEE Computing Society Press.

[24] G. Lanzola and M. Stefanelli. A specialized framework for medical knowledge based systems. *Computers and Biomedical Research*, 25:351–365, 1992.

[25] G. Lanzola and M. Stefanelli. Inferential knowledge acquisition. *Artificial Intelligence in Medicine*, 1993. to appear.

[26] R. Neches, R. Fikes, T. Finin, T. Gruber, R. Patil, T. Senator, and W. R. Swartout. Enabling technology for knowledge sharing. *AI Magazine*, pages 36–56, 1991. Fall.

[27] B. Hayes-Roth. A blackboard architecture for control. *Artificial Intelligence*, 26(3):251–321, 1985.

[28] M. Linster. Special issue on Sisyphus 91-92 "Models of Problem Solving". *Knowledge Acquisition*, 1993. forthcoming.

Artificial Intelligence in Medecine
S. Andreassen et al. , Eds.
IOS Press, 1993

A Framework for Modular Knowledge Bases in the Domain of Hypertension Diseases

Barbara Heller, Sonja Schlegelmilch

University of Bielefeld, Faculty of Technology, P. O. Box 10 01 31, 33501 Bielefeld, Germany

Abstract

To manage medical diagnosis and treatment in extremely involved knowledge domains we consider particular aspects of structuring medical knowledge into knowledge modules. In our approach we arrange these modules in a three-dimensional structure. The three dimensions are defined by the degree of knowledge abstraction, specifity of domain knowledge and system-technical form of knowledge description. Furthermore we propose an idea of how to manage the transfer of knowledge among modules. To achieve an appropriate modular model of our knowledge domain we explain the decomposition of domain knowledge into knowledge modules. Finally, an example illustrates the knowledge transfer among modules.

Keywords

Knowledge-Based Systems, Hypertension, Modularization, Conceptualization of Diagnostic and Therapeutic Knowledge, Management of Knowledge Modules, Decomposition of Knowledge

1. INTRODUCTION

This paper describes a conceptual view on the modularization of medical knowledge. It outlines how this approach can be applied to the framework of the HYPERCON system (HYPERtension CONsultation). In the project HYPERCON [1] the main task is a comprehensive modeling of knowledge about diagnostic and therapeutic aspects for managing hypertension diseases. One of the difficulties of modeling the medical domain lies in the high interdependency of domain knowledge which is characterized by different levels of abstraction and domain specifity. This difficulty and the large scale of the knowledge domain are a strong motivation for modularization. We arrange the domain knowledge in smaller units called knowledge modules. They are characterized by:

- self-contained specific knowledge (e. g. modules containing associative anamnestic knowledge, causal anamnestic knowledge or associative knowledge about laboratory data)
- the transparency of modeled knowledge
- the ability to transfer knowledge via a well-defined interface.

Further advantages are to be seen in a better system maintenance and an easier control of knowledge access. To support our idea of a modular knowledge based system and to reach an appropriate framework it is necessary to account for the distribution and redundancy of domain knowledge.

2. CRITERIA OF MODULARIZATION IN HYPERCON

2.1. Domain Specific Characteristics

The main tasks of research in the project HYPERCON include the conceptualization and structuring of extremely involved knowledge domains. In order to cope with this we need new concepts on knowledge-related modularization. Referring to the specific phenomena of knowledge acquisition and modeling in the medical domain we develop new approaches to the topic of hypertension.

The necessity of a modular design will be obvious by a close look at the characteristics in the domain of hypertension. Hypertension is a chronic, multifactorial disease which is characterized by qualitatively different phases in the course of its development. The phases are characterized by specific intensities of symptoms as a result of fundamental changes at different pathophysiological levels [2]. In contrast to acute diseases, time courses are a subject of observation in the case of chronic diseases. Since therapy has to start during ongoing monitoring of diagnostic data, evaluation of symptoms must take into account presumed diagnoses and the previous and actual therapy protocol.

In case of hypertension qualitatively new states can only be identified on the basis of a long-time observation of individual patient data. Their interpretation by means of pathological and pharmacological knowledge and epidemiological data requires knowledge about [2]:

- anamnesis
- physical examinations
- laboratory tests
- specific examinations
- therapeutic treatment.

The goal of HYPERCON is to incorporate into a modular knowledge-based system diagnostic and therapeutic knowledge on different abstraction levels [3].

2.2. A Framework for HYPERCON

As introduced in the previous part, the domain is characterized by a high interdependency among the different partial problem-solving spaces (e.g. an–amnesis and physical examination). Reflecting the perpective of developing knowledge modules separately by different team members, we consider the following main components:

(1) the dialog component **(DC)**
(2) the manager component **(MC)**
(3) the hypertension consultant component **(HCC)**.

ad (1): The DC translates the user's cognitive model of the domain to the model of the HCC. This translation process is performed bidirectionally. Because of the scope of this paper we cannot take a close look at this point.

ad (2): The MC controls all dialog activities between the user and the HCC. Corresponding to the part 'Control Maintenance', which is explained in chapter 3. The manager interprets, evaluates, defines and distributes tasks between knowledge modules of the HCC. This is to be seen against the background of the global problem-solving process and the shared local knowledge of the modules.

ad (3): The hypertension consultant component reflects the knowledge of the medical experts in the domain of hypertension diseases. The HCC includes knowledge modules that are differentiated on the basis of three dimensions:

- the degree of specifity
- the degree of abstraction
- the quality of structural and strategic knowledge seen from the viewpoint of systems technology.

2.3. Conceptualization of Knowledge Modules

Figure 1 presents the conceptual framework of HYPERCON. The high interdependency and the unknown status of the given knowledge domain make it necessary to assign the diagnostic and therapeutic knowledge units to separate modules [1].

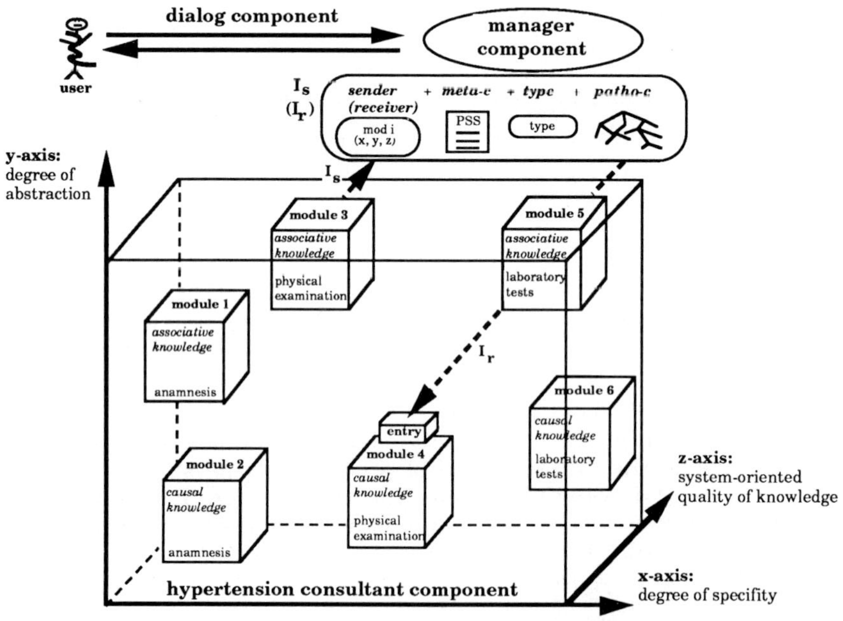

Figure 1. The conceptual model of the HCC and the MC.

As shown in figure 1, the modules are arranged in the suggested three-dimensional structure as follows:

- The x-axis shows the degree of specifity of the hypertension knowledge where e.g. 'anamnesis' modules are less specific than 'physical examination' modules and these are in turn less specific than 'laboratory tests' modules.

- Along the y-axis, the modules are arranged with respect to their degree of abstraction. This means e.g. for the data that they are divided into associative and causal elements corresponding to the local problem-solving process [4]. Subsequently, they are bundled in separate modules. Modules in the y-dimension are arranged accordingly: associative modules are of a higher abstraction degree than ones of causal knowledge [3].
- The third dimension (z-axis) is required for representing the different qualities of structural and strategic characteristics of the knowledge modules. This system-oriented dimension is important for the communication between the MC and a module. For the MC it is essential to have information about the technical quality status (e.g. representation of knowledge units in form of rules or methods) of the domain knowledge represented in a module.

The task of the MC with respect to the hypertension consultant component is to interpret the actual information in form of a tuple sent by a module (I_S). According to the tuple I_S (sending information tuple) the MC's decisions are based on:

- the location (mod_i (x, y, z)) of the sending module (*sender*) in the three-dimensional structure
- the meta-concept (*meta-c*) which is here defined as a problem-solving situation (PSS) describing both the inference status of a module and the processed actions
- the *type* for identifying the contents as fact, concept or knowledge structure
- the pathological concept (*patho-c*) which adapts and describes the actual status of a patient in form of a knowledge structure.

The information tuple I_r contains the information for a receiving module in the same internal structure as described above.

3. CONTROL MAINTENANCE

3.1. The Manager Component

By way of illustration consider medical experts with shared medical competences (i. e. medical student, medical assistant, assistant medical director). The most successful form of organization to achieve a common goal in a problem-solving process could be a manager (medical superintendent) who knows about the shared competences. On this basis the manager should be able to define and distribute new tasks to the respective specialist without the necessity of having deep knowledge about the solving process of specific problems [5].

With this metapher in mind we suggest a component which is capable of:

- adapting and interpreting the information sent by a module
- evaluating the information as a contribution for the common problem-solving process
- defining the next adequate task for a module whereas the meaning of 'task' is decribed in [6]
- delegating the task to the most adequate knowledge module.

First the manager component adapts the sent tuple, then interprets and evaluates it on the basis of the global problem-solving goal. In accordance with the actual problem-solving situation, the next adequate task and the most adequate of the possible competent modules are decided. Hence a new receiving information tuple I_r is created and transferred as an entry to the focused receiving module.

3.2. Transferring Knowledge among Modules

Another important aspect of modularization is to be seen in the control of the knowledge transfer among modules. In HYPERCON, the transferred knowledge does not consist of *facts* as single data or *expressions* as combined data. But in our approach a module needs and gets more information about the status of the global problem-solving process than can be provided by simple facts. Therefore the transferred information has to include more complex contents like *concepts* or combined concepts in form of a *knowledge structure*.

As a consequence of the exchanging of knowledge structures we could also imagine to transfer strategies between modules. Concerning the characteristics of knowledge modules the essential feature lies in their individual problem-solving capability. Therefore the more challenging aspects within the communication process are to be seen in connection with the transfer of concepts, knowledge structures, problem-solving situations and the local task of a given knowledge module. Each module contains its specific knowledge. To make communication feasable, the transfer process needs a standardized common basis of information exchange. The corresponding information tuples for sending (**I_s**) and receiving (**I_r**) information are described below.

I_s (sender, problem-solving situation (PSS), type, contents)
I_r (receiver, problem-solving situation (PSS), type, contents)

sender:	sending module
receiver:	the adequate receiving knowledge module
PSS:	actual status of problem-solving process (s. figure 2)
type:	kind of contents
contents:	fact, expression, concept, knowledge structure.

structure of PSS

actual_p:	< true, false >
hypothesis:	< tentative >
status_hyp:	< singular, competitive, multiple >
main_task:	< local task assignment >
activities:	< processed inference steps >

instance of PSS

actual_p:	true
hypothesis:	prim_hyperaldosteronism
status_hyp:	competitive
main_task:	confirm_laboratory_tests
activities:	(serum_potassium serum_cholesterol 24h_urine_potassium)

Figure 2. PSS - An actual status of the problem-solving process.

What is missing in the sending information tuple is the specification of the receiving knowledge module. This is impossible for a sending module because of the specifity of its knowledge. What is more the task of defining the next adequate receiving module underlies the management component.

4. INTERDEPENDENCY OF KNOWLEDGE

4.1. Knowledge Decomposition

A major task to modularize large knowledge domains takes the following general aspects into account:

- the increasing complexity of domain knowledge
- the resulting interdependency of knowledge to be accounted for
- the transparency of complex knowledge domains
- the maintenance problem in the development of a large knowledge-based system and
- the reusability of knowledge bases.

The discussion of such objectives has mostly been limited to a technical level. Nevertheless the modularization of knowledge-based systems reflecting domain criteria is of great interest [7]. For modularization it is essential that a knowledge domain is not monolithic even if it is difficult to grasp, as it is obviously the case within the medical domain of hypertension research.

For the modular design of large scale knowledge-based systems it is necessary to take the conventional idea of a module into account. It views a module as a functionally complete unit which communicates with the environment via a well-defined interface [8]. With regard to knowledge engineering it seems inevitable to modify the notion of functional completeness and communication over interfaces, since the high interdependency of domain knowledge does not allow a decomposition on functionality aspects in general.

The interdependency of a domain is given by the number of relations between different problem-solving situations. These problem-solving situations are related to partial problem-solving spaces (PPSP). Hence the partial problem-solving spaces are not separable. In addition, we cannot speak about the functionality of a knowledge unit. Moreover, a knowledge unit is an atomic knowledge source which is applied to a problem-solving situation.

On the basis of similar knowledge units which contribute answers to the same sort of question, specific problem-solving situations can be identified. For decomposing the acquired knowledge of a problem-solving space, the degree of its interdependency is made transparent by the following steps:

A reflection of problem-solving situations (**PSS**) on the basis of knowledge units (**KU**)
B abstraction of the definite problem-solving situations to problem-solving types (**PST**)
C extraction of partial problem-solving spaces (**PPSP**) from the problem-solving types
D specialization of PST in PPSP to PSS
E characterization of knowledge units to be applied to PSS.

Figure 3 illustrates the decomposition process as described above.

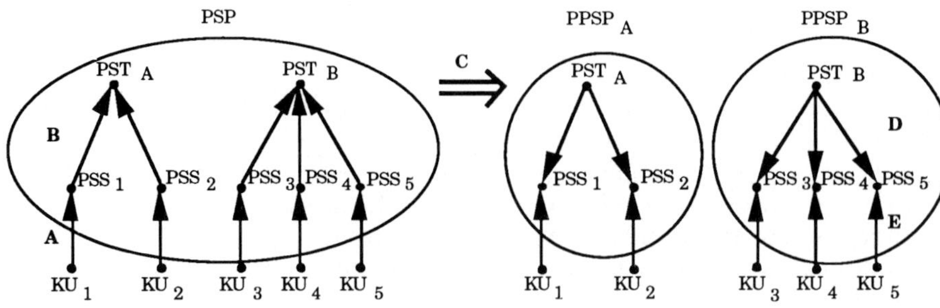

Figure 3. Decomposition process on a problem-solving space (**PSP**).

Two difficulties arise during the decomposition process. First, it is possible that no well-defined relation of PSS_i to a problem-solving type PST_A can be found due to their interdependency during the abstraction step. Second, the difficulty in the specialization step consists in the concretization of problem-solving situations and therefore in the allocation of knowledge units. The problem of completion which arises is reflected in the next section.

4.2. Knowledge Encapsulation

We consider a problem-solving space PSP with a number of different problem-solving situations PSS_i (i=1, ..., n), within which knowledge units KU_j are to be identified. Suppose for each KU_j that the specific knowledge for solving PSS_i has been obtained and therefore the PSS_i can be related accordingly. In the case of similar KU_j ($1 \leq j < n$) the corresponding PSS_i can be bundled first. The above-mentioned process is also performed on the set of knowledge units KU_k ($j < k \leq n$) obtained in this way. Two cases can now be distinguished:

(1) A KU_k and a KU_j as well can be applied to a PSS_i ($KU_j, KU_k \rightarrow PSS_i$).
(2) A KU_j respectively KU_k can be applied to a PSS_{i_1} as well as to a PSS_{i_2}, where $i_1 \neq i_2$ ($KU_j \rightarrow PSS_{i_1}, PSS_{i_2}$), ($KU_k \rightarrow PSS_{i_1}, PSS_{i_2}$).

In the first case, different specific knowledge units can be applied to one specific problem-solving situation, while these are appropriate to solve it. In the second case, one knowledge unit will be applicable to different specific problem-solving situations. The frequency of the occurrence of (1) and (2) defines the degree of interdependency within the PSP. Whereas in case of (1) the interdependency can be reduced by distribution of ($KU_j, KU_k \rightarrow PSS_i$) to ($KU_j \rightarrow PSS_i$) and ($KU_k \rightarrow PSS_i$), the interdependency in case of (2) has to be minimized by redundant assignment of ($KU_j \rightarrow PSS_{i_1}, PSS_{i_2}$) to ($KU_j \rightarrow PSS_{i_1}$) and ($KU_j \rightarrow PSS_{i_2}$). Figure 4 shows the decomposition process for both cases.

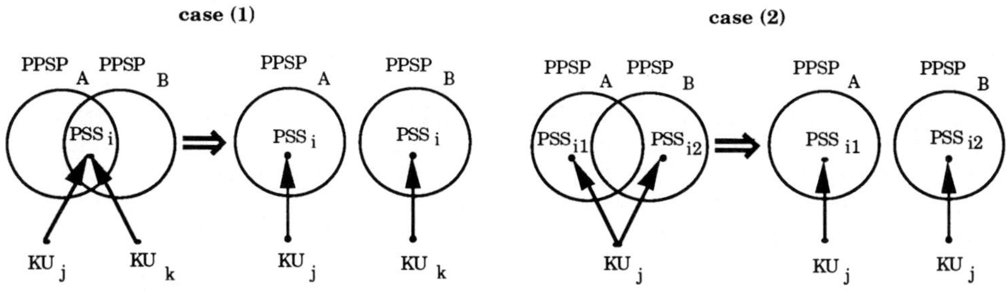

Figure 4. Decomposition of a PSP with interdependency.

Redundant decomposition allows the extraction of separate partial problem-solving spaces. Therefore the knowledge units related to partial problem-solving spaces can be encapsulated in knowledge modules.

5. AN EXAMPLE

Now we present a short excerpt of the knowledge transfer among the modules in HYPERCON (the medical example is taken from the previous project HYPERTON [2]). The following background is given: A middle-aged woman consults a physician (a general practitioner, for example). The physician has not met the patient before.

By means of the physician's input concerning the patient data the MC constructs the adequate pathological concept. (Text written in Geneva script indicates user-input and text written in *italics* indicates system explanations).

Pathological concept:

History:	female, 37 years old, height 164 cm, weight 79 kg, smoker, not pregnant, uses oral contraceptives, alcohol and salt intake unknown, hypertension in the past, no other recurring illnesses in the family.
Hypertension degree:	semi-critical hypertension.
Physical examination:	not currently complaining of vegetative disturbances such as headaches or sweat attacks, other findings normal.

Hypothesis: semi-critical hypertension caused by smoking, obesity and oral contraceptives.

(1) **MC:** must decide which module(s) is (are) the best one(s) for the given status of the patient reflecting this hypothesis.

By means of the present associative (history) data the MC checks the hypothesis with the help of the corresponding causal knowledge module. This may confirm or reject the given hypothesis. There is the possibility of discovering a competitive hypothesis as well.

PSS (I_S):

actual_p:	true	hypothesis:	hypertension_by_risk_facts
status_hyp:	singular	main-task:	confirm_by_causal_anamnesis
activities:	nil		

First the MC sends the adequate I_r to the 'causal anamnesis' module. Because, however, an earlier diagnosted hypertension was determined for the patient, the hypothesis of the physician, namely that smoking, obesity and oral contraceptives are the sole causes of the hypertension, cannot be confirmed absolutely. Since the module concludes that a primary hyperaldosteronism (i.e. an over-functioning of the kidney wall) could be a probable cause of semi-critical hypertension, additional data such as laboratory results (and here especially the 24h potassium secretion in urine) are requested. The over-functioning of the kidney wall results in an increased production of the mineral cortisone aldosteron. The increase in aldosteron causes an increased production of serum potassium and results in hypokalemia.

PSS (I_r): actual_p: true hypothesis: prim_hyperaldosteronism
status_hyp: competitive main-task: confirm_by_causal_anamnesis
activities: (confirmed_hypothesis refinement competition)

The 'causal anamnesis' module sends a PSS to the manager component containing a further hypothesis: Primary hyperaldosteronism as a probable tentative diagnosis.

(2) MC: receives the adequate I_S. While interpreting this tuple it recognizes that the pathological concept had not been modified by the 'causal anamnesis' module. To refine the pathological concept it is necessary to gain more information about the probable presence of a primary hyperaldosteronism.

The problem-solving situation shows that up to this time only the module with the associative knowledge about laboratory findings is able to infer about the hypothesis of primary hyperaldosteronism [9].

(3) MC: sends the I_r to the 'associative laboratory tests' module.

PSS (I_S): actual_p: true hypothesis: prim_hyperaldosteronism
status_hyp: competitive main-task: refine_by_associative_laboratory
activities: nil

The patient's laboratory data indicate a low potassium level and high serum cholesterol level. The 24h determination of potassium in the urine is also increased. These facts are connected to the pathological concept by the MC.

Pathological concept (refinement):

Laboratory data: low serum potassium level, high serum cholesterol level, increased 24h urine potassium level

The module's conclusion that a low serum potassium level could be a possible cause of the hypertension ushers in further questions about hypokalemia.

PSS (I_r): actual_p: true hypothesis: prim_hyperaldosteronism
status_hyp: competitive main-task: refine_by_associative_laboratory
activities: (serum_potassium serum_cholesterol 24h_urine_potassium)

Since there is no more associative knowledge to get more details about hypokalemia the communication between the MC and the 'causal laboratory tests' module has to be processed as mentioned above. The causal knowledge on hypokalemia must take a possible biogastrone treatment of the patient into consideration, because the chemical structure of biogastrone is similar to the structure of steroids and can lead to serum hypokalemia under certain conditions.

(4) MC: receives the I_S from the 'causal laboratory tests' module.

PSS (I_r): actual_p: true hypothesis: prim_hyperaldosteronism
status_hyp: competitive main-task: confirm_by_causal_laboratory
activities: (confirmation question_on_biogastrone_treatment)

The physician is questioned once more and subsequently the pathological concept can be refined by the data that the biogastrone therapy was terminated three months before the examination.

Pathological concept (refinement):

Therapy data: terminated biogastrone therapy three months before examination.

With this knowledge the 'therapy' module concludes that the hypothesis that the hypokalemia was caused by treatment with biogastrone can only be confirmed with a less certainty by the answers to the further questions regarding biogastrone treatment. The preliminary conclusion that the cause of the hypertension could be primary hyperaldosteronism is strengthened because the cause of the hypokalemia could not be adequately explained until now.

For further differential diagnostic steps in the direction of primary hyperaldosteronism the pathological concept of the patient should be transferred to more specific modules. In our example this will be the 'special examinations' module which contains causal knowledge about the physiological model of the renin-angiotensin-aldosterone cycle (RAA-cycle). The model can be questioned to find explanations about the pathological status of the patient in the way as shown above.

6. CONCLUSIONS

We can summarize our approach on modularization in HYPERCON as follows:

For receiving encapsulated partial problem-solving spaces decompose the entire problem-solving space in the case there is reasonably little redundancy. This means that parts of the RAA-model are represented in different knowledge modules and on the basis of different abstraction levels (causal specific examination module and associative specific examination module). You should also take into account that there is a communication process among the obtained knowledge modules referring to the actual problem-solving situation.

Furthermore there will be a manager component which controls all interactions between the medical expert (user) and the knowledge modules, between the knowledge modules. The latter are arranged in a three-dimensional structure. In our opinion this three-dimensional arrangement of knowledge modules is an adequate structure to support the design of a modular knowledge-based system. This conclusion is based on our considerations of hybrid knowledge representation and the different abstraction levels of knowledge in the domain of hypertension diseases.

7. ACKNOWLEDGEMENTS

We would like to acknowledge many helpful discussions concerning this research with Ipke Wachsmuth, Josef Meyer-Fujara and Krystina Kauffmann. This research has been supported in part by the North-Rhine Westfalia Ministry of Research and Technology (MWF grant IVA6-400 015 92) and the University of Bielefeld, Faculty of Technology.

8. REFERENCES

1 Wachsmuth, I., Heller, B., Meyer-Fujara, J.: *HYPERCON: Modulare Wissensbasen für Hypertonie-Konsultation.* Research Proposal, University of Bielefeld, Faculty of Technology, 1992.

2 Heller, B., Kauffmann, K., Wetter, Th.: *HYPERTON- Method of Argumentation and Status of Implementation.* IBM Scientific Center, Heidelberg, 1989.

3 Bylander T., Chandrasekaran, B.: Generic Tasks for Knowledge-Based Reasoning: the "Right" Level of Abstraction for Knowledge Acquisition. *International Journal of Man-Machine Studies* 26:231-243, 1987.

4 Simmons, R. G.: The roles of associational and causal reasoning in problem solving. *Artificial Intelligence* 53 (2,3):159-207, 1992

5 Newell, A.: The Knowledge Level. *Artificial Intelligence* 18 (1):1-20, 1982.

6 Benjamins, R.V., Abu-Hanna, A., Jansweijer, W.: *Dynamic Method Selection in Diagnostic Reasoning.* 12th Scientific Conference, Vol. 1: 153-164, Avignon, 1992.

7 Wachsmuth, I.: *On structuring domain specific knowledge.* LILOG Report 12, IBM Scientific Center, Stuttgart, 1987.

8 Parnas, D. L.: On the criteria to be used in decomposing systems into modules. *Communications of the ACM* 15 (12): 1053-1058, 1972.

9 Clancey, W. J.: Heuristic Classification. *Artificial Intelligence* 32 (3):333-377, 1987.

Artificial Intelligence in Medecine
S. Andreassen et al. , Eds.
IOS Press, 1993

KAVAS-2: Knowledge Acquisition, Visualisation and Assessment System

J. Brender[a], J. Talmon[b], P. Nykänen[c], R. O'Moore[d], P. Drosos[e], P. McNair[f #)]

[a]Medical Informatics Laboratory ApS, Stengaards Allé 33d, DK-2800 Lyngby, Denmark. [b]University of Limburg, P.O.Box 616, 6200 MD Maastricht, The Netherlands. [c]Technical Research Centre of Finland, P.O.Box 316, SF-33101 Tampere, Finland. [d]FDVH/St. James Hospital, P.O.Box 795, Dublin 8, Ireland. [e]ALPHA S.A.I., 72-74 Salaminos St., Kallithea, 17675 Greece. [f]Hvidovre Hospital, DK-2650 Hvidovre, Denmark.

The KAVAS-2 (A2019) AIM project develops a toolbox, named KAVIAR, with which the domain expert can formulate (capture) his/her own knowledge and/or derive domain models (socalled "learning") on the basis of example cases on the clinical problem under focus. Key issues for the global learning process within KAVIAR are 1) quality assessment of the derived domain models, 2) controlling the domain model generation in a desired direction, and 3) coupling of machine learning techniques with knowledge elicitation techniques. Other main issues addressed in KAVAS-2 are the cognitive aspects in the display of information and knowledge, the refinement of an evaluation methodology for KBS, and elucidation of problems inherent in the transfer of medical data, information and knowledge and hence, of dissemination of medical KBS.

1. INTRODUCTION

KAVAS-2 (A2019), which is an R&D project within CEC's AIM Telematics in Health Care Program, is based on its feasibility study KAVAS (A1021), carried out within the AIM Exploratory Action 1989-1990 [1]. KAVAS-2's main objective is to provide medical experts with a computer-based toolbox, named KAVIAR ("Knowledge Acquisition, VIsualisation Assessment and Refinement"), for making the domain knowledge explicit as well as for assessment and refinement.

The process in KAVIAR compares to an iterative learning process containing the below five steps in a (circular) sequence. These operational steps correspond to the conceptual steps for tasks' accomplishment in general: goal clarification, selection of means, carrying out the task, and subsequently assessing fulfilment of the task:

1) Goal definition for the learning process, i.e. among others the elicitation of the conditioning information (see below) and formulation of the medical problem approached.
2) Selection (and parameter setting) of appropriate tools and techniques to be applied among others on the basis of the medical problem focused on and the conditioning information.
3) Application of the selected tool(s).

#) Further, also involved actively in the project technical work are the key persons: M. Demeester, Premium (Belgium); J. Grimson, Trinity College Dublin (Ireland); H.-K. Johansen, CRI A/S (Denmark); A. Rossi-Mori, CNR (Italy); S. Weber, Risø National Laboratories (Denmark); W. Wilhelm, SIG Services BV (The Netherlands).

4) Measuring and exploring aspects of quality and characteristics of the domain models,
5) Validation of domain models against the defined goals, leading to either a new learning cycle iteration or to an implicit/explicit acknowledgement or rejection of the outcome.

It is elements of this learning cycle that the present paper outlines together with a discussion of the relevance of KAVIAR. Not mentioned elsewhere here is that emphasis is put on taking into account the cognitive aspects of the user interaction.

2. THE KAVAS-2 PROJECT

The toolbox KAVIAR contains several tools for knowledge elicitation and for machine learning based on different paradigms. Innovative elements of KAVIAR are the following key functionalities: 1) built-in quality assessment of semantic aspects of knowledge [2], 2) features for controlling the machine learning process in order to make it focus on the desired qualities, a process called Conditioning [3, 4], and 3) coupling of machine learning techniques with knowledge elicitation techniques to integrate these paradigm techniques, thereby enabling the support of the user in varying clinical situations where different data and knowledge sources are available. Further, important issues dealt with by KAVAS-2 are the evaluation of KBS and transferability of medical data, information and knowledge.

2.1. Knowledge Capturing

Medical research aims at improving clinical practise. Improvements may be achieved by applying information technology on different medical domains and problems with the purpose of producing practical, clinically useful and acceptable solutions. Medical experts apply many different types of knowledge at different cognitive and epistemic levels. Therefore flexible and well integrated methods are needed to tackle all aspects of the clinical situations: dynamic, causal, goal-structured and context-related knowledge, as well as basic biomedical knowledge.

The knowledge capturing part in the KAVAS-2 project integrates different methods for the analysis, structuring, modelling and representation of different types of knowledge into a toolbox usable by a domain expert. The methods presently dealt with are extended conceptual graphs for conceptual analysis and state-transition diagrams with rule-editors for qualitative, structure/function, task-oriented and strategy models. The generic type of problem solving tasks, uses and roles of knowledge in clinical situations give the criteria to select more methods into the toolbox under development.

2.2. Machine Learning

The starting point for the KAVAS project was the growing data pollution currently experienced in medicine. One feasible approach is to introduce protocols (in terms of decision trees) in e.g. laboratory medicine in order to avoid generation of data items which in the context provide no further information to the clinical problem elucidation for the case at hand [5]. Hence, major emphasis has been put on further developments of an existing induction algorithm [6]. The added-value are State-of-the-Art features like management of missing values and noise, different data types, quality measures, etc.

Other machine learning tools presently dealt with are: 1) a neural network building tool using feed forward networks (trained by back-propagation) in particular experimenting with quality measures, and 2) new machine learning technique, called density inference, which provides the most appropriate class label on the basis of a probabilistic analysis of neighbours in an N-dimensional space.

2.3. Quality Assessment

KAVAS-2 has developed a framework for the assessment of semantic aspects of knowledge based (see [2]). Semantic is here used in the sense of meaning of something as opposed to the formalism related with its representation. This framework provides guidance for the construction of and the selection among different classification models. To support the user in assessing the quality of the models derived, metrics for various quality measures are developed and implemented in KAVIAR.

2.4. Conditioning

We use the term *conditioning* for the processes involved in eliciting user requirements (the goal setting) regarding the domain classification models to be created as well as in setting the parameters of the machine learning algorithms on the basis of these requirements. In case the tool selected is not able to adjust to the specified requirements a priori, these requirements may be applied in stead for the selection among various models generated [3].

2.5. Evaluation of medical KBS

The KAVAS project developed a methodology for the evaluation of medical knowledge-based decision support systems which divides the entire KBS life cycle into four phases: the Preliminary Exploration, Validity, Functionality and Impact phases. The evaluation in each phase addresses different aspects of the system's properties. In KAVAS-2 the objective is to experiment with the methodology in practise and refine it. Within this experimentation it is intended to develop methods, metrics and measures for system's evaluation within each phase.

The particular value of the methodology comes from the enforcement of applying a stringent, systematic approach to KBS development thereby supporting quality management.

2.6. Transferability of medical data, information and knowledge

At present telematics is mainly dedicated to an exchange of data. Implicit in the interpretation of these data at the receiver's site is their context (terminology, methodology applied, etc.). Hence, a prerequisite for safe exchange of information within telemedicine is that the data, information and the related knowledge have exactly the same meaning at the sender and receiver ends. The problems within this transfer of data, information and knowledge originate from differences in e.g. terminology (symptoms, signs, diagnoses, etc.), methodologies applied for their assessment, local epidemiology, and cultural aspects [7, 8].

The key philosophy is that what is implicit should be dealt with explicitly. The aim in KAVAS-2 as regards transferability is to experiment further to elucidate the factors hampering transferability. From the experience gained we will formulate user requirements as regards telematics application in medicine. Draft user requirements are formulated in [9].

3. DISCUSSION

The status of the KAVAS-2 project is that a pre-prototype KAVIAR toolbox is being integrated for a first demonstration of its functionality as described above.

The relevance of KAVIAR shall been seen in view of the need for optimising and rationalising the Health Care scenario. KAVIAR is a toolbox for making (and assessing) decision making medical protocols in the broadest sense, e.g. clinical protocols for patient management or protocols for control of the analytical production in a clinical laboratory to optimize the data production in an information efficient manner. The knowledge capturing techniques are means for making the user's own knowledge explicit. Besides having a value on their own they serve as a frame of reference within the assessment of domain models and vice versa.

Further, KAVIAR shall be seen as a means for transfer of KBS: the knowledge capturing tools address deep knowledge models of the domain, while the machine learner tools provide shallow classification models based on data from the real world. It is anticipated that the deep models in general are much less vulnerable to differences in culture, terminology and methodology, and hence, that they may be moved from one organisation to another and then be verified/quantified/refined by means of local data covering the problem area of interest.

ACKNOWLEDGEMENTS

This work was partly funded by the Commission of the European Communities under the AIM Exploratory Action (KAVAS (A1021) Project) and the AIM Telematics in Health Care Program (KAVAS-2 (A2019) Project).

REFERENCES

1. Brender J, McNair P, Nykänen P, Talmon J, et al. KAVAS: Knowledge Acquisition, Visualization and Assessment Study. In: Noothoven van Goor J, Pihlkjær Christensen J, eds. Advances in Medical Informatics. Results of the AIM Exploratory Action. Amsterdam: IOS Press, 1991:199-206.
2. Brender J, Talmon J, Egmont-Petersen, Schiøler T, McNair P. KAVAS's Framework for quality assessment of medical knowledge. (see elsewhere in this volume)
3. Brender J, Karthaus V, Talmon J, Thygesen H, et al. KAVAS's Conditioning of the Induction Algorithm. (see elsewhere in this volume).
4. Talmon JL, Braspenning P, Brender J, McNair P. Machine Learning in data rich domains - Some experiences from the KAVAS project. In: Stefanelli M, Hasman A, Fieschi M, Talmon J, eds. Lecture Notes in Medical Informatics 1991;**44**;283-293.
5. McNair P, Brender J. Information Enhancement in Clinical Decision Making by Controlled Data Generation. Scand J Clin Lab Invest 1990;**50 suppl. 202**:112-119.
6. Talmon JL. A multiclass nonparametric partitioning algorithm. Pattern Recogn Letters 1986;**4**:31-38.
7. Nolan J, McNair P, Brender J. Factors influencing the transferability of medical decision support systems. Int J Biomed Comput 1991;**27**;7-26.
8. Schiøler T, Talmon J, Nolan J, McNair P. Transferability of knowledge based systems. Information technology factors. AIM 1993 (in press).
9. McNair P, Brender J. KBS in a telematics prospective - needs and challenges. In: Barahona P, ed. Proceedings of the EPISTOL Working Conference on CKD-Techniques. Munich:AIM-MEDWIS. 1993: (in press).

Artificial Intelligence in Medecine
S. Andreassen et al. , Eds.
IOS Press, 1993

KAVAS's Framework for quality assessment of medical knowledge

J. Brender[a], J. Talmon[b], M. Egmont-Petersen[c,d], T. Schiøler[a,e], P. McNair[e]

[a]Medical Informatics Laboratory ApS, Stengaards Allé 33d, DK-2800 Lyngby, Denmark. [b]University of Limburg, Dept. of Medical Informatics, P.O.Box 616, 6200 MD Maastricht, The Netherlands. [c]CRI A/S P.O.Box 173, DK-3460 Birkerød and [d]DASY, Copenhagen Business School, Copenhagen, Denmark. [e]Hvidovre Hospital, Dept. of Clinical Chemistry 339, DK-2650 Hvidovre, Denmark.

The KAVAS framework for assessment of semantic aspects of knowledge is outlined. It is composed of a set of orthogonal perspectives (each containing several concepts), of which a subset will be presented. Although it was designed for the assessment of Knowledge-Based Systems in medicine it is generally applicable. It has a close relation with the work item 2.10 of CEN/TC251/WG2, named "Certification of KBS development and evaluation".

1. INTRODUCTION

One of the key issues in the development (and subsequent application) of medical knowledge is the assessment of the quality of the derived knowledge models of the user domain. The KAVAS and KAVAS-2 AIM Projects have developed a framework for the assessment of quality of (executable) classification models [1, 2]. The KAVAS framework for quality assessment has the purpose of managing and making measurable the quality of classification models in the semantic sense. By semantic we refer to the "meaning" of something as opposed to the formalism for representing it.

The framework is closely related with the KAVAS Evaluation Methodology [3]. It may be applied within this framework for the assessment of validity of the outcome of KBS application on example cases.

2. THE QUALITY ASSESSMENT FRAMEWORK

The KAVAS Framework for quality assessment constitutes a high level semantic description of quality management. It is composed of a set of orthogonal perspectives [4] containing several concepts. Only a subset of these perspectives and concepts will be addressed here:

a) the perspective of Quality Management,
b) the conceptual hierarchy in measurements,
c) conceptual viewpoints on the semantic aspects of quality of knowledge.

2.1. Concepts within Quality Management

Quality Management (QM) is the act of dealing with quality in a goal oriented and structured way. Within QM there are three concepts constituting a layered operational structure: quality assurance (QA), quality control (QC) and quality inspection (QI). QA is concerned with the strategic (objectives, premises) and planning activities (e.g. selection of methods) to ensure the desired level of quality. QC is concerned with operationalization of the strategic aspects on the concrete problem case by means of the selected methods. QI is concerned with practical aspects in the measurement of individual measures. These three aspects function in a conceptual hierarchy of increasing abstraction, in which each level is operationally linked to the other levels. The above description highlights the establishment part of QM, however, there is a similar follow-up part of the QA ,QC and QI: the most simple quality assessment constitutes the measurement part of the QI alone, i.e. providing measures only. QI together with a frame of reference for the quality measures lead to the level of QC. When the interpretation of the measures is related to the question of "good enough for the purpose?" the level of QA emerges.

2.2. Conceptual Hierarchy of Measurements

The conceptual hierarchy within the concept of measurements comprises *methodology, methods, metrics and measures*. *Methodology* constitutes the global approach (goal definition and strategics) together with a consistent and coherent set of methods from which one may select and combine a subset to achieve the goal; *method* is a formalized description (including theories, application range and assumptions) for accomplishing a task; *metric* is a formalized procedure or technique for measuring a quality or characteristic, therein also its basic theoretical framework; and *measure* is a named concept that may bear a value.

The idea is that for each of the quality concepts identified (defined preliminary in [1, 2]) there shall exist a methodology for establishing and interpreting their value, by means of the methods, their operational formula (the metrics) and the measures to which they give a value.

2.3. Conceptual Viewpoints on the Semantic Aspects of Quality

Already from the definition of *correctness*[1] is it seen there are at least two viewpoints in semantic aspects of quality of knowledge: i) the success characteristics ("general validity of the system's output when applied on a population of cases of interest"), and ii) the assumptions characteristic ("it concerns only those cases that are classified").

In clinical biochemistry, biostatistics and other domains that formally apply metrology, it is also common practice to express characteristics of failures, for example in terms of the measures of dispersion (a measure for randomness in measurement) and bias (a measure of systematic error) (see e.g. [5]).

Hence, it is obvious also to look for a third viewpoint in semantic aspects of quality of knowledge: iii) failure characteristics.

An example may be taken from statistics: in linear regression analysis the variation

1) **Correctness** is defined as *the general validity of the system's output when applied on a population of cases of interest. Correctness* is meaningless, when items of input information are mutually conflicting or when the knowledge is not applicable, and hence, it concerns only those cases that are classified.

around a regression line expresses how good the model fits the data, i.e. it constitutes a success estimate which of course is highly dependent of the underlying data. The existence (and nature) of a pattern within the residual variation indicates the failure of fitting the model chosen (e.g. a 2nd order polynomial) with the data, i.e. a failure characteristic. An assumption is that the error of an individual datum is normally distributed.

3. EXAMPLE OF QUALITY ASSESSMENT

KAVAS-2 has experimented with metrics and measures for quality estimates among others in neural networks [6] e.g. the success characteristic *correctness* and the failure characteristic *bias*:

The Contingency Table in Table I illustrates an outcome for a classifier. It may be viewed as a matrix with 3 rows and columns. The metrics for correctness and bias can easily be expressed in terms of this matrix: the overall correctness equals the sum of figures in the diagonal divided by the sum of figures in all cells. The (true) class conditional correctness for e.g. class C equals the figure in column C row c divided with the sum of the figures in column C. The label conditional correctness for e.g. label b equals the figure in column B row b divided by the sum of figures in row b.

	A	B	C
a	15	0	0
b	2	132	23
c	0	0	27

Table I. Contingency Table displaying the distribution of cases according to the (true) class belonging (A, B, C) against their label (a, b, c) as categorized by a classifier.

Also bias (a measure for systematic errors) may be expressed overall or conditioned for one particular class or label. Table I shows a severe bias: all misclassifications are carrying label b, and especially class C cases are mislabelled, i.e. there is a bias in labelling C class patients as label b.

There is an assumption for applying the contingency table approach: that the classifier categorically labels each case, i.e. a probabilistic classifier requires another metric.

Further, note that the metrics applied to achieve these measures are not constrained to the 2*2 contingency table usually applied within medicine [9].

4. RELATION TO STANDARDISATION WORK

The CEN/TC251/WG2 deals with standardisation of terminology, classifications and knowledge-based systems. One of the work items is the 2.10 "Certification of KBS development and evaluation". The motivation given for this work item places the work presented here in a proper context [7]: "An imperative prerequisite for certification of a subject is to decide on what "quality" is, and establish criteria for assessment of an object, herein which aspects to measure, establish metrics to perform the measurement and procedures for definition and assessment of knowledge. Irrespective of technology, two major aspects of quality are: i) syntactics related, like consistency and redundancy in rule-based systems, and ii) semantics related like correctness, sensitivity and specificity. Within the development of large information systems ISO 9000 has been established as a standard for quality assurance procedures of the systems development. Similarly, approaches dedicated to quality assurance procedures for the development of KBS may be identified, i.e. establishment of a formal user evaluation methodology.".

The Approach for work item 2.10 of CEN/TC251 is delimited to the following aspects [7]: 1) certification of the organisation developing KBS, therein certification of the overall evaluation approach, and 2) certification of quality assurance/control parameters. The former may take an approach similar to ISO 9000 series and within that include elements from e.g. KAVAS's Evaluation Methodology. The latter corresponds very well with the framework for quality assessment of semantic aspects of knowledge-based systems as presented here [8].

ACKNOWLEDGEMENTS

This work was partly funded by the Commission of the European Communities under the AIM Exploratory Action (KAVAS (A1021) Project) and the AIM Telematics in Health Care Program (KAVAS-2 (A2019) Project).

REFERENCES

1. Brender J, McNair P, Raun H, Nolan J, et al. Meta-knowledge as a Means for Quality Management in Knowledge-Based Systems. In: O'Moore RR, et al. eds. Lecture Notes in Medical Informatics 1990;**40**:360-367.
2. Brender J, McNair P, Raun H, Nolan J, Vingtoft S. Meta-knowledge Concepts, 2nd ed. Technical Report META-1.1, KAVAS (A1021) AIM Project, 1990.
3. Clarke K, O'Moore R, Smeets R, Talmon J, et al. A Methodology for Evaluation of Knowledge-Based Systems In Medicine. AIM 1993 (in press).
4. Brender J, Talmon J, Schiøler T, McNair P. Framework for Validation of Semantic Aspects of Knowledge. (in preparation). 1993
5. Magid E, ed. Some concepts and principles of clinical test evaluation. Classification, analytical performance, monitoring and clinical interpretation. Scand J Clin Lab Invest 1992;**52(suppl. 208)**.
6. Egmont-Petersen M, Talmon J, Brender J, McNair P. On the Quality of Neural Net Classifiers. (submitted for publication) 1993.
7. Directory of the European standardisation requirements for health care informatics and programme for the development of standards. European Standardisation Committee (CEN), Technical Committee 251. 1993;Draft version 1.7.
8. Brender J. CEN/TC251/WG2, Standards for evaluation of KBS. In: Talmon J, ed. Proceedings of ATIM Workshop, Lanaken, Belgium, 24-25th May 1993: (in press).
9. Gerhardt W, Keller H. Evaluation of test data from clinical studies; I. Terminology, graphic interpretation, diagnostic strategies, and selection of sample groups; II. Critical review of the concepts of efficiency, receiver operated characteristics (ROC), and likelihood ratios. Scan J Clin Lab Invest 1986;**46 suppl.181**.

Artificial Intelligence in Medecine
S. Andreassen et al. , Eds.
IOS Press, 1993

KAVAS's Conditioning of the Induction Algorithm

P. McNair[a], V. Karthaus[b], J. Talmon[b], H. Thygesen[c], T. Schiøler[c], J. Brender[c]

[a]Hvidovre Hospital, Dept. of Clinical Chemistry 339, DK-2650 Hvidovre, Denmark. [b]University of Limburg, Dept. of Medical Informatics, P.O.Box 616, 6200 MD Maastricht, The Netherlands. [c]Medical Informatics Laboratory ApS, Stengaards Allé 33d, DK-2800 Lyngby, Denmark.

Conditioning refers to the specification of users' goal as regards quality and other characteristics of the classification model(s) aimed at by the application of machine learning tools. The KAVAS-2 AIM Project has identified and implemented the elicitation of a set of medical concerns and their transformation into directives to be used in the machine learning algorithms.

1. INTRODUCTION

The induction algorithms all optimize their outcome with respect to some performance criteria which has to do with the stopping criteria and pruning techniques [1]. However, these techniques mainly address the mathematical, statistical or similar technical criteria. We have demonstrated [2, 3] that classification trees have to be optimised along other criteria as well which are of a medical origin. This originates from the fact that it is not equally important (e.g. efficient with respect to time or certainty, etc.) to distinguish class A from class B as it is to distinguish class B from class A. Take the example of three outcome classes of an in-depth diagnostic investigation, *normals, cancer, otherwise (benign) diseased*, in which it is unethical to leave the normals uncertain for a long time or to let them go through risky examinations. Hence, the first step should be to separate as many *normals* and *otherwise diseased* from the potential cancer cases as possible and let only a few cases be examined more in depth. Further, it is unethical to overlook an early (treatable) cancer by a false negative classification, while it harms less with a few false positive outcomes which may later be correctly classified.

This type of user knowledge has to be incorporated and taken into account by the machine learning process. The KAVAS-2 project applies the concept *Conditioning* for the process of eliciting and incorporating the user knowledge in a goal-oriented strategic description of the model solution.

This paper illustrates briefly the potential effects of Conditioning and outlines a few approaches for achieving the desired guidance of one machine learning technique, an induction algorithm based on [4, 5] and recently extended with additional functionalities like allowing for both multiple and binary splits, and the handling of missing data.

2. ELICITATION OF CONDITIONING INFORMATION

Conditioning comprises a goal specification for the learning process. It is composed of the following two step process: 1) elicitation of the users' constraints/preferences as regards quality and other properties of the classification model in spe, and 2) transformation of these into directives (tool parameters) that can be used by the machine learning tools for guiding the learning process in the desired direction. The means for testing the degree to which the constraints/preferences for a given classification tree is fulfilled may be achieved by means of computation of its *utility*, (being) a linear weighted combination of quality measures.

There are two major issues of concern, medical and organisational aspects. We will focus on the medical aspects and ignore the organisational aspects except one. The medical issues are primarily concerned with different aspects of ethics:

* balancing false negative and false positive outcomes against the correctly classified,
* balancing the number of uncovered (with the outcome "unclassified") against the classified,
* time aspects, e.g. by focusing on a quick identification of normals followed by a thorough discrimination between different types of sickness),
* risky and unpleasant examinations are postponed and used only for specific purposes and for limited groups of patients,

etc.

The organisational aspect of cost (or similar availability) of given examinations should be included also as a minimum requirement to be incorporated in the Conditioning: some examinations takes seconds or minutes to perform, another examination takes days or it is performed on an equipment that needs booking three weeks in advance.

3. CONTROLLING THE INDUCTION ALGORITHM

There is not one generic and global solution for how to control and guide the learning process. A number of techniques have to be applied and combined to achieve a classification tree with the desired characteristics. The key issue is how the user requirements can be utilized during the various phases of constructing and assessing the classification models. For the induction algorithm there is the following three phases: tree construction, tree pruning and model comparison. During the tree construction one has the possibility to influence the criteria that are used to find the optimal tree, while after the tree construction one has the possibility of selecting among those generated for instance by applying a multicriteria analysis.

KAVAS-2 has experimented with several of the mentioned approaches for conditioning the induction algorithm, however, the present paper shall outline only the following:

* node labelling during the tree construction,
* attribute selection during the tree construction, and
* pruning of classification trees.

Neural networks also have potentials for conditioning. This is however, beyond the scope of the present paper.

3.1. Node Labelling

Very often the induction algorithm provides a classification tree like the one in Figure 1, where a number of end nodes contain more than one class. It obvious that the number of false positive and false negative outcomes will depend on the strategy for the labelling of these nodes (irrespective of whether this labelling is performed manually or automated). If false positive outcomes for B are to be avoided then all of the ambiguous nodes should have the label A, and so on. Trade-off curves (similar to ROC curves) for the relevant quality aspects may be a useful means in this respect.

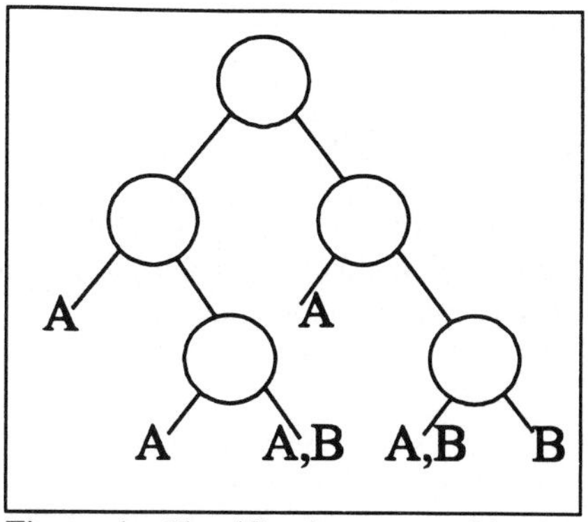

Figure 1: Classification tree with two outcome classes, A and B.

3.2. Attribute Selection

Another aspect of concern in the Conditioning is the ethical concerns. It may be acceptable to perform a certain investigation only when this is used for the ultimate discrimination between two particular class outcomes irrespective of the discriminative power of the investigation, e.g. liver biopsy or other unpleasant or risky investigations.

In this case the technical solution is to suppress the application of a particular attribute within the learning process until a given relevant criterion allows for its use for that particular (circumscribed) application range.

3.3. Pruning

In the induction algorithm we make use of two completely different techniques to handle pruning. The original reason for pruning is to prevent classification tree to become overly large, due to overfitting of noisy data. The most obvious way to accomplish this is to stop the tree from growing while building it [4]. This is referred to as *prepruning*. In general, we can say that the resulting trees are less complex and have an increased predictive power.

The other technique, *postpruning*, makes direct use of (a subset of) the users' constraints and preferences. The approach can be summarized in terms of two steps: firstly, we generate the maximal possible classification tree, i.e. we grow the tree until all terminal nodes cover only cases of one class. Secondly, we use the constraints specified (translated into usable parameters for the algorithm) to prune the tree.

In the current implementation, we discern hard constraints and an optimisation function. The constraints are expressed as class conditional correctness measures (see this concept in [6]), while the optimisation function compares the correctness against coverage. The classification tree needs to fulfil the constraints, while the optimisation function will balance the improvement in one measure against the loss in the other. The general strategy followed in the pruning algorithm is to check whether any constraint is violated. If that is the case, nodes will become labelled as "unclassified" until all constraints are fulfilled. Next, the optimisation function is utilized to maximize the performance of the classification tree by deleting subtrees, modification of the labelling of terminal nodes, and/or merging of brother nodes.

This pruning can be done at a global tree level or at a level where each individual terminal node must meet the constraints. The local approach puts stronger conditions on the quality of the tree than the global variant.

4. DISCUSSION

The experience from previous work has been that the predominant approach used (optimization along mathematical/statistical criteria) is insufficient for clinical application [2, 3]. This is further illustrated from the examples above. The relevance of Conditioning comes with the need for safe and efficient (cost, time) protocols for clinical decision making, as also indicated.

KAVAS-2 has implemented the Conditioning of the mentioned aspects and is experimenting with others. At present we are in the process of fully integrating and documenting the impact of Conditioning on the overall performance and behaviour of the induction algorithm.

ACKNOWLEDGEMENTS

This work was partly funded by the Commission of the European Communities under the AIM Exploratory Action (KAVAS (A1021) Project) and the AIM Telematics in Health Care Program (KAVAS-2 (A2019) Project).

REFERENCES

1. Mingers J. An empirical comparison of selection measures for decision-tree induction. Machine Learning 1989;**3**:319-342.
2. Talmon JL, Braspenning P, Brender J, McNair P. Machine Learning in data rich domains - Some experiences from the KAVAS project. In: Stefanelli M, Hasman A, Fieschi M, Talmon J, eds. Lecture Notes in Medical Informatics 1991;**44**;283-293.
3. Talmon JL, Braspenning P, McNair P, Brender J. Machine learning in medical domains: some experiences of the KAVAS project. In: Lun K, Degoulet P, Piemme TE, Rienhoff O, eds. Proceedings of the Seventh World Congress on Medical Informatics 1992. Amsterdam: North-Holland. 1992:447- 453.
4. Talmon JL. A multiclass nonparametric partitioning algorithm. Pattern Recognition Letters 1986;**4**:31-38.
5. Talmon J. The effect of noise on the performance on machine learning algorithms. Technical Report KAFE-3.1 (deliverable 5) of the KAVAS (A1021) AIM project 1990.
6. Brender J, Talmon J, Egmont-Petersen, Schiøler T, McNair P. KAVAS's Framework for quality assessment of medical knowledge. (see elsewhere in this volume)

Artificial Intelligence in Medecine
S. Andreassen et al. , Eds.
IOS Press, 1993

Clinical decision-support in the field of TETANUS serology using an associative storage model implemented in LISP

J. P. Schröder[1], P. Henne[2], W. D. Kuhlmann[3]

1 Department of Medical Informatics, Federal Armed Forces Medical Office, Platanenweg 29, 53222 Bonn, Germany

2 German National Research Center for Computer Science (GMD), I3-KI 53757 Sankt Augustin, Germany

3 Department of Immunology, Ernst-Rodenwaldt-Institut, PO Box 7340, 56065 Koblenz, Germany

ABSTRACT

Vaccination without the knowledge of the immune status run the risk of complications to vaccination to a high degree. Therefore a quantitative serological detection of TETANUS-antitoxin is recommended before booster-vaccination. The diagnostic interpretation of results can be improved by including extensive knowledge using a neural-network-system implemented in LISP. This system constitutes of a general associative storage-model, which can be used for the implementation of a variety of purposes, for instance simple perceptrons, associative sequences or semantic nets. The latter is done using context-sensitive association, where an output is obtained from input together with an additional context-form. The essential characteristics of the structure of that knowledge base as well as examples are presented.

INTRODUCTION

The necessity for a booster vaccination can be easily determined by means of a serological analysis of tetanus antitoxin [1]. Vaccinations without knowledge of the immune status carry a high risk of postvaccinal complications. An examination of the vaccination status is above all indicated in the case of an unclear vaccination anamnesis so that hyperimmuno-reactions can be largely avoided, if the immune-protection is still adequate. In that connection the knowledge of the vaccine protection titer level, measurable in IU/ml, serves as a decision-making aid as to whether or not a booster vaccination is indicated [2].

It was the objective of the work to improve the diagnostic interpretation in the field of the Tetanus serology by applying extensive knowledge. Furthermore, we wanted to get more insight of the involved parameters in the decision making process of vaccination serology by means of a neuronal network.

Representing knowledge on a computer can be done using production-rules where the rule-left-hand-sides observe facts and the rule-right-hand-sides generate new facts without the need of specific knowledge about the semantics of the link between the two sides, this is an associative connection. Processing of this representation is performed by an interpreter which incorporates several adequate strategies for using the rule-coded knowledge as for instance forward- or backward-chaining or intelligent techniques to select the next acting rule from a set of possible rules and so on.

Production-rule-systems are successfully used for the implementation of expert-systems for medical or technical diagnoses, for classification- and interpretation-tasks and are sometimes told to be "AI's FORTRAN". As in the case of FORTRAN used for "formula translation" there are some severe disadvantages in using production-rule techniques for processing associative knowledge: Any associative link (any "rule") has to be hand-coded making it almost impossible to efficiently implement knowledge with more then some hundred highly interconnected facts. Currently valid facts associate connected facts during a time-consuming computation of the interpreter-program which matches the valid facts against (all) rule-left-hand-sides. The possible speed of associative reasoning is not obtained in favorite of the possibility of more elaborate logical tests on the valid facts.

It was the aim of our work to construct a System which performes reasoning by addressing pieces of knowledge directly from other associativly connected pieces of knowledge without the need for a global interpreter [3,4]. Furthermore, these pieces of knowledge should not be restricted to rule-conditions and rule-consequences.

METHODS

The software ASM, an associative storage model, is based on a general construction tool for artificial neural networks implemented in LISP. This system constitutes a general associative memory-model, which can be used for the implementation of a variety of purposes, for instance simple perceptrons, associative sequences, rule-based systems or semantic nets. The latter is done using context-sensitive association, where an output is obtained from input together with an additional context-form. This scheme is also used to remind data-triplets of the format (object attribute value). Thus object-oriented systems can be constructed, where only the instances are explicitely known and the class-descriptions are obtained on demand by determination of features common to a set of instances. In contrast to a pure rule- or object-based system, where the abstract knowledge is explicitely programmed into the machine, in our attempt the instances or examples are the input and the abstract knowledge is evaluated by the system, thus representing a kind of learning behavior.

The system enables a kind of machine-learning by means of examples. We undertook two ways of implementing knowledge:
1. Looking for similarities and combination of similarities
2. Generation of class-descriptions from instances on demand.

Some explanations about the generalized model:
- outside-world-entities (facts) are represented by concept-nodes
- concept node has an activation, a value describing its validity
- a concept node may be (associatively) linked to other nodes
- a triplet (OBJECT ATTRIBUTE VALUE) is represented by a special node-structure which retrieves all VALUES for a given ATTRIBUTE-OBJECT-pair and all OBJECTS for a given ATTRIBUTE-VALUE-pair (see Figure 1).

The system is entirely written in Allegro Common LISP and implemented on sparc stations and APPLE Macintosh.

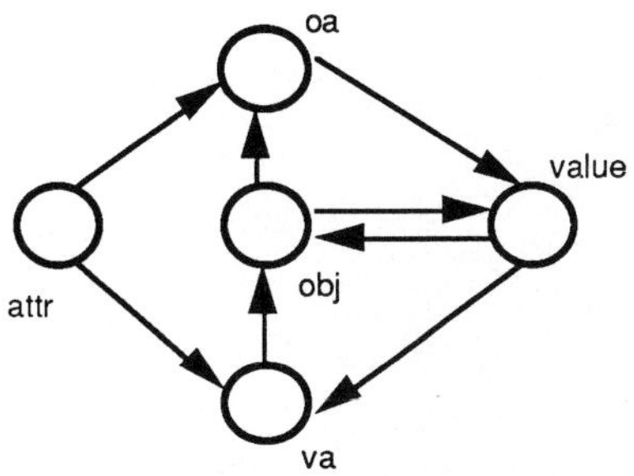

Figure 1. A neural assembly for the representation of (object-attribute-value)

RESULTS

On the basis of the knowledge base structure for the interpretation of tetanus-antitoxin titers by making use of a LISP-based associative storage model (ASM), the diagnostic interpretation of constellations of tetanus-antitoxin has been improved. On the one hand, the interpretation of tetanus-antitoxin titers is based on the results of the applied methods, i.e. ELISA or TR-FIA. It is further based on interfering characteristic as age, number of vaccinations, amount of IgE, appearance of hyperergic-reactions in the history and on inferences defined as a function of certain value constellations.

Figure. 2 shows a part of node-framework representing some object knowledge. It indicates that the assessment of the goals immunosuppression and booster immunization require knowledge about sex, age, Tetanus-titer, previous vaccinations and any relevant findings.

DISCUSSION

The indication for a booster vaccination can be easily objectified by means of the quantitative measurement of Tetanus antitoxin [1,2]. Inspite of the vaccination programs offered, there are gaps in the Tetanus vaccine protection, particulary in the older population. A serological review of the vaccination status is also indicated in order to avoid hyperimmunoreactions in sufficiently immunized individuals. Due to the varying degrees of response of the individual immunological system to vaccinations and an unforseeable reaction of the person to be vaccinated, a precise documentation of the vaccination times on the one hand and a stricter indication for booster vaccinations than commonly applied so far on the other hand seem to be expedient [1]. In doing so, the level of the Tetanus-antitoxin titer, measurable in IU/ml of serum can serve as a decision-making aid [2].
The possiblilities of a knowledge-based support for diagnostics have been proven sucessfully in the field of laboratory medicine in various specialist areas as well as in other disciplines of medicine so that from the original prototypes programs have developed which are employed in routine operations as well [5,6,7].

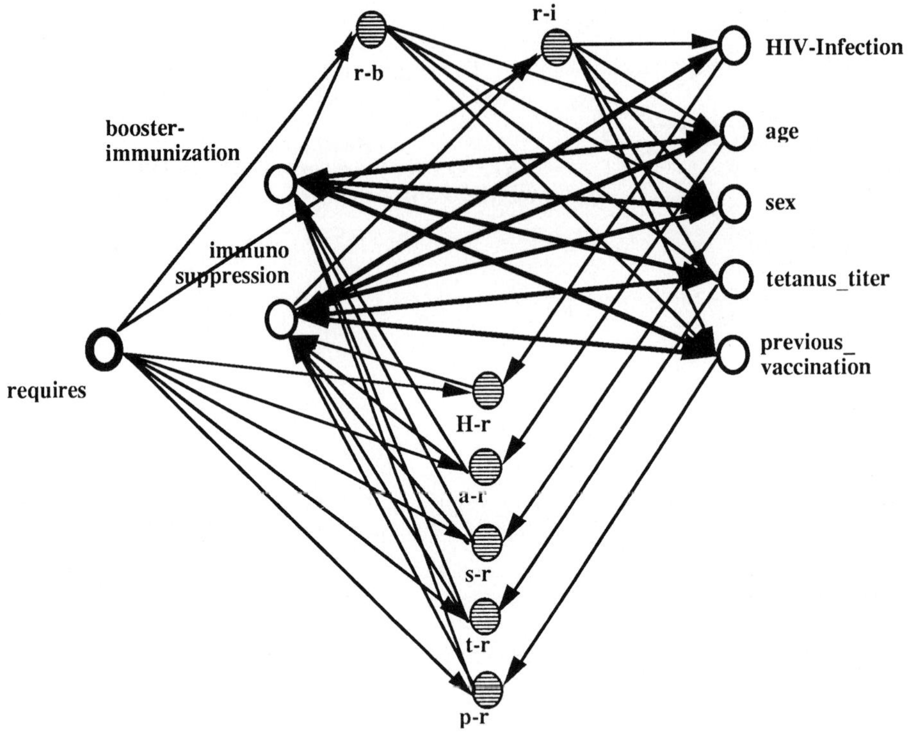

(save3 booster-immunization requires age)
(save3 booster-immunization requires sex)
(save3 booster-immunization requires tetanus_titer)
(save3 booster-immunization requires previous_vaccination)
(save3 immunosuppression requires age)
(save3 immunosuppression requires sex)
(save3 immunosuppression requires tetanus_titer)
(save3 immunosuppression requires previous_vaccination)
(save3 immunosuppression requires HIV-infection)

Figure 2. Part of a Node-Framework representing some object-knowledge

The development of our system was strongly influenced by the experiences of the medical project Pro.M.D. on the one hand and the artificial intelligence project TASSO on the other hand [7,8,9]. As the representation of knowledge using the production-rules of the Pro.M.D.-shell did not fully meet our expectations we began to focus our work on a case-based approach using an associative storage model (ASM) implemented in LISP.

Our system provides the basis for a value-dependent interpretation of the tetanus-antitoxin titer for assessing the prospective duration of immuno-protection and for recommending the time for another booster immunization. Previous postvaccinal complications are taken into consideration by the treatment proposal.

The inferences of the system can be logically comprehended by means of automatically generated class-descriptions relevant to the respective findings. The system enables the listing of the diagnostically relevant characteristic quantities for the findings and the interpretation of the values. This approach makes it possible to achieve a standardization and a constantly high quality of later medical findings.

CONCLUSION

A programmed uniform static network built from only one type of base-cells - the 5-node-save3-structure - allows storage and processing of qualified associative knowledge. Necessary search is reduced to the addressing of labelled nodes in the net whereas the basis inferencing-process is performed by the local behaviour of the nodes itself without any global interpreter. For this reason an implementation of this model even on a sequential computer gives much faster response than an equivalent production-rule-system. The evaluation of the findings present the interpretations of the Tetanus-antitoxin titers in a more transparent way and in a technically well-founded manner so that an improved basis has been provided in order to objectify the indication for revaccination and to avoid vaccinations without knowing the serum-antitoxin concentration and possible complications associated therewith. The TETANUS associative storage model (ASM) is comprehensive, runnable, useful, modifiable by anyone who works with LISP and who is able to provide medical knowledge in this special field. The system base does, however, not claim to be complete.

REFERENCES

1. Schröder, J. P. und W. D. Kuhlmann, The Lancet Vol, 340 (1992) 379
2. Schröder, J. P. and W. D. Kuhlmann. J, Clin. Microbiol., 29 (1991) 1504
3. Palm, G.: Neural assemblies - An alternative approach to Artificial Intelligence - Springer Verlag, Berlin 1982
4. Rumelhart, D. E., McClelland, J. L. (ed.): Parallel distributed processing - Vol. 1+2, MIT Press, Cambridge 1986
5. Puppe, B., Puppe, F., Meth. Inf. Med., 27 (1988) 10
6. Shortliffe, E. H.,West Jour Med., 145 (1986) 830
7. Trendelenburg, Chr. und Pohl, B. Pro.M.D.Medizinische Diagnostik mit Expertensystemen. Georg Thieme Verlag, Stuttgart-New York, 1988.
8. Henne, P.: Ein experimentelles Assoziativspeicher-Modell. Tasso-Report 15, (1990)
9. Henne, P., Schmitgen, G.: Graphisches Suchsystem SKaGra: Konzepte und Realisierung. Tasso-Report 49, (1993)

Artificial Intelligence in Medecine
S. Andreassen et al. , Eds.
IOS Press, 1993

Model based learning support to knowledge acquisition: A clinical case study

K. Morik[a], G. Potamias[b], V. Moustakis[b,c], and G. Charissis[d]
[a]University Dortmund, Dept. Computer Science, Dortmund, Germany
[b]Institute of Computer Science, FORTH, Heraklion, Greece
[c]Department of Production and Management Engineering, Technical University of Crete, Greece
[d]Director, Pediatric Surgery Clinic, University of Crete, Heraklion, Greece

Abstract

This paper presents a methodology to support knowledge acquisition based on the integration of pre-established domain knowledge with knowledge induced (i.e., learnt) from past clinical cases. Integration is achieved via filtering of clinical cases using pre-established domain knowledge and the enhancement of pre-established knowledge using clinical cases. We demonstrate our methodology by way of a 'real-world' clinical domain involving therapy planning of maldescensus testis.
Keywords: Machine learning, model based learning, maldescensus testis.

1. INTRODUCTION

Over the last few years machine learning, (ML), has been extensively applied to medical domains, supporting diagnosis, therapy planning and monitoring [1, 3, 11]. Most of these approaches operate on a repository of past medical cases and apply learning heuristics to support the derivation of discriminant or characteristic descriptions, modeling diagnostic, therapeutic and patient monitoring decisions. However, a major drawback of these approaches is that they do not take into account contextual factors influencing expert decision making [4]. This calls for enhanced learning procedures capable of uncovering hidden patterns in clinical data, thought to be carriers of contextual influence, and capable of modeling inconsistency in clinical decision making. Such learning procedures should be able to support cooperative feedback between pre-established domain knowledge and knowledge induced (i.e., learnt) from past clinical cases. Specifically, we may use pre-established domain knowledge to guide learning from cases and filter out noisy or inconsistent data, and cases to enhance domain knowledge and model contextual influence.

This paper presents a methodology to support knowledge acquisition based on the integration of domain knowledge and knowledge induced (i.e., learnt) from clinical cases. We demonstrate our methodology by way of a 'real-world' clinical domain involving therapy planning of maldescensus testis. We organize the paper in the following manner: in section 2 we delineate our methodology and briefly present Mobal - the machine learning system upon which our work is based - in section 2.1; in section 3 we present the maldescensus testis domain and in section 4 we present and discuss the results derived from the application of our methodology on the maldescensus testis domain. We conclude the paper in section 5 by further elaborating upon the significance of our work and by suggesting areas for further work on the subject.

2. METHODOLOGY

We view our methodology as a heuristic process, namely:
Given :

1. Pre-established domain knowledge represented by way of IF...THEN rules; we denote such knowledge by R_0, where each member r_{0j} of R_0 takes the following representation:

$$r_{0j} : \&_{i=1}^{m} P_i(x, v_i) \rightarrow T_j(x, R_0) \tag{1}$$

where $m \leq\mid M \mid$, M denotes the total number of attributes used to represent the domain, x is the case identifier, P_i the predicate names used to represent domain attributes and $T_j(x, R_0)$ the decision T_j suggested by rule r_{0j} for a case x.

2. Clinical cases which have been dealt with in the past represented as a collection of facts in first-order logic format, namely:

$$\&_{i=1}^{m} P_i(x, v_i) \& T_j(x, D) \tag{2}$$

where m, x and P_i are defined as in (1) and $T_j(x, D)$ the decision T_j taken for case x and recorded in the data set D.

Find :

- A set of rules capable of explaining decision making inconsistency between decisions derived using R_0 elements and decisions recorded in D.

Procedurally, the methodology proceeds in the following manner:

1. Apply R_0 to D and derive the set of cases E_k whose members imply decision making inconsistency. Formaly E_k is defined in the following manner:

$$E_k = \{x \in D / \&_{i=1}^{m} P(x, v_i) \& T_j(x, R_0) \& T_j(x, D), T_j(x, R_0) \neq T_j(x, D)\} \tag{3}$$

where m, x, P_i, $T_j(x, R_0)$ and $T_j(x, D)$ are defined as in (1,2). In other words, E_k stores all the cases in which R_0 derived and D recorded decisions are not identical.

2. If $E_k = \emptyset$ it means that there is no discrepancy between pre-established domain knowledge and actual decision making. However, if $E_k \neq \emptyset$ then it means that for at least one case there exists a deviation between what should be done (domain knowledge; $T_j(x, R_0)$) and what is actually done (case decision; $T_j(x, D)$).

3. When $E_k \neq \emptyset$ we attempt to explain (i.e. to learn) the reasons for the deviation. The first alternative is to try to induce rules that link $T_j(x, R_0)$ with $T_j(x, D)$ decisions via specific factors realized by the conjuction of domain attribute-values. Failing to induce such rules it means that the information recorded in the data set is not enough to explain the deviation and so some additional information is needed. This represents a case of learning from inconclusive data; a data set of examples expressed in terms of attributes is said to be inconclusive if there exist no set of rules utilizing only the given attributes that classifies all possible examples perfectly [10].

4. Additional context depended attributes are introduced which are targeted to uncovering hidden patterns in D that are associated with E_k set case members; we denote the set of additional attributes by A:

$$A = \{a_i(x, v_i)\} \tag{4}$$

where a_i is the name of the attribute and v_i its value for the x case.

5. We try to induce rules that link the conjuction of elements in A with the $T_j(x, D)$ on the basis of one or more factors. By this means the original R_0 set is expanded and when applied to D (step 1) may cover consistently more cases. In other words, step 5 forwards to the begining of this process and implements an iterative use of it.

6. We stop either when $E_k = \emptyset$ (strong condition) or if $| E_k | \leq \tau$, where τ is a satisfactory threshold value ($| E_k |$ denotes the cardinality of set E_k).

The methodology presented above operates in a cooperative mode between theoretical (pre-established) and practical (case) knowledge and encompasses both deduction (2) and induction (3,5) steps realizing in a sense a Select and Test hypothesis Model - STM [9], in the course of knowledge acquisition. Within this methodology the role of domain experts remains active and inquiring and knowledge acquisition processes become more vivid and more realistic. Following such a methodology we try to produce more knowledgable results in a way of enhancing the knowledge base with more contextual factors which influence the decision making process in the domain at hand.

2.1 Learning : the Mobal system

To support the acquisition of theoretical and practical knowledge in terms of rules and cases a learning system should be able to: effectively represent and handle cases and rules; deductively apply rules to cases; inductively learn rules from cases; detect inconsistencies and restrict the set of hypotheses to focus learning.

The Mobal learning system [6, 13], meets the above requirements. With Mobal, cases are represented as a collection of facts in first-order logic; for example: `age(x,"0-6months")`, `etiology(x,congenital)`, `status(x,sliding_inguinal)`, `size(x,abnormal)`, `actual(x,hormonal)`.

Furthermore, the built-in inference engine of Mobal can immediately execute the rules that have been entered to show the consequences on existing input. The built-in *model-based relational learning algorithm*, RDT (Rule Discovery Tool), induces rules from cases [5]. Rule schemata are used to restrict the hypothesis space for learning. Rule schemata allow the user to describe sets of rules that he or she wants the system to test. For instance, if the user wants to know which combination of two predicates determines a particular classification `c`, the following rule schema is appropriate: `P1(X,Y)` & `P2(X,Z)` → `c(X)`.

All domain specific predicates where their arguments fit the structure are then used to instantiate the predicate variables `P1` and `P2`. An instantiated rule schema is a rule which is tested, for verification or not, against the facts and user-defined criteria.

The application described in this paper uses RDT, the inference engine, and parts of the knowledge revision tool all integrated into the computational enviroment of the application.

3. MALDESCENSUS TESTIS

Maldescensus Testis (MT) refers to a problem in male infants where one or both of the testicles do not properly descend from their inner-body positions after birth. If untreated, this leads to non-functional (atrophied) testicles that may even become malignant (cancerous) in adulthood [2]. In general there are no ideal MT treatment scenarios. The pediatrist decides whether to use `hormones`, `operate`, or remove the testicle based on personal judgement on, for instance, the size relationship between the affected and the healthy testicle. In many cases the pediatrist may decide to `follow up` the case. In summary, each MT case may be classified into one of the three classes (treatments), `follow_up`, `hormonal`, `surgical`.

Each MT case is represented by means of five attributes all of them treated as nominal variables: `age (10)`, `etiology (2)`, `status (15)`, `size (3)` and `actual (3)` the class attribute (in the parentheses the number of attributes's values). The data set consisted of 151, 'real-world' patient cases, collected from the Pediatric Surgery Clinic of University Hospital of Crete, Greece.

Pre-established domain knowledge is represented in the form of rules devised by medical experts, for example: `status(x,ing_ing)` & `not(age(x,0_6months))` → `expert_decision(x,hormonal)`

R_0 [see methodology, (1)] consisted of thirteen such rules. The `expert_decision` predicate represents the treatment classification as suggested by the rules and is to be contrasted with predicate `actual` which holds the treatment classification recorded in the patient's case report.

4. THE CASE STUDY

In the first experiment we started by testing the completeness and correctness of pre-established domain knowledge. Storing expert rules and activating Mobal's inference engine we were able to deduce an `expert_decision` fact for **all** data cases (methodology, step 1). This result proves the completeness of pre-established domain knowledge with respect to the recorded case data.

The next question is whether the rule base is correct with respect to the cases (methodology, step 2). For this, we introduced into Mobal rules capable of identifying conflict between `actual` and `expert_decision` classifications, namely:

```
expert_decision(x,follow_up) & actual(x,hormonal)
→ expert-data-inco(x,follow_up_hormonal)
```

Mobal was queried for each conclusion and a total of 25 `expert-data-inco` facts were deduced; 7 `actual=hormonal` cases were classified as `expert_decision=follow_up` ; 6 `actual=follow_up` cases were classified as expert_decision=hormonal and 12 actual=surgical cases were classified as expert_decision =hormonal.

In order to explain these conflicts we introduced into Mobal special rule schemata like the following (methodology, step 3):

One predicate:
expert_decision(x,follow_up) & P(x,c) → actual(x,hormonal)
Two predicates:
expert_decision(x,follow_up) & P1(x,c1) & P2(x,c2) → actual(x,surgical)

We activated Mobal's Rule Discovery Tool using the above rule schemata. In each case, predicates P_i were instantiated with all domain predicates (according to schema structure) and the resulted grounded rules were tested for confirmation. In all cases the results were negative, no rules were confirmed. This result indicates an inability to explain conflict.

We now know that some information which could explain the difference between rule-derived and actual classification may be missing (inconclusiveness, leading to decision making inconsistency). Since inconsistency may be seen as a "fact of life" in clinical decision making, an attempt to control, i.e., "modeling of inconsistency" it would be far more practical as compared to an attempt to eliminate it. Drawing towards this direction, the 151 MT cases were provided to four medical experts who where the same persons who generated (treated) the cases in the first place. The experts were requested to assign three different treatment decisions to each case: what treatment they should prescribe; what treatment they might prescribe and what treatment they would avoid to prescribe (methodology, step 4). These judgements were used as additional attributes for the description of cases and represent a kind of "problem-solving" approach to clinical decision making, see also [7]. Each of the should, might, avoid attributes take as values one of the original treatment classifications. Expert judgements were combined in a single classification using only cases in which a consensus was achieved. This led to the reduction of the initial 151 case set to 147.

The results of the expert inquiry match the actual classification quite well: in 128 cases (87% of the total) the should treatment matches the actual one; in 16 cases (10.88% of the total) the might treatment matches the actual one and in 7 cases (4.76% of the total) the avoid treatment matches the actual one. The reason for no perfect match between pre-established domain knowledge - in the form of should-might-avoid patterns - and case data classifications (at least between should or might and actual treatments) is rest in the presence of tolerance between the different MT therapeutic treatments. In MT decision making the physician conceives a case with a pattern of treatment priorities and then tries to identify factors that confront with this pattern, to select a specific (i.e., 'customized') treatment with due regard to patient and decision making context. Patient and/or decision making context may relate to non-medical factors (e.g. social factors, habitance of the patient, education level and awareness of parents, etc); such factors are, most often than not, not captured in patient cases yet are used in clinical decision making. This leads to inconclusiveness.

The task now is to identify factors, allready recorded in the domain description, explaining the actual therapy decisions on the basis of the treatment priority patterns. We are looking for one or more predicates which represents a reason for an actual classification given a should-might-avoid pattern. In order to generate only those hypotheses that could lead to such an explanation, we introduced into Mobal rule schemata (methodology, step 5) for inducing rules able to explain inconsistencies between decision priority patterns and actual decisions. These rules may incorporate one or more such factors recorded in the original domain description and represented with the used predicate names:

One predicate:
should(x,S) & might(x,M) & avoid(x,A) & P(x,c) → actual(x,ACT)
Two predicates:
should(x,S) & might(x,M) & avoid(x,A) & P1(x,c1) & P2(x,c2) → actual(x,ACT)

For S, M, A,and ACT variables a constant was introduced from the set of the original treatment classification names. These rule schemata were then instantiated by all domain predicates (that fits schema's structure) using Mobal's RDT. With this procedure we were able to induce a total of 69 rules like the following ones:

One predicate:
`should(x,follow_up) & might(x,hormonal) & avoid(x,surgical) & status(x,norm_slid)`
`→ actual(x,hormonal)`
Two predicates:
`should(x,hormonal) & might(x,surgical) & avoid(x,follow_up) & status(x,slid_ing)`
`& etiology(x,congenital) → actual(x,follow_up)`

The second of the rules above indicates that the specific expert's treatment priority pattern result into a `follow_up` decision on the basis of the factors `status(x,slid_ing)` (the pathology status of the testicles is sliding_inguinal) and `etiology(x,congenital)` (the testicles's pathology is of congenital cause). The 69 induced rules cover a total of 128 cases (87% of the original 147) which was considered as an acceptable stoping threshold (τ) value (methodology, step 6) given MT domain characteristics. These rules link theory and practice; such linking could not be achieved by relying on the case data alone. Learned rules *enhance* the expert-given rule set and make it more precise and "context" depended by refering to the `should-might-avoid` patterns.

5. CONCLUSIONS

The importance of revisions and on-going efforts of enhancing a rule set have been stressed by the work on the Mobal system. A particular way of integrating revision and learning is supported by a knowledge revision tool [14] and a concept formation tool [12]. A similar approach to restrict rules because of contradictions is discussed in [8]. Provided that the information recorded in the data cases is sufficient to support revision and/or invention of new concepts, these tools could be used. This was not the case with the available MT data cases.

In this paper, we have described a different approach. Instead of restricting particular rules of the expert-given rule set, additional rules are learned that link the classifications of the expert inquiry, the case data, and the actual classification. This approach does not require sophisticated knowledge revision tools. It can be followed with any system that offers some *deductive* capabilities so that the conflicts between derived and given classifications can be detected. The method also requires *inductive* learning to extract additional (i.e., context dependent) rules that link differentiated expert classifications with actual respective ones.

Furthermore, this approach shows that machine learning tools can provide an effective vehicle towards the integration of clinical data (case data; the agent of reality and of bias) with medical knowledge possesed by the expert and/or the literature (pre-established knowledge; the agent of clinical theory). This approach can be readily generalized in any domain in which one suspects differences in predicted and actual decisions and when tolerance between decisions is present.

Work was enabled by the inference engine and the Rule Discovery Tool (RDT) of Mobal. The services of the inference engine were important for the detection of completeness, inconsistency, and conflict.

Acknowledgements

This paper is an extented and revised version of a paper presented at the "Real World Applications of Machine Learning" workshop held in the context of European Conference of Machine Learning - ECML 93. The work has been performed in the context of the Machine Learning Toolbox - MLT (ESPRIT, P2154) and GAMES-II (AIM, A2034) projects, both funded by the CEC. The learning system Mobal has being developed at the German National Research Center for Computer Science, GMD and is available via anonymous FTP from ftp.gmd.de, directory pub/gmd/mlt, for non-commercial academic use.

References

[1] A. Babic, E. Krusinka, JE. Stromberg. Extraction of diagnostic rules using recursive partitioning systems: A comparison of two approaches. *Artificial Intelligence in Medicine*, 4, pages 373 – 387, 1992.

[2] W.E. Grupe. Abnormalities of the genital tract. In M.E.Avery and H.W. Taeusch, editors, *Schaffer's Diseases of the Newborn*, pages 402 – 411. Saunders, 1984.

[3] M. Hadzikadic. Automated design of diagnostic systems. *Artificial Intelligence in Medicine*, 4, pages 329 – 342, 1992.

[4] E.T. Keravnou, F. Dams, J. Washbrook, R.M. Dawood, C.M. Hall and D. Shaw. Background knowledge in diagnosis. *Artificial Intelligence in Medicine*, 4, pages 263 – 279, 1992.

[5] J. Kietz and S. Wrobel. Controlling the complexity of learning in logic through syntactic and task-oriented models. In Stephen Muggleton, editor, *Inductive Logic Programming*, chapter 16, pages 335 – 360. Academic Press, London, 1991. Also available as Arbeitspapiere der GMD No. 503, 1991.

[6] K. Morik. Acquiring domain models. *Intern. Journal of Man Machine Studies*, 26:93–104, 1987. also appeared in Knowledge Acquisition Tools for Expert Systems, volume 2, J. Boose, B. Gaines, eds., Academic Press, 1988.

[7] V. Moustakis, G. Potamias, L. Gaga, M. Blazadonakis, P. Vassilakis, and G. Charissis. Bias identification using inductive learning techniques - a medical case study. In B.G. Silverman, editor, *Expert Judgement, Human Err or, and Intelligent Systems Workshop*, pages 117 – 123. ECAI 92, 1992.

[8] S. Muggleton and M. Bain. Non-monotonic learning. The Turing Institute, Glasgow, Scotland, 1990.

[9] M. Ramoni, M. Stefanelli, L. Magnani, and G. Barosi. An epistemological framework for medical knowledge based systems. *IEEE Trans. Syst. Man and Cybernetics*, 22(6), pages 1361 – 1375, 1992.

[10] S. Spangler, U .M. Fayyad and R. Uthurusamy. Induction of decision trees from incoclusive data. *Proc. of the 6th International Workshop on machine learning - 89ML*, pages 146 – 150, 1992.

[11] G.I. Webb, J.W.M. Agar. Inducing diagnostic rules for glomerular disease with the DLG machine learning algorithm. *Artificial Intelligence in Medicine*, 4, pages 419 – 430, 1992.

[12] S. Wrobel. Automatic representation adjustment in an observational discovery system. In D. Sleeman, editor, *Proc. of the 3rd Europ. Working Session on Learning*, pages 253 – 262, London, 1988. Pitman.

[13] S. Wrobel. Demand-driven concept formation. In K. Morik, editor, *Knowledge Representation and Organization in Machine Learning*, pages 289–319. Springer, Berlin, Tokio, New York, Jan. 1989.

[14] S. Wrobel. On the proper definition of minimality in specialization and theory revision. In Pavel Brazdil, editor, *Procs. of the European Conference on Machine Learning*, 1993.

Artificial Intelligence in Medecine
S. Andreassen et al. , Eds.
IOS Press, 1993

MODELS FOR MEDICAL KNOWLEDGE REPRESENTATION AND MEDICAL REASONING IN A C.A.I SYSTEM

Ch. RIOU [a], P. LE BEUX [a], P.LENOIR [a], D.LECLET [b]

[a] Department of Medical Informatics - RENNES University School of Medicine, FRANCE

[b] University of Compiegne - Computer Science and Engineering Department, FRANCE

Abstract
We present in this paper a model for medical knowledge representation in a computer Assisted Instruction system. Entities used in medical reasoning and relations between these objects are described. We explained the difficulties in modeling medical diagnosis in order to help students to structure their reasoning.

1. INTRODUCTION

The objective of an intelligent Computer Assisted Instruction (CAI) system in medicine is to provide the students with a tool enabling the acquisition of decision strategies for medical diagnosis and therapy.

An intelligent CAI system includes four components [1] :

- -The expert module which has a representation of the medical knowledge and is able to solve problems.
- - The student module which contains the informations about the student
- - The pedagogical module which manages the student knowledge acquisition
- - The user interface.

A combination of the different techniques for knowledge representation is used in the medical knowledge-bases [2] and the systems which already exist : rules and frames in GUIDON-NEOMYCIN [3] and SPHINX [4], objects rules and algorithms in CONSULT-EAO [5] or ILIAD [6], objects and rules in DIABOLO [7], objects and fuzzy rules in ANTIB-ES [8].
An existing CAI system called AEDM has been improved in Rennes School of Medicine [9]. It has been developped using the ADM knowledge base [10]. This system provides informations about diseases and helps the practitioner to make diagnosis. The approach taken is the guided simulation of clinical cases. The simulation of cases is divided in five steps. The first step consists in extracting pertinent information from a textual clinical case description. In the second step the student has to define the clinical situation and then he must ask for clinical complementary data with regard to the situation. In the third step he makes syndromic groupings, identifies physiopathological mechanisms and anatomical structures which can be related to the case, and consequently define several pathological frames. In the fourth step, for each frame defined in the previous step, he evokes the diseases which can be possible diagnosis. The fifth step considers differential diagnosis. The student must ask complementary tests in order to find the right diagnosis.
Presently, we introduce new knowledge representation in order to modelize the student and the teacher knowledge, and to manage a dialogue with the student.

2. KNOWLEDGE BASE : ORGANISATION

We describe the entities used in medical reasoning (signs, syndroms, diseases, diagnosis and physical examination, complementary examinations, treatment), some concepts are used in reasoning (clinical situation, anatomical structure, physiopathological mechanism).
Within each type of entities, objects are usually described in a hierarchy (for example :diseases, complementary tests). Classes of clinical signs can be created from a general concept. Therefore the object oriented modeling seems to be appropriate.

2.1. The methods used for knowledge representation

An object-oriented modeling has been choosen where each field can be described by attributes and methods. Relationships between objects of different classes are defined. Each class will be instanciated in a case study. We will take examples from a knowledge base for rheumatology.

2.2. The entities of the domain

2.2.1. Clinical examination

It is described with fields which are objects too. As our purpose is not to teach how make a clinical examination we developped only the examinations which occur in the definition of physical signs. We create a "mother" class named ***clinical examination*** . This class has several sub-classes which inherit fields from the mother class. With the field named *examination-type* we define implicitly the relations between several instances of the same class, this field can have two values : a generic or a precise term. During the dialogue with the student, it will be asked him to specify his or her question or to consider a more general knowledge.
As examples of instances of joint mobilization class we have :

- A precise instance which is : *passive hip motion in abduction*
  - *title* : passive hip motion in abduction
  - *examination-type* : precise
  - *type* : passive
  - *joint name* : hip
  - *direction* : abduction
- A generic instance which is : *hip motion*
  - *title* : hip motion
  - *examination-type* : precise
  - *type* : no precision
  - *joint name* : hip
  - *direction* : no precision

In such a way we improve the semantic knowledge about the physical signs related with joint examination and the system will be able to make better inference on clinical cases.

2.2.2. Complementary tests

Similary, using the object oriented approach we can describe also Complementary tests as objects included in a taxonomy. At the top the object-class *complementary test* is shown below.

The fields are :

- the knowledge which the physician requires when asking for complementary tests (invasive character which is implied by the procedure, waiting period, cost)
- the result classes which are possible for a test
- the linguistic type is explained on one hand by the test-class. *Single test class* (ie : *standard X ray* class where no field can be multiple). *Composite test class* (ie : *hematology-count* where the field named *element* can be multiple). On the other hand it is specified by the instance when there is a composite class : *elementary test* (ie : platelet-count where a single element is considered) or *composite test* (ie : blood-count where several blood elements are specified).

2.2.3. Complementary tests results

Four types of results can be defined : quantitative result, qualitative result, text-result, object-result. There is a lot of object-results, they are specific to a test-class. They are composed of several fields which are sometimes objects themselves. Such classes are called aggregate classes, so that all the results observed for a test can be grouped together.
We give here an example concerning the class named ***joint x-ray result*** :

class *joint x-ray result*

Fields	joint-space name :
Joint-space : object --------->Fields	lesion-presence :
	lesion type :
	lesion place :
Bone density : object --------> Fields	where :
	outline :
	shape :
	size :
	lesion :
....	

2.2.4. Signs and symptoms

All the sign sub-classes will inherit from the head class sign. The class sign is composed of the following fields : title, number, medical type, linguistic type, presence. We have adopted two models for the representation of the signs.
In the first one, a common concept or a common semantic term define a sub-class, it is the case for all the functional signs (ie : pain, functional disability, and several physical signs (ie : heart murmur, hepatomegaly). In the second one, the sub-class is defined with 2 other objects : *way to obtain the sign* and attributes defining the result,this is the case for some physical signs (ie : joint mobility) and test results [11].

2.2.5. Syndroms

A syndrom is an association of signs. Rules are composed of disjunction of conjonctions of signs (ie : syndrom named **femoral neuralgia** *was evidence of* (anterior thigh pain and absent patellar reflex) *or* (anterior thigh pain and decreasing of quadriceps's muscular strength).

2.2.6. Diseases

In order to represent the diseases we required simple attributes (title, frequency, nosology, prognosis) and also two types of relationships : between diseases and signs and syndroms (*is-expressed-by*), between diseases : class hierarchies (*is -a* , *specifies*) and others (*has-an-etiology* , *has-a-complication* , *has-a-linked-disease*).

2.2.7. Diagnosis

The class diagnosis includes only relationships, which are on one hand relations between diagnosis and signs or syndroms (*is-evoked-by* , *is-asserted-by* , *is-eliminated by*), and on the other hand between diagnosis and complementary tests (*is-oriented-by* , *is-confirmed-by*).

2.2.8. Treatments

The head class has several relations from which the sub-classes will inherit (medical treatment, surgical operation, physical therapy).We have three relations between treatment and disease; their names are : *is-appropriate-for* , *is-contra-indicated* , *has-for-complication* .

The other objects have been created in order to help the student in diagnosis evocation. Considering a patient history, the student will have to define a clinical situation for which he will have to follow a questionning plan and an examination plan in order to collect complementary informations. In a second phase he will give the anatomical structures and the physiopathological mechanisms which can be involved in.These objects are important due to their relations with the other objects (signs, syndroms, diseases).The representations of these objects are given further.

2.3. Relationships between objects

The different objects are connected by relations which build a network. There are several kinds of relations :

- the taxonomy relations : *is-a* , *is-specified-in* , they are used to describe the links between diseases or complementary tests
- the meronomy relations : *is-broken up-into* , they are used in the model of anatomical structure, for example joint *is-broken-up-into* cartilage, synovia and ligament
- the other relations connect objects belonging to different taxonomies.

We show some examples which will give an idea of the complexity of the representation.
The relation *evoke-structure* between an instance of the class *clinical situation* and instances of the class *anatomical structure* is relatively simple, it joins a clinical situation and a disjunction of anatomical structures.The relation *evoke-disease* is more complex because it joins two instances of different classes, in fact a conjunction between an instance of the class *anatonical structure* and an instance of the class *physiopathological mechanism*, and a conjunction of disease's instances.The relation *is-asserted-by* between an instance of *diagnosis* and a disjunction of signs's conjunction or syndroms's conjunction is still more difficult to implement. It links a diagnosis and the association of signs which allows to assert it.

3. DISCUSSION

The choice of a model in order to represent medical knowledge has confronted us with several problems. Medical vocabulary is very rich, so it is difficult to be homogeneous in the representation. The U.M.L.S semantic network was not adapted for our system. It is used essentially for information retrieval in bibliographic database and not for description of symptoms [12].
With an object-oriented model we must create a large number of classes and sub-classes. We have not yet developped all the associated procedures. The relationships between objects of different classes are difficult to implement. So it is important to use several techniques. The implementation is made on PC using Pascal Object Oriented programming language. Relationships are represented with pointers and lists of entities. Because of the complexity of the representation we had to reduce the number of classes. The representation was too precise and this level of accuracy is not necessary for the explanation the system will have to give to the students. Most of the entities were modeled at the beginning in order to analyze free text. We decided to converse with the student principally with menus, so we did not need such a precise description of objects. Presently we have been working on natural language interface and we attempt to introduce conceptual graphs in the interface module of the ADM system. We expect that we will be able in the future to allow the student to talk with the system in natural language. In our system the entities are described with more precision than in the ILIAD system [6], but on the other hand ILIAD is structured according to the Bayes model.

4. CONCLUSION

The objects we have built are included in an Intelligent Tutoring system intended for clinical medicine learning [13]. One of the purposes of this system is to help students to structure their reasoning used for diagnostic . The model we have chosen will contribute to improve the explanation given to the student and will provide him or her a real guided tutorial system.
In the future the lessons could be built automatically. A first evaluation of the knowledge base has been made [14] then we will have to validate the model with experts and then to assess the performance of the system with students.

5. REFERENCES

1. Nicaud J.F., Vivet M. Les tuteurs intelligents : réalisations et tendances de recherches. Techniques et Sciences Informatiques, 1988, Vol.7, n°1, 21-45
2.Stary C., Fasching K. : UnPatient: A knowledge base for medical diagnostic expert systems Tenth International Congress on Medical Informatics, Vienna, 1991, Springer-Verlag, 629-633
3. Clancey W.J. Neomycin: Reconfiguring a rule-based expert system for application to teaching. 7th IJCAI, 1981, 829-836
4. Fieschi D. Contribution au système expert SPHINX : application à l'enseignement médical Thèse de doctorat 3ème cycle, Paris VI, 1984
5. Aegerter P. Consult-EAO : Etude et réalisation d'un système expert d'aide à l'enseignement de la médecine : Application aux pays en développement. Thèse de Doctorat, UTC Compiègne, 1988
6. Lepage E., Bouhaddou O., Tredaniel J., Chassany O., Warner H., Warner H.R. ILIAD: an expert system for diagnostic assistance and teaching: implementation in France Tenth International Congress on Medical Informatics, Vienna, 1991, Springer-Verlag, 629-633
7. Mahé H., Altman J.J. DIABOLO : Un système expert d'aide à la thérapeutique et à l'éducation du diabétique insulino-dépendant. MARI-COGNITIVA 87, Paris, 18-22 Mai 1987
8. Palmer G., Morlat P., Pillet J.C, Labroille G., Tilly B., Nejjari C., Luguet J., Aubertin J., Medahoui A., Hassar M., Salamon R. AntibES/Rabat - A fuzzy computer-aided instruction on the treatment of infectious diseases designed for Morocco medical students and medical practitioners. Tenth International Congress on Medical Informatics, Vienna,1991, Springer-Verlag, 434-438
9. Meadeb J., Chales G., Lenoir P. : Apprentissage du diagnostic médical par simulation sur ordinateur (AEDM). MED.INFORM. (1986),vol 11,n°2, 167-175
10. Lenoir P., Bourel M., Roger J.M, Chalès G., Système d'aide au diagostic médical: méthodes utilisées, Med. Inform., 1980, vol 5, n° 4, 291-307
11. Riou C., Le Beux P., Lenoir P. , La représentation des connaissances dans le système d'aide à la décision ADM, In Informatique et Santé, 1992, (5) : 95-107
12. Miller P.L., Wright L.W., Frawley S.J., Clyman J.I. and Powsner S.M. Selecting relevant informations resources in a network-based environment : The UMLS information sources map, In MEDINFO 92, North Holland
13. Leclet D., Fontaine D., Riou C., A plan-based approach for the teaching of musculoskeletal medicine, Proceedings, AVIGNON 93, Ed. EC2
14. Denier P., Le Beux P., Lenoir P., Simulated case-patients to evaluate the ADM computer assisted diagnosis system, proceedings of MIE 93, Jerusalem, April 1993, p661-666

Artificial Intelligence in Medecine
S. Andreassen et al. , Eds.
IOS Press, 1993

Case Based Reasoning in Clinical Evaluation

Klaus Goos

Universität Würzburg
Lehrstuhl für Künstliche Intelligenz
Allesgrundweg 12
97218 Gerbrunn

Stefan Schewe

Universität München
Medizinische Poliklinik
Pettenkofferstraße 8a
80336 München

email: goos@informatik.uni-wuerzburg.de, FAX: ++ 49 931 70 561 20

Abstract: Most case based classification systems take little advantage of expert knowledge. They use as input for problem solving only a very large set of cases. We show a case based approach where expert knowledge can be incorporated into the similarity measure. We describe a successful application of this approach to clinical rheumatology and report on its evaluation.

1 Introduction

Case based reasoning for knowledge based systems has received much attention during the last few years. The idea is to overcome the bottleneck of knowledge acquisition for heuristic expert systems by reasoning directly on known cases without abstracting generic knowledge like correlations or rules from them.

Case based reasoning in general records a set of exemplar cases and then compares the actual case to the exemplar cases by determining the degree of similarity of the new case to the given ones. Systems such as PROTOS [Porter et al. 90] use fixed similarity measures, e.g. the Euclidian distance. Others like PATDEX [Wess93] use parameterized similarity measures which only yield acceptable results if a very large set of cases is given for determining the parameters.

In this paper we show that good performance can be achieved by using the similarity measure itself as an input parameter of the system. The knowledge acquisition is significantly simplified by treating the set of exemplar cases and the similarity measure, i.e. the expert knowledge, as two completely separate entities, which can be acquired independently of each other. In particular, new cases or additional similarity knowledge can be added at any time.

It is assumed that the importance of features is not given statically but is inferred dynamically depending on the reasoning context and the expert knowledge. Dynamic computation of the similarity measure already occurred e.g. in HYPO [Ashley 88]. The possible context in HYPO consists of assumptions which are independent of the considered cases. In case based classification, the context consists only of the features (in the following we use the medical term finding) of the cases to be compared and the solution of the known cases.

The incorporation of expert knowledge in a similarity measure requires that the similarity measure is expressive, easy to understand and easy to enter into the system. To achieve this aim we have designed a representation to describe similarities and implemented a case comparison component named CcC+ [Puppe&Goos 91]. It is integrated in the expert system shell D3 [Gappa et al. 93, D3 91]. The graphical knowledge acquisition of D3 was extended in a way that similarities can be acquired, too.

We first explain the knowledge representation. Then we report about the successful application of CcC+ to the area of clinical rheumatology and its evaluation. A discussion of possible further improvements concludes this paper.

2 Knowledge Representation

Cases are stored as a vector of findings together with a solution. A new case is a vector without solution. In case based classification a solution to a new case is found simply by taking over the solution of a known case, if the similarity between both cases is strong enough.

To keep case comparison structurally simple, the knowledge representation only allows comparison of the values of corresponding findings. So finding combinations typical for rules are impossible. To compensate this restriction, the ranges of findings may be much more complex than yes/no alternatives like in INTERNIST [Miller 82]. These more complex ranges include (see also [Puppe et al. 91]):

- scalar types with numerical ranges
- set/subset types with comparison of general and specific values of a finding (e.g. localisations of findings like "abdominal pain" versus "abdominal pain in right upper quadrant")
- one or multiple choice types with the range consisting of one or a list of items without an internal structure

For the different ranges we have schemes for computing partial similarities between findings´ values.

We not only allow static weights to determine the importance of a finding but also allow to consider the particular diagnostic situation. It is possible to modify the importance of findings by the solution (one or more diagnoses) of a compare case, e.g. the static weight of a finding may be modified dynamically to express special causalities or correlations between findings and diagnoses. In the following we describe the mechanisms of the knowledge representation in detail:

(1) computing partial similarities between findings´ values
(2) dynamic weighting
(3) dealing with finding abstractions

ad 1: To compute partial similarities between two values A and B of a finding, the knowledge representation provides three basic schemes:

- **individual** (for all types): *if A = B then 1 else 0.*
- **functional** (for scalar types only): $f(A)/f(B)$[1] or $1 - |f(A) - f(B)| / K$, where the function f and the constant K are given in the similarity specification by an expert. In the simplest case for a numerical range, f is the identity function. If a constant is used and the formula produces a negative result, it is set to 0. In a frequent special case, f is a stepwise linear function defined by a list of points and K is the distance between the lowest and the highest y-coordinate of the points. A slightly modified version of this is used for ordinal one-choice ranges, where a number (corresponding to an y-coordinate) is assigned to each item of the range.
- **grouped** (for checklist types only): *if A = B then 1, else if A and B belong to the same group, then x else 0.* If the range is multiple-choice and *A* and *B* denote several items, each item group is treated separately and the singular results are averaged to one number.

ad 2: While for some findings a static weight (relative importance) might be sufficient, other findings should get a dynamic weight depending on the diagnosis. E.g. abnormal findings are weighted higher than normal ones. Thus, we account for the fact that especially in troubleshooting but also in other classification domains most measurements are normal and only the few abnormalities are important for classification.

Dynamic weights may also be used for representing special relationships between findings and diagnoses. Supposing a diagnosis D occurs only together with finding value S(V). While in general the finding S might be unimportant and could have a low weight, the special value

[1] $f(A)$ is assumed to be smaller than $f(B)$.

S(V), however, must be highly weighted for inferring the diagnosis D. Apparently such dynamic weights cannot be represented in pure case based approaches. In CcC+ there are two ways for expressing such knowledge: Solution-dependent weight-modifications and similarity-modifications with each diagnosis.

ad 3: Several findings may be interdependent, e.g. a certain value may lead to diagnosis D only in case the patient has the age of a child, otherwise it is unimportant. For such higher order conclusions CcC+ provides a simple rule language, which also allows arithmetic operations. However, it must be avoided to produce contradictions by using the pure findings on their own and additionally possible existing abstractions.

Therefore each finding may be labelled with an appropriate abstraction layer. At problem solving time an abstraction layer is selected by the user and only findings on this layer are considered. Also different views of cases may be developed.

3 Evaluation

In an earlier project [Gappa et al. 93] a considerably large heuristic knowledge base in rheumatology was acquired. The goals of this project were to systematize the collection of data of medical history of patients for assisting non-specialist physicians in rheumatology, to document the cases and to automatically generate a case report. This knowledge base containing 69 diagnoses and 197 findings (historical data, physical examination, laboratory tests and various technical investigations) was used in the evaluation reported here.

Separate similarity knowledge was acquired by a rheumatologist for a first prototype of a case based expert system using graphical methods.

To evaluate our case based reasoning system, we accumulated a database of 408 rheuma cases prospectively examined cases with joint complaints using the data input mechanisms of our expert system shell D3 to get the historical data of the patients. Then the results of the physical examination, laboratory and radiology test were added to the database using the expert system. Finally the results of the heuristic expert system and the physicians´ documented diagnoses were included. The patients in the database came from two sources with different patient sets and different diagnostic strategy:

(1) 305 out-patients with joint complaints from the Medizinische Policlinic of the University Munich.

(2) 103 patients (in-patients n=50, out-patients n=53) hospitalized in the public Krankenhaus in Baden-Baden.

The in-patients of the second clinic often had complicated symptoms: The consequences of the operative and pharmacological therapy sometimes disguised the characteristic symptoms of the basic illness.

We applied the case comparison to about 100 cases from the database, tested at least one case per diagnosis. Knowing the physicians´ diagnoses of every test-case, the similarity measures were adjusted. Afterwards the findings of 102 new patients were prospectively acquired using the expert system to get the history of present joint complaints. The physicians´ examination, radiology and laboratory results were also documented without knowing the physicians´ diagnoses.

These 102 test-cases were used to evaluate both the heuristic problem solver [Puppe&Gappa92] and the case comparison component. During the evaluation neither the heuristic nor the case based knowledge base was changed. For evaluation, the heuristic result and the results of the three most similar cases were compared with the physicians´ diagnoses. The overall results are shown in table 1.

In 14 cases there was no exact final clinical solution. From the remaining 88 cases 70 (79,5%) had a correct or nearly correct solution in the case based system versus 77 (87,5%) in the heuristic system. This is a none significant difference between the two problem solving methods (chi-square = 2,023; t = 0,15; DF = 1).

In 10 of 14 cases without a clinical solution the heuristic system also had no solution, whereas the case based system in each comparison found similar cases but with a very low similarity.

	case comparison system		heuristic system	
Diagnoses completely correct	48	47,0%	62	60,8%
Diagnoses partially correct	22	21,6%	15	14,7%
Diagnoses partially incorrect	15	14,7%	8	7,8%
Diagnoses incorrect	3	3,0%	3	3,0%
No diagnoses	14	13,7%	14	13,7%

Tab. 1: The overall results of the evaluation with 102 cases. "Diagnoses completely correct" means that the physicians´ diagnoses are identical; "Diagnoses partially correct" means there are additional diagnoses to the physicians´ result. "Partially incorrect" or "Incorrect" means that part or all of the diagnoses in the system's result were incorrect. "No diagnoses" means that the system produced no solution and there was also no clinical diseases.

4 Discussion and Outlook

There are two reasons for the slightly poorer results of the case comparison compared to the heuristic system: (1) In order to handle multiple diagnoses it would be necessary for the database to include at least one case for each possible combination of diagnoses. The current available database is still to small to meet this necessity. Instead the diagnoses of the most similar cases could be combined. (2) It turned out that a lot of finding abstractions should be acquired to rate characteristic combinations of findings indicating similar diseases. Nevertheless that is quite expensive. Therefore a more explicit mechanism than finding abstractions is necessary to allow this.

An advantage of the case based approach is significant less time was used to acquire the additional case comparison knowledge (about 1/6 of the working time during 2 months). For building the heuristic knowledge base much more time (about 1/6 of the working time during 1 1/2 years) was needed.

A general problem in medicine for any problem solving method is that different physicians will diagnose the same disease with the same findings but use a different terminology for this disease. This discrepancy will always lead to inevitable disagreements between system's and the physicians´ diagnoses.

References

Ashley, K. and Rissland, E (1988). Waiting on Weighting: A Symbolic Least Commitment Approach, AAAI-88, 239-244, 1988.

D3 (1991). Bamberger, S., Gappa, U., Goos, K., Meinl., A., Poeck, K., & Puppe, F.: Die Diagnostik-Expertensystem-Shell D3. Handbuch. Institut für Logik, Komplexität und Deduktionssysteme der Universität Karlsruhe.

Gappa, U., Puppe, F., and Schewe, S. (1993). Graphical knowledge acquisition for medical diagnostic expert systems. Artificial Intelligence in Medicine, 5:pp 185-211, 1993.

Miller, R., Pople, H., and Myers, J. (1982). INTERNIST1, an Experimental Computer-Based Diagnostic Consultant for General Internal Medicine, New England Journal of Medicine 307, 468-476, 1982.

Porter, B., Bareiss, R., and Holte, R. (1990). Concept Learning and Heuristic Classification in Weak-Theory Domains, AI-Journal 45, 229-263, 1990.

Puppe, F. and Gappa, U. (1992). Towards knowledge acquisition by experts. Industrial and Engineering Applications of Artificial Intelligence and Expert Systems, 5th International Conference IEA/AIE-92, Paderborn, Belli, F., & Radermacher, F. J. (Eds.), pp 546-555, Lecture Notes in Artificial Intelligence 604, Springer.

Puppe, F. and Goos, K. (1991). Improving case based classification with expert knowledge. 15. Fachtagung für Künstliche Intelligenz, GWAI-91, Christaller, Th. (Ed.), 196-205, Informatik-Fachberichte 285, Springer.

Puppe, F., Legleitner, T., and Huber, K. (1991): DAX / MED2 - A Diagnostic Expert System for Quality Assurance of an Automatic Transmission Control Unit, in Zarri, G. (ed.): Operational Expert Systems in Europe, Pergamon Press, 1991.

Wess, S. (1993). PATDEX–ein Ansatz zur wissensbasierten und inkrementellen Verbesserung von Ähnlichkeitsbewertungen in der fallbasierten Diagnostik. 2. Deutsche Tagung Expertensysteme (XPS-93), Puppe, F., Günter, A., (Hrsg.), 42-55, Springer.

Artificial Intelligence in Medecine
S. Andreassen et al. , Eds.
IOS Press, 1993

'Object-oriented mentality : the most suited paradigm for medical knowledge-based systems.'

J.-L. Mommaerts

Object-Orientedness (OO) is not just the latest 'nouvelle vague' in software development. In fact, it transcends software alltogether, even in analysis and design stages. It is a way of thinking, a philosophy that goes back a very long time. Platonism, the 'superclass' of all other philosophies, has as its central focus the postulated existence of 'Ideias'. These 'Ideias' can be seen as abstract classes from wich other classes and objects are more and more objective derivatives.
What is new is that these concepts now and for the first time in history are getting practical and visible. That of course makes a very big difference. It can even lead to the verification of old philosophical disputes and theories that were until now mystified and completely unclear.
For OO in software and especially AI, this philosophical connection means that one can benefit from millennia of thinking practice, a very vast source of knowledge!

More recently, in the field of psychology, two streams of thought can be compared :
-cognitive psychology, especially information-processing theories. These have a view on human psyche much like a conglomerate of knowledge systems, a composite of modules, each consisting of still smaller modules.
-Gestalt psychology. This views human psyche much as a neural network.
The fact the the same system, namely our own mind, can be seen at the same time as a neural network and as a composite of modules, indicates that mother nature has chosen for us at least a very close integration of different paradigmata of knowledge representation and inferences. As I will discuss, such integrations can benefit very much from the characteristics that make up an OO mentality.

Object-orientedness brings mainstream software and AI closer together in different ways :
-It makes 'intelligence-business' more comprehensible by providing a relatively (!) simple (because in reality very simplified) framework for everybody to think about what terms like 'artificial intelligence' and 'machine knowledge' can denote.
-It brings the opportunity for object-oriented mainstream programs to attract principles from AI to one or some of its objects, without interference to or from other objects. 'Normal' objects, being encapsulated, are protected from the inner workings of objects that start behaving more or less intelligently within the same program structure.
-Likewise, AI programs can benefit from object-oriented mainstream software techniques in much more direct ways than with other software paradigms, for instance by using very efficient object-base techniques or multimedia-modules developed outside the AI community. Encapsulation can give a closer fit while at the same time providing less interference between objects. Thus the brute but very forcefull mainstream techniques can intertwine

more complexely with the elegant and flexible, but not always very efficient (programmatically) AI techniques.

Object-orientedness has by now well proven its worth in mainstream programming. Many practical systems, of which also very big ones, are testifying the fact that it provides a major jump forward in efficiency of analysis, design, programming and maintenance, as well as in the coordination of all these. But apart from those very important contributions, there are, for the world of AI, still greater fruits to reap from the object-tree. In my opinion, this stems from its being in the first place an important philosophy. The consequences are and will not be just 'philosophical', but very practical indeed. I will focus on two practical aspects that can be much improved through the use of the object-oriented philosophy, namely : prototype based development of knowledge systems and the integration of formalisms for knowledge representation.

PROTOTYPE BASED DEVELOPMENT

The object-oriented paradigm very much facilitates a prototype based development of software systems in general, through techniques that are called together 'fast prototyping.' This kind of development is very typical and, I dare say, necessary for knowledge systems, mainly for the following reasons :

- The lack of possible specifications of a knowledge system project makes it very useful to have user feedback from the first stages of analysis. Users can think much better about their own requirements if they can visualize the intended system. This is especially the case for complex software like knowledge based systems, while they are much more difficult to conceptualize and understand on paper. It is still more so if users don't have informatical background, as is mostly the case with medical personnel.
- Developers of knowledge systems often mistakenly think that a grown-up, commercial system is nothing more than their scaled-up prototype. Therefore a waterfall model of system development with only one or two prototypes often fails in discerning sufficiently early in the project the many pitfalls that have to be avoided. The parts of the domain that researchers tackle in their single prototypes, usually are the most easily formalized parts. Scaling up means not doing more of the same thing, but looking for other ways, diversifying, integrating. In human medical decision making, such a diversification has been psychologically proven : commonsense and pattern recognition come along with many forms of more formal, theoretical decision taking.

The facility with which object-prototypes are made and changed gives the opportunity of semi-direct implementation of one's thoughts, thereby learning from mistakes and developing the knowledge system in an organic way. Several parts of a systems can be OO prototyped indepently and incrementally as needed. Afterwards, the results of these efforts can be integrated in one building, and it works! In non-OO, one would be left with ruins.

- The introduction of knowledge systems in a specific situation as for instance a medical consultation, can change some of its fundamental attributes. The introduction of the system itself can change the environment for which the system was written. E.g. bringing expertise about economical factors of medical decisions can make doctors more personally involved in how the resources of the community can be used for a better health care for everybody.

With the use of OO rapid prototyping, these changes can be appreciated in earlier stages

of the development and this can be of influence on what the systems ultimately look like.
- The interface of a knowledge system is specifically important because it is the 'forum of interplay' between the two thinking entities : user and system. Doctors do not accept, and with very good reasons, that their cognitive actions are replaced by artificial systems. After all, the doctor remains the only responsible for the decisions made. To accomplish this, the interface must be as flexible as possible, while remaining easy to understand and work with. The interface therefore is one of the main reasons to build prototypes for knowledge systems in the first place. Object-oriented programming is especially well equipped for these requirements. If the main system-objects can be visualized in some way on the screen, this also much stimulates an understanding of all potential users about what goes on in and around the artificial reasoning faculties. This modelling, in 'real-life', of objects on the screen, is relatively easily done with object-oriented modules.

INTEGRATION OF FORMALISMS FOR KNOWLEDGE REPRESENTATION

As is well known, different knowledge representation paradigms exist and are used, mainly separately, in different knowledge based systems (R.Davis, H.Shrobe & P.Szolovits '93). Real intelligence however, artificial or not, does not lie in one or another magic bullet, but in the complexity of using different paradigms of knowledge representation and inferencing in the same system, each providing, in formalized ways or ideosyncratically, the kind of thinking that is most appropriate in the specific micro-situations. Medical decision taking also derives much (most?) of its power from being very flexible (cf. supra), according to the available internal resources and the particular situations it has to deal with.

R.Davis et al. describe five different knowledge representation paradigms. Implemented in different objects, they can be used, as described before, closely fitted and at the same time independent from each other. This makes the overall system at the same time more complex and easily understood. What gives this already significant lever even much more power, is the fact that objects can be used to implement, with great advantage, each of the five paradigms :

-The logical paradigm. Logic can be implemented within objects. Furthermore, an object and an attribute can be seen as predicate (the attribute) and argument (the object). The attribute can be just another object. A multi-argument predicate can be an object (attribute) that is composed of more than one objects.

-The frames paradigm. The relationship between frames and objects is very close and even more blurring as time passes. In fact, frames can really be seen as just one kind of objects. Even frame-demons can easily be implemented as special object-functions. In medicine, frames are specifically appropriate for representing patterns like syndromes, diseases or working diagnoses. Thus a significant part of medical knowledge can be declared with the use of frames - in conjunction with other representation formalisms.

-The connectionist paradigm. Objects are used by several authors (e.g. T.Masters '93) to implement neural networks. One advantage of objects in this case is the possibility to make a hierarchy of neural net paradigms and letting them inherit many resembling characteristics from abstract classes. Another advantage is the use of 'minimal objects.' These are very simple objects with just a summation-input, a weight on this input, an activation function and an output. Thus objects can be used as the neuron-like units of a neural network.

-The causal networks paradigm. Objects can perform the roles of nodes and links which the causal network is made of. This gives the network maximum flexibility. At the same time, it provides maximal reusability of nodes and structures of nodes that are equal or resemble each other in one way or the other. The network itself can also be implemented as an object not very different from each node. This gives the advantage of maximal extendibility of the network, as well as understandability : Every node potentially can be seen as a causal network on a deeper level. With a causal network on the screen, one just has to point on a node to make the underlying network appear. In OO technology, this is already a well established technique.
-The rational agents paradigm. Rational agents are structures that can be seen as having some responsibility for their own doings. Therefore they need to have a complex structure. In object-oriented programming, this is solved through the use of complex objects, being conglomerates of objects acting as one. From the outside, i.e. from the viewpoint of other objects, it makes no difference if the composite object is composed of many small objects, or is just one object with the same functionality. The complexity is achieved through simplicity. A further implication of this is that objects can always be made more 'rational' (complex, intelligent) as the context requires, without effecting the rest of the program.

In a complex domain, the interactions that come from the simultaneous use of these and other paradigms is a necessity. Philosophical and psychological considerations indicate that general human decision making has many flaws. In medical decision making, it is not a bit different. But in spite of this we can make fairly accurate (though frequently still flawed in a normative way) end decisions in most of the cases. The reason lies in our own flexibility of using different ways of thinking to bootstrap each other. My only hope is to have made the point that OO is mainly a paradigm that widely transcends informatics, or even knowledge technology in a broad sense. This is in my opinion the clearest indication that for knowledge systems on very complex domains like medicine, OO is the one and only road to take.

Literature
-Mark Mullin ('89). Object-Oriented Program Design
-D.A.Taylor ('92). Object-Oriented Information Systems
-J.D.McGregor & D.A.Sykes ('92). Object-Oriented Software Development
-J.Martin & J.Odell ('92). Object-oriented Analysis and Design
-B.Meyer ('88). Object-Oriented Software Construction
-D.Berry & A.Hart ('90). Expert Systems. Human Issues
-T.Masters ('93). Practical Neural Network Recipes in C++
-Hayes-Roth, Waterman & Lenat ('83). Building Expert Systems
-P.S.Churchland & T.J.Sejnowski. ('92) The Computational Brain
-A.C.Gillies ('91). The Integration of Expert Systems and Mainstream Software
-L.Steels ('92). Kennissystemen
-H.Heathfield ('91). Object-Oriented Design and Programming in Medical Decision Support ; Computer Methods and Programs in Biomedicine
-B.Thuraisingham ('89). From Rules to Frames and Frames to Rules ; AI Expert
-R.Davis,H.Shrobe & P.Szolovits ('93).What is a Knowledge Representation?;AAAI News

Applications Based on Neural Nets

Artificial Intelligence in Medecine
S. Andreassen et al. , Eds.
IOS Press, 1993

Classification of protein patterns using neural networks: pixel based versus feature based approach

J.R. Vargas[ab], G. Bologna[ab], R.D. Appel[a], D.F. Hochstrasser[a] and C. Pellegrini[b]

[a]Numeric Imaging Group, Geneva University Hospital
24, rue Micheli-du-Crest, CH-1211 Genève 14, Switzerland

[b]Computer Sciences Department, Geneva University,
24, rue Général Dufour, CH-1211 Genève 4, Switzerland

Abstract

We present a new approach for classifying images produced using two-dimensional polyacrylamide gel electrophoresis (2D-PAGE). In traditional approaches, features representing proteins are first detected in the images and quantified. The corresponding features are then matched across the images. In a final step, classification programs are used on the matched features. Protein detection, quantification, and matching are usually considered to be the problem areas of the classification process because they are subject to many errors and imprecisions. The approach described in this paper is original in that *feature extraction and matching are not needed*. Classification is carried out using artificial neural networks in a three steps process. First, the 2D-PAGE images are aligned with each other using a polynomial warping method. Second, a multiresolution pyramid is generated for each aligned image. Third, one resolution level is selected and fed into a neural network. Results and performance are discussed and compared with other methods.

1. INTRODUCTION

Two-dimensional polyacrylamide gel electrophoresis (2D-PAGE) is a biochemical technique for separating proteins in biological samples [12,20]. This technique produces images containing up to 3000 spots. The position of a spot in the image is defined by the isoelectric point and the molecular weight of the corresponding protein (Figure 1).

In recent years, the interest in computer assisted analysis of 2D-PAGE has grown dramatically within the medical community. In particular, the study of similarities and differences between samples from patients with various diseases has helped in finding new disease markers [13,14]. Classification tools have been developed which have given promising results [3-6]. However, due to the imprecise nature of the biochemical technique, these classification programs rely on complex feature extraction methods and sophisticated matching tools. Feature extraction and matching are subject to many errors and imprecisions which bias the analysis and hence constitute the main problem areas in computer assisted classification of 2D-PAGE. At the Numerical Imaging Group of the University Hospital and the Computer Sciences Department of the University of Geneva, we are searching simpler and more robust classification approaches.

This paper presents a new approach in which feature extraction and matching are no longer needed. The image itself is used instead of its feature values. Therefore, matching can be reduced to image alignment, which is performed by the polynomial warping method using a set of control points (landmarks) [21]. Then, a multiresolution pyramid is generated for each aligned image using the Burt method [7]. Finally, classification is carried out by selecting one resolution level in the pyramid and feeding the corresponding image data to a neural network.

In this paper, we first present the polynomial image warping method. Next we describe the multiresolution pyramid image construction technique and our model of artificial neural networks. Finally, results are discussed and compared with those obtained by traditional methods.

2. POLYNOMIAL WARPING

Polynomial image warping is currently considered the approach of choice for aligning two images in which the source and degree of misalignment are unknown. The warping is performed in four stages. First, control points or landmarks are selected (manually or automatically) on one image (the reference image). Second, corresponding control points are given manually in the second image (data image). Third, the warping transformation is determined by solving the equation (2). Given a set of control points, we solve this equation using least square minimisation. In the fourth stage, warping is performed on the data image using the following transformation:

$$(x, y) \rightarrow (u(x, y), v(x, y)), \tag{1}$$

where (x,y) are the pixel coordinates in the original data image, (u,v) are the pixel coordinates in the resulting warped data image aligned to the reference image. u(x,y) and v(x,y) are two polynomial functions (one for each axes) determined by the least squares method in order to minimize the distance between the transformed control points in the data image and those in the reference image.

To do this we need to solve the following two systems of linear equations (u and v are linear with respect to a_i and b_i):

$$u = \sum_{i=0}^{n} \sum_{j=0}^{i} a_{ij} x^i y^{j-i} \qquad v = \sum_{i=0}^{n} \sum_{j=0}^{i} b_{ij} x^i y^{j-i}, \tag{2}$$

where (x,y) are the landmark positions in the reference image, (u,v) are the positions of the corresponding points in the data image, and a_i and b_i are the polynomial coefficients to be determined. The polynomial order n is specific to the problem. For M control points and polynomial functions of order n, the coefficients a_i and b_i are determined by two systems of M linear equations with T variables, where $T = (n+2)(n+1)/2$. The least squares method may be used to solve these equations only if $M \geq T$.

The image warping is performed by applying the spatial mapping functions and interpolating the resulting points (Figure 1).

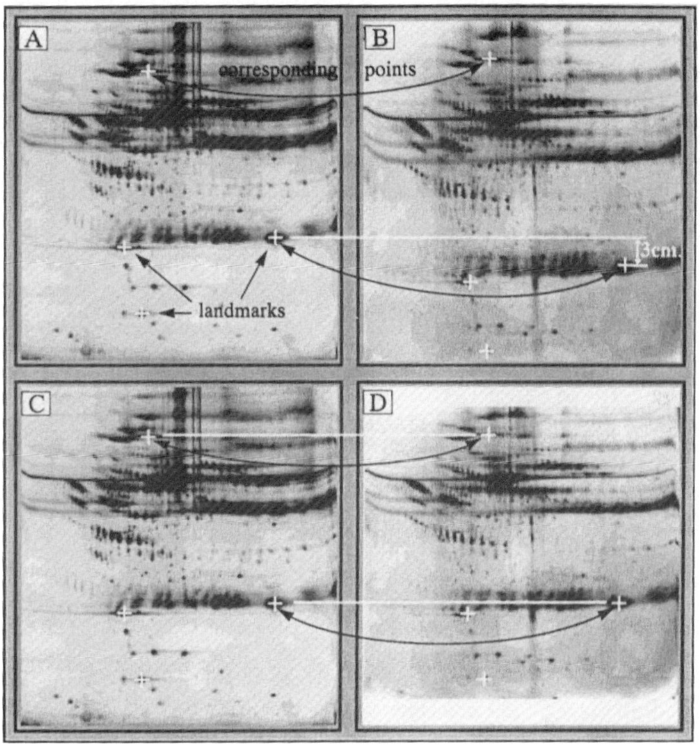

Figure 1: (A) and (C) 2D-PAGE reference image, (B) data image to be warped, (D) mapped data image after warping using two second order polynomial functions, nine landmarks and bilinear interpolation.

3. MULTIRESOLUTION PYRAMID

The 2D-PAGE images produced in our laboratory have a resolution of about 2000x2000 pixels (4 million pixels). This is far too much input data to be fed into an artificial neural network which commonly uses at most around one thousand inputs per pattern. The pyramid resolution is a hierarchical structure for representing images at multiple resolutions, varying from a fine to a coarse one [18]. These images are calculated by combining scale-space and sub-sampling techniques according to two operators: *reduction*, which produces a coarse image from a finer one, and *projection*, which produces finer resolutions from coarse ones. Typically, the sub-sampling between levels is 2x2.

Given an image I, we can define I(i,j) as the pixel at position (i,j) in image I. Therefore, we have:

- $I_0(i,j)$, $0 \le i,j \le 2^N - 1$, where I_0 is the image at the initial (finest) level and

- $I_p(i,j)$, $0 \le i,j \le 2^{N-p} - 1$, where I_p is the image at level p.

Passing from level p-1 to level p is a sub-sampling process. This is performed by low pass filtering to prevent aliasing. The multiresolution pyramid is calculated by applying a generating kernel filter defined further.

Let W(i,j) be a KxK generating kernel filter. The multiresolution pyramid is defined as follows:

$$I_p(i,j) = \sum_{m=0}^{K-1}\sum_{n=0}^{K-1} W(m,n)\, I_{p-1}(2i+K-1-m, 2j+K-1-n), \tag{3}$$

with $0 \le i,j \le 2^{N-1} - K/2$.

In general the generating kernel is separable:

$W(i,j) = w(i)\, w(j)$,

where w is a one-dimensional kernel with the following properties:

- normalisation: $\sum_{i=0}^{k-1} w(i) = 1$,
- symmetry: $w(i) = w(K-1-i)$,
- unimodality: $0 \le w(i) \le w(j)$, $i \le j < K/2$,
- equal contribution: $\sum_{i=0}^{k-1} w(i+2m) = \frac{1}{2}$, $m = 0, 1$.

We are using the gaussian low pass filter pyramid proposed by Burt [7]. The generating kernel w(i,j) is a 5x5 gaussian filter with the one-dimensional kernel w defined by:

- $w(0) = w(4) = \frac{1}{4} - \frac{\alpha}{2}$,
- $w(1) = w(3) = \frac{1}{4}$,
- $w(2) = \alpha$.

Then equation (3) becomes:

$$I_p(i,j) = \sum_{m=0}^{4}\sum_{n=0}^{4} w(m)\, w(n)\, I_{p-1}(2i+m, 2j+n). \tag{4}$$

Finally, the Burt gaussian pyramid is calculated using equation (4). The application of this equation to a 2D-PAGE image generates a 2D-PAGE multiresolution gaussian pyramid (Figure 2).

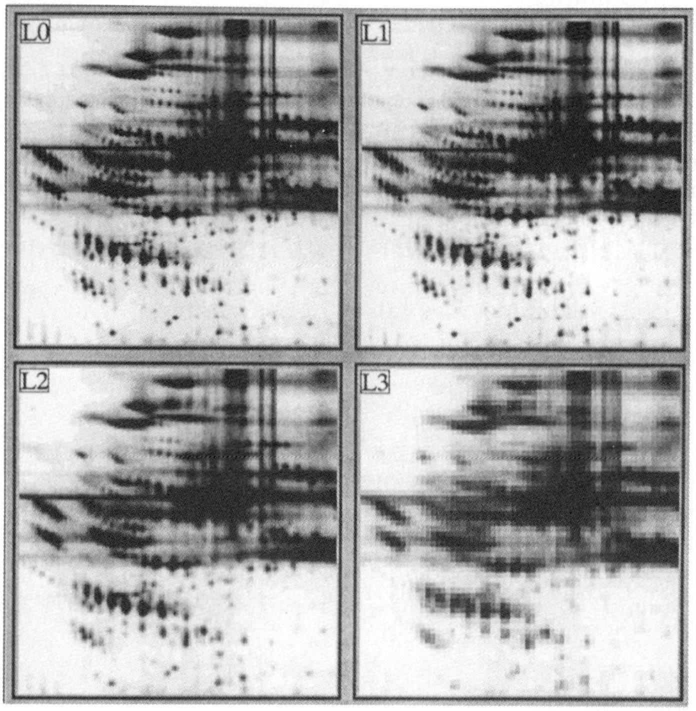

Figure 2: Levels zero L0 (finest level, 512x512 pixels) to three L3 (64x64 pixels) of the low pass multiresolution gaussian pyramid calculated using the Burt gaussian kernel with $\alpha = 0.4$.

4. ARTIFICIAL NEURAL NETWORK

Neural networks are able to solve classification problems that are difficult to solve with classical methods. They learn first using a set of patterns and then generalise to find correct answers for a large portion of unlearned patterns. Several neural network models are commonly employed: Perceptron [19], Back-propagation [22], Kohonen feature maps [17], Counterpropagation [11], Hopfield nets[15], Simulated Annealing [16] and ART [8]. Some of them (like the Perceptron, Counterpropagation, and Hopfield nets) cannot learn every set of patterns. Others (like Kohonen feature maps, Simulated Annealing and ART) need a very long time to classify complex objects such as 2D-PAGE images if implemented on monoprocessor computers. The Back-propagation network is an acceptable compromise. It learns every training set of patterns and in general, training time is reasonable compared to other models. Several learning algorithms have been derived from Back-propagation to speed up the training [9,10]. Nevertheless, their generalisation power is, in most cases, very close to that of Back-propagation.

4.1. The Dystal model

A new neural model, called Dystal [2], inspired from neurobiological observations in the hippocampus brain region of the rabbit [1], shows some similarities with Kohonen feature maps and ART. This model is trained by associative learning. It has three important properties: *learning time linearity* (training time is directly proportional to the number of connections, whereas the previous models have at least a quadratic learning time), *dynamic learning* (new units are created during training), and *cumulative learning* (new patterns can be learned without forgetting the previous ones).

The basic structure of the Dystal model is composed of several elements (Figure 3), including:

- conditioned stimuli neurons called CS-neurons (x_1, x_2),
- unconditioned stimuli neurons called UCS-neurons (y'_1),
- inter-neurons (s_1, s_2),
- patches (p_1, p_2, p_3, p_4),
- output-neurons (y_1).

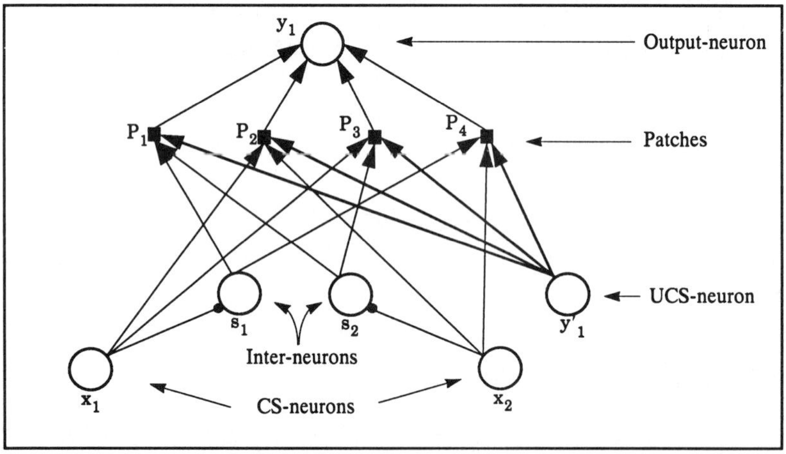

Figure 3: Dystal architecture for two logical function variables.

Input neurons are CS-neurons and UCS-neurons. CS-neurons represent conditioned stimuli, UCS-neurons represent unconditioned stimuli (i.e. the association to be learned with CS-input). There is the same number of UCS-neurons as of output neurons. Every CS-neuron is associated with an inter-neuron: it is activated when there is no signal on the CS-neuron. Patches are the long term local memory, reflecting patterns of activity on the input neurons (in Figure 3, the patch P_1 detects when s_1 and s_2 are active, the patch P_2 detects when x_1 and x_2 are active, etc.). When an input pattern is presented to CS-neurons, the best similar patch carries the signal, shunting all other patches. A UCS-neuron receives a kind of teaching value and fires into all patches associated with an output neuron, together with all CS-neurons and inter-neurons. Only one weight is associated with a patch. In this way, input signals are learned together rather than individually from each input. Weight values depend on the stimulation frequency during training, reflecting how well the patch pattern association is learned.

During the learning phase, teaching patterns (e.g. expected output values) are presented to UCS-neurons, and patterns to be learned to CS-neurons. Prior to training, no patches belong to any output neural elements. All patches will be created at learning time. Their number depends on a threshold criterion: the Patch Creation Threshold (PCT). A local (non-Hebbian) learning rule is applied on all weights: weight changes are neither dependent on the output of the post-synaptic neuron nor on a global error term.

The model shown on Figure 3 has a binary patch sensitivity (i.e. CS-neurons and inter-neurons fire into patches). We can then generalise it to a discrete patch sensitivity by imagining every CS-neuron associated with a discrete number of inter-neurons. An inter-neuron will be activated only if the value presented to the CS-neuron corresponds to its sensitivity range. Finally we generalise the model to continue patch sensitivity.

4.2. The extended Dystal model

Since the description of Dystal in 1990 [2], several improvements have been carried out on the model. We are using it with a continuous patch sensitivity [23]. The training algorithm can be described as follows.

When an input pattern is presented, a similarity measure S_i is computed between the CS pattern and each patch P_i (for instance the Euclidean distance between P_i and S_i). Also, the UCS input is compared to the expected value of the UCS U^i, in order to find the set of k patches $\{P^k\}$ and their similarity $\{S^k\}$. The largest value S_{max} is then chosen.

In the next step, either a new patch is created or an existing patch is updated, depending on the value of S_{max}. If this value is less than the predefined criterion value PCT, then the incoming association is not sufficiently similar to an existing association stored in a patch. As a result, a new one is created by storing both the vector of CS input values and the value of the UCS input. If S_{max} is greater than PCT, the corresponding patch is modified. The patch vector and expected UCS are adjusted to increase their similarity to the CS and UCS patterns, respectively.

At the end of the training cycle each patch will contain a vector reflecting a kind of mean of training patterns which have stimulated it and a kind of UCS mean. The output of a neural element equals of the similarity between the CS and the most similar patch (S_{max}), times the expected value of the UCS of the most similar patch (U_m).

The number of parameters in the Dystal model is larger than the number of parameters in the Back-propagation model. The most sensitive parameter is the Patch Creation Threshold (PCT) which determines the number of patches created during training. Its optimal value is application dependent and there are no rules to find it. A random choice cannot guarantee that the training set will be fully learned.

5. RESULTS AND DISCUSSIONS

The above described method was tested on a set of 118 2D-PAGE images made from human physiological fluids samples (56 from ascitic fluid and 62 from pleural fluid). These images were preprocessed in five stages. First, nine control points were selected in one image (a reference image). Second, the corresponding control points were determined in the other images. Third, each image was aligned to the reference image using the second order polynomial warping method described in section 2. In the fourth stage, one region of interest (512x512 pixels) was selected and extracted from all images. Finally a resolution pyramid was generated for each image using the 5x5 Burt gaussian kernel with $\alpha = 0.4$, as presented in section 3.

A Dystal network was constructed using 4096 input neurons (64x64 pixels, level L3 of the 2D-PAGE pyramid in Figure 2) and one output neuron. The training sets were built by choosing a given number of images from the two classes. The remaining images were used for testing. A series of experiments were performed on the same data sets, testing various values for the important parameters.

In the first experiment we selected 1000 different training sets, each of which contained 20 images from the ascitic class and 20 images from the pleural class. Only 2 patches were created (one for each class). The learning phase took about 20 seconds on a Sun Sparcstation-10. Table 1 (L3) shows the mean, variance, minimal, and maximal percentages of the correct classifications for the 1000 testing sets. Each testing set contained 78 images.

Table 1
Statistical measurements of the correctly classified images in two testing sets having 1000 members. The corresponding resolutions levels are illustrated in Figure 2

Pyramid resolution	L3: 64x64 pixels	L2: 128x128 pixels
Mean	70.69	71.92
Variance	42.11	24.50
Minimum	33.33	47.44
Maximum	84.62	85.90

The variance is large for vector patches, as they are often attracted to non representative regions of the pattern space. This explains why bad classifications (33.33% of correctly classified images) were found in some testing sets. This also explains why during the training phase the rate of correctly trained patterns never exceeded 87.50%.

In the second experiment data was taken from level L2 of the resolution pyramid (128x128 pixels, level L2 of 2D-PAGE pyramid in Figure 2). The architecture of the neural network was modified accordingly. Since the patterns were 4 times larger, the learning time increased by a factor 4.

It appears from Table 1, that the variance in L2 is better than that of L3. This suggests that more discriminating information is present due to the higher resolution. Unfortunately, the mean values are comparable. To save computation time, other experiments were carried out with the 64x64 resolution (L3).

In the third experiment, 100 training sets were run with different PCT values. The network created respectively 40, 10 to 20, and 4 to 12 patches (Table 2).

Table 2
Statistical measurements for the training and testing sets using different PCT.

PCT values	1	5	8
Number of created patches	40	10 to 20	4 to 12
Mean	71.55	70.96	66.25
Variance	29.68	23.46	26.25
Minimum	55.13	56.41	26.69
Maximum	84.62	82.05	78.21

Tests showed that a reasonable compromise between low computation time and high success rate of training set and testing set patterns can be obtained with PCT=5.

In the last experiment, various sizes of training sets were used. Statistical measurements were computed from 200 selections of each size of training set. Table 3 shows results with PCT=5. As expected, the mean improves when the number of training patterns increases.

Table 3
Statistical measurements of correct classifications varying the training set size.

Training set size	20 (10 + 10)	40 (20 + 20)	60 (30 + 30)
Mean	67.27	70.63	73.28
Variance	28.09	28.49	25.57
Minimum	47.96	55.13	58.62
Maximum	78.57	80.77	84.48

Although the mean of correctly classified images lies around 70%, the results obtained by the classification method presented here are considered good, as the two classes of images used (2D-PAGE of pleural versus ascitic fluid) are not easily distinguishable by visual inspection.

As a comparison, the Back-propagation model [22] was run on our protein patterns. The network was configurated with 4096 inputs, 100 hidden neurons and two output neurons (one for each class). The learning process cycle took about 800 minutes. Because of time constraints, the performance of this network was only tested on 10 training sets. Table 4 shows the mean, variance, minimal, and maximal percentages of the correct classifications for the Back-propagation and Dystal model.

Table 4
Statistical measurements of the correct classifications by two neural network models using 100 selections of testing sets, 60 patterns and 1330 inputs.

	Back-Propagation NN model	Dystal NN model
Mean	71.40	73.47
Variance	24.17	22.04
Minimum	60.00	61.67
Maximum	83.33	86.87

We see that the performances of the Back-propagation model are similar to those of the Dystal model. Nevertheless, the training speed of the Dystal model outperforms the Back-propagation model.

6. CONCLUSION

To our knowledge, this is the first published attempt to classify 2D-PAGE images prior to feature extraction and matching. This approach might drastically improve further feature detection and image matching if the detection and matching are performed after classification.

The pixel based approaches for classifying 2D-PAGE images with neural networks may be compared to feature based classifications. Both Dystal and Back-Propagation methods were tested in earlier works on similar images [4,6]. In these works, the input patterns were obtained by quantifying the detected proteins on the 2D-PAGE images. While the results were close to those described in this paper, the pixel based classification approach constitutes a promising alternative.

7. AKNOWLEGEMENTS

We wish to thank A. Goodman for the helpful comments on the paper and J-C. Sanchez and C. Pasquali for the 2D-PAGE images.

8. REFERENCES

1 D.L. Alkon, Memory storage and neural system, Sci. Am., July (1989) 42.
2 D.L. Alkon, K.T. Blackwell, G.S. Barbour, A.K. Rigler, T.P. Vogl, Pattern recognition by an artificial network derived from biologic neuronal systems, Biol. Cyber., No. 62 (1990) 363.
3 R.D. Appel, D. Hochstrasser, C. Roch, M Funk, A.F. Muller, C. Pellegrini, Automatic classification of 2 dimensional gel electrophoresis pictures by heuristic clustering analysis: a step toward machine learning, Electrophoresis 9 (1988) 132.
4 R.D. Appel, G. Bologna, D.F. Hochstrasser, Classification tools for diagnostic rule formation from protein maps, MIE93 Conf. Proc., (1993) 40.

5 S. Bakir, MEHDINET: Etude et réalisation de réseaux de neurones artificiels, avec une interface X11/Motif, pour la classification de gels d'électrophorèse bidimensionnelle, Master Thesis, University of Geneva, 1991.

6 G. Bologna, DYSTAL, Etude et implantation d'un modèle de réseaux de neurones, Master Thesis, University of Geneva, 1991.

7 P.J. Burt and E.H. Adelson, The Laplacian pyramid as a compact image code, IEEE Trans. Comunications, No. 31, 4, (1983) 532.

8 G.A. Carpenter, S. Grossberg, ARTMAP: Supervised Real-Time Learning and Classification of Nonstationary Data by a Self-Organizing Neural Network, Neural Networks, 4 (1991) 543.

9 S.E. Fahlman, Faster-learning variations on back-propagation: An empirical study, In: Connectionist Models Summer School, San Mateo, Morgan Kaufmann (eds.), CA, 1988.

10 S.E. Fahlman, C. Lebiere, The Cascade-Correlation Learning Architecture. In: Advances in Neural Information Processing Systems 2, Morgan Kaufmann (eds.), 1990.

11 R. Hetch-Nielsen, Counterpropagation networks, IEEE First intl. Conf. on Neural Networks II (1988) 19.

12 D.F. Hochstrasser, A. Patchornik, C.R. Merril, Development of polyacrylamide gels that improve the separation of proteins and their detection by silver staining, Anal Biochem. No. 173 (1988) 412.

13 D.F. Hochstrasser, R.D. Appel, J.R. Vargas, R. Perrier, F. Ravier, M. Funk, C. Pellegrini, A.F. Müller and J.-R. Sherrer, Clinical Molecular Scanner: The Melanie Project, Hawaii Jan 1991: Proc HICSS-24, Hawaii International Conference on System Sciences, (1991) 626.

14 D.F. Hochstrasser, J.-D. Tissot, Clinical application of high-resolution two dimensional polyacrylamide gel electrophoresis, In: Advances in Electrophoresis, vol. 6. VCH Publishers 1993 (in press).

15 J.J. Hopfield, Neural networks and physical systems with emergent collecive computational abilities, Proc. Natl. Acad Sci. USA 79 (1982) 2254.

16 G.E. Hinton, T.J. Sejnowski, D.H. Ackley, A Learning Algorithm for Boltzmann Machines, Technical Report CMU-CS-84-119, May 1984.

17 T. Kohonen, Self-organization formation of topologically correct feature maps, Biol. Cyb., No. 43 (1982) 56.

18 P. Meer, E.S. Baugher and A. Rosenfeld, Frequency domain analysis and synthesis of image pyramid generating kernels, IEEE PAMI, 4, July, (1987) 512.

19 M. Minsky, S. Papert, Perceptron, Cambridge, MA: MIT Press. 1969.

20 P.H. O'Farrell, High resolution two-dimensional electrophoresis of proteins, J. Biol. Chem. No. 250 (1975) 4007.

21 W.K. Pratt, Digital image processing, Second edition, WILEY publishers, NY., 1992.

22 D.E. Rumelhart, J.L. McClelland, Parallel distributed processing: explorations in the microstructure of cognition, vol I: Foundations; vol II: Applications, MIT Press, Cambridge, 1986.

23 T.P. Vogl, K.L. Blackwell, S.D. Hymann, G.S. Barbour, D.L. Alkon. Classification of hand-written digits and Japanese Kanji. IJCNN 91, I (1991) 97.

Artificial Intelligence in Medecine
S. Andreassen et al. , Eds.
IOS Press, 1993

Evaluation of an epidemiological data set as an example of the application of neural networks to the analysis of large medical data sets

T. Waschulzik[1], K. Quandt[1] , M. Lewis[2,3], A. Hörmann[1], R. Engelbrecht[1], W. Brauer[4]

[1] GSF-Institut für medizinische Informatik und Systemforschung, Ingolstädter Landstr.1, Neuherberg, Postfach 1129, 85758 Oberschleißheim, Germany

[2] GSF-Institut für Epidemiologie, Ingolstädter Landstr.1, Neuherberg, Postfach 1129, 85758 Oberschleißheim, Germany

[3] Zentralklinikum Augsburg Stenglinstr. 2, 86156 Augsburg, Germany

[4] Technische Universität München (Institut für Informatik), Arcisstr.21, 80290 München 2, Germany

Abstract

The objective of this paper is to assess the suitability of neural networks for the analysis of large medical data sets. For this purpose, we used an epidemiological data set from the Augsburg MONICA study (MONItoring trends and determinants in CArdiovascular diseases). The method of perceptron analysis and the interpretation of the model established by the network are explained. The results of a predicition of survival or death of patients who suffered acute myocardial infarction show that even simple perceptrons yield good classification quality. Further, the analysis of the connections within the neural network leads to information about relations between input and output data which are of interest for future epidemiological research. The results of these investigations can also be applied to other medical data sets like data on the segmentation of CTs and ECG data for the diagnosis of myocardial infarction.

1. Introduction

The last few years have seen an enormous increase in the availability of medical information. Hospitals have introduced and extended hospital information systems, computer systems have appeared in the offices of general practitioners [6], and health insurances have established administrative data bases which are often used for epidemiologic research [2]. The results of medical examinations like electrocardiogram (ECG), electrophoresis or sometimes even X-ray examinations are digitised. In some standard diagnostic instruments like computer tomography (CT) or nuclear magnetic resonance (NMR), the computer is an integrated component in the data acquisition and data preparation process. The exchange of information, in some fields even the use of local area networks, makes more and more information available for medical data analysis. This information is often up to date, well prepared and of high quality.
These are excellent circumstances for the introduction of information tools that can systematically analyse large data sets. Particularly the idea of constructing an example-driven knowledge base with neural networks is intriguing. These systems with neural components can be used in two different ways:

- When new information is introduced to these systems the facilities of the neural networks can be used to determine the presence of new unknown associations between complex variables.
- The resulting network structure can be analysed to determine the internal model of the domain constructed by the neural network. This knowledge can be transformed into a comprehensible description which is useful for the training of medical staff.

Neural networks have a powerful potential for the analysis of examination results and for the integration of fuzzy knowledge. When analysing large data sets, the appropriate choice of the used artificial neural network model reduces time requirements and uses the advantage of massive parallel execution. The choice of the neural network model is also restricted by the requirement that the internal representation must be interpretable.
Other projects have evaluated the possibility of applying artificial neural networks to examination results [1,4], but there have been, to our knowledge, no applications of neural networks in the domain of epidemiology. There are some special problems in applying neural networks in epidemiology:

- Data sets consist of a mixture of numerical and categorial variables
- Specific complex classifications, like the often used International Classification of Diseases (ICD9-Code) [3], need to be presented.
- Data sets often contain missing values

Our project, which is described in detail in [10,11], was initiated to address the following questions:

- Is it possible and efficient to evaluate data from epidemiologic studies with neural networks?
- If the data are assessed adequately, how can the internal structures of the networks be interpreted?

- Is it possible that relations between data can be found with neural networks which are not within the scope of conventional statistical methods?
- Since in epidemiologic studies some information can not be raised for all persons, is it possible to estimate incomplete data on certain variables of interest with the help of neural networks?

We used data from the Augsburg component of the MONICA project which is organized by the World Health Organization. The precise objective was to forecast the survival or death of patients suffering from myocardial infarction by using inputs like age, sex and ICD-coded prior medical conditions. Once a good predictive performance was reached, it was assumed that the network had learned the underlying connections between input and output data. The next step was to analyse and interpret the associations on which the network based its classifications.

2. The MONICA project

The main objective of the WHO MONICA project is the analysis of the trends in cardiovascular mortality, morbidity and case fatality over 10 years in defined populations and the explanation of these trends. The global study is conducted in 40 participating centres all over the world. The data used in this work came from the coronary event register of the MONICA collaborating centre Augsburg, Germany [7].

3. Methods

The neural network used was a fully connected feed-forward perceptron [12] with one input- and one output-layer (no hidden units). The units in this model were frequency-coded i.e. their activities are between 0 and 255. The weights ranged from -32768 to 32767, initialised to 0. The unit's sigmoid activation function was approximated by a semi-linear activation function.

The formula for the output function and the forced learning procedure are described below:

$$a_i(t) = net_i(t) = \sum_j w_{ji}(t-1)o_j(t-1)$$

$$o_i(t) = \begin{cases} 0 & \text{, if } a_i(t) \le thr\_low_i \\ \dfrac{a_i(t) - thr\_low_i}{\dfrac{thr\_high_i - thr\_low_i}{255}} * 255 & \text{, if } thr\_low_i < a_i(t)_i < thr\_high_i \\ 255 & \text{, if } a_i(t) \ge thr\_high_i \end{cases}$$

Forced learning: $\Delta w_{ji}(t) = a_j(t)\, \eta_{ij}(t)$

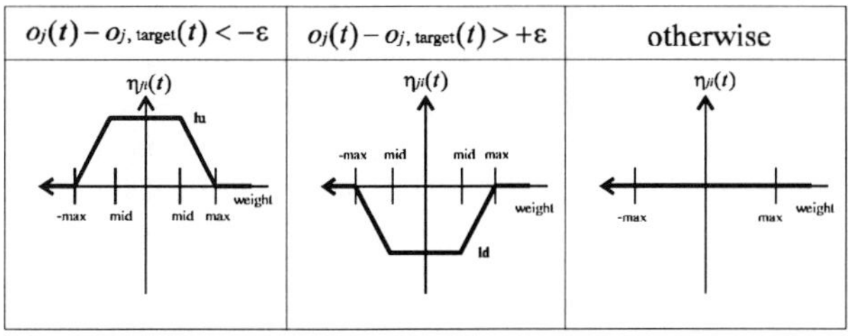

$a_i(t)$: activity of unit i,
$o_i(t)$: output of unit i,
$w_{ji}(t)$: weight from unit j to i,
$net_i(t)$: sum of input to unit i,
ε: smaller differences treated as equal,
thr_low (thr_high): lower (higher) bound of activation function,
max: higher bound of weights,
mid: point of decreasing rate of change of weights,
ld: upper bound of decreasing a weight,
lu: upper bound of increasing a weight

Figure 1: Output function formula and forced learning procedure

The unit's model and the basic neural network have been previously described in [14,15]. The categorical variables selected from the extensive MONICA-data set on 4285 patients are shown in table 1. Also included were three ICD-coded diagnoses [3] on clinical condition or cause of death (CLIND1-3) for each patient and data on date of birth and date of onset of the event as well as on residence.

Table 1: Input variables from the MONICA data for the neural network

Name of variable	Values	Number of patients
SEX	1 male	3039
	2 female	1246
PREMI	5 previous myocardial infarction	1008
	7 no previous myocardial infarction	2896
	9 insufficient data	381
HISIHD	1 history of chronic heart disease	2439
	2 no history of chronic heart disease	1371
	9 insufficient data	475
SURVIV	1 patient survived	1864
	2 patient died	2421

The input patterns were generated by a specially written program. Most variables were categorical i.e. the given data represent one of several possible, clearly separated categories. These variables were coded in one neuron per category with the neuron representing the given data being active and all others non-active. All categorical input variables and the target variable SURVIV were coded in this way.

Medically diagnosed conditions were coded with the 4-digit International Classification of Diseases, 9th revision (ICD9). We altered the network encoding procedure to provide a more adequate representation of the medical condition (CLIND) and to reflect the structure of the ICD classification, which currently contains over 30.000 specific conditions. The algorithm developed increased coding precision according to the number of patients suffering from a given condition. ICD provides for 17 major disease categories comprising general diagnoses like "conditions of the respiratory organs". If more than a specified number of patients had a given condition, this disease was also represented in a sub-group (i.e. a slightly more precise diagnosis). If yet more patients had that condition, another neuron for the 3-digit ICD9-code was provided, and finally, for the most prevalent conditions among these patients, a neuron for the 4-digit ICD9-code was allocated. In this way, only 230 units were required to represent all medical conditions occurring in these patients.

The three diseases per patient given by the MONICA data were represented in the same neurons. CLIND1, supposed to be the most important disease, was taken into account with 45% weight, CLIND2 with 30% and CLIND3 with 25%.

The age of the patients was computed from the date of onset of infarction and date of birth. Since the age is a continuous variable it was represented by topologically distributed encoding [5,6]. Since data were raised only for persons between 24 and 74 years, 50 neurons were made available for encoding the age. Later this number was reduced to three units without any effect on classification rates. This is in accordance with the number of groups found appropriate for age in statistical analysis of this data set. One of the main advantages of topologically distributed encoding was that no boundaries between the groups had to be defined.

The network was trained by dividing the available data from 4285 patients suffering from myocardial infarction into a training (2856) and a test set (1429). Training took place by first choosing randomly the class of fatal or non-fatal cases and then randomly picking a pattern from this class for training. This assures the same frequency for training of both classes. Otherwise, the relative frequency of patterns from the two classes might lead the network to put all patterns into the more frequent class to achieve a relatively good classification quality.

Performance was scored as correct if the target output unit had maximum activation. Classification quality was computed by assuming both classes as being of the same frequency. An exit criterion developed to interrupt the training algorithm at the point with its best classification ability was based on the misclassification patterns encountered within a specified number of training cycles. If the number of misclassified patterns per cycle did not improve for a defined number of cycles, training was stopped.

The remaining third of all patterns (test set) was used for testing classification quality of the network with the best classification ratio per cycle in training. Over-adaption was recognized by comparing the difference between the classification quality of the training and the test sets.

4. Results

In a first training session all input variables were used to train the network for predicting the variable SURVIV. Thus the input layer consisted of 291 units, the output layer of two units. The network correctly diagnosed 86,33% of all patterns from the training data set. The classification ability with the test data set was

85,12%. This was better than the epidemiological expert had expected, suggesting that data artefacts were present. The following picture (figure 2) shows the weights of all connections in the network:

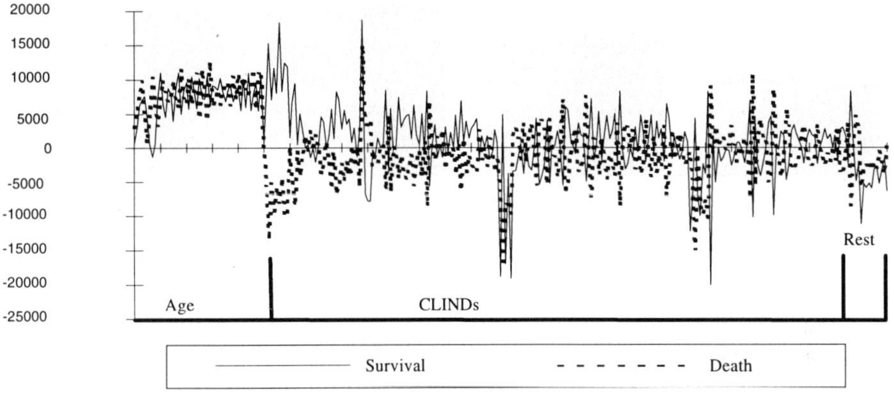

Figure 2: Weight structure

The network distinguished between three separate groups of association patterns (figure 2). These consisted of age, clinical conditions and the remaining set of categorical variables. Comparisons between these groups need to be treated with caution, because the first 50 units representing the age on one hand and the units for the categorical variables on the other hand were used by the network to fix a working level. Within-group comparisons are possible, however. The fact that the weights of the CLIND-units are of opposite sign indicates that classification is based largely on information from the medical conditions. This conjecture was confirmed by another training session where the CLINDs were excluded from the input for the network. The classification ability of this network decreased by more than 20%. Excluding one of the other input variables showed hardly any effect on the original classification ability (Figure 3).

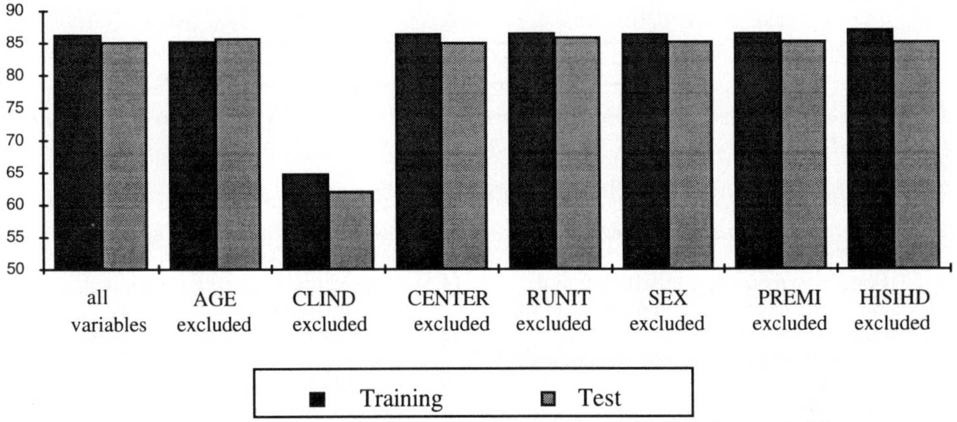

Figure 3: Classification results excluding one of the different input fields

In a second experiment we were surprised by the classification ability of 72,52% (test data set) that was shown by a network which was trained with only 17 input units and with the CLINDs as the only input (Figure 4). This time the diseases were coded only by their main-group and still the result was much better than expected.

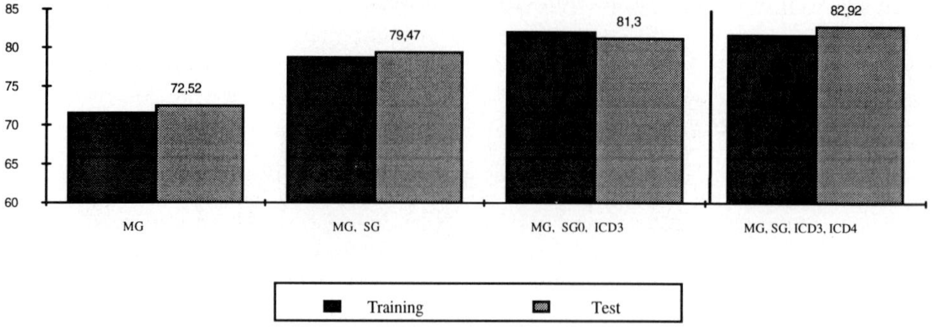

Figure 4: Classification results relative to coding for medical conditions (MG=Main Group; SG=Subgroup)

Evaluation of the weights of these connections showed that particularly conditions not related to cardiac disorders or myocardial infarction were associated with improved survival chance of a patient (figure 5). Thus a diagnosis of a nutritional and metabolic disorder appeared to have a positive influence on the survival of a patient following myocardial infarction.

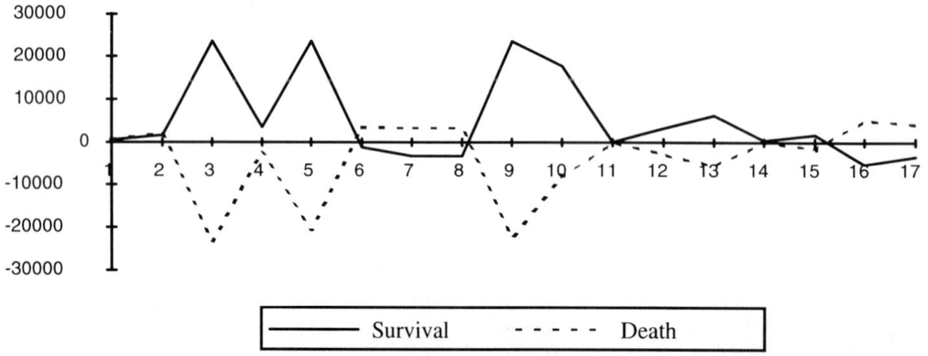

Figure 5: Coeffitions of the network trained only with the 17 Main ICD groups (Non-fatal, Fatal)

The numbers indicate the following organ groups:

1 Infectuous and parasitic disorders
2 Neoplasms
3 Endocrine disorders, nutritional and metabolic disorders, and disordes of the immune system
4 Disorders of the blood and hematological systems
5 Psychiatric disorders
6 Disorders of the nervous system and sensory organs
7 Disorders of the circulatory system
8 Disorders of the respiratory system
9 Disorders of the gastrointestinal system
10 Disorders of the urinary and the reproductive system
11 Complikations during pregnancy, delivery and postnatal period
12 Disorders of the skin and subcutaneous tissue
13 Musculoskeletal disorders
14 Congenital disorders
15 Disorders originating during the perinatal period
16 Symptoms and
17 Injuries and poisonings

The network´s behaviour can be explained as follows: If a patient died because of myocardial infarction, all diseases he suffered from are taken from the death certificate which states the reason for death and other grave diseases. Information about diseases of a surviving patient are raised for the MONICA project from the discharge charts which also include mild diseases like lipid disorders. The network clearly recognizes this data collecting artefact (due to a posteriori information), and achieves this high classification quality because a deceased patient hardly ever has "unimportant" conditions as perceived by the coroner. It is very unlikely that complex relations like this can be readily established with the conventional methods of data analysis in epidemiology.
Other training sessions showed that it is possible to read positive or negative influences of an input variable from the weights of the trained network and even to set up a ranking order of influence for the different input variables by evaluating the weights of their units. A cursory comparison to discriminant analysis showed that the classification yielded by the neural network was somewhat better.
Unprecise or missing values can also be estimated by a neural network by training the net on predicting this variable with a complete data set and then presenting the network with the incomplete patterns. This method yields an estimated value for the variable for each pattern which is given by the output activation of the network. It also yields a probability for the quality of the estimation which can be seen in the classification quality of the training data set.

5. Application of the same methodology to other domains

The results of the analysis of the MONICA data set are based on a methodology for neural network engineering. This methodology called NNET (Neural Network Engineering Technique) was improved during this study and the concerning tools where extended. It is based on the SEtec-Method [7] which is often used especially in economical applications. NNET can be applied to very different fields of application. It supports modular design, training and testing of neural networks. NNET is assisted by a set of tools for the preparation of data, the configuration of the network and automatic training and test.
For example, we have applied NNET to the development of feature detectors for the segmentation of CT's [4]. The feature detectors yield the following results for a CT of a patient with a kidney stone:

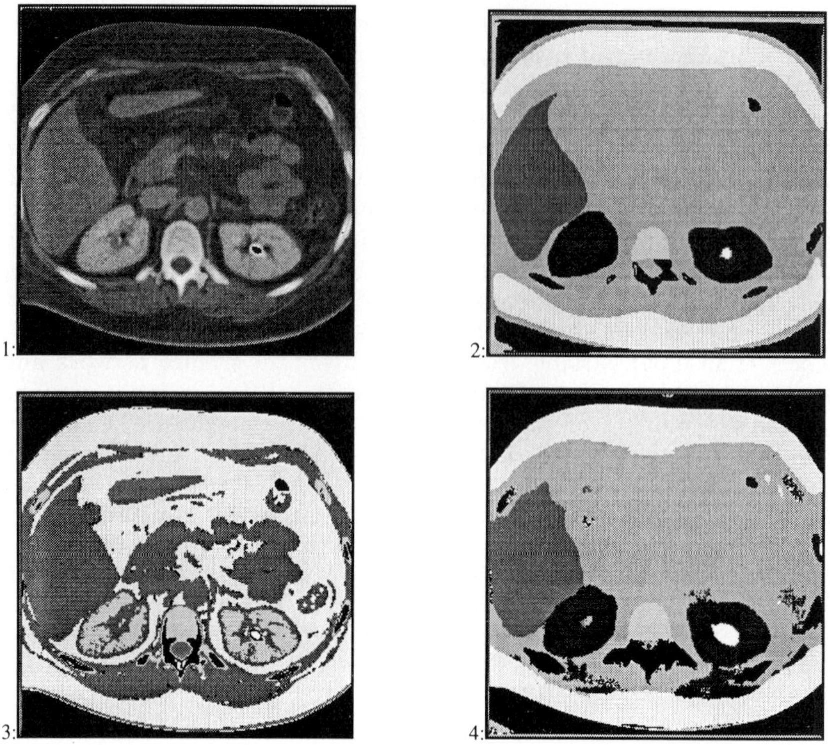

Figure 6: *1: original picture,*
2: result of the manual segmentation,
3: segmentation with grey hues,
4: segmentation with the feature detector

The methodology was also used for an analysis of pre-processed ECGs for the diagnosis of myocardial infarction. This application includes 256 different numeric input variables to be examined. The first steps of the analysis brought also encouraging results.

In NNET we use perceptrons, competitive learning and other common techniques, but we don't use networks trained with back-propagation (BP) [13,16] for different reasons:

- Compared to other training algorithms like delta rule [12], BP is very time-consuming and a lot of user interaction and parameter adjustment is necessary to train a network.
- If comparisons of results of different input variables are necessary, it is not clear if the input variable that yielded the best result really is the "best variable" or if the parameter settings (number of hidden layers and number of neurons in these layers) just fitted better for the training of the variable. This problem normally does not occur when using simple perceptrons.
- The number of input neurons that can be trained conveniently with a perceptron is much larger than the number of inputs for BP.

- In normal projects an "XOR type" problem hardly ever occurs. In case, usually the information was coded inadequately for a neural network. Every "XOR type" or "encoding" problem can be solved with a simple perceptron, if the right coding for the information is used. From our experience it is much cheaper, faster and according to the results better to think about the right representation rather than to use BP.
- The networks that result from a training with BP cannot be analysed adequately because the function of the neurons in the hidden layer cannot be determined. This is very important for the quality control of the resulting system. Every component has to be tested by the glass-box and black-box method. This does not mean that no subsymbolic representation should be used in neural networks, since this would lead to a tremendous loss of advantages of neural networks. For example neurons trained with competitive learning are subsymbolic and can also be interpreted and analysed.

6. Conclusion and future plans

This paper shows that data from epidemiological studies and other medical applications can be evaluated with simple neural networks and that the weight structure of these networks can be interpreted if caution is exercised. Besides confirming associations known to exist in the data set, the network analysis provided interesting new aspects which either generate the hypotheses for future studies or which - by indicating data artefacts - may lead to improvements in the design of studies of the same type. Especially if no prior knowledge of the data exists, neural networks provide a screening method revealing input variables of interest as well as associations between variables to enhance modelling.

The encoding of the variables is an important factor for the performance and the quality of the network results. Too exact coding of a variable in too many units might lead to an over-adaptation which also aggravates the interpretation of the network's structure. A poor ability to generalise is signalled by a large difference between the classification ability for the training and the test data set.

This method can also be applied to totally different tasks like segmentation of CT's or the analysis of ECG's. It works with very simple networks that can be easily combined with other neural networks or conventional systems to get a powerful hybrid system.

The automatic system for coding the data, configuring, training and testing a neural network which has been extended and improved in this project will be combined with an expert system. The expert system will be designed to support an expert of the domain (like epidemiology, CT-segmentation, ECG-analysis) to develop a neural system by defining the representation of information and selecting variables "of interest" and combinations of variables. The expert system should support the expert and help him with the interpretation of the structure found by the network.

References

[1] Baxt W.G.: Use of an Artificial Neural Network for Data Analysis in Clinical Decision-Making: The Diagnosis of Acute Coronary Occlusion.- In: Neural Computation 2, p.480-489 (1990)

[2] Bright RA., Avorn J., Everitt DE.: Medicaid data as a resource for epidemiologic studies: strength and limitations. J Clin. Epidemiol. 1989; 42: 937-945

[3] Bundesministerium für Jugend, Familie und Gesundheit: Internationale Klassifikation der Krankheiten, Verletzungen und Todesursachen.- Verlag W. Kohlhammer GmbH, Köln Stuttgart Berlin Mainz

[4] Däschlein R.: Segmentation von Computertomogrammen mit Hilfe neuronaler Netze.- Diploma thesis at the Technische Universität München, Institut für Informatik, Lehrstuhl Prof. W. Brauer (1993)

[5] Eldracher M., Waschulzik T.: A Topologically Distributed Encoding to Facilitate Learning.- To appear in: Journal of Systems Engineering

[6] Geiger H.:Storing and Processing Information in Connectionist Systems.- In: R. Eckmiller, editor, Advanced Neural Computers, p. 271-277. Elsevier Science Publishers B.V. (North Holland) (1990)

[7] Hesse W., Merbeth G., Fröhlich R.: Software-Entwicklung - Vorgehensmodelle, Projektführung Produktverwaltung. Oldenbourg (1992)

[8] Jick H., Jick SS., Derby LE.: Validation of information recorded on general practitioner based computerised data resource in the United Kingdom. Br med J 1993; 302: 766-768

[9] Lewis M., Löwel H., Winter C., Zimmermann G., Pitschi P., Göpfert E., Luhitsch D., Schwarzwälder I., König W., Bolte H., Hörmann A., Schneider A., Janku D., Kaup U., Keil U.: MONICA-Augsburg, Herzinfarktregister, Handbuch zur Registrierung von Krankenhauspatienten.- GSF-Bericht 25/90, GSF-Institut für Medizinische Informatik und Systemforschung

[10] Quandt K.: Auswertung einer Herz-Kreislauf-Studie mit Hilfe strukturierter neuronaler Netze.- Diploma thesis at the Technische Universität München, Institut für Informatik, Lehrstuhl Prof. W. Brauer (1992)

[11] Quandt K., Waschulzik T., Lewis M., Hörmann A., Engelbrecht R., Brauer. W.: Evaluation of epidemiological data with neural networks.- Accepted at WCNN 1993

[12] Rosenblatt F.: The perceptron: A Probabilistic model for information storage and organisation in the brain.- In: Psychol. Rev. 65, p.386-408 (1958)

[13] Rummelhart, D. E., Hinton G. E., Williams R. J.: Learning Representations by Back-Propagating Errors. Nature 323;p.533-536 (1986)

[14] Waschulzik T.: Optische Mustererkennung in neuronalen Architekturen.- Diploma thesis at the Technische Universität München, Institut für Informatik, Lehrstuhl Prof. W. Brauer (1988)

[15] Waschulzik T., Geiger H.: Eine Entwicklungsmethodik für strukturierte konnektionistische Systeme.- In: G. Dorffner, editor, Informatik Fachberichte 252, Konnektionismus in Artificial Intelligence und Kognitionsforschung, p. 202-206. Springer Verlag, Berlin (1990)

[16] Werbos P.: Beyond Regression: New Tools for Prediction and alysis in the Behavioral Sciences. Ph.D. Theses, Harvard University (1974)

Artificial Intelligence in Medecine
S. Andreassen et al. , Eds.
IOS Press, 1993

A Neural Network Modular System for Object Classification in Brain MR Images

P.Blonda §, *A.Carella* ¶, *R.DeBlasi* ¶, *F.Dicuonzo* ¶, *V.LaForgia* §, *D.Milella* ¶, *G.Pasquariello* §, *G.Satalino* §.

§ Istituto Elaborazionc Segnali ed Immagini CNR-IESI,
Via Amendola 166/5 - 70126 Bari - Italy

¶ Cattedra di Neuroradiologia - Universita' di Bari
P.za G. Cesare, 11 - 70124 Bari - Italy

Abstract

In this paper we present a modular system for segmentation and classification of brain Magnetic Resonance (MR) images. It consists of two Neural Network architectures, a Self Organizing Map and a Multilayer Perceptron. The objective of the work is to evaluate the effectiveness of a Neural Network approach for automatic recognition of anatomic structures in MR images. The system has been useful to discriminate 20 different anatomic classes.

1. INTRODUCTION

The number of recent paper reporting very good results of Neural Networks (NN) approaches is growing rapidly. However, few papers have appeared about the application of this technology in the field of medical image processing. The utilization of one specific architecture, such as a Multilayer Perceptron, an Hopfield Network and a Probabilistic Network, for the interpretation of magnetic resonance cerebral images (MR) is reported in [1],[2] and [3]. Both supervised and unsupervised architectures used in those papers have produced, as result, the recognition of few categories: background, white matter, gray matter, Cerebral Spinal Fluid (CSF) and fat. The same result is obtained in [4], with a traditional statistical methodology.

In this work an integrated approach based on a Neural Network modular system supported by a set of rules from an *expert* neuroradilogist is proposed for anatomical objects recognition in MR brain images. The modularity is introduced, as suggested in [5], to decompose the recognition problem in a two stage procedure for feature extraction and feature labelling. The first stage is performed, in this work, by a Kohonen Self-Organizing network [6], that is an unsupervised algorithm for data clustering. The second one is realized by a supervised Multilayer Backpropagation network [6]. In paragraph 2 is illustrated the data analysis procedure. In 3 results are presented.

2. DATA PROCESSING

Magnetic resonance imaging have the peculiarity of providing multicontrast images of human tissues by the adjustment of parameters which define the experiment. Because of this characteristic MR images can be analyzed as a multiband data set.

In this work the proton density-weighted, the T1 and T2 weighted images of a preselected brain section with no pathology, have been used. The images were obtained on a plane passing through the optic nerves and tracts, the substantia nigra and red nucleus, the optic radiations and cortex. The size of the three images, referred as band in this paper, is 256-by-256 pixels. The grey level values, originally ranging between 0 and 4096, have been rearranged between 0 and 255, by a threshold linear transformation.

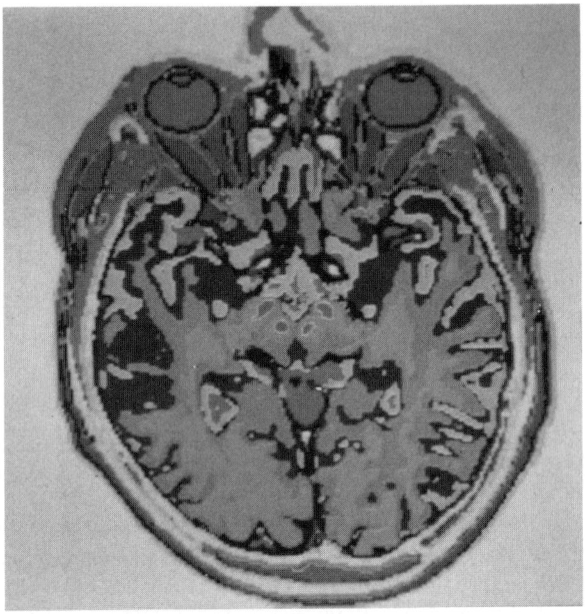

Figure 1. Segmented image

2.1. The unsupervised module

The SOM is a neural network model characterized by the capability to map pattern's features on the output layer [6]. The system is self-organizing by an unsupervised learning process that permits to each output neuron to become sensitive to a class of the input pattern space. In this work, the SOM module consists of 27 neurons in the input layer and 36 neurons in the output layer. In training, the input to the network are the 3 band values of each pixel in all the 3-by-3 windows, extracted from the 256-by-256 input grid, by shifting the coordinates of the central pixel one column per line. The output layer perform an oversegmentation of the input data in 36 regions, whereas about 20 anatomical classes should be recognized, as desired goal, in the last stage. The result of this analysis step is presented in fig. 1.

According to the expert neuroradiologist, this output seems to produce a correct distinction of tissues, that are histologically different, in well separated and homogeneous regions. The attention has been focused on some regions more populous, in terms of pixels, and more interesting from a neuroradiologic point of view.

For a correct training of the next MLP module the radiologist has suggested the introduction of positional information. In order to distinguish the same region corresponding to some kind of tissues in different anatomic objects. Moreover it is correct to merge two or more regions to completely characterize an anatomic structure. In this work, the positional information to recognize the 20 classes in table 1. have been explicited. A code 0-1 for five vertical and five horizontal area in a grid, located by the *expert*, on the image has been used.

2.2. The MLP module

The MLP architecture used for the classification step is a *feed-forward NN*. Given an input, the corresponding net outputs, can be computed feed-forwarding the input values through the network. The net is trained with the *Back Propagation* learning algorithm, based on the minimization of an energy function. The network used in this work consists of an input layer of 46 input nodes: 36 are to mark the input region, while the remaining 10 units stay for the relative position coding. The hidden layer and the output layer consist of 46 and 20 units, respectively. In the learning phase, the module receives as input, the label of some selected regions, the code for those positions defining an object and the corresponding object's label. Once trained, the network has been used to produce the classified image. Each pixel from the Kohonen map has provided to the MLP and labelled, in output, as one out of the 20 selected anatomical classes.

3. RESULTS AND CONCLUSIONS

The SOM algorithm has been found to perform robustly a segmentation of the input images in a map of very homogeneous regions. According to the radiologist, the regions correspond to different tissues of the brain, such as CSF, fat, white and grey matter, or to the complex interfaces existing among them. CSF results in one main region, according to its distribution in cisterns or in open subarachnoid spaces. Substantia nigra and red nucleus were assigned to the same region and require some topographic rules to be recognized by the MLP classifier. The segmentation of grey (GM) and white matter (WM) is probably the more interesting result of the SOM network: GM and WM were considered in different but near regions, and their distribution along the brain cortex and the optic radiations corresponds to the realty. Moreover an intermediate region of interest has been attributed to the interface between grey and white matter and the reticular present in mesencephalon. The MLP module has produced an output image whose quality depends on the "goodness" of the reference grid used to explicit the positional rules. The discontinuities in some structures and most of the misclassifications, in the median anterior part of the image, corresponding to the front of basal gyri, are due to this grid. In fig. 2 is presented the final output of the system.

A quantitative measure for the "goodness" of recognition is very difficult, because of the lack of any reference map. In this work the performance evaluation is based on human expertise. The MLP classifier has performed a satisfactory recognition of the objects of interest, but much work has to be done to automatize the process and to generalize the whole system. The improvement of the rules should help the system to overcome the current limits.

Table 1
List of classes

grey matter;
interface;
sclera;
vitreous body;
optical nerve;
lateral cistern;
hypothalamus;
optic radiations;
mesencephalon;
grey matter;
substantia nigra;
red-nucleus;
mamillar bodies;
ventricular bodies;
sylvian artery;
interpedunc. cistern;
fat tissue;
periaqueduttal grey;
straight sinus;
white matter.

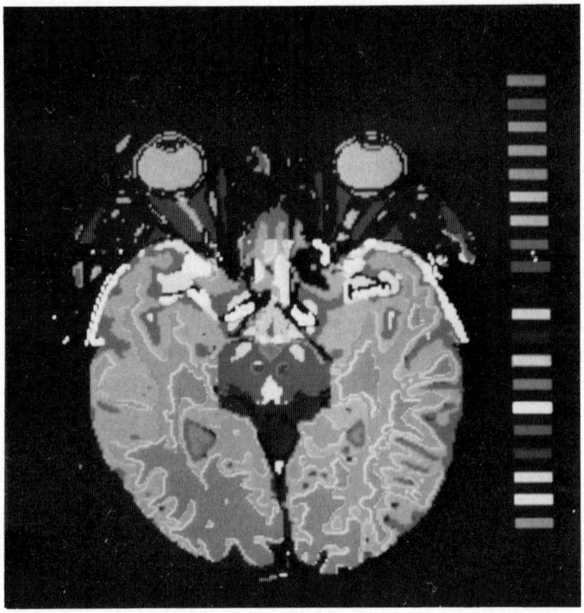

Figure 2. Output classified image: the colour scale corresponds from top to bottom, to the classes in Table 1.

5. REFERENCES

[1] D.L. Toulson and J. Boyce,*Segmentation of MR images using Neural Nets,* Image and vision computing, vol. 10, no. 5, june 1992.

[2] S.C. Amartur et al.,*Optimization Neural Networks for the Segmentation of Magnetic Resonance Images,* IEEE Trans. on Medical Imaging, Vol. 11, No.2, June 1992.

[3] M. Morrison and Y. Attikiouzel, *A probabilistic Neural Network based image segmentation Network for Magnetic Resonance Images,* Proc. of IJCNN-92, June 7-11, 1992, Baltimore, Maryland.

[4] G. Gerig, et al., *Automating Segmentation of Dual-Echo MR Head Data,* Proc. of 12th Conf. on Information Processing In Medical Imaging, July 7-12, 1991, Wye, UK.

[5] T. Hrycei, *Supporting supervised learning by self-organization,* Neurocomputing 4, (1992), 17-30.

[6] J. Hertz, et al., *Introduction to the theory of Neural Computation,* Addison-Wesly, 1991.

Artificial Intelligence in Medecine
S. Andreassen et al. , Eds.
IOS Press, 1993

A Neural Network Identifies Faces with Morphological Syndromes

R. Herpers, H. Rodax and G. Sommer*

GSF - Medis Institut
Institut für medizinische Informatik und Systemforschung
Ingolstädter Landstr. 1 D-85764 Oberschleißheim
Email: herpers@gsf.de

Abstract

The diagnosis of craniofacial dysmorphic signs has a high medical importance. Physicians specialized on human genetics need to get quick reliable information about dysmorphic syndromes characterized by facial abnormalities to give a prognosis about the risk of incidence for following children. In numerous cases of dysmorphic syndromes no chromosomal aberration can be found. Therefore the dysmorphic diagnosis is based on an extensive phenotyp analysis of craniofacial signs. In this study we investigate an artificial neural network approach to identify face images with morphological abnormalities. Different full-connected multi-layer perceptrons (MLP) are trained only with a small set of observations using back-propagation as learning algorithm. The gray level images are sampled, preprocessed and scaled to a size of 55 x 72 pixel. The best results are achieved with a network architecture of 4 hidden and 2 output units. The individual classification error of each investigated network architecture is calculated by the leaving-one-out method. The average classification error was 5 %, the best percentage of correct identifications of one network architecture reached 100 %. The presented results show that classifications generated by aritificial neural networks based on small sets of training examples are able to support a dysmorphic diagnosis.

1. Introduction

The human ability to recognize, identify or distinguish faces is very remarkable. This skill is quite robust and very accurate, despite several visual changes due to viewing conditions, facial expressions, aging and so on. As a consequence the visual processing of human faces has fascinated philosophers and scientists for centuries.

The recognition of minor facial abnormalities are important to identify dysmorphic syndromes [1]. Most dysmorphic signs are affecting the face but, by definition, do not lead to functional disturbances. A syndrome is a grouping of two or more signs into a characteristic constellation that allows a medical prediction of a disorder [2]. These constellations are occasionally very complex, so that no accurate or reliable definition can be found to charaterize the underlying syndrome.

---

*Present address: Institut für Informatik, Lehrstuhl Kognitive Systeme, Universität Kiel, Preußerstr. 1-9, D-24105 Kiel

The study reported here shows an approach identifying gray level face images of children with dysmorphic signs by training an artificial neural network. Full connected multi-layer perceptrons (MLP) are known to perform well complex recognition tasks, like sex-recognition in faces by assumption of a sufficient amount of training examples [3]. The aim of this research was to find appropriate network architectures performing this identification task by a small set of training examples.

2. Methods

The presented approach works on frontal viewed face images of young children. The small database consists of 10 dysmorphic and 21 non dysmorphic, 512 x 512 high resolution, gray level images. All the face images have to be scanned and preprocessed before using as input for the networks.

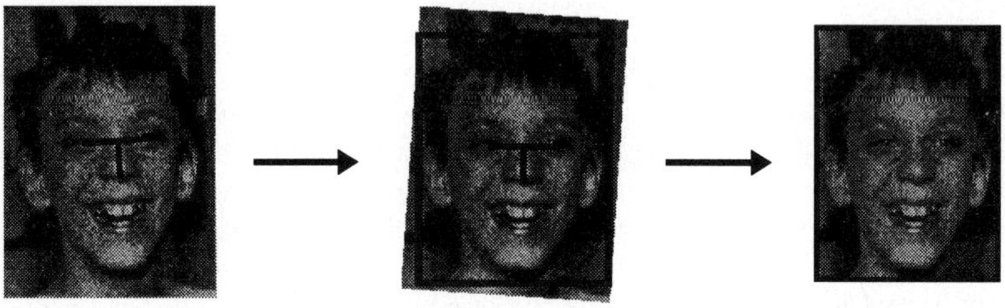

Figure 1: Preprocessing of the face images. After locating the eyes the images were rotated, scaled and cropped.

The preprocessing and the modelling of the network architectures are based on investigations of B. A. Golomb et al., who identify the sex from human faces [3]. After locating the eyes, the 8-bit digitized images are rotated to align the line joining the eyes (Figure 1).

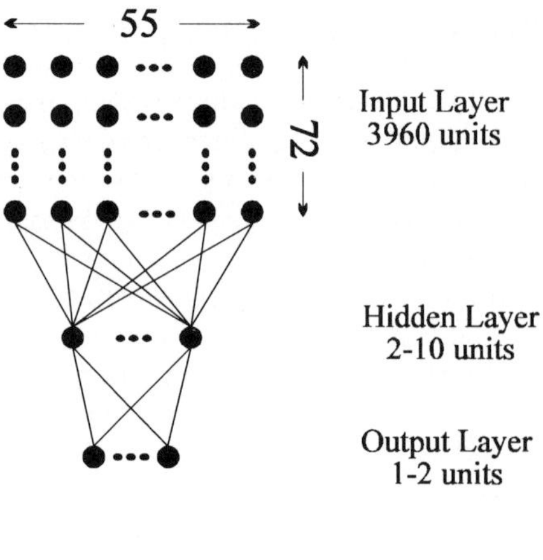

Figure 2: Design of used network architectures

We use a gaussian convolution kernel to reduce the image size and the resulting parts are cropped and scaled to a size of 55 x 72 pixel. Thus, the input is limited to 3960 units and the natural proportion of the human head is taken into account. Furthermore, all the images are adjusted to the same average brightness. We use various network configurations to train and classify different image sets. The number of units in the hidden layer is varied from 2 to 10 units. The amount of hidden units serves the network to generalize, while the number of output units is responsible for the classification result. One output unit coded "1" for dysmorphic, "0" for non-dysmorphic and two output units coded "0; 1" and "1; 0" for the different classification results are alternatively used (Figure 2).

For the realization of this study we choose the Stuttgart Neural Network Simulator [4] because of the fast computation and batch programming properties. The different networks are trained with 7 to 30 preprocessed face images of the database using standard backpropagation as learning algorithm [5] with a sigmoid activation function and a learning rate of 0.2 or 0.3. The learning process is supervised and determined after right identification of all trained samples. We use the leaving-one-out method [6] for training and testing all examined networks because of the small number of the considered images (Figure 3).

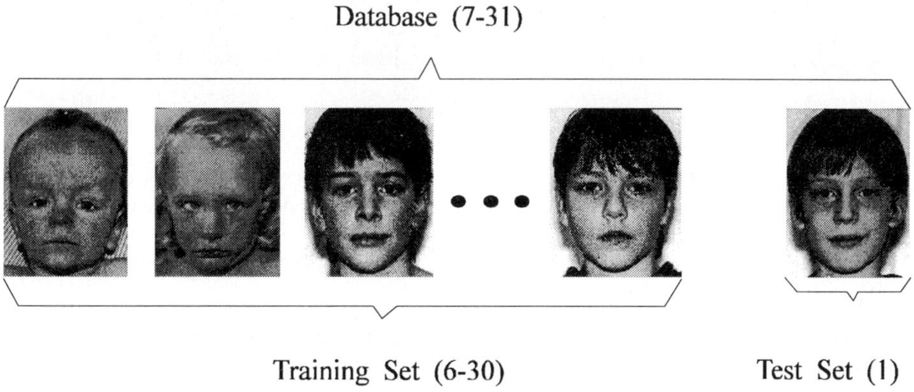

Figure 3: Leaving-one-out method for training and testing the different network configurations

Only one unknown test image of each sampling set is used for testing the network. The test image is changed until each image of the sampling set was used. The network is trained respectively with the remaining ones. Thus, we train repeatedly one network configuration with different training sets of one sampling set. The average classification error of each configurated network architecture is calculated by the amount of misclassifications of all considered examinations.

3. Results

The small sampling set of available observations effects a reduced ability of generalization of each examined network architecture. The average classification error calculated by counting the misclassifications of 8 samples per network configuration reaches about 25 %. Using all available face images (30 training + 1 testing sample respectively) and classifying dysmorphic and non-dysmorphic faces the percentage of misclassification decreases down to 5 %. In our best considered investigation the percentage of correct identifications reaches 100 % configurating the network with 4 or 6 hidden and 2 output units (Figure 4).

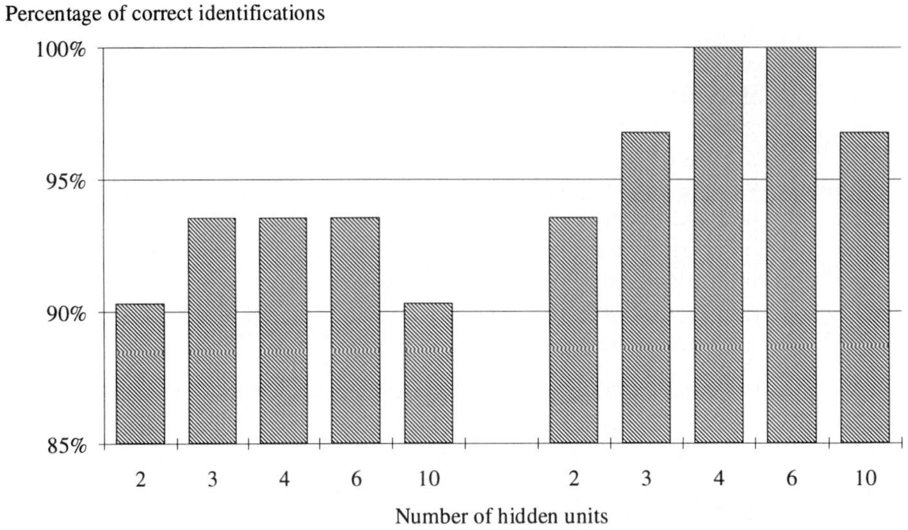

Figure 4: Diagram of the percentage of correct identifications to the number of used hidden units of two different network architectures.The first group is configurated with one output unit, the second with two output units.

The increasing of the amount of hidden units doesn't enhance the classification result but reduces the generalization properties of the network. In comparison to a network configuration with two output units the classification error improves for a network configurations with only one output unit, because the discrimination properties of the output layer cannot be trained so exactly. With these conditions of available observations an identification of different subsamples of dysmorphic face images wasn't possible.

4. Discussion

We have shown that the complex visual pattern recognition task of identifying face images with dysmorphic signs can be adequately performed by artificial neural networks without a large number of training examples. The evaluation of the neural network classifier by estimation of the average classification error using the leaving-one-out method offers robust performance and allows to transfer the results to similar problems. Dependent on the amount of training examples an optimal network architecture can be found so that the percentage of correct identifications reaches 100 %. By using only few hidden units the network has good generalization qualities.

However, the features being responsible for the classification cannot be reconstructed without paying attention to the underlying dysmorphic signs. It is intended to examine the face images on local facial features of morphological abnormalities. The local charateristic dysmorphic signs will be detected automatically by an attentional mechanism [7] and processed by specialized algorithms [8]. The extracted local features might build an understandable and reasonable basis for a sophisticated image processing system.

Acknowledgements

We are indebted to Prof. Dr. S. Stengel-Rutkowski and Dr. C. Apacik, Institut für Soziale Pädiatrie und Jugendmedizin, Abteilung Genetik der Universität München, for providing the images used in this study and giving helpful medical suggestions.

References

[1] S. Stengel-Rutkowski, P. Schimanek and A. Wernheimer, *Anthropometric definition of dysmorphic facial signs*, Hum. Genet. 67, pp. 272-295 (1984)

[2] P. R. Dyken and M. D. Miller, *Facial features of neurologic syndromes*, St. Louis, Missouri, C. V. Mosby Company (1980)

[3] B. A. Golomb, D. T. Lawrence and T. J. Sejnowski, *Sexnet: A neural network identifies sex from human faces*, R. P. Lippmann (eds.) Advances in Neural Information Processing Systems 3, pp. 572-577 (1990)

[4] A. Zell et al., *SNNS Stuttgart Neural Network Simulator Vers. 3.0*, Report No. 3/93, Institut für parallele und verteilte Hochleistungssysteme, Stuttgart (1993)

[5] D. E. Rumelhart and J.L. McClelland, Parallel Distributed Processing, volume 1, MIT Press (1986)

[6] G. Deichsel and H. J. Trampisch, *Biometrie, Clusteranalyse und Diskriminanzanalyse*, Gustav Fischer Verlag (1985)

[7] R. Herpers, H. Kattner and G. Sommer, *GAZE: An attentional mechanism for the extraction of prominent facial features*, In this proceedings (1993)

[8] M. Michaelis and G. Sommer, *Characterization of key-points in images*, accepted by Int. Symp. on Subst. Ident. Techn. ´93, Innsbruck (1993)

Artificial Intelligence in Medecine
S. Andreassen et al. , Eds.
IOS Press, 1993

Grading of Gliomas in Stereotactic Biopsies with Neural Networks

v.WANGENHEIM A.[1], VINCE G.H.[2], KOLLES H.[2], RICHTER M.M.[1], FEIDEN W.[2]

[1] Artificial Intelligence Working Group of the University of Kaiserslautern; D-67653 Kaiserslautern. Germany.

[2] Department of Neuropathology Medical School of the University of the Saarland. D-66421 Homburg. Germany.

Summary

The stereotactically gained glioma biopsies are graded using four stereological-morphometrical parameters with the help of an image analysis system and a backpropagation neural network. These parameters enable quantifying the essential characteristics of malignant gliomas: growth pattern, cellularity, proliferation index, and nucleus polymorphism. Employing these parameters neural networks were trained with a varying number of samples from a total of 679 measured fields. Subsequently, the network was checked with all of these measurements, so that presently the system can offer its own glioma graduation.

1. Introduction

The exact grading of a glioma is an important factor determining the prognosis of the tumour disease. In this connection the term „grading“ refers to the histological evaluation of the tumours dignity. Structure parameters visible under an ordinary light microscope are weighted and the results are arranged in a scale with 3 or 4 grades of increasing malignancy. To date, various grading propositions exist, whereby their prognostic validity is usually founded on the respective survival rates calculated by the Cox-regression model.

Since the choice of therapy dramatically depends on the grading of the tumour, this information is of decisive value in the array of diagnostical parameters. However, the complexity of the structure parameters leads to a certain subjectivity in the grading. Objective grading seems only to be possible on the condition that exact morphometrical and stereological parameters are available. New developments in immunohistochemical staining enabling for instance comfortable calculation of the proliferation index should also be included in modern research work.

2. Material and Method

The basis of our study are stereotactically gained glioma biopsies of 86 patients. As a rule numerous biopsy cylinders are taken along a stereotactical trajectory through the tumour. Despite the minute size of these biopsies it was possible to evaluate the cell nuclei in 4 consecutive fields using combined morphometrical and stereological techniques. The cell nuclei were stained with a new combination of Feulgen and Ki-67 immunostaining, whereby non-proliferating nuclei are coloured pale red and proliferating nuclei appear dark blue. However, the cytoplasm of the cells and the matrix background remain colourless so that automatic discrimination of the nuclei is possible.

The following morphometrical and stereological parameters were determined with the image analysis system :

- relative nuclei area of the proliferating cells; an indicator of the proliferation activity [1]
- volume weighted nuclei volumes, an indicator of nuclear size and pleomorphism.
- minimal spanning trees (MST) based on the x and y coordinates of the centre of gravity of the nuclei enabling quantification of the growth pattern [2]

All gliomas were graded histologically according to the WHO-Scale, the Daumas-Duport-Scale [3] and according to a new, morphometric-based, three-step grading scale (referred to as „HOM“-Scale), which was determined by cluster analysis . These parameters of 679 measured fields are fed into a backpropagation neural network, are trained and then tested. The system is based on the network simulator NEURALTALK [4], run on a Sun SPARC workstation. Aditionally, discriminant analysis was caried out. The classification results of both approaches are compared.

3. Results and Discussion

The mean minimal spanning trees (MST) as well as the variation of MST decrease with increasing degree of malignancy. High nuclear pleomorphism and large nucleus size are characteristic of high-grade gliomas in the Daumas-Duport and WHO-schemes. These parameters are of little importance in the structure-orientated HOM-scale. Proliferation activity only increases significantly within the WHO-scale. In the Daumas-Duport and the HOM-scale this parameter is less influential.

Using discriminant analysis, a correct automatic grading rate of 93% is possible with the HOM-Scale, while with the WHO-Scale only 55%, and with the Daumas-Duport only 49% of the cases are classified correctly. Neural networks with one hidden-layer

(10 units), trained with samples (about 10% of the total data set), showed following learning and generalisation capabilities:

Table 1.
Learning and generalisation results for all grading scales.

Scale	Learning of sample set	Generalisation
WHO	97%	61%
Daumas-Duport	93%	49 %
HOM	100%	97%

Good results for the HOM-scale were to be expected, due to the nature of data generated by cluster analysis. The poor results with the WHO and Daumas-Duport scales may lie in the complexity of data, which cannot be expressed by the simple neural architecture used in these initial experiments. To overcome this problem, a parallel version of the network simulator was implemented, and simulations are at the present time being executed on a nCUBE2 supercomputer, with bigger training sets and more complex network architectures. The generation of specially representative, non-random training sets is also in preparation.

4. Literature

1. SCHRÖDER R., BIEN K., KOTT R., MEYERS I., VÖSSING R.: The relationship between Ki-67 labeling and mitotic index in gliomas and meningeomas: demonstration of the variability of the intermitotic cycle time. Acta Neuropathol. (1991) 82: 389-394.
2. DUSSERT C., RASIGNI G., LLEBARIA A.: Quantization of directional properties in biological structures using the minimal spanning tree. J.Theor.Biol (1988) 135: 295-302.
3. DAUMAS-DUPORT C., SCHEITHAUER B., O'FALLON J., KELLY P. : Grading of Astrocytomas. Cancer (1988) 62: 2152-2165.
4. RITZER H.: NEURALTALK: Ein Simulator für neuronale Netze in SMALLTALK-80, Projektarbeit, Universität Kaiserslautern, 1990.

Artificial Intelligence in Medecine
S. Andreassen et al. , Eds.
IOS Press, 1993

Self Organizing Maps for the Evaluation of High Resolution ECG

Barbi Schulz[1], Erich Pelikan[1], Jiri Silny[2], Martin Sigmund[3], Günter Rau[2]

1: Institut für Medizinische Informatik und Biometrie, RWTH Aachen (Direktor: R.Repges)
2: Helmholtz-Institut für Biomedizinische Technik an der RWTH Aachen (Direktor: G.Rau)
3: Medizinische Klinik I der RWTH Aachen (Direktor: P. Hanrath)

Abstract:
An approach for an all-embracing ECG signal analysis is introduced. Self organizing maps are applied to spatial high resolution multilead ECG recorded during the acute phase of myocardial infarction to detect characteristic changes. The algorithm deals with the measurement of similarity between different pathological signal types.

1. Introduction

One of the most important aids in diagnosis of heart deseases is still the 12 lead ECG technique. Additionally to enhance diagnostic quality multi-lead approaches known as "Body surface-ECG" or "Mapping" have been developed by several groups to gain more information from the potential deviation onto the thorax. For example in acute myocardial infarction (AMI) the therapy is determined by criterias such as age of patient, infarct size and infarct phase. Within the first six hours after the onset of symptoms efforts for a limitation of infarct size are promising. Due to rapid changes in ECG-signal shape especially the infarct size can not be derived reliably from standard ECG and mapping during the acute phase. About 72 hours after AMI a valuation is possible by means of both 12 lead ECG (Selvester Scoring System [Sel85]) and mapping. These methods require a calming of the ECG-changes and use only single points [Awa80, Ike87, Mar80, Yus79] or sections of the signal [Hor85, Hul92,

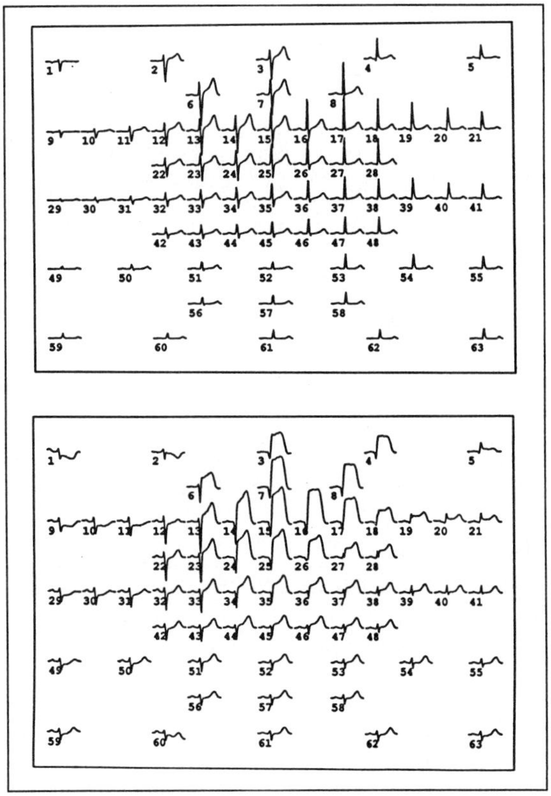

Fig. 1: High resolution ECG from a healthy case (top) and an AI-case (bottom)

Kub85, Mon84, Sta86, Iga87] for estimation. The introduced approach is based on the whole ECG-signal derived from the acute phase. It estimates their similarity to signal prototypes of different pathological kinds. For this task a self organizing map [Koh84, Rit91] has been chosen.

2. Materials and Methods

High resolution ECG data was recorded during acute myocardial infarction using a 63 precordial lead mapping system developed at the Helmholtz-Institut Aachen [Hin85]. Data was obtained from 39 patients with anterior myocardial infarction (AI) and 52 patients with posterior myocardial infarction (PI). Enzymatic changes (CK, α-HBDH) which could be used for estimation of infarct size were available in 16 (28) cases. Additionally high resolution ECG from 78 healthy subjects was recorded. Figure 1 shows a high resolution ECG of a healthy person and a patient with AI.

The capabilities of a self organizing map for valuation of similarity has been studied. Its important features of dimension reduction and support of neighbourhood relationship are used

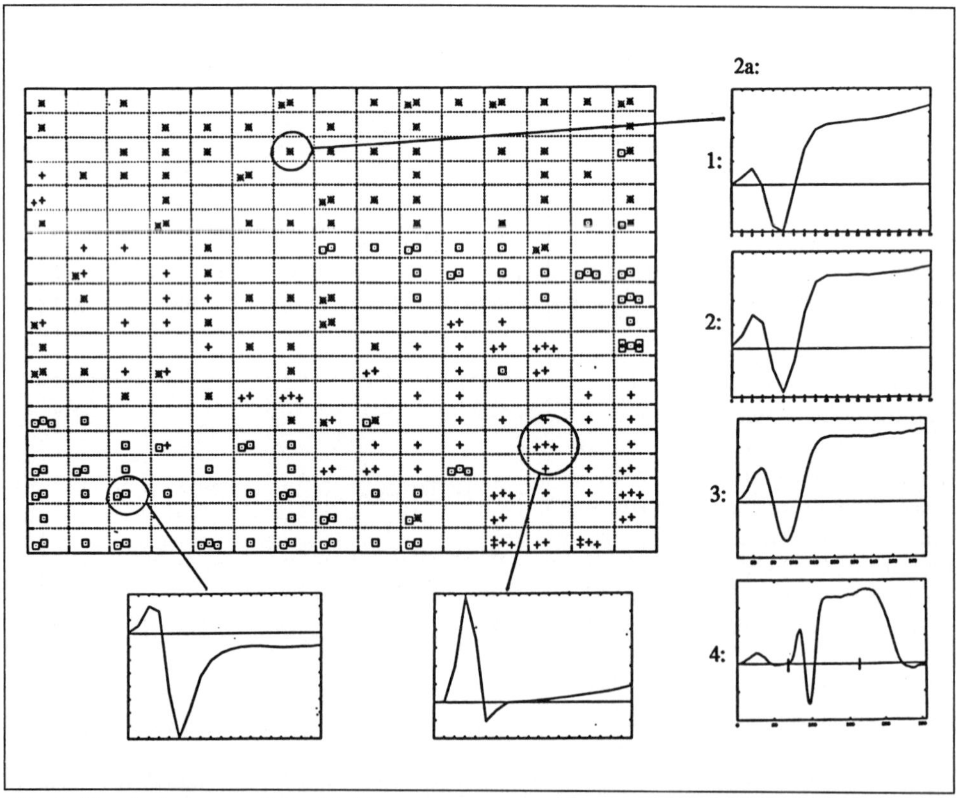

Fig. 2: Topological map of size 15x19 vectors and examplary map vectors of its different areas. (healthy: + posterior myocardial infarction: □ anterior myocardial infarction: *).
Fig. 2a: map vector (1), feature vector (2) and ECG (3,4).

to perform a continuous signal classification represented by the arrangement of input signals on the topological map. Therefore the input data was derived from 28 central leads out of the 63. To represent the whole signal between Q-wave and T-wave for every lead 20 values corresponding to an equidistant sampling were arranged in a feature vector. A training set was constructed containing the 28 sampled ECG-signals from 3 AI (*), 3 PI (□) and 3 healthy cases (+). This set was used for the training of a self organizing map with a size of 15x19 vectors shown in figure 2.

3. Results

Each map vector represents a prototype of different QRS-complex types or ECG-sections. This is shown in figure 2a. A map vector, his corresponding feature vector and the real ECG are depicted. It is important to mention that a continuous representation is provided by the map.

For classification tasks a test set was created containing cases different from those used in the training set. Figure 3 shows a classification of an AI-case based on the topological map from figure 2. The feature vectors were placed in an area covered by the AI-cases of the training set. Accordingly figure 4 shows classifications for a PI-case.

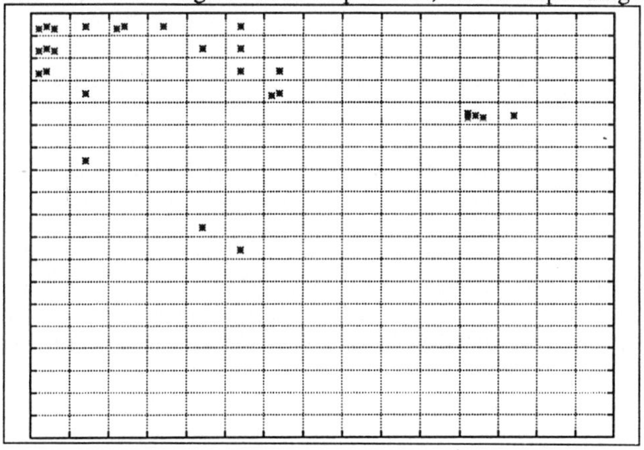

Fig. 3: Classification of an AI-case with the topological map from Fig. 2.

A clustering indicating different pathological appearances can be observed. A visualization of the map vectors explains this behaviour. These results show, that the algorithm is able to classify ECG-signals of different infarct types even from the acute phase. At the end of the training phase an interpretation e.g. a grading of the results must be added by a physician because the self organizing map is an unsupervised classification algorithm.

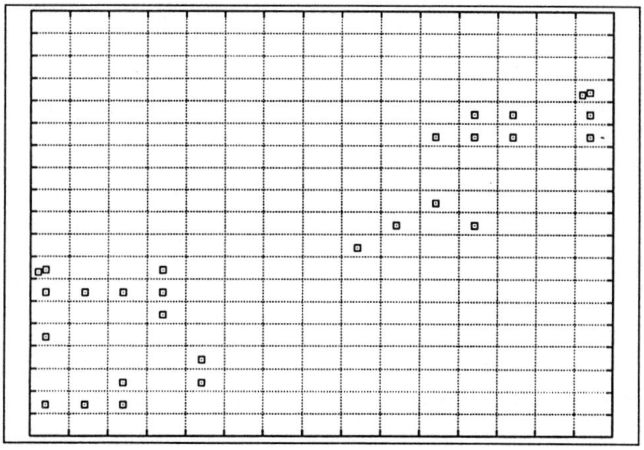

Fig. 4: Classification of a PI-case with the topological map from Fig. 2.

4. Conclusions

The described approach provides an all-embracing signal representation as basis for classification. The classification based on Euclidean distance as similarity measure leads to an approximately continuous set of signal prototypes. In opposite to statistical approaches the results are transparent and in the sense of medical meaning an interpretation of the topological map can be given. The property of unsharp membership is modelled by the two-dimensional arrangement of the feature vectors. Accordingly the underlying pathological findings are projected onto the topological map. Further research has to prove in what extent the presented approach is advantageous for the clinical routine diagnostic in cardiology.

References

[Awa80] Awan, N.A., Vera, Z., Mason, D.T.: Determination of MI Size and LV Performance by Precordial Q-Wave Mapping Quantification of Myocardial Ischemia. In: Advances in Clinical Cardiology Vol.1 , 32, (H.W.Heiss eds.), 1980

[Hin85] Hinsen, R.: Ein Beitrag zur Methodik und Anwendung der Hochauflösenden Thorax-Elektrokardiographie. Dissertation, Fakultät für Elektrotechnik, RWTH Aachen, 1985

[Hor85] Horan, L.G., Sridharan, M.R., Hand, R.C., Flowers, N.C.: Variation of the Precordial QRS Transition Zone in Normal Subjects. J Electrocardiol 21, 25, 1985

[Hul92] Hulin, I., Slavkovsky, P.: Special computer graphical method for detection of myocardial infarction. Comp Methods and Programs in Biomedicine 39, 85, 1992

[Iga87] Igarashi, A., Kubota, I., Ikeda, K., Tsuiki, K., Yasui, S.: Determination of the Site of Myocardial Infarction by QRST Isointegral Mapping in Patients with Abnormal Ventricular Activation Sequence. Jap Heart J 28, 165, 1987

[Ike87] Ikeda et al.: Temporal Changes in Body Surface Peak R Isochrone Maps and Left Ventricular Function in Patients with Myocardial Infarction. J Electrocardiol 20,121, 1987

[Koh84] Kohonen, T.: Self-Organisation and Associative Memory. Springer Series in Information Science 8, Heidelber, 1984

[Kub85] Kubota, I., et al.: Noninvasive Assessment of Left Ventricular Wall Motion Abnormalities by QRS Isointegral Maps in Previous Anterior Infarction. Am Heart J 109, 464, 1985

[Mar80] Maraoko, P.R., DeBoer, L.W.V.: Usefulness of Precordial Electrocardiographic Mapping in Assessing the Effect of Interventions in Myocardial Ischemic Damage. In: Advances in Clinical Cardiology 1, 39, (H.W.Heiss eds.), 1980

[Mon84] Montague, T.J., et al.: Temporal Evolution of Body Surface Map Patterns Following Acute Inferior MI. J Electrocardiol 17, 319, 1984

[Rit91] Ritter, H., Martinetz, T., Schulten, K.: Neuronale Netze. Addison Wesley, Bonn, 1991

[Sel85] Selvester, R.H., Wagner, G.S., Hindman, N.C.: The Selvester QRS Scoring System for Estimating the Myocardial Infarct Size - Development and Application of the System. Arch Intern Med 145, 1877, 1985

[Sta86] Startt, R.H., Selvester, R.H., Solomon, J.C., Pearson, R.B.: Body Surface Map Criteria for Quantitating Infarct as Direved from Computer Simulations. In: Electrocardiographic Body Surface Mapping, 49, (van Dam, van Oosterom eds.), Martinius Nijhoff Publishers, 1986

[Yus79] Yusuf, S., Lopez, R., Maddison, A., Maw, P., Ray, N., McMillan, S., Sleight P.: Value of Electrocardiogramm in Predicting and Estimating Infarct Size in Man. British Heart J 42, 286, 1979

AUTHOR INDEX